DINTINO

THERAPEUTIC MODALITIES

THE ART AND SCIENCE

THERAPEUTIC MODALITIES

THE ART AND SCIENCE

KENNETH L. KNIGHT
DAVID O. DRAPER

Kenneth L. Knight, PhD, ATC, FACSM
Jesse Knight Professor of Exercise Sciences
Department of Exercise Sciences
College of Health and Human Performance
Brigham Young University
Provo, Utah

David O. Draper, EdD, ATC, LAT
Professor of Exercise Sciences
Department of Exercise Sciences
College of Health and Human Performance
Brigham Young University
Provo, Utah

Wolters Kluwer | Lippincott Williams & Wilkins
Health
Philadelphia · Baltimore · New York · London
Buenos Aires · Hong Kong · Sydney · Tokyo

Acquisitions Editor: Emily Lupash
Managing Editor: Meredith Brittain
Freelance Development Editor: Betsy Dilernia
Marketing Manager: Christen Murphy
Production Editor: Julie Montalbano
Designer: Terry Mallon
Photographer: Mark A. Philbrick
Graphic Artist: Kim Battista
Cartoonist: Cornel Rubino
Compositor: Maryland Composition, Inc.

351 West Camden Street   530 Walnut Street
Baltimore, MD 21201   Philadelphia, PA 19106

9 8 7 6 5 4 3 2 1

Library of Congress Cataloging-in-Publication Data

Knight, Kenneth L.
   Therapeutic modalities : the art and science / Kenneth L. Knight, David O. Draper.
      p. ; cm.
   Includes bibliographical references.
   ISBN-13: 978-0-7817-5744-7
  1. Physical therapy. 2. Orthopedic surgery—Patients—Rehabilitation. I. Draper, David
O. II. Title.
   [DNLM: 1. Physical Therapy Modalities. 2. Orthopedic Procedures—methods. WB 460 K69t 2008]
   RM700.K555 2008
   615.8′2—dc22

                                 2007106569

DISCLAIMER

To purchase additional copies of this book, call our customer service department at **(800) 638-3030** or fax orders to **(301) 223-2320**. International customers should call **(301) 223-2300**.

Visit Lippincott Williams & Wilkins on the Internet: http://www.lww.com. Lippincott Williams & Wilkins customer service representatives are available from 8:30 am to 6:00 pm, EST.

To our students, patients, and colleagues—for stretching our thinking

Preface

The use of therapeutic modalities, like clinical practice in all the health professions, is an art—an art influenced by experience and tradition as well as by science and theory. It would be easier if using therapeutic modalities were based entirely on scientific fact, but this is not the case. When research is inadequate, the clinician must rely on tradition and experience to guide application. Hence we have subtitled this textbook *The Art and Science*.

Clinicians need to understand both the how and the why of therapeutic modality use to be thinking, decision-making professionals rather than technicians. Although there is a theoretical basis for each modality application, the robustness of the theories varies. Some theories have a solid science base, whereas others are derived mostly from tradition. The lack of a scientific basis does not mean a theory is wrong, but that it might be uncertain. We have made a great effort to help readers understand the basis of the theories without overwhelming them with detail and depth. Studying the development of various theories will help students sharpen their critical-thinking skills. Only then will they become professionals and have the ability to make proper decisions about which modality to use when, to keep up with future developments, and to evaluate intelligently the claims of manufacturers.

The Audience

This introductory text is intended primarily for undergraduate students and others new to therapeutic modalities. We feel, however, that the book has much to offer to graduate students, clinicians, and those who may not be current with all the latest research and techniques in the field.

Why We Wrote This Book

We are passionate about therapeutic modalities. We have devoted our professional lives to understanding and teaching therapeutic modalities and injury rehabilitation. There isn't another topic that we would rather think about, write about, research, or speak on (except our families). And we feel we have information that has not yet been integrated into current texts.

We wrote this book from the perspective of a combined total of 60 years of teaching therapeutic modalities, 34 years of clinical experience, and 52 years of laboratory research on therapeutic modalities. With this background, we can introduce how, why, and when modalities should be used and stimulate deeper thinking by presenting cutting-edge research, much of which we have performed ourselves. In addition, we have developed some unique perspectives that we want to share with colleagues.

Our Writing Approach

We attempted to tell a complex story simply by sharing in-depth information in a way that novices can easily grasp. We wrote the text as if we were carrying on a conversation with the reader. Although there are many new and technical terms, we avoided using "stuffy" words, which can distance the learner from the teacher. (Why use a $50 word when a $5 word works as well?)

The text will appeal to a variety of learning styles. Many pedagogical (learning) aids—charts, tables, graphs, photographs, and drawings—will facilitate visual learners. Clinical application tips and practice techniques are included for those who prefer, or perform best from, hands-on activities (kinesthetic learners). The conversational tone of our writing may assist those who are auditory learners.

Our extensive teaching, clinical, and laboratory research experience guided our writing. This text integrates our research and ideas into a composite whole.

Another basic principle that guided us is that patients and injuries are unique, so applications must be tailored to individual situations. This requires critically thinking clinicians who understand the theory and science of injuries and possible interventions and adapt their applications accordingly. Hence we have theory and the evidence for that theory in our writing.

This book was a totally collaborative effort. Although we divided the responsibility of writing the first drafts of chapters, we reviewed and challenged each other's work before submitting each chapter for review. The process of challenging and defending concepts significantly strengthened the work.

Structural Organization

The book is divided into seven parts. Each part begins with an overview to help readers see the big picture and to understand how the chapters are related. This is not a mystery novel. We don't want readers wondering "who did it" as they read.

Each chapter begins with an outline of the chapter's topics, to help readers anticipate what is to come. We then present an "opening scene," a brief vignette featuring a fictional therapeutic modalities student in a situation related to the chapter content. A "closing scene" at the end of the chapter completes the story. Each chapter is richly illustrated with tables, illustrations, charts, and photographs. They also contain "critical thinking" exercises, "modality myths," and "application tips." Chapters conclude with "chapter reflections," a series of open-ended questions about the material covered. Most chapters included a reference numbered to correspond to citations in the text. We include these references both to document the material and to guide readers who want to explore a topic further. Sets of multiple-choice questions come at the end of each part.

We present standard operating procedures for the modalities so there is no question in the reader's mind about how to properly apply each modality. In addition, we present enough theory and background so the clinician can critically choose the appropriate modality for a specific situation. Armed with this information, the clinician can also educate his patients about why a particular modality is being used, facilitating the placebo effect and improving patient compliance.

Part I, "In Perspective," consists of three foundational chapters. In Chapter 1, we define therapeutic modalities and their role in the bigger picture of injury rehabilitation, including which of the major rehabilitation goals therapeutic modalities can help achieve. Having a perspective of overall rehabilitation makes therapeutic modality use more effective and, therefore, enhances patient care. Clinical decision making is introduced as well as the need to make decisions based on scientific evidence. Chapter 2 introduces the concept of general application procedures,

including a specific five-step process. Readers are urged to master the elements of the five-step process so they can use it as an outline for applying all therapeutic modalities, adding specifics as needed for each specific modality. Chapter 3 presents five reasons for keeping good treatment records, beginning with enhanced patient care. Other types of patient records are briefly discussed because we feel students should be introduced to these concepts early in their careers (when a course in therapeutic modalities is generally taught) rather that at the end of their program, when administration issues are usually taught.

Part II, "Orthopedic Injury, Immediate Care, and Healing," also consists of three chapters. In Chapter 4, we discuss the inflammatory response, which always occurs after an orthopedic injury and is essential to healing. Swelling and edema are differentiated, and a theoretical basis for their development and resolution is presented. In Chapter 5, we outline, in detail, the protocol of rest, ice application, compression, elevation, and stabilization (RICES). Chapter 6 explains the effects of various therapeutic modalities on injury repair.

Part III, "Pain and Orthopedic Injuries," consists of two chapters. Because pain is the primary symptom that causes people to seek treatment, a successful clinician must understand it thoroughly. In Chapter 7, we review basic neuroanatomy and neurophysiology so readers have a solid basis for understanding pain theories. We review the major pain theories of the past as a basis for discussing the latest and most comprehensive and complex theory, the neuromatrix theory of pain. Three general approaches for relieving orthopedic injury pain are then discussed.

In Chapter 8, we go into specific detail about pain relief, including both the philosophy and the principles of pain relief, such as Dehne's spinal adaptation syndrome, resetting central control during rehabilitation, and the placebo effect. Tools for relieving pain are also discussed in this chapter, including exercise, counterirritants, thermotherapy, electrotherapy, and cryotherapy. Techniques for monitoring and assessing pain relief during rehabilitation are also described.

Part IV, "Electrotherapy," also contains two chapters. The major sections of Chapter 9 are a review of the physics of electricity, electrical equipment, the generation of electricity, output current characteristics, tissue responses to electrical stimulation, and therapeutic uses of electrical stimulation. Chapter 10 includes an overview of electrotherapy application and research as well as the five-step application procedures for transcutaneous electrical nerve stimulation (TENS), interferential current therapy for pain relief (IFC), neuromuscular electrical stimulation (NMES), iontophoresis for transcutaneous drug delivery, and high-volt pulsed current (HVPC) stimulation for wound healing. Microcurrent electrical nerve stimulation (MENS) is also briefly reviewed.

Six chapters are in Part V, "Therapeutic Heat and Cold." Chapters 11 and 13 are theory, Chapters 12 and 14 are application, and Chapters 15 and 16 contain both theory and application. In Chapter 11, we define heat, its contraindications, differentiate between deep and superficial heat, and then discuss transferring heat to and from the body, the therapeutic use of heat, radiant energy and electromagnetic waves, and the difference between radiation and acoustic waves. Chapter 12 begins with a discussion of superficial thermotherapy and then presents the five-step application procedures for whirlpool, hot packs, and paraffin bath. The applications of infrared lamps, electrical heating, and portable superficial heating devices are briefly discussed.

Chapter 13, is our second chapter on cryotherapy theory. We are unique in this regard. Cryotherapy is not a single modality; it is used quite differently the day after an injury than it is immediately after injury occurs. Both the reason for using it and the way it is applied vary, a point that many do not understand. By separating the coverage, we hope to reduce the confusion. This chapter examines different physiological effects from those discussed in Chapter 5. Here, additional effects are described and their implications on rehabilitation are explored. The facts and fallacies of cold-induced vasodilation are presented, and we hope to put to rest the idea that therapeutic cold applications result in increased blood flow. We compare the use of heat and cold for rehabilitation and give specific recommendations for when to use each. In Chapter 14, we apply the principles discussed in Chapter 13. Applications of cryotherapy for numerous situations are presented, including the five-step application procedure of cryokinetics for joint sprains and cryostretch for muscle injuries.

Chapter 15, on ultrasound, and Chapter 16, on diathermy, take similar approaches. Both chapters include the science, theory, and application of the device, including the physics of the unit, components of the device, thermal and nonthermal effects, treatment parameters, case studies, and a comparison of the two modalities. Clinical applications of each one are presented in the five-step application format.

Part VI, "Other Modalities," collects three modalities that do not have a unifying principle or shared features: therapeutic massage, spinal traction, and laser and light therapy. The science of therapeutic massage, facts and misconceptions about massage, and the difference between therapeutic massage and a rubdown are reviewed in Chapter 17. The five common strokes used in sports massage and the application of a comprehensive therapeutic massage are explained and illustrated. Myofascial release is briefly discussed.

In Chapter 18, we review the anatomy of the intervertebral disk, and cervical and lumbar pain. The physiological effects of traction, commonly used traction devices, and guidelines for applying various forms of cervical and lumbar traction complete the chapter.

Characteristics of laser and light therapy (LED and SLD) devices and their use in medicine are explored in Chapter 19. Treatment parameters and the application of light therapy are reviewed. Ultraviolet radiation is briefly discussed.

Part VII, "Putting It All Together," is a unique feature of this text. It consists of two chapters. The intent of these chapters is to bridge the gap between understanding modalities and using them most effectively for treating patients. In Chapter 20, we attempt to reverse the reader's thinking about the material in the previous chapters. Throughout the book we use the traditional approach in presenting modalities. Each modality is discussed in isolation—what it is, what it can do, and the types of injuries it is typically used to treat. In real life, however, a patient does not approach a clinician with a request to apply a specific modality; rather, the patient presents with a problem, and the clinician must choose—from a variety of options—the modality that will be most effective in treating the problem. The last chapter consists of a series of case studies to help readers integrate their knowledge about individual therapeutic modalities by challenging them to select specific modalities or protocols for particular situations.

Two elements follow the last chapter: an appendix with the answers to the multiple-choice review questions (at the end of each part) and a glossary of the boldface terms found throughout the text.

Special Features

Special features are incorporated to enhance the usability of the text and the clinical application of the material.

- "Application Tips" are integrated throughout most of the theory chapters. Obviously, a chapter on application is, by definition, full of tips. Often, however, as we discuss the scientific basis of modalities, we offer a tip to help readers understand the application of the scientific principle being taught.
- "Modality Myths" appear in most chapters. By debunking some widely held, but false, misconceptions, we hope to reduce their influence on clinicians' thinking.
- "Critical Thinking" exercises serve three purposes: (1) They help readers engage with the material, (2) they provide another check for comprehension, and (3) they

help teach students to think critically. How will they learn critical thinking if they never do it? At the end of each chapter, we provide our response to these exercises.

- Analogies are used in almost all chapters to help clarify new concepts.
- The five-step application procedure is a template for the application of modalities. It benefits clinicians by providing a standardized process to help them organize the information needed to apply a specific modality. A second benefit is that novices will be able to learn numerous applications more quickly using a consistent approach. Some might argue that outlining specific application protocols could encourage students to become mechanical technicians rather than critical thinkers about modality application. Novices, however, need a cookbook at the start. And in most cases, it's not the specific application that requires critical thinking, it is the decision about which procedure to use. We have integrated specific step-by-step application protocols with sufficient theoretical and research information to allow students to critically choose when to use the procedure.
- Special-topic boxes, which appear in many of the chapters, cover a range of subjects that add value without interrupting the flow of the chapter's text. For example, boxes contain anecdotes about great pioneers (such as Ernst Dehne) or specific interactions with patients to illustrate a principle. Boxes can also be used to review information that some students may have learned in other courses (such as the chemistry and physics of electricity).
- "Chapter Reflections" and review questions are two types of self-quizzes. Open-ended questions and tasks appear at the end of each chapter and multiple-choice questions can be found at the end of each part. The different types of questions will appeal to different learning styles, and all readers can benefit from both. The answers to the multiple-choice questions are given in the appendix.
- A research basis characterizes our text. In fact, we have performed much of the research ourselves. Therefore, much of the information presented is firsthand.
- Original photographs complement the text and demonstrate many of the techniques. The photos were specifically set up and taken for this book.

For the Therapeutic Modalities Instructor

We understand the demand on an instructor's time, so to help make your job easier, you will have access to Instructor Resources upon adoption of *Therapeutic Modalities: The Art and Science*. The instructor's resource center at www.thePoint.lww.com/knight includes the following materials:

- A test generator with approximately 500 multiple choice, true–false, and fill-in-the-blank questions
- PowerPoint slides for Chapters 1–19
- An image bank that contains all of the figures and tables from the textbook

In addition, *Clinical Activities to Accompany Therapeutic Modalities: The Art and Science* (ISBN 9780781793193), sold separately, contains the following student materials that correspond with the book content:

- 18 discovery activities
- 16 modality application proficiency activities

Final Thoughts and Thanks

Writing this textbook is our dream come true. Each of us has wanted to do this for many years, but other responsibilities took priority. Although the process has been difficult at times, overall it's been a joy to discover new ideas and approaches in response to comments and queries from each other, our editors, and reviewers. We have grown tremendously in the process. New concepts and ideas have emerged, which we trust will result in improved patient care.

We want to thank many people whose direct and indirect contributions to the book have been enormous. Thinking does not occur in a vacuum. Many individuals have stimulated our thinking about therapeutic modalities, for which we are grateful. First, our thanks go to the thousands of patients whose pain and suffering first introduced us to therapeutic modalities and whose questions and desire to get better quicker stimulated our first critical thinking about our use of the modalities. Each of us was driven to research because of clinical questions we could not answer.

Second, many of our students have challenged our thinking about why and how various therapeutic modalities are used and, in some cases, not used. We have been blessed with an abundance of students whose zest and quest for learning about therapeutic modalities have kept us on our toes. To our former students at Weber State, the University of Missouri–Columbia, SUNY–Brockport, Indiana State, Northern Illinois, Illinois State, Illinois Wesleyan, and Brigham Young University—thanks.

We have enjoyed a rich, rewarding association with many professional colleagues. Our interactions with them concerning their research and thinking as well as their comments and challenges to our research have increased our understanding. We especially appreciate the contributions of our colleague Ty Hopkins, who stepped in at a crucial time to help us with Chapter 19. His background and experience with laser and light therapy was invaluable.

We must also acknowledge and thank Pete Darcy and our development team at Lippincott Williams & Wilkins. Pete convinced us that LWW's ideas for this text were compatible with our ideas, and they delivered. Betsy Dilernia, a master wordsmith, helped clarify our thinking and presentation. And we have thoroughly enjoyed working with Robyn Alvarez, Emily Lupash, and Meredith Brittain, who managed this project with insight and care.

Our peer reviewers were indispensable to this project. Their comments solidified our resolve in many places; but of greater help were comments that made us realize that we were not adequately communicating our thoughts.

Thanks to Gaye Merrill and Kevin Morris of BYU for making their athletic training clinics, and themselves, available for our photo shoot. We also appreciate other members of the athletic training clinical staff and the numerous athletic training students and BYU athletes who volunteered to be subjects for our photographs. Mark Philbrick, BYU photographer is not only very talented but also a joy to work with. We also appreciate Robyn Alvarez and Emily Lupash of LWW for help in organizing and administering the photo shoot.

We also want to acknowledge our wives and families. Shari and Nancy are the salt of the earth. They, as well as our children, have made sacrifices for this text. Thanks for your love and support.

It is plain to see that even though we are listed as the authors of this work, many others have contributed. It takes a village to write a good book, and we are grateful for our village. We'll wait for your opinions to see if it is good.

User's Guide

This User's Guide introduces you to the many features of Therapeutic Modalities: The Art and Science. Taking full advantage of these features, you not only read about therapeutic modalities, you become engaged in activities that help you learn and put your knowledge into practice.

The authors have loaded the chapters with features that help you understand the key points and apply your new skills in choosing and implementing therapeutic modalities.

Opening Scenes start each chapter with a short scenario posing a situation related to the chapter contents.

Closing Scenes at the end of the chapter complete the vignette, helping you see how content is put into practice.

Modality Myths present common misunderstandings and then set the record straight.

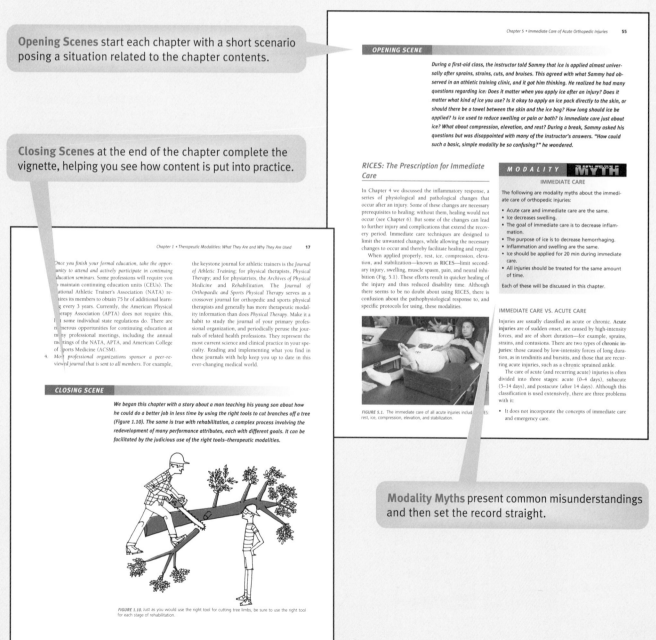

OPENING SCENE

During a first-aid class, the instructor told Sammy that ice is applied almost universally after sprains, strains, cuts, and bruises. This agreed with what Sammy had observed in an athletic training clinic, and it got him thinking. He realized he had many questions regarding ice: Does it matter when you apply ice after an injury? Does it matter what kind of ice you use? Is it okay to apply an ice pack directly to the skin, or should there be a towel between the skin and the ice bag? How long should ice be applied? Is ice used to reduce swelling or pain or both? Is immediate care just about ice? What about compression, elevation, and rest? During a break, Sammy asked his questions but was disappointed with many of the instructor's answers. "How could such a basic, simple modality be so confusing?" he wondered.

RICES: The Prescription for Immediate Care

In Chapter 4 we discussed the inflammatory response, a series of physiological and pathological changes that occur after an injury. Some of these changes are necessary prerequisites to healing; without them, healing would not occur (see Chapter 6). But some of the changes can lead to further injury and complications that extend the recovery period. Immediate care techniques are designed to limit the unwanted changes, while allowing the necessary changes to occur and thereby facilitate healing and repair.

When applied properly, rest, ice, compression, elevation, and stabilization—known as RICES—limit secondary injury, swelling, muscle spasm, pain, and neural inhibition (Fig. 5.1). These efforts result in quicker healing of the injury and thus reduced disability time. Although there seems to be no doubt about using RICES, there is confusion about the pathophysiological response to, and specific protocols for using, these modalities.

FIGURE 5.1. The immediate care of all acute injuries includes: rest, ice, compression, elevation, and stabilization.

MODALITY MYTH

IMMEDIATE CARE

The following are modality myths about the immediate care of orthopedic injuries:

- Acute care and immediate care are the same.
- Ice decreases swelling.
- The goal of immediate care is to decrease inflammation.
- The purpose of ice is to decrease hemorrhaging.
- Inflammation and swelling are the same.
- Ice should be applied for 20 min during immediate care.
- All injuries should be treated for the same amount of time.

Each of these will be discussed in this chapter.

IMMEDIATE CARE VS. ACUTE CARE

Injuries are usually classified as acute or chronic. **Acute injuries** are of sudden onset, are caused by high-intensity forces, and are of short duration—for example, sprains, strains, and contusions. There are two types of **chronic injuries**: those caused by low-intensity forces of long duration, as in tendinitis and bursitis, and those that are recurring acute injuries, such as a chronic sprained ankle.

The care of acute (and recurring acute) injuries is often divided into three stages: acute (0–4 days), subacute (5–14 days), and postacute (after 14 days). Although this classification is used extensively, there are three problems with it:

- It does not incorporate the concepts of immediate care and emergency care.

Once you finish your formal education, take the opportunity to attend and actively participate in continuing education seminars. Some professions will require you to maintain continuing education units (CEUs). The National Athletic Trainer's Association (NATA) requires its members to obtain 75 hr of additional learning every 3 years. Currently, the American Physical Therapy Association (APTA) does not require this, but some individual state regulations do. There are numerous opportunities for continuing education at many professional meetings, including the annual meetings of the NATA, APTA, and American College of Sports Medicine (ACSM).

4. *Most professional organizations sponsor a peer-reviewed journal that is sent to all members. For example,* the keystone journal for athletic trainers is the *Journal of Athletic Training;* for physical therapists, *Physical Therapy;* and for physiatrists, the *Archives of Physical Medicine and Rehabilitation.* The *Journal of Orthopaedic and Sports Physical Therapy* serves as a crossover journal for orthopedic and sports physical therapists and generally has more therapeutic modality information than does *Physical Therapy.* Make it a habit to study the journal of your primary professional organization, and periodically peruse the journals of related health professions. They represent the most current science and clinical practice in your specialty. Reading and implementing what you find in these journals with help keep you up to date in this ever-changing medical world.

CLOSING SCENE

We began this chapter with a story about a man teaching his young son about how he could do a better job in less time by using the right tools to cut branches off a tree (Figure 1.10). The same is true with rehabilitation, a complex process involving the redevelopment of many performance attributes, each with different goals. It can be facilitated by the judicious use of the right tools—therapeutic modalities.

FIGURE 1.10. Just as you would use the right tool for cutting tree limbs, be sure to use the right tool for each stage of rehabilitation.

Charts, Tables, and Graphs summarize and serve as a quick reference to key information.

Critical Thinking Exercises move you beyond rote memorization to deepen your understanding of each chapter.

Application Tips give you tips for practice and understanding.

Original Photographs taken specifically for this text demonstrate how to perform many of the techniques.

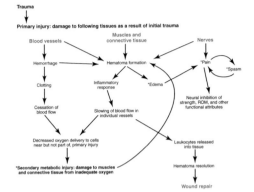

Chapter 4 • Tissue Response to Injury: Inflammation, Swelling, and Edema **49**

FIGURE 4.16. A summary of the inflammatory response to acute trauma. *, phases of the response that benefit by cold application to the injury; ROM, range of motion. See text for details (see also Chapter 5).

Changes in Capillary Filtration Pressure After Injury

With injury there is a change in the average capillary filtration pressure, caused by an increase in TOP.[26] The changes in capillary filtration pressure after an injury are presented in Table 4.2 and Figure 4.18. Because TOP pulls fluid into the tissue, edema and swelling result. Tissue oncotic pressure increases because of increased free protein. As a part of the inflammatory response, tissue debris from primary injury, secondary metabolic injury, and hemorrhaged whole blood is broken down into free protein by macrophages. In addition, some free protein escapes from the circulatory system during the period of hemorrhaging (if a vessel was damaged) or as a result of the increased permeability. The increased tissue free protein upsets the capillary filtration balance, and fluid (edema) builds up in the tissue (Fig. 4.19). The greater the injury, the greater the amount of free protein and eventually edema.

CRITICAL THINKING 4.2 Because the source of most swelling is excess free protein in the tissue, what must happen to remove the swelling? What effect, if any, does ice have on swelling once it has occurred?

This process accounts for the delayed nature of most incidences of swelling after acute injury. Both secondary injury and the breakdown of tissue debris by macrophages occur over an extended period of time. Edema, therefore, begins minutes to hours after the injury and continues to develop over many hours. The swelling that occurs immediately after the injury is caused directly by hemorrhaging.

Secondary injury results in increased edema, and increased edema can contribute to increased secondary metabolic injury. Two mechanisms are involved. First, as

✔ **APPLICATION TIP**

USE A COMPRESSION WRAP FOR AN ACUTE INJURY. Always apply a compression wrap for the first day or so after acute injury, even if the injury appears minor and there is no swelling. Swelling is often delayed. Once it occurs, you cannot turn back the clock. And there is no harm in wearing a compression bandage overnight in situations in which swelling would not occur. It is better to be safe than sorry.

Chapter 5 • Immediate Care of Acute Orthopedic Injuries **69**

as gel packs, but they are much more flexible than refrozen crushed ice packs. Because of their nylon covering, artificial ice packs are not as effective in cooling tissue as is crushed ice, but they are more effective in cooling than a gel pack because they undergo a phase change. They are preferred for home use because they can be safely applied after cooling in a kitchen freezer, are flexible, and go through a phase change as they warm.

Crushable Chemical Pack

A **crushable chemical pack** consists of a thin-walled vinyl pouch of a liquid packaged within a stronger, larger vinyl pouch of dry crystals. When squeezed with sufficient force, the smaller pouch is broken, leaking its fluid into the larger, outer pouch. The fluid and crystals combine in a chemical reaction that cools the fluid. Crushable chemical packs are not recommended because they neither get the body cold enough nor last long enough to be used in place of crushed ice.[60] There also is a danger of chemical burns if the contents of such a pack leak onto the skin. Crushable chemical cold packs should be used only as a last resort.

APPLICATION DIRECTLY TO THE SKIN

In general, crushed ice packs are applied directly to the patient's skin (Fig. 5.16).[61,62] A towel or elastic wrap between the ice pack and the body insulates against the full effect of the cold, thereby making the treatment less effective.[60,63–65] If used for <60 min, most cold packs do not

cause frostbite. Frozen gel packs are an exception, however, and should not be applied directly on the skin. Their temperature may be many degrees below zero and could cause frostbite.

✔ **APPLICATION TIP**

KNOW WHEN NOT TO APPLY COLD PACKS DIRECTLY TO THE SKIN. Some types of cold packs are too cold to be applied directly to the skin because they will damage the skin. These include frozen gel packs and crushed ice packs using ice frozen in a refrigerator or freezer. Most crushed ice packs are made from ice from an ice machine, which stores the ice just below freezing (30°F or −1°C). But ice from a freezer and gel packs are in the range of −2°F to −5°F (−16°C to −19°C). This is much too cold for the skin and often results in tissue damage.

Placing a towel or elastic wrap between the skin and the cold pack, as many recommend,[7,66] insulates the skin against the cold, decreasing the effectiveness of the cold pack (Fig. 5.17).[60,61–65] Using wet [7,67] or frozen[68] elastic wraps between the skin and the cold pack is preferable to using dry ones, but not as beneficial as application directly to the skin.[61–65]

Most first-aid texts recommend against applying ice packs directly to the skin.[7,66] This is beginning to change,

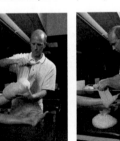

FIGURE 5.16. **(a)** Apply cold packs directly to the skin. **(b)** A towel or wrap between the cold pack and the skin will decrease the effectiveness of cooling.

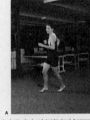 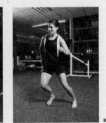

FIGURE 14.9. Jogging begins slowly and straight ahead. It progresses to **(a)** lazy S and **(b)** sharp Z patterns. Speed increases until the patient is jogging.

The Five-Step Application Procedure

The application of all therapeutic modalities should follow a standard procedure to ensure that all essential elements occur and to prevent rogue applications (Fig. 2.3). Although there is a wide range of therapeutic modalities, each one can follow a general application process. Our **five-step application procedure** eliminates the need to learn SOPs for each modality.[1] After learning the five-step framework, you can plug in specifics for each therapeutic modality. By learning and applying this system, you will be more organized and effective in delivering therapeutic modality treatments.

STEP 1: FOUNDATION

A. Definition. A description of the modality and the basics of how it operates (Fig. 2.4).
B. Effects. The physiological and/or pathological changes the modality evokes, both locally and systemically (throughout the body).
C. Advantages. The benefits of the modality that make it more effective in treating injuries than other modalities.
D. Disadvantages. The possible negative effects the modality might cause as well as the benefits that might be lost from using this modality over another.
E. Indications. Situations in which the modality should be used or for which it is a suitable treatment or remedy for the condition.
F. Contraindications. Situations in which the modality should not be used—that is, situations in which it may do more harm than good.
G. Precautions. Situations that could cause harm if the clinician is not careful—for example, failure to move

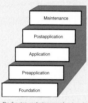

Maintenance

Postapplication

Application

Preapplication

Foundation

FIGURE 2.3. The five-step application procedure is a standardized framework for applying any therapeutic modality. It is rigid enough for quality control, yet flexible enough to allow the clinician to use modalities in the context of a critical thinking approach to rehabilitation.

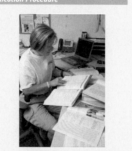

FIGURE 2.4. Before a therapeutic modality can be properly applied, you must have foundational knowledge about the modality and how specific types of injuries respond to the various ways of applying it.

the soundhead during ultrasound treatment could damage tissue or cause extreme pain.

MODALITY MYTH

THERE ARE RELATIVE AND ABSOLUTE CONTRAINDICATIONS

Some clinicians inappropriately use the terms *absolute contraindication* and *relative contraindication* to refer to contraindications and precautions, respectively. The term *absolute contraindication* is redundant. *Contraindication* means "do not use," so it is already absolute. The term *relative contraindication* contradicts itself. It is impossible to "relatively" not use a modality. Use the more precise terms, contraindication and precaution.

STEP 2: PREAPPLICATION TASKS

A. Selecting the proper modality
 1. Determine the pathological and physiological changes associated with the injury by doing the following:
  a. Evaluate (or reevaluate) the injury or problem.
  b. Review the patient's response to any previous treatment (Fig. 2.5).

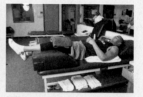

FIGURE 2.5. Patient interaction is an essential preapplication task. Detailed questions about how the patient responded to previous treatments help you decide whether to continue with the present modality or to select another one. Explaining the purpose, the expected outcome, the body's physiological response, and what the patient should feel help prepare the patient psychologically for the treatment.

 2. Establish the objectives (goals) of the therapy.
 3. Match your therapeutic goal with a modality that will help you achieve that goal; consider the effects, advantages, disadvantages, indications, contraindications, and precautions of all the possible modalities you could use to reach your goals.
 4. Make sure the modality is not contraindicated for the injury or condition in question.
B. Preparing the patient psychologically. This step entails more than just good bedside manners. As we will discuss in Chapter 7, there is a strong connection between emotions and physiological responses. The patient's psychological state modifies tissue responses to the therapy.
 1. Explain the purpose and expected outcome of the procedure.
 2. Describe the body's basic physiological response to the treatment, if the patient is interested.
 3. Explain what the patient should expect to feel—for example, tingling, pins and needles, or gentle warmth.
 4. Demonstrate the procedure on yourself if the patient is apprehensive.
 5. Warn the patient about precautions.
C. Preparing the patient physically
 1. Remove clothing as necessary.
 2. Remove bandages, braces, and so on, as necessary.
 3. Position the patient in a manner that will be comfortable, yet allow accessibility to the modality. Have an ample supply of pillows or bolsters (supports) to use in positioning the patient (Fig. 2.6).

FIGURE 2.6. Pillows and bolsters are helpful in positioning a patient for treatment. You can never have too many pillows and bolsters in an athletic training clinic.

D. Preparing the equipment
 1. Set up the equipment.
 2. Check the equipment operation.
 3. Perform a safety check.

STEP 3: APPLICATION PARAMETERS

A. Procedures
 1. Turn on the unit (if necessary).
 2. Adjust the output parameters as needed.
 3. Check the patient's response and readjust the output as needed.
B. Dosage
C. Length of application
D. Frequency of application
E. Duration of therapy

STEP 4: POSTAPPLICATION TASKS

A. Equipment removal; patient cleanup
B. Equipment replacement; area cleanup
C. Instructions to the patient. *Note:* These should be written if they are extensive or complicated.
 1. Schedule the next treatment.
 2. Instruct the patient about the level of activity and/or self-treatment she should administer before the next formal treatment.
 3. Instruct the patient about what she should feel after treatment.
D. Record of treatment, including unique patient responses (Fig. 2.7).

STEP 5: MAINTENANCE

A. Regular equipment cleaning
B. Routine maintenance
C. Simple repairs

Five-Step Application Procedure Templates streamline how you organize the information needed to apply a modality, helping you quickly learn new modalities.

The body often mishandles pain. It has a great memory for what it wants to do, but not for why it is doing it.[2,3] Thus pain often persists long after the cause of the pain is resolved. It's that annoying relative who you thought was coming to visit for a few days but who stayed much longer than anticipated. You must respect pain—use it to guide you—but be tough on it when necessary so that it does not take on a life of its own.

NO PAIN, NO GAIN?

When it comes to conditioning, "no pain, no gain" is absolutely right. But this adage does not apply to rehabilitation. During rehabilitation, the mantra is twofold:

• Ignore the pain equals no brain.
• Pandering to pain propagates pain.

Together these statements explain how to both respect pain and be tough on it during rehabilitation. To ignore pain is not smart because it often leads to more pain and disability. On the other hand, if you eliminate all activity to avoid causing any pain, the pain will take on a life of its own, meaning that it will take much less stimulus than normal to evoke a pain response (even minor aches and pains will seem worse than they are).

DEHNE'S SPINAL ADAPTATION SYNDROME

The **spinal adaptation syndrome** is a theory based on a 20-year study of sprains by Ernst Dehne (Box 8.2).[2-5] The logic of the theory is summarized as follows:

• Afferent nociceptive impulses arising from traumatized tissues or tissue in the process of repair alter the integration of central nervous system (CNS) excitation at the spinal cord level.
• These alterations result in decreased response to volitional stimuli and increased response to otherwise subliminal peripheral stresses, resulting in involuntary muscle action.
• The altered muscle response through the mediation of vasomotor reaction (dilation or constriction of blood vessels) determines the local chemical environment that produces the process of repair.
• The process of repair is a highly sensitive state. It responds adversely to additional stress and favorably to the reestablishment of central control.
• The spinal adaptation syndrome seems to operate in all conditions connected with inflammation or repair. Covering such a broad spectrum, it is not specific to any one condition. It appears that all tissue in the process of repair has an extremely sensitive nociceptive potential and reacts violently to all additional stress as well as to stress that would be subliminal in the normal

BOX 8.2 DEHNE: AN ORTHOPEDIC VISIONARY

Ernst Dehne[2-5] is often considered the father of modern orthopedic rehabilitation. Although he is relatively unknown, his observations and revolutionary thinking set the stage for the great advances in rehabilitation during the past 30 years. His ideas seemed way out in the 1950s and 1960s, but they are now standard thinking; although few clinicians are aware of how Dehne has influenced their practices.

Dehne was a German orthopedic surgeon who in the 1930s recognized that the standard practice of long-term cast immobilization (often up to 16 weeks) after orthopedic injury and surgery was detrimental to full recovery.[6,7] Through the years, his idea of less immobilization and quicker active use of orthopedically injured limbs grew, even without the support of the mainstream medical community. Markey[8] who served a residency under Dehne, tells of Dehne's frustration with the lack of cooperation by the nursing staff. They were reluctant to follow the surgeon's orders to get the patients out of bed and walking immediately after surgery. It was so bad that Dehne would sometimes pound on a desk, an empty hospital bed, or a table with a baseball bat as he urged the staff to follow his orders.

Although Grant[9] and Hayden[10] do not mention Dehne in their classic papers on cryokinetics (see Chapter 13), they worked one floor below him at Brook Army Hospital in San Antonio, Texas, and treated many of his patients. Their experiment with ice and early active exercise grew, no doubt, from

state. The competitive influence of volitional impulses tends to inhibit and eventually to terminate the nociceptive interference at the spinal cord level.

In short, the theory holds that nociceptive impulses from traumatized tissue inhibit motor functions and tissue repair but that voluntary activity can reestablish central control and prevent this inhibition. In other words, prolonged inactivity after an injury will lead to neural inhibition that could become permanent.

RESETTING CENTRAL CONTROL DURING REHABILITATION

Removing the pain sensation after injury is not enough; you must also get rid of the effects of the pain—that is,

Special Topic Boxes cover a range of interesting topics such as anecdotes about great pioneers and interactions with patients that illustrate key principles.

Special Study Tools

These special study tools enhance your learning and your success of applying therapeutic modalities in the future.

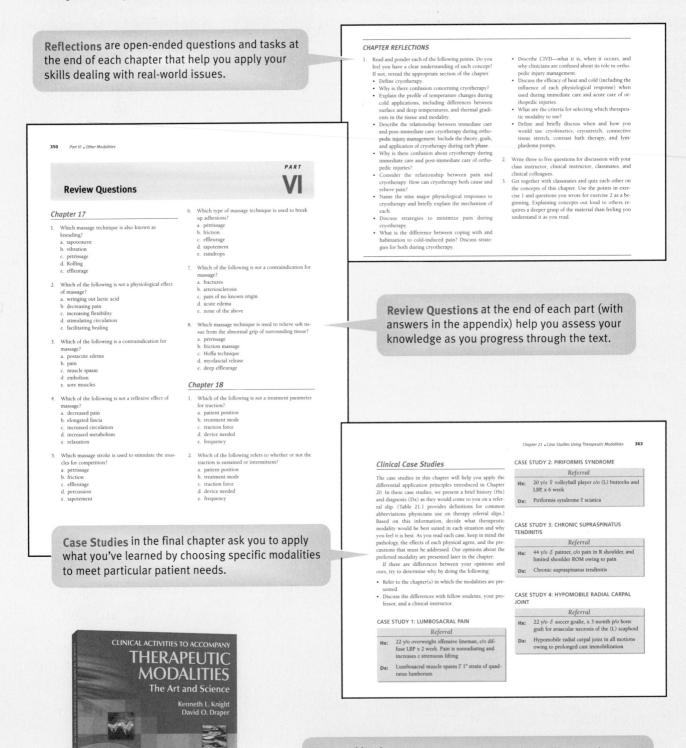

Reflections are open-ended questions and tasks at the end of each chapter that help you apply your skills dealing with real-world issues.

Review Questions at the end of each part (with answers in the appendix) help you assess your knowledge as you progress through the text.

Case Studies in the final chapter ask you to apply what you've learned by choosing specific modalities to meet particular patient needs.

Your workbook, *Clinical Activities to Accompany Therapeutic Modalities: The Art and Science,* offers 18 discovery activities and 16 modality application proficiency activities in which you apply new concepts and skills. Working through the activities in the workbook will help ensure your understanding.

---

350   *Part VI • Other Modalities*

Review Questions

PART VI

Chapter 17

1. Which massage technique is also known as kneading?
   a. tapotement
   b. vibration
   c. pétrissage
   d. Rolfing
   e. effleurage

2. Which of the following is *not* a physiological effect of massage?
   a. wringing out lactic acid
   b. decreasing pain
   c. increasing flexibility
   d. stimulating circulation
   e. facilitating healing

3. Which of the following is a contraindication for massage?
   a. postacute edema
   b. pain
   c. muscle spasm
   d. embolism
   e. sore muscles

4. Which of the following is *not* a reflexive effect of massage?
   a. decreased pain
   b. elongated fascia
   c. increased circulation
   d. increased metabolism
   e. relaxation

5. Which massage stroke is used to stimulate the muscles for competition?
   a. pétrissage
   b. friction
   c. effleurage
   d. percussion
   e. tapotement

6. Which type of massage technique is used to break up adhesions?
   a. pétrissage
   b. friction
   c. effleurage
   d. tapotement
   e. raindrops

7. Which of the following is *not* a contraindication for massage?
   a. fractures
   b. arteriosclerosis
   c. pain of no known origin
   d. acute edema
   e. none of the above

8. Which massage technique is used to relieve soft tissue from the abnormal grip of surrounding tissue?
   a. pétrissage
   b. friction massage
   c. Hoffa technique
   d. myofascial release
   e. deep effleurage

Chapter 18

1. Which of the following is *not* a treatment parameter for traction?
   a. patient position
   b. treatment mode
   c. traction force
   d. device needed
   e. frequency

2. Which of the following refers to whether or not the traction is sustained or intermittent?
   a. patient position
   b. treatment mode
   c. traction force
   d. device needed
   e. frequency

CHAPTER REFLECTIONS

1. Read and ponder each of the following points. Do you feel you have a clear understanding of each concept? If not, reread the appropriate section of the chapter.
   • Define cryotherapy.
   • Why is there confusion concerning cryotherapy?
   • Explain the profile of temperature changes during cold applications, including differences between surface and deep temperatures, and thermal gradients in the tissue and modality.
   • Describe the relationship between immediate care and post-immediate care cryotherapy during orthopedic injury management. Include the theory, goals, and application of cryotherapy during each phase.
   • Why is there confusion about cryotherapy during immediate care and post-immediate care of orthopedic injuries?
   • Consider the relationship between pain and cryotherapy: How can cryotherapy both cause and relieve pain?
   • Name the nine major physiological responses to cryotherapy and briefly explain the mechanism of each.
   • Discuss strategies to minimize pain during cryotherapy.
   • What is the difference between coping with and habituation to cold-induced pain? Discuss strategies for both during cryotherapy.
   • Describe CIVD—what it is, when it occurs, and why clinicians are confused about its role in orthopedic injury management.
   • Discuss the efficacy of heat and cold (including the influence of each physiological response) when used during immediate care and acute care of orthopedic injuries.
   • What are the criteria for selecting which therapeutic modality to use?
   • Define and briefly discuss when and how you would use cryokinetics, cryostretch, connective tissue stretch, contrast bath therapy, and lymphedema pumps.

2. Write three to five questions for discussion with your class instructor, clinical instructor, classmates, and clinical colleagues.

3. Get together with classmates and quiz each other on the concepts of this chapter. Use the points in exercise 1 and questions you wrote for exercise 2 as a beginning. Explaining concepts out loud to others requires a deeper grasp of the material than feeling you understand it as you read.

Chapter 21 • Case Studies Using Therapeutic Modalities   **363**

Clinical Case Studies

The case studies in this chapter will help you apply the differential application principles introduced in Chapter 20. In these case studies, we present a brief history (Hx) and diagnosis (Dx) as they would come to you on a referral slip. (Table 21.1 provides definitions for common abbreviations physicians use on therapy referral slips.) Based on this information, decide what therapeutic modality would be best suited in each situation and why you feel it is best. As you read each case, keep in mind the pathology, the effects of each physical agent, and the precautions that must be addressed. Our opinions about the preferred modality are presented later in the chapter.

If there are differences between your opinions and ours, try to determine why by doing the following:

• Refer to the chapter(s) in which the modalities are presented.
• Discuss the differences with fellow students, your professor, and a clinical instructor.

CASE STUDY 1: LUMBOSACRAL PAIN

Referral	
Hx:	22 y/o overweight offensive lineman, c/o diffuse LBP x 2 week. Pain is nonradiating and increases c strenuous lifting
Dx:	Lumbosacral muscle spasm c̄ 1° strain of quadratus lumborum

CASE STUDY 2: PIRIFORMIS SYNDROME

Referral	
Hx:	20 y/o ♀ volleyball player c/o (L) buttocks and LBP, x 6 week
Dx:	Piriformis syndrome c̄ sciatica

CASE STUDY 3: CHRONIC SUPRASPINATUS TENDINITIS

Referral	
Hx:	44 y/o ♂ painter, c/o pain in R shoulder, and limited shoulder ROM owing to pain
Dx:	Chronic supraspinatus tendinitis

CASE STUDY 4: HYPOMOBILE RADIAL CARPAL JOINT

Referral	
Hx:	22 y/o ♂ soccer goalie, x 3 month p/o bone graft for avascular necrosis of the (L) scaphoid
Dx:	Hypomobile radial carpal joint in all motions owing to prolonged cast immobilization

---

CLINICAL ACTIVITIES TO ACCOMPANY

THERAPEUTIC MODALITIES

The Art and Science

Kenneth L. Knight
David O. Draper

Wolters Kluwer | Lippincott Williams & Wilkins

*the*Point

Reviewers

Jeromy M. Alt, MS, ATC
Field Service Assistant Professor
University of Cincinnati
Cincinnati, OH

J. C. Andersen, PhD, ATC, PT, SCS
Assistant Professor and Director, Athletic Training
Program
The University of Tampa
Tampa, FL

Amanda K. Andrews, PhD, ATC
Assistant Professor
Troy University
Troy, AL

Jennifer Austin, PhD, ATC
Assistant Professor
Colby-Sawyer College
New London, NH

Barbara Belyea, PT, MS, CSCS
Clinical Associate Professor
Ithaca College
Ithaca, NY

Jay A. Bradley, MEd, LAT, ATC
Clinical Assistant Professor
IUPUI
Indianapolis, IN

Debbie Bradney, DPE, ATC
Program Coordinator for Athletic Training & Exercise
Physiology
Assistant Professor
Lynchburg College
Lynchburg, VA

Scott Bruce, MS, ATC
Lecturer/Assistant Athletic Trainer
University of Tennessee at Chattanooga
Chattanooga, TN

John Burns, MS, ATC, LAT
Clinical Education Coordinator
Washburn University
Topeka, KS

Mary Carbaugh, SMS, MT, CPFT, SMT
Assistant Professor
Ivy Tech Community College
Fort Wayne, IN

BC Charles-Liscombe, EdD, ATC
Associate Professor
Greensboro College
Greensboro, NC

Gwen Cleaves, MA, ATC Professional
Clinical Education Coordinator
Kean University City
Union, NJ

Keith A. Clements, ATC/L
Head Athletic Trainer—Men's Athletics
University of Tennessee
Knoxville, TN

Matthew J. Comeau, PhD, LAT, ATC, CSCS
Associate Professor
Arkansas State University
State University, AR

Vincent M. Conroy, PT, DScPT
Assistant Professor
Department of Physical Therapy & Rehabilitation Science
University of Maryland School of Medicine
Baltimore, MD

Earl R. "Bud" Cooper, EdD, ATC, CSCS
Associate Professor
Georgia College & State University
Milledgeville, GA

Rev. Deacon Carl Cramer, EdD, RKT, ATC, LAT
Professor
Barry University
Miami Shores, FL

Jim Crawley, MEd, ATC, PT
Athletic Training Program Director
Dominican College
Orangeburg, NY

Alyson Dearie, MS, ATC
Clinical Coordinator of Athletic Training
State University of New York at Cortland
Cortland, NY

Gianluca Del Rossi, PhD, ATC
Assistant Professor
University of South Florida
Tampa, FL

Amy Everitt, EdD, ATC
Associate Professor
Salem State College
Salem, MA

Brian K. Farr, MA, ATC, LAT, CSCS
Director, Athletic Training Education Program
The University of Texas at Austin
Austin, TX

Xristos K. Gaglias, MA, ATC
Curriculum Director/Assistant Professor
Athletic Training Education Program
School of Health Technology & Management
Stony Brook University
Stony Brook, NY

Kara Gange, MAEd, ATC
Instructor
North Dakota State University
Fargo, ND

Kevin Gard, DPT, OCS
Clinical Associate Professor
Associate Director
Drexel University
Philadelphia, PA

Traci Gearhart, PhD, LAT, ATC
Assistant Professor
Wingate University
Wingate, NC

Brian T. Gerry, MS, ATC
Program Director Athletic Training
Augustana College
Sioux Falls, SD

Bonnie M. Goodwin, MESS, ATC
Director, Athletic Training Education Program
Assistant Professor, Assistant Athletic Trainer
Capital University
Columbus, OH

Hugh W. Harling, EdD, LAT, ATC
Associate Professor
Methodist University
Fayetteville, NC

Dawn Hammerschmidt, MEd, ATC
Assistant Professor
Minnesota State University Moorhead
Moorhead, MN

Jerald D. Hawkins, EdD, ATC, FACSM
Professor
Lander University
Greenwood, SC

Jolene M. Henning, EdD, ATC, LAT
Assistant Professor
University of North Carolina at Greensboro
Greensboro, NC

Paul Higgs, MEd, ATC, LAT
Head Athletic Trainer
Georgia College and State University
Milledgeville, GA

Bill Holcomb, PhD, ATC
Associate Professor
University of Nevada, Las Vegas
Las Vegas, NV

Timothy G. Howell, EdD, ATC, CSCS
Assistant Professor
Athletic Training Education Program Director
Alfred University
Alfred, NY

Tricia J. Hubbard, PhD, ATC
Assistant Professor
The University of North Carolina Charlotte
Charlotte, NC

Shawna Jordan, PhD, ATC, LAT
Assistant Professor
Athletic Training Education Program Director
Kansas State University
Manhattan, KS

Owen Keller, ATC
Associate Professor
Athletic Trainer
Ohio Northern University
Ada, Ohio

Robin E. Kennel, MS, LAT, ATC, CSCS
ATEP Director/Assistant Athletic Trainer
Mars Hill College
Mars Hill, NC

Casey Kohr, MS, PT, ATC, LAT
Instructor of Athletic Training
Clarke College
Dubuque, IA

Mark Lafave, PhD (ABD), MSc, CAT(C)
Department Chair and Instructor
Mount Royal College
Calgary, Alberta

Rifat Latifi, MD, FACS
Professor of Clinical Surgery
The University of Arizona College of Medicine
Tucson, AZ

Christine A. Lauber, EdD, LAT, ATC
Associate Professor
University of Indianapolis
Indianapolis, IN

Barbara H. Long, MS, VATL, ATC
Chair, Health & Exercise Science
Bridgewater College
Bridgewater, VA

Susan Lowe, PT, DPT, MS, GCS
Associate Clinical Professor
Northeastern University
Boston, MA

William T. Lyons, MS, ATC
Director of Athletic Training Education
University of Wyoming
Laramie, WY

Brendon P. McDermott, MS, ATC
Laboratory Instructor/Research Assistant
University of Connecticut
Storrs, CT

Tsega A. Mehreteab, PT, MS, DPT
Clinical Professor
New York University
New York, NY

Mark A. Merrick, PhD, ATC
Associate Professor & Director
Division of Athletic Training
The Ohio State University
Columbus, OH

Angela Mickle, PhD, ATC
Associate Professor
Radford University
Radford, VA

Charles Miller, MS, ATC, CSCS, PES
Athletic Trainer
West Liberty State College
West Liberty, WV

Matthew Miltenberger, MS, ATC, CSCS
Instructor
East Stroudsburg University
East Stroudsburg, PA

Kyle Momsen, MA, ATC
ATEP Clinical Education Coordinator
Gustavus Adolphus College
St. Peter, MN

Brad Montgomery, MAT, ATC
Head Athletic Trainer/Instructor
The University of West Alabama
Livingston, AL

Patricia Morganroth, MSN, RN, CDE
Program Chair—Health and Fitness
Cincinnati State Technical and Community College
Cincinnati, OH

Derek Suranie, MEd, ATC
Assistant Professor
North Georgia College & State University
Dahlonega, GA

Erik E Swartz, PhD, ATC
Associate Professor and Clinical Coordinator
Athletic Training Education Program, Department of
Kinesiology
University of New Hampshire
Durham, NH

LesLee Taylor, PhD, ATC, LAT
Assistant Professor
Texas Tech University Health Sciences Center
Lubbock, TX

Adam J. Thompson, PhD, ATC, LAT
Associate Professor
Indiana Wesleyan University
Marion, IN

Brian Udermann, PhD, ATC, FACSM
Associate Professor
University of Wisconsin—La Crosse
La Crosse, WI

Heather L. VanOpdorp, MSEd, ATC
Instructor/Athletic Training Room Coordinator
University of Tampa
Tampa, FL

Ben Velasquez, DA, ATC, LAT
Associate Professor
University of Southern Mississippi
Hattiesburg, MS

Gary Ward, MS, ATC, PT
Assistant Professor and Program Director
Department of Sports Medicine and Athletic Training
Missouri State University
Springfield, MO

Scot A. Ward, MS, ATC
Clinical Coordinator/Athletic Trainer
Keene State College
Keene, NH

Tony Ward, MS, ATC, LAT
Assistant Professor
Director
Athletic Training Education Program
Shawnee State University
Portsmouth, OH

Susie Wehring MS, ATC, LAT
Associate Professor
Loras College
Dubuque, IA

Chuck Whedon, MS, ATC, CSCS
Coordinator of Athletic Training Services
Instructor, Health and Exercise Science
Rowan University
Glassboro, NJ

Jackie Williams, PhD, LAT, ATC
Director of Athletic Training Education
University of Idaho
Moscow, ID

Scott Woken, MA, ATC
Director of Sports Medicine
North Dakota State University
Fargo, ND

Michael Scott Zema, MEd, ATC
Assistant Professor/Football Athletic Trainer
Slippery Rock University of Pennsylvania
Slippery Rock, PA

Contents

Part V: Therapeutic Heat and Cold

Part VI: *Other Modalities*

Part VII: *Putting It All Together*

IN PERSPECTIVE

What are therapeutic modalities? Why are they used? How do they relate to therapeutic exercise? How do you know what therapeutic modality to use and when to use it? The objective of Part I is to answer these questions and thus establish an overall perspective for therapeutic modality use. We define therapeutic modalities and help you understand their place in orthopedic injury management and explain how they relate to total rehabilitation. We also present a rationale for using a standardized systems approach to therapeutic modality application. Finally, we present a case for proper record keeping, indicating how doing so can strengthen both the efficacy of your treatments and the quality of your health care. Thus Part I is a foundation for the rest of the book.

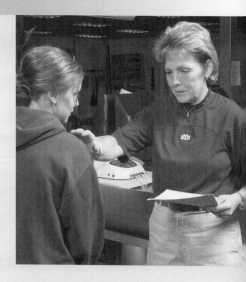

Part I consists of three chapters:

1   Therapeutic Modalities: What They Are and Why They Are Used

2   General Application Procedures

3   Injury Record Keeping

Therapeutic Modalities: What They Are and Why They Are Used

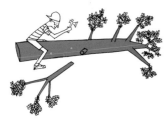

A father enlisted his young son to help remove a dead tree from their yard. The eager boy got a small hatchet from the garage and began feverishly chopping away at tree limbs (Fig. 1.1). Although he worked very hard, his progress was slow. The father appeared with a power saw and quickly cut off the limbs and trunk. He said, "Son, it's important to work hard—but it's even more important to work smart. We could use that little hatchet and work hard all day chopping up these limbs, or we could work smart and use the right tool to finish the same job in just minutes."

FIGURE 1.1 You can get the job done with the wrong tool, but it takes longer and the result might not be successful.

Many clinicians believe that their hands and exercise are the best tools for treating orthopedic injuries. However, these aren't the only tools, and integrating therapeutic modalities as part of a treatment regime often facilitates the hands-on treatment. For example, cryokinetics involves numbing a joint with cold, followed by active exercise. If the patient did not ice the ankle before exercise, pain and inhibition would compromise the exercise, thereby making it less effective. In this case, ice is the tool that causes numbing, so the patient can perform a higher level of exercise. The exercise alone is good, but using numbing and exercise together is smart.

In **physical medicine**, a therapeutic modality is a tool for bringing about a desired therapeutic response. In this book, you will learn why, how, and when to use several tools in your treatment regimens.

Defining and Classifying Therapeutic Modalities

A **therapeutic modality** is a device or application that delivers a physical agent to the body for therapeutic purposes. The most common **physical agents** used in treating orthopedic injuries are:

- Heat
- Cold
- Light
- Electricity
- Exercise

The **therapeutic purposes** of these agents are to promote or improve:

1. Wound healing
2. Pain relief
3. Flexibility and range of motion
4. Muscular strength
5. Muscular endurance
6. Muscular speed
7. Muscular coordination or skill
8. Power
9. Agility
10. Cardiorespiratory endurance

There are several systems of classifying therapeutic modalities. They can be classified according to the physical agent used, such as hydrotherapy, thermotherapy, and electrotherapy. They can be classified according to tissue responses, such as deep heating, superficial heating, and cooling. However, these categories are not exclusive, and many therapeutic modalities fit into more than one category. For example, ultrasound can be classified as thermotherapy, mechanical, or deep heating. Contrast therapy is both cryotherapy and thermotherapy. General classifications are shown in Table 1.1. Modalities in italics are classified in more than one category.

Which of the classification systems is preferred? None of them. Because so many modalities fit into multiple categories, trying to force one particular classification system is an exercise in futility.

Maximizing the Effectiveness of Therapeutic Modalities

Therapeutic modalities can be powerful tools for caring for and rehabilitating orthopedic injuries, or they can contribute little to the process. They are effective only when the proper modality is applied in the proper way to injured tissue. There is little value in using the wrong modality properly or in using the right modality improperly. Consider the following ideas as you develop your personal philosophical basis for using therapeutic modalities.

TABLE 1.1	*General Classifications of Therapeutic Modalities**	
CLASSIFICATION	**DESCRIPTION**	**EXAMPLES**
Cryotherapy	Use of cold (usually between 32°F and 70°F, or 0°C and 21°C)	Ice massage, ice packs, *ice slush/ice immersion,* part of contrast therapy, cold *whirlpool,* vapocoolant sprays
Thermotherapy	Use of superficial and deep heat (usually between 98.6°F and 109.4°F, or 37°C and 43°C)	Moist heat packs, warm *whirlpool,* paraffin wax baths, ultrasound, *pulsed shortwave diathermy,* ultraviolet
Hydrotherapy	Application of water	*Whirlpool* and aquatic therapy pools, *ice slush/ice immersion*
Electrotherapy	Use of electricity	Electrical muscle stimulation, iontophoresis, TENS, *diathermy*
Light therapy	Use of electromagnetic radiation	Laser, light therapy, *infrared*
Mechanotherapy	Use of motion, force, or pressure	Massage, mobilization, intermittent compression, continuous passive motion, traction, *whirlpool,* *ultrasound*
Exercise	Activities the patient performs to bring about a desired response	Various

*Modalities in italics are classified in more than one category.

ART AND SCIENCE

The use of therapeutic modalities, like all practices in the health professions, is an art—an art influenced by experience and tradition and by science and theory (Fig. 1.2). It would be ideal if the use of therapeutic modalities were based entirely on scientific fact. But this is unrealistic for two reasons. First, the human body is quite complex and there has not been enough research to fully explain its response either to injury or to the application of therapeutic modalities. Second, many clinicians are not current with the modality research that has been done; therefore, their use of modalities is outdated.

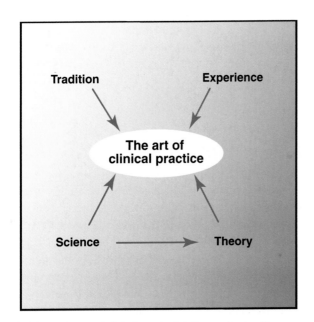

FIGURE 1.2. The art of clinical practice is influenced by tradition, experience, science, and theory.

Your initial use of therapeutic modalities will be influenced heavily by the traditions and theories of your clinical instructors. They may or may not agree with the concepts presented in this text. We have heard horror stories over the years of clinics in which most patients were treated the same way, regardless of their injury. For example, in one clinic 95% of patients were "hum'd," treated with hot packs, ultrasound, and mobilization. Regardless of the approach of your initial clinical instructors, strive to gradually increase the scientific and theoretical influence of your own clinical practice.

KNOBOLOGY

Knobology is a tongue-in-cheek term for the study of application without theory. One of our colleagues uses the term *knobologist* for students and clinicians who want to know only which knobs on a therapeutic modality to turn and are uninterested in why they are doing so (Fig. 1.3). Not only would there be little advancement in medicine if all clinicians were knobologists but patients would suffer from inadequate treatment. Don't be a knobologist!

 CRITICAL THINKING 1.1 *List some ways that knobologists can harm the health professions.*

THEORY VS. APPLICATION

The ideal is that all application is based on scientifically derived evidence and theory. Yet this is not possible, because application almost always precedes theory, and there is often a lack of valid research. A clinician frustrated with a particular case, or group of similar cases, tries something new to help her patients. It seems to work, so she modifies

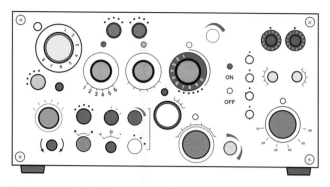

FIGURE 1.3. Knobologists know the knobs but not why they use the knobs.

the approach, talks to colleagues, talks to patients, fine-tunes some more, and shares the approach with others. As the popularity and acceptance of the technique grow, people begin trying to explain why the application works. These explanations become a theory. In time, scientists test the theory with research. The research either strengthens or alters the theory, and often results in adjustments to the application. Thus application, theory, and research are intertwined, each stimulating the other.

It is critical for a clinician to learn both application and theory. She must adjust the application and its theoretical basis as new knowledge becomes available. This practice may even provide opportunities for participating in the discovery of new approaches.

CLINICAL DECISION MAKING

Clinical decision making is the process of determining how to treat patients. It is an ongoing, dynamic process that should occur before every therapeutic modality application. It requires critical thinking and evaluation of the evidence available for the specific injury, patient, availability of therapeutic modalities, and other therapeutic interventions (such as drugs and therapeutic exercise). The process begins with a thorough evaluation of the patient and the specific injury or condition. Analysis of the subjective and objective data leads to a tentative diagnosis. A plan of action is then outlined, which prescribes how the patient will be treated, including the role of therapeutic modalities.

Following are the four main sources of information that clinicians draw on when formulating plans of action:

1. *Tradition.* The way it has always been done; techniques and procedures that have been handed down from one clinician to the next to the next.
2. *Experience.* The result of successes and failures with similar patients and similar conditions.
3. *Research.* The result of scientific investigation, ranging from general to specific evidence (explained later in this chapter).

4. *Theory.* The best guess of what is going on, based on a logical evaluation of experience and evidence. The strength of a theory is determined by the strength of the evidence on which it is based and the care with which the evidence is tied together.

TYPES OF RESEARCH EVIDENCE

There are many types of research evidence, each of which has a role in clinical decision making. Although their relative value varies, each is essential, if used properly. These types are as follows:

- *Physiological responses of healthy, uninjured humans to specific interventions.* This research is easy to do, and it provides good, but limited, information. The greatest limitation is that healthy, uninjured tissue often does not respond to specific interventions the same way injured tissue does.
- *Pathophysiological responses of injured animals to specific interventions.* Injury or diseased states can be modeled with this type of research, but the value of the results depends on how closely the animal's responses mimic human responses.
- *Case studies or nonrandomized clinical trials.* This research involves carefully recording the details of specific interventions. It does not involve control subjects.
- *Randomized clinical trials.* Positive clinical trials provide the best evidence because they involve patients with the specific injury or condition. Negative clinical trials must be interpreted cautiously, however.

EVIDENCE-BASED CLINICAL PRACTICE

Evidence-based practice is health care that is based on scientific evidence. Its goal is to improve the quality and effectiveness of health care.[1,2] The concept grew out of a 1972 book by a British epidemiologist, Archie Cochrane,[3] who stressed the importance of basing health care decisions on evidence from randomized clinical trials because these were likely to provide much more reliable information than other sources of evidence. **Randomized clinical trials (RCTs)** are controlled research of a specific medical intervention on patients who have a specific injury or disease. Cochrane's work led to setting up the Cochrane Collaboration,[4] now a worldwide endeavor to collect, evaluate, synthesize, and maintain a database of RCTs in all areas of medicine.

Evidence-based practice has also become a major initiative of the U.S. Department of Health and Human Services, the American Medical Association, and America's Health Insurance Plans.[5] So far, 12 evidence-based practice centers, housed in major medical schools, have been established to conduct systematic reviews of the scientific literature related to specific diseases or health problems. The goal is to determine whether specific **interventions** (treatments) for a specific condition work. Guidelines are then written for treating the problem, including statements concerning the strength of clinical evidence for the intervention. The guidelines from these reviews are housed in a national database for use by medical and health-related personnel to use. The database[5] is not limited to reports from the evidence-based practice centers. Reports from many other professional and private organizations are also referenced. This is a great source of information for the clinician who wants to provide the best care possible to his patients.

Another database that is particularly useful to orthopedic injury care is the Physiotherapy Evidence Database (PEDro),[6] an initiative that began with the Australian Physiotherapy Association. The PEDro Scale was developed to help evaluate the quality of published clinical trials and thereby help determine the validity of the data.

CRITICAL THINKING 1.2 *Log on to the National Guideline Clearinghouse (www.guideline.gov) and enter a topic related to sports medicine. Read one of the guideline summaries returned. If by chance there are no hits, try another condition. How could referencing this site in the future contribute to your education?*

EVIDENCE OTHER THAN RANDOMIZED CLINICAL TRIALS

Some have misinterpreted Cochrane's plea as meaning that other forms of evidence were of limited value and that all research should involve randomized clinical trials. Not true. Positive clinical trials provide the best evidence, but the only conclusion that can be made from negative clinical trials is that the treatment was of no value as it was applied. For example, an RCT of the use of 10 min applications of ice packs for acute sprained ankles would probably be negative. Does this mean that ankle sprains should not be treated with ice packs? No. It means only that 10 min applications are ineffective. Had the clinical trial been done with 30 min applications, the results would probably have been overwhelmingly positive.

We must have a combination of research. Case studies and research on uninjured humans and on animals help develop theory and get scientists into the ball park by eliminating way-out ideas and establishing treatment parameters with some degree of potential for success. Can you imagine how much time and money it would take to test every possible way of treating every possible injury in every possible type of patient?

It is important when reviewing research to recognize the difference between the concept that something *proves* the theory and the idea that something *is consistent* with the theory. Only RCTs are capable of providing definitive proof of a specific treatment. But other types of research evidence can get us close to the truth.

Selecting a Therapeutic Modality

Who selects the modality to treat patient X? On what criteria is that decision based? In this section we discuss the philosophy and general principles of modality selection.

WHOSE DECISION?

Who selects which therapeutic modality to use when treating a patient? The athletic trainer? A physical therapist? The team physician? The patient's family physician? The decision depends on your specific state's practice act, which usually stipulates that athletic trainers apply therapeutic modalities under the direction of a physician. This can be problematic, however, when physicians do not provide specific guidelines and leave clinicians to determine the treatment. For instance, if a physician prescribes "therapy for Melvin Laird owing to pain and swelling of the left ankle," the clinician must choose the specific modality to use.

Physical therapists (PTs) and athletic trainers (ATs) sometimes work under the direction of a **physiatrist**, an MD who is a specialist in **physical medicine and rehabilitation**, the medical subspecialty relating to the treatment and rehabilitation of physical conditions. Physiatrists usually provide clear prescriptions, so the clinician knows exactly what modality to use. But most PTs and ATs receive prescriptions from physicians who either have not been trained in the use of therapeutic modalities or are not up to date concerning their use. What then? Does the athletic trainer make his own decision and ignore the physician? This is not only against the law, it is unethical. Instead, you must help the physician understand why and when to use various therapeutic modalities so that he can adequately direct their use.

SELECTION CRITERIA

To responsibly decide which modality to use, you should:

1. Have a correct diagnosis, which results from analysis of the subjective and objective data obtained during a thorough evaluation of the patient and the specific injury or condition.
2. Have a definite concept of the pathological and physiological changes associated with the injury.

3. Outline an overall treatment plan that includes long-range, medium-range, and short-range therapeutic goals.
4. Understand the modality's effects, indications, and contraindications, including the type and strength of evidence supporting this information.
5. Match your therapeutic goal with a modality that will help you achieve that goal.

Rehabilitation and Therapeutic Modalities

Many will question having a section on rehabilitation in a therapeutic modality text. A proper understanding of the role of therapeutic modalities depends, however, on understanding the overall orthopedic injury rehabilitation process. The definition of rehabilitation (given in the next subsection) will help you appreciate how therapeutic modalities fit into the rehabilitation process. You must begin now to understand that therapeutic modality use is part of rehabilitation, not something that precedes it.

In this and subsequent sections, we discuss some erroneous concepts about rehabilitation, present some basic principles to guide rehabilitation, develop a rationale for a systems approach to rehabilitation, and discuss some of the psychological factors that can optimize rehabilitation.

REHABILITATION DEFINED

Rehabilitation means restoring to a former capacity by providing training or therapy.[7,8] (The term is derived from the Latin *rehabilitare*, "to make fit again.") The entire process of returning an injured patient to her preinjury status, including the use of therapeutic modalities, is rehabilitation.

FOUR ERRONEOUS CONCEPTS ABOUT REHABILITATION

Four commonly used concepts about rehabilitation are erroneous, and applying them might compromise proper and complete rehabilitation. Clinicians should try to avoid letting these ideas become part of their thinking about rehabilitation.

Misconception 1: Treating Injuries, Then Rehabilitating Them

Some clinicians think treating injuries is separate from rehabilitation. They "treat" their patients with modalities and then "rehabilitate" them with exercise. This is inconsistent with the definition of rehabilitation. Rehabilitation is the entire process of returning an injured person to her normal habits. So treatment with modalities is part of rehabilitation, not something that precedes it.

Does it matter how you define these processes? Yes. If you define treatment and rehabilitation as separate processes, you would be inclined to use therapeutic modalities and therapeutic exercise sequentially, rather than together. As you will see throughout this text, therapeutic modalities and therapeutic exercise complement each other and in many cases should be used together.

The next two erroneous concepts are part of the reason that some clinicians think treatment and rehabilitation are separate. Tie each of these concepts back to this one as you read.

Misconception 2: Rehabilitation as Reconditioning

Injury rehabilitation is often called **reconditioning**, meaning "conditioning again." The two processes do share some common principles, but there are also some fundamental differences. Rehabilitation includes conditioning, but it also involves the promotion of healing and pain relief. For instance, a patient who has torn a tendon cannot begin a reconditioning program until the tendon has healed. Pain relief is also part of rehabilitation. Because pain activates neural mechanisms that inhibit strength, flexibility, and so on, pain must be addressed before reconditioning can begin.

Another difference is that the speed at which physical attributes redevelop during rehabilitation can be much faster than during original conditioning.[9] Thus rehabilitation can be much more aggressive than conditioning.

Misconception 3: Working with Weights

Although the "rehab area" of many athletic training and sports medicine clinics is the area that contains the weight-training equipment, the terms *rehab, working with weights,* and *strength training* are not synonymous. Rehabilitation is not complete if the patient works only with weights, regardless of how creative and intense the work.

Misconception 4: The Cookbook Approach

In the **cookbook approach to rehabilitation**, the clinician follows a specific recipe, or protocol, for treating each injury. The protocol includes phases with specific time periods and therapeutic interventions. For instance, phase 2 might last from 2 to 6 weeks postinjury and include thermotherapy, isokinetic exercises, isotonic exercises, StairMaster, cycling, swimming, and light running. The appeal of the cookbook approach is that it is easy to follow because there is a specific protocol for each injury. Its limitation is that all patients with the same or similar injury are treated the same, without regard for individual differences.

Variables that are disregarded in the cookbook approach include:

- The patient's genetic makeup, general health, preinjury state of conditioning, psychological profile, and work ethic
- The severity of the injury and associated problems
- The rate of progress (patients respond differently to the same interventions)
- The difference in demands placed on the injured body part during sport participation (a runner must spend more time developing muscular endurance than a golfer; a football player must develop more muscular speed than a distance runner)
- The time of the season (demands on a patient are greater during the sport season than during the off-season)

Every patient and every injury is different, so rehabilitation programs must be individualized. Optimal rehabilitation is not planned by the calendar and not achieved by specific exercises.

This erroneous concept developed because application techniques generally precede theory; clinicians tend to use treatments or rehabilitation techniques before they know why they are effective. As a result, many professionals have a bag of tricks, an assortment of techniques, that have not been brought together under an overall theoretical umbrella. This is changing, however; professionals are more often looking at the entire process and taking a systems approach to rehabilitation.[10,11]

A Systems Approach to Rehabilitation

The guiding philosophy of the **systems approach to rehabilitation** is that each patient and each injury is unique, and therefore treatment must be individualized, dynamic, and interactive. Therapeutic intervention is based on the patient's initial signs and symptoms customized to the patient's needs and adjusted according to patient progress. The systems approach is based on 11 principles of rehabilitation and directed by 10 core goals related to the independent but interrelated physical **performance attributes**, such as pain-free movement, muscular strength, and motor control. Because injury disrupts one or more of the performance attributes, rehabilitation consists of systematically reestablishing the attributes. The principles and core goals are discussed in the next two sections.

PRINCIPLES OF ORTHOPEDIC INJURY REHABILITATION

This section covers the 11 essential principles of rehabilitation. All of them apply, regardless of the type of injury being rehabilitated. These principles provide the theoretical framework for decision making during rehabilitation.

The SAID Principle

Rehabilitation is dominated by the **SAID principle**, an acronym for "specific adaptation to imposed demands." Stated another way, the body responds to a given demand with a specific and predictable adaptation. For a specific adaptation to occur, a specific demand must be imposed. For example, if you want to develop endurance in a particular muscle group (the specific adaptation), you must require that particular muscle group to repeatedly contract over a longer time (the imposed demand).

An athletic trainer (or other clinician) must identify and use training to specifically address each performance attribute to be redeveloped (or developed if the patient was not properly conditioned before the injury). A patient can achieve total rehabilitation only if the athletic trainer works with him to redevelop each aspect of conditioning through individual specific imposed demands.

Therapeutic Goals

Therapeutic goals establish your aim or desired result. To put the SAID principle into practice, you must establish therapeutic goals and then select a therapeutic regimen that elicits the physiological and psychological responses required for achieving those goals. Goals help you determine the specific demand to impose on the patient. Plan your work and then work the plan.

Plan specific goals for a variety of time frames. Daily goals should lead to short-range goals, which in turn should progressively lead to helping the patient attain long-range goals. Be flexible in adjusting or adding goals as the rehabilitation progresses and the needs of the patient change.

Another advantage of goal-oriented rehabilitation is that by directing the rehabilitation using numerous specific goals, patients can see regular progress as they achieve those goals.[12] The satisfaction in achieving the goals gives patients a psychological boost. Use goals liberally during rehabilitation.

Continual Evaluation

Proper application of the SAID principle does not end at determining a specific adaptation and planning goals after the initial diagnosis of the nature and severity of the injury. Reevaluation is necessarily almost daily to determine the patient's response to the therapeutic regimen and progress toward her goals (Fig. 1.4).

Overload and Progression

Overload is the concept of challenging the body to greater function by pushing it beyond its comfort zone to near its limits. The body likes to have a reserve, so when you demand near-total functioning by a system, the body attempts to develop a reserve. Of course, if your demands

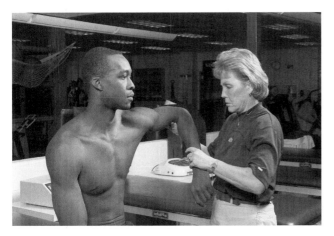

FIGURE 1.4. Constant evaluation of the anatomical and pathological changes induced by the injury are essential to establishing therapeutic goals and selecting the appropriate modality.

are too great, you will injure the system. (Fig. 1.5). Once the body adapts to the overload, you increase the challenge and thus require additional adaptation.

Weight training is a good example of this concept. If a muscle's maximal strength is 50 lb and a person trains by lifting 40 lb for a few sessions, the muscle will adapt so that it can lift 55 lb. Training at 45 lb will result in an additional strength increase. Continuing the process with incremental increases once the body has adapted is known as **progression.**

Functional Progression

Functional progression, also known as *progressive reorientation,* is accomplished by **graded exercise**, or the performance of functional activities in an ordered sequence, begin-

ning with simple, easy activity and progressing to full sport or work activity.[13] It is based on the concept of progressive resistive exercise (PRE) to regain strength during rehabilitation, developed by Delorme and Watkins.[14] Functional progression facilitates the acquisition or reacquisition of skills required for the safe and effective performance of complex skills.[13] Patients usually progress from:

- unloaded activities to
- loaded activities to
- overloaded activities

And from:

- single-plane activities to
- multiple-plane activities

Both of which progress from:

- slow speed to
- normal speed to
- high speed

And with:

- slow transition to
- normal transition to
- very quick transition

The Absence of Pain

All therapeutic exercise should be relatively pain free. If the activity is more than mildly uncomfortable, this is a signal from the body that something is wrong. The rehabilitation exercise or activity should not evoke pain. If it does, the activity is too vigorous and should be simplified.

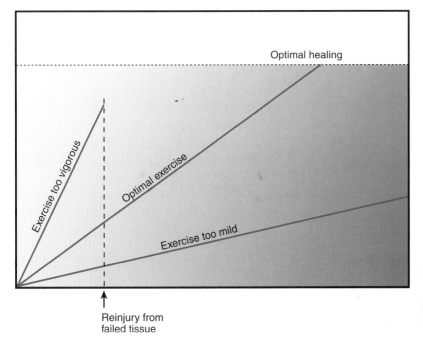

FIGURE 1.5. Healing occurs when an injured body part is exercised. Optimal healing requires a balance between exercise that is so vigorous that it might cause further injury and exercise that is so mild that healing is delayed. Reinjury (vertical dashed line) can result from exercise that is too vigorous.

APPLICATION TIP

REHABILITATION MUST BE PAIN-FREE. "No pain no gain" does not apply to rehabilitation, but "Ignore the pain equals no brain" does.

Biofeedback

Biofeedback is a process of measuring a biological mechanism using some objective means and then telling the patient his scores. The feedback helps the patient progress more quickly. Although there are commercial biofeedback devices that measure variables such as electrical activity in a muscle or the temperature in a finger, biofeedback does not require these devices. The concept is much greater in scope and simpler to use than a machine. For instance, when you are trying to develop elbow flexibility, you could tell the patient, "Move your arm so that your fingers touch the wall during extension and my hand during flexion." Tell the patient to perform a specific number of repetitions, say 10. Count each repetition out loud so the patient hears you. If a repetition is incomplete, (does not reach both the wall and your hand), tell the patient the repetition does not count. You can provide further biofeedback by timing the patient's performance: "Let's see how long it takes you to perform 10 complete repetitions." Tell the patient the time and then ask, "Do you think you can perform 10 more repetitions faster than before?" The second set of repetitions will almost always be faster than the first.

Do you think Sir Roger Bannister would have broken the 4 min mile if he just went out and ran without keeping track of his time? Of course not. Performance improves when the patient or athlete is given specific feedback concerning his performance.

Use your imagination to determine specific performance goals for every therapeutic exercise you have the patient do. Then measure the performance and report the results to the patient.

CRITICAL THINKING 1.3 Try the following biofeedback exercise. Think of a number between 1 and 100. Ask a friend to guess the number. Unless she is very lucky, she will guess wrong. Say, "Wrong." Continue this process until she eventually gets lucky and guesses the number. Repeat the process, perhaps with someone else, but this time give more effective feedback; say, "lower [or higher]" after each guess. The specific feedback should cause the friend to guess the number much more quickly. Why?

Early Exercise

Early exercise is essential to rehabilitation. Not only does the proper use of exercise speed the healing process[15–19]

but a lack of exercise during the early stages of rehabilitation can result in permanent disability.[20] Caution is essential, however, because exercise that is too vigorous can also result in permanent disability.[20] The optimal conditions for healing depend on a fine balance between protection from too much stress and a return to normal functioning at the earliest possible time[12] (see Fig. 1.5).

A classic series of studies by Jarvinen and associates[15–19] support this theory. Immediate mobilization after contusions to the legs of rats led to a more pronounced macrophage reaction, quicker hematoma resolution, an increased vascular ingrowth, quicker regeneration of muscle and scar tissue, and increased tensile strength of the healed muscle. Immobilization for only 2 or 5 days, on the other hand, delayed contraction and maturation of the scar when measured 42 days later. Exercise during rehabilitation also results in stronger ligaments and tendons.

Relatively Rapid Rate of Reconditioning

As mentioned, many physical attributes can be redeveloped much more quickly than they were developed originally. Much of the loss of performance with injury is the result of pain-induced inhibition. Rehabilitation involves systematically removing the inhibitions rather than developing the attribute from the beginning.

Timeliness

Rehabilitation should begin immediately after the injury occurs and end only when the patient can fully participate in her sport, with no limitations imposed by the injury. Obviously the complexity of rehabilitation will depend on the magnitude and type of injury sustained as well as the requirements of the sport. A runner with a sprained finger usually will not have to worry about it as much as a quarterback would. But even for a quarterback, rehabilitation of a sprained finger would not be as complicated or take as long as rehabilitation of a sprained ankle. Whether the process is simple or complex, it should follow the same general process to ensure complete rehabilitation.

It is important to accomplish the rehabilitation process as quickly as possible. Many negative consequences result from prolonged absence from participation. Inactivity can lead to atrophy of specific muscle groups, loss of overall conditioning, skills becoming rusty, loss of the patient's sixth sense, and emotional trauma. Often an injury is accompanied by feelings of frustration, discouragement, and self-doubt that become greater the longer the patient is unable to participate.

Prioritizing

The return of the patient to full performance is the priority, and the motivating force, of early rehabilitation. No matter how valuable an athlete is to the team, the interests of neither the team nor the coach should take precedence over the health of the patient.

THE 10 CORE GOALS OF ORTHOPEDIC INJURY REHABILITATION

The fundamental goal of orthopedic injury rehabilitation is to return the patient to full, unhindered activity. For an athlete, this means the ability to fully perform his sport. Injury results in torn tissue and/or pain, both of which cause **neural inhibition** (decreasing or stopping) of performance attributes. Thus during rehabilitation you must be concerned with healing damaged tissue, removing pain, and reestablishing each of the performance attributes.

The 10 core goals of rehabilitation are listed in Table 1.2. Goals 3–10 are performance attributes necessary for an athlete to be successful. Goals 1 and 2 are prerequisites for the last 8. When a healthy athlete develops these attributes, he is conditioning; when a patient redevelops them after injury, he is being rehabilitated. Think of these 10 core goals as long-term goals.

The 10 core goals are somewhat sequential. With two exceptions, each attribute builds on the previous attributes. For example, because muscle power is a combination of strength and speed, both muscular strength and speed must be redeveloped before muscle power. Goals 1–4 must be developed in sequence. Goals 5–7 can be developed in any order or at the same time but before goals 8–10. Goals 8–10 can be developed in any order or at the same time.

A thorough evaluation of the patient's injury and the limitations imposed on the patient by the injury must precede rehabilitation. Functional activities are often part of the evaluation. Not all injuries involve torn tissue, and pain is sometimes not present until the patient exceeds a specific level of performance. You then select the appropriate core goal to begin working on, establishing specific short-range goals to guide the patient in meeting the core goal. You then select specific therapeutic modalities and techniques that will help the patient progressively meet the core goal. Once the patient achieves the core goal, you repeat the process for the next core goal.

Goal 1: Structural Integrity

Structural integrity refers to the health of a patient's anatomical structures, such as bones, muscles, ligaments, and tendons. Any disrupted structure has to be repaired before its function can be rehabilitated. In general, both surgery and immobilization are necessary for repairing a severely injured musculoskeletal structure. Immobilization and/or rest are used to protect less seriously injured structures during the healing process.

Although immobilization is often necessary, it can cause problems.[21,22] It frequently increases neural inhibitions, thereby resulting in decreased neuromuscular function. Exercising the immobilized part helps minimize neural inhibition, but it must not be so vigorous that it disturbs the structure that is healing.

Thermotherapy is often used during healing. It increases circulation and metabolism, thus speeding the healing process (see Chapter 5).

Goal 2: Pain-Free Joints and Muscles

Immobilization, therapeutic modalities, cryotherapy, and exercise are all used to reduce pain. Graded exercise (functional progression) is especially important in pain reduction, by helping the patient overcome neural inhibitions and by gradually readjusting or reorienting the body part to full pain-free activity.

It is important to monitor pain throughout the rehabilitation process. Pain accompanying an activity indicates the activity is too difficult, and the patient should revert to a lower level of activity. **Residual pain**, or pain the next day, is a signal that the previous day's activity was too demanding and the current day's activity needs to be adjusted accordingly. Activities that cause pain during rehabilitation will compromise the rehabilitation by invoking neural inhibition.

Goal 3: Joint Flexibility

The ability of a joint to move through its full range of motion is known as **joint flexibility**. Impaired joint flexibility is the result of muscle spasm, pain, and/or neural inhibition secondary to acute injury or from connective tissue adhesions and contractures secondary to surgery and/or immobilization. Therapeutic exercise is essential to restoring flexibility, and its effects are enhanced by applications

TABLE 1.2	The 10 Core Goals of Rehabilitation*
GOAL	**DESCRIPTION**
1	Structural integrity
2	Pain-free joints and muscles
3	Joint flexibility
4	Muscular strength
5	Muscular endurance
6	Muscular speed
7	Motor skill
8	Muscular power (strength and speed)
9	Agility (speed and skill)
10	Cardiorespiratory endurance

*Goals 1–4 should be developed sequentially, followed by goals 5–7 and then goals 8–10. Goals 5–7 and 8–10 can be developed in any order or at the same time with others in their group.

of hot packs and cold packs. Cold packs are generally more effective in treating muscular conditions, and hot packs are preferred when connective tissue is involved.[23]

During periods of immobilization, limited motion can help limit the loss of joint flexibility. After the immobilization period has been completed, static stretch and **proprioceptive neuromuscular facilitation (PNF)** techniques, such as hold–relax (static stretch interspersed with isometric contraction of the involved muscle) and contract–relax (static stretch interspersed with isometric contraction of the antagonistic muscle), are effective. Flexion and extension exercises to range-of-motion limits and riding a stationary bike are other good ways to restore flexibility.

For acute muscle spasm, the two most effective modalities are the cryostretch technique (see Chapter 14), which combines cold applications with hold–relax, and electrical muscle stimulation (EMS), if applied to cause successive maximal tetanic contractions (see Chapter 10). Heating a joint capsule with pulsed shortwave diathermy before joint mobilizations is effective for restoring range of motion to stiff, frozen joints (see Chapter 16).

Goal 4: Muscular Strength

Muscular strength is a measure of the ability of a muscle to exert force. Some type of progressive resistive exercises must be performed on a regular basis by the involved muscles if an increase in strength is desired (Fig. 1.6). Elastic tubing exercises will help some, but weight training is more effective. Manufacturers of strength equip-

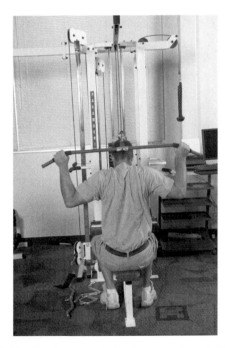

FIGURE 1.6. Muscular strength development is important early in the rehabilitation process to establish a basis for developing performance attributes such as endurance, speed, skill, agility, and power.

ment constantly assert the merits of their products, but the strengthening program used is more important than the equipment.

The **daily adjustable progressive resistive exercise (DAPRE) technique** is a four-set, isotonic muscle strengthening technique that leads to rapid strength gains during rehabilitation (Tables 1.3 and 1.4).[9,24,25] An individual's strength can be redeveloped more quickly than it was originally developed. The DAPRE technique maximizes this because patients are required to perform maximal repetitions during their third and fourth sets, and the number of repetitions is used as a basis for adjusting the resistance during the fourth set and on the next day, respectively.

It is essential to exercise both sides of the body independently, which prevents the injured side from depending on the uninjured side. You must also establish a strength development goal for the uninjured side. The uninjured limb will lose strength after the injury, so if its strength is not reestablished, you have not set a proper goal.

Once the strength of the injured side reaches 90–95% of the strength in the noninjured side, the program is changed from strength development to strength maintenance, and the rehabilitation goal changes to developing muscular endurance. Muscular strength can usually be maintained with one or two weekly workouts at near maximal resistance.

Goal 5: Muscular Endurance

Muscular endurance refers to the ability of a muscle to contract repeatedly without becoming fatigued. Some athletic trainers use a stationary bike to redevelop muscular endurance (Fig. 1.7). Although this is effective, running (or an equivalent upper body exercise for upper extremity injuries) is more specific to most sports and is therefore preferred. For example, the patient should jog 400 m the first couple of days and increase this distance 200–400 m each day as tolerance increases. Pain or soreness indicates the previous day's activity was too much and the distance should be decreased for a few days. After the patient can run a distance appropriate for his sport (say, 1600 m for a football player), start working toward other goals. But distance running should continue, reaching a level proportionate to the needs of the patient's sport.

Weight lifting is not recommended for developing muscular endurance. Repetitions of more than 100–300 would be necessary for reaching significant endurance levels, and this is impractical.

Goal 6: Muscular Speed

Muscular speed is the speed at which a muscle contracts. A good way to develop muscular speed is participation in

TABLE 1.3	*The DAPRE Technique*	
SET	**PORTION OF WORKING WEIGHT USED**	**NUMBER OF REPETITIONS**
1	$^1/_2$	10
2	$^3/_4$	6
3	Full	Maximum*
4	Adjusted	Maximum[†]

*The number of repetitions performed during the third set is used to determine the adjusted working weight for the fourth set, according to the guidelines in Table 1.4.

[†]The number of repetitions performed during the fourth set is used to determine the adjusted working weight for the next day, according to the guidelines in Table 1.4.

Adapted with permission from Knight.[26]

team drills at half-speed, then three-quarters speed, and finally at full speed, focusing on explosive-type activities (short duration, maximal power). Isokinetic exercise also successfully develops muscular speed, but it is not needed if the patient develops near maximal strength and then progresses through team drills at increasing speed.

Goal 7: Motor Skill

Motor skill is the integration and coordination of many muscles acting together to produce a desired movement. Practicing sport-specific skill patterns, such as increasingly complex drills, will develop both motor skills and muscular speed (Fig. 1.8). The athletic trainer or clinician should observe the patient closely to ensure the correct performance of the activities. It is often necessary to isolate a particular part of the skill pattern and work on it individually. This involves restarting, with a focus on flexibility development while performing the specific part of the skill pattern; then progressing through strength, endurance, and speed development with the particular muscles involved in the isolated part of the skill pattern.

Goal 8: Muscular Power

Power is a measure of the rate of doing work. **Muscular power** is a combination of strength and speed of movement, so it must be developed after those attributes. It can be developed with an isokinetic device or with high-speed resistive exercises with traditional weights. Traditional weights, or weight machines, are recommended because they are less expensive and more accessible.

Goal 9: Agility

Agility is a combination of muscular speed and coordination, and it is developed in the course of performing skill patterns quickly. As with redeveloping motor skill, sport-specific drills can be used to redevelop agility.

Goal 10: Cardiorespiratory Endurance

Cardiorespiratory endurance is the ability of the heart and lungs to supply exercising muscles with adequate oxygen to produce the energy needed to maintain the activity. The exercises used to develop muscular endurance may stimulate some cardiorespiratory endurance develop-

TABLE 1.4	*General Guidelines for Adjusting Weight When Using the DAPRE Technique*	
NUMBER OF REPETITIONS PERFORMED DURING SET	**ADJUSTMENT FOR THE FOURTH SET***	**WORKING WEIGHT FOR THE NEXT DAY[†]**
0–2	Decrease 2–5 kg and repeat the set	
3–4	Decrease 0–2 kg	Keep the same
2–7	Keep the same	Increase 2–5 kg
8–12	Increase 2–5 kg	Increase 2–7 kg
13+	Increase 5–7 kg	Increase 5–10 kg

*The number of repetitions performed during the third set is used to determine the adjusted working weight for the fourth set, according to the guidelines in this column.

[†]The number of repetitions performed during the fourth set is used to determine the adjusted working weight for the next day, according to the guidelines in this column.

Adapted with permission from Knight.[26]

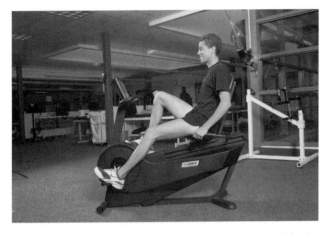

FIGURE 1.7. A stationary bike is a versatile tool that can be used for developing range of motion, endurance, and power.

ment. Other sport-specific conditioning drills should be used, gradually at first and then increasing in difficulty.

If it looks like it will take more than 2 weeks to complete the total rehabilitation program, the clinician should try to minimize the patient's loss of cardiovascular endurance. The method depends on the body part injured. If the injury does not compromise the patient's ability to perform normal conditioning activities, it's fine to continue with them. For instance a football player with an arm injury can still run. If the injury prevents running, a substitute activity should be used. A football player with a thigh injury, for example, can run in a swimming pool in chest-high water or ride a stationary bike.

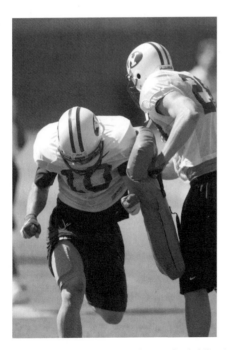

FIGURE 1.8. Team drills are an essential part of rehabilitation if used properly and at the right time.

Modality Effectiveness in Achieving the Core Goals

When using a systems approach in rehabilitation, you must have some basis for choosing certain therapeutic modalities when working toward specific goals. The correct therapeutic modality must be matched with the therapeutic goal. For instance, a whirlpool treatment is clearly not the best choice for improving cardiorespiratory endurance.

Table 1.5 presents various therapeutic modalities rated according to their effectiveness in achieving each of the 10 core goals of rehabilitation. The most commonly used modalities are given one of three ratings for each of the core goals on which they have some effect. Here are the three ratings:

1. The modality has a direct effect and is a good choice for this rehabilitation goal.
2. The modality can be effective if used in a specific way. For example, performing several hundred isotonic resistive exercises three times per week would be effective in developing muscular endurance, but performing 10–15 repetitions would not develop significant muscular endurance.
3. The modality is somewhat effective but not the best choice for this rehabilitation goal.

As you look at Table 1.5, notice that the body of the table forms an L shape. What does this tell you about the use of therapeutic modalities during rehabilitation? They are most effective during the earlier stages of rehabilitation, when trying to promote healing, relieve pain, and restore full range of motion and flexibility. Achieving the core goals of strength and beyond requires mostly therapeutic exercise.

Through most of the text we will talk about a specific modality and its **indications**. In the real world you start with a problem, not with the modality. The scenario is "Here is a problem, here are my therapeutic goals, so which of the myriad modalities should I use?" In Chapter 20, we will reverse the process of the bulk of the book and begin with specific injuries and phases of injury/healing and discuss the best modality choices for treating them. In essence, we will expand Table 1.5.

The Psychology of Rehabilitation

Rehabilitation is usually discussed in terms of physiological aspects, but the psychological side is important as well. In fact, some say that rehabilitation is 75% psychological and 25% physiological. Some patients seem to give up after being injured and must be regularly encouraged to reach their rehabilitation goals (Fig. 1.9a). The clinician has to constantly check on them to make sure they comply. Other patients can be overly aggres-

TABLE 1.5   The Efficacy of Various Therapeutic Modalities When Used to Achieve Each of the 10 Core Goals*

MODALITY	Structural Integrity	Pain-Free Joints and Muscles	Joint Flexibility	Muscular Strength	Muscular Endurance	Muscular Speed	Motor Skill	Muscular Power	Agility	Cardio-respiratory Endurance
Cold packs		1	2							
Ice massage		1	2							
Whirlpool, cold		1	2							
Whirlpool, hot	1	1	2							
Hot packs	1	1	2							
Paraffin baths	1	1	2							
Contrast baths	1	1	2							
Infrared	1	1	2							
Laser	1	1	2							
Ultrasound	1	1	2							
Diathermy	1	1	2							
LV muscle stimulation	?	1	3	2						
HV muscle stimulation	2	1								
TENS		1								
Traction		1	2							
Massage		1	2							
Joint mobilization		1	1							
EXERCISE										
Passive		2	1							
Assistive		2	3	?						
Active										
Range of motion	2	2	3							
Jogging (or EUBA)†		2		3	1					1
Running (or EUBA)†		2		3	2	1				1
Agility drills		2		3	2	1		1		2
Team drills		2		3	2	2		1		2
Team practice		2		3	2	2		1		2
Resistive										
Manual				2						
Isometric				2						
Isotonic										
Free weights				1	2	2		3		3
Machine, weight stack				1	2	2				3
Machine, cam	2			1	2	2				3
Isokinetic				1	2	2				3

*1 = good choice, 2 = effective under certain conditions, 3 = somewhat effective; not the best choice.

EUBA, equivalent upper body activity; HV, high volt; LV, low volt; TENS, transcutaneous electrical nerve stimulation.

sive and must be held back to avoid overworking and possible reinjury (Fig. 1.9b). Both types of patients require the same amount of time and effort during rehabilitation.

Another psychological aspect of rehabilitation is the direct connection that exists between the mind and the body's physiological functioning. The way a person thinks is manifested in the way her body performs. There apparently is power in positive thinking. During rehabilitation, the clinician needs to make every effort to ensure that the patient doesn't give up on herself or her ability to recover from the injury and perform again. Pointing out even the smallest sign of progress can help.

Preparation for Using Therapeutic Modalities

Ideally, anyone who is properly trained in the correct theory and application and remains up to date with current research is qualified to use therapeutic modalities. However, many clinicians do not find the time to stay current with research. Regardless, state regulations determine who can legally administer therapeutic modality treatments, so you need to be aware of the laws in the state in which you are employed.

To prepare yourself to use therapeutic modalities, keep the following in mind:

1. *Be an active learner.* This is not a spectator sport. You will not learn therapeutic modalities simply by reading the text, listening to classroom lectures, cramming for exams, and spitting out the answers. You must do these things, but also you must make this information part of yourself. How do you do that? You interact with the information by:
   - Writing questions as you read and then discussing the questions with classmates, other students, professors, clinical instructors, and even patients
   - Writing reflectively about the material
   - Experimenting with various forms of application
2. *Aside from classroom experiences, try to use the various modalities every day.* A model of education that combines academics in the morning and clinical work in the afternoon or evening is powerful. During your clinical experiences, question, consider, and reflect on what you have been taught in the classroom. Experiment on yourself. For example, put your foot in a plastic container of ice water and record how many minutes it takes for your foot to go numb. When treating patients, think about whether there is a better way to do something and discuss it with both your clinical instructor and your classroom teacher.

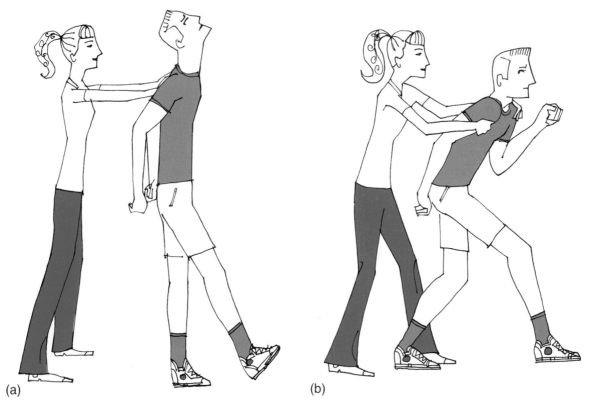

(a)   (b)

FIGURE 1.9. **(a)** Some patients must be prodded and cajoled. **(b)** Others need to be held back from risking reinjury.

3. *Once you finish your formal education, take the opportunity to attend and actively participate in continuing education seminars.* Some professions will require you to maintain continuing education units (CEUs). The National Athletic Trainer's Association (NATA) requires its members to obtain 75 hr of additional learning every 3 years. Currently, the American Physical Therapy Association (APTA) does not require this, but some individual state regulations do. There are numerous opportunities for continuing education at many professional meetings, including the annual meetings of the NATA, APTA, and American College of Sports Medicine (ACSM).

4. *Most professional organizations sponsor a peer-reviewed journal that is sent to all members.* For example, the keystone journal for athletic trainers is the *Journal of Athletic Training*; for physical therapists, *Physical Therapy*; and for physiatrists, the *Archives of Physical Medicine and Rehabilitation*. The *Journal of Orthopaedic and Sports Physical Therapy* serves as a crossover journal for orthopedic and sports physical therapists and generally has more therapeutic modality information than does *Physical Therapy*. Make it a habit to study the journal of your primary professional organization, and periodically peruse the journals of related health professions. They represent the most current science and clinical practice in your specialty. Reading and implementing what you find in these journals with help keep you up to date in this ever-changing medical world.

CLOSING SCENE

We began this chapter with a story about a man teaching his young son about how he could do a better job in less time by using the right tools to cut branches off a tree (Figure 1.10). The same is true with rehabilitation, a complex process involving the redevelopment of many performance attributes, each with different goals. It can be facilitated by the judicious use of the right tools–therapeutic modalities.

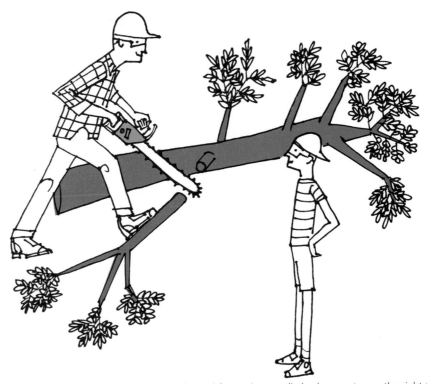

FIGURE 1.10. Just as you would use the right tool for cutting tree limbs, be sure to use the right tool for each stage of rehabilitation.

CHAPTER REFLECTIONS

1. Read and ponder each of the following points. Do you feel you have a clear understanding of each concept? If not, reread the appropriate section of the chapter.
   - Define therapeutic modality, physical agent, and therapeutic purpose.
     - Explain the concept of knobologist.
     - Describe the relationship between the theory and the application of therapeutic modalities.
     - Identify the various therapeutic modality classification systems.
     - Discuss the roles of physicians and athletic trainers in determining which therapeutic modality is used; discuss the selection criteria.
     - Define rehabilitation and the relationship between therapeutic modalities and rehabilitation.
   - Discuss each of the four erroneous concepts of rehabilitation. What effect do these misconceptions have on therapeutic modality use?
   - Describe the 11 principles of rehabilitation.
   - Describe the 10 core goals of rehabilitation.

2. Write three to five questions for discussion with your class instructor, clinical instructor, classmates, and clinical colleagues.

3. Get together with classmates and quiz each other on the concepts of this chapter. Use the points in exercise 1 and questions you wrote for exercise 2 as a beginning. Explaining concepts out loud to others requires a deeper grasp of the material than feeling you understand it as you read.

CRITICAL THINKING RESPONSES

Critical Thinking 1.1

Knobologists can harm the health professions in several ways:

1. They lack the theory and scientific background to be able to modify or modulate the treatment to cater to the specific needs of their patients.
2. Their patients do not heal as well or as quickly.
3. They may not be able to answer questions asked by their patients.
4. They do not stay current with changes and updates in their profession.
5. They give their profession a bad name or poor image because they are perceived as robots or technicians.

Critical Thinking 1.2

Were you surprised at the number of links you got and the amount of information contained in the National Clearinghouse Guidelines? The wealth of information on this Web site is growing each day, and you should begin to think of it as being as important as your dictionaries. (You do have two dictionaries, don't you—a general one and a medical one?) Consult this Web site often during your formal educational career and during your lifetime learning career.

Critical Thinking 1.3

When performance is evaluated and the performer is given specific feedback regarding that performance, she is able to make corrections. For example, in the number-guessing game, if your friend chose 55 and was told it was wrong, her next choice would be one of 99 numbers. Telling her lower, however, reduced the choices to one of 54 numbers. With each guess and response, she gets closer to the right answer. The same is true when you give performance goals, such as a specific place to move a limb; when you time an event or a series of events; and when you count the number of repetitions performed.

REFERENCES

1. Hootman JM. New section in JAT: Evidence-based practice. J Athl Train 2004;39:9.
2. Steves R, Hootman JM. Evidence-based medicine: What is it and how does it apply to athletic training? J Athl Train 2004;39:83–87.
3. Cochrane AL. Effectiveness and Efficiency. Random Reflections on Health Services. London: Nuffield Provincial Hospitals Trust, 1972 (rpnt. London: Royal Society of Medicine Press, 1999).
4. The Cochrane Database of Systematic Reviews. Available at: www.cochrane.org. Accessed Aug 2005.
5. Agency for Healthcare Research and Quality. National Guideline Clearinghouse. Available at: www.guideline.gov. Accessed Aug 2005.
6. Centre for Evidence-Based Physiotherapy. PEDro Physiotherapy Evidence Database. Available at: www.pedro.fhs.usyd.edu.au. Accessed Sept 2005.
7. Mish FC, ed. Merriam-Webster's 11th Collegiate Dictionary. Springfield, MA: Merriam-Webster, 2003.
8. MSN Encarta. Dictionary. Available at: encarta.msn.com/encnet/features/dictionary/dictionaryhome.aspx. Accessed 20 Aug 2005.

9. Knight KL. Quadriceps strengthening with the DAPRE technique: Case studies with neurological implications. Med Sci Sports Exerc 1985;17:646–650.

10. Knight KL. Guidelines for rehabilitation of sports injuries. Clin Sports Med 1985;4:405–416.

11. Knight KL. Total injury rehabilitation. Phys Sportsmed 1979;7:111.

12. DePalma MT, DePalma B. The use of instruction and the behavioral approach to facilitate injury rehabilitation. J Athl Train 1989;24: 217–222.

13. Kegerreis S. The construction and implementation of functional progressions as a component of athletic rehabilitation. J Orthop Sports Phys Ther 1983;5.

14. Delorme TL, Watkins AL. Technics of progressive resistance exercise. Arch Phys Med 1948;29.

15. Kvist H, Jarvinen M, Sorvari T. Effect of mobilization and immobilization on the healing of contusion injury in muscle. A preliminary report of a histological study in rats. Scand J Rehabil Med 1974;6: 134–140.

16. Jarvinen M. Immobilization effect on the tensile properties of striated muscle: An experimental study in the rat. Arch Phys Med Rehabil 1977;58:123–127.

17. Jarvinen M. Healing of a crush injury in rat striated muscle. 3. A micro-angiographical study of the effect of early mobilization and immobilization on capillary ingrowth. Acta Pathol Microbiol Scand [A]. 1976;84:85–94.

18. Jarvinen M. Healing of a crush injury in rat striated muscle. 4. Effect of early mobilization and immobilization on the tensile properties of gastrocnemius muscle. Acta Chir Scand 1976;142:47–56.

19. Jarvinen M. Healing of a crush injury in rat striated muscle. 2. A histological study of the effect of early mobilization and immobilization on the repair processes. Acta Pathol Microbiol Scand [A] 1975;83: 269–282.

20. Dehne E, Torp RP. Treatment of joint injuries by immediate mobilization. Based upon the spinal adaptation concept. Clin Orthop 1971;77:218–232.

21. Enwemeka CS. Inflammation, cellularity, and fibrillogenesis in regenerating tendon: Implications for tendon rehabilitation. Phys Ther 1989;69:816–825.

22. Morrissey MC. Reflex inhibition of thigh muscles in knee injury causes and treatment. Sports Med 1989;7:263–276.

23. Sapega AA, Quedenfeld TC, Moyer RA, Butler RA. Biophysical factors in range-of-motion exercise. Phys Sportsmed 1981;9.

24. Wadey VM, Knight KL. Four week training of quadriceps strength with electrical muscle stimulation and the isotonic DAPRE technique. J Can Athl Ther Assoc 1989;16:14–20.

25. Knight KL, Ingersoll C, Bartholomew J. Isotonic contractions may be more effective that isokinetic contractions in developing muscle strength. J Sport Rehabil 2001;10:124–131.

26. Knight KL. Knee rehabilitation using an adjustable progressive resistive exercise technique. Am J Sports Med 1979;7:336–337.

General Application Procedures

Jennie, a new student, is in her 5th day of clinical observation/experience. She has noticed that patients with similar injuries are treated the same, with little regard to how they respond to the treatment. She reflects on the three times she sprained her ankle during her high school athletic career. Even though she was told with each one that it was a lateral sprain, her response to the injuries was different in each instance. With one, her ankle hurt constantly for the 1st week; with another, she had pain only when she tried jumping or running. As she talked to the patients, she learned they were responding differently to the treatments. Then why were they all being treated the same way?

Jennie is also amazed at the number of different therapeutic modalities and the variety of their knobs, switches, and applicators. And the clinic has three machines called "electrical muscle simulators" that appear to be quite different modalities. She asks, "How long will it take me to master the use of all of these machines? What if I get mixed up and use the procedures of one modality when applying another modality?"

Jennie's two concerns are the basis of this chapter. How do you modify treatment to the specific needs of the patient? How do you learn the application of so many different modalities and keep them straight?

Application Approaches

Therapeutic modalities can be either powerful rehabilitation tools or a waste of time. What makes the difference? Using the right tool in the right way. Successful application requires more than knowing which knob to turn or what button to push (being a knobologist). You must know how to apply the modality, but you must also know:

- What your specific goals are
- That the modality you have chosen is the proper modality for achieving those goals
- What other therapy, such as therapeutic exercise, is beneficial and should be applied in combination with the modality

The application must be part of a carefully thought out, goal-driven rehabilitation plan. This is sometimes called the rifle approach, as contrasted to the shotgun approach. The following analogy helps explain these two approaches.

When a hunter fires a shotgun, hundreds of small round pellets are emitted from the gun. If a few of these pellets hit the target, they might kill a small animal, even though many pellets missed. On the other hand, when a hunter shoots a rifle, only one bullet comes out of the barrel. The hunter must take careful aim or else the target

will be missed. With the **shotgun approach**, the patient is treated with every possible modality, with the hope that one will be effective. The **rifle approach** is more focused; the patient is treated with one or two specific modalities, targeted to achieve a particular goal (Fig. 2.1).

In Chapter 1 we discouraged the use of a cookbook approach to rehabilitation, and we repeat that advice here. The cookbook approach is rigid; it follows a specific recipe. In contrast, the critical thinker approach is more flexible. Just as some clinicians fall into the habit of using the same rehabilitation protocol for every injury, some also use the same modalities (and settings) when treating several different types of injuries. Although the one-recipe-fits-all approach to modality application is easier to learn and use, it is not in the best interest of patients. No two patients or injuries are alike, and not everyone responds the same way to all treatments. With the cookbook approach, clinicians often treat the symptoms rather than the cause of the injury.

CRITICAL THINKING 2.1 *Can you think of some ways that you might be a better clinician by applying the rifle approach when you use therapeutic modalities? List several, then turn to the end of the chapter and compare your responses with ours.*

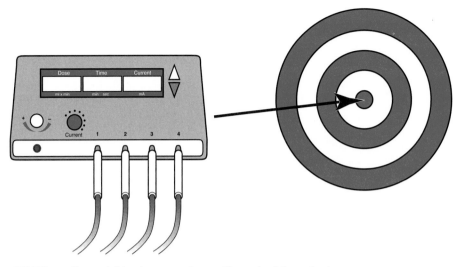

FIGURE 2.1. Use modalities that target the specific needs of the patient.

THE CRITICAL THINKER APPROACH

The **critical thinker approach to rehabilitation** uses an organized procedural outline that includes fairly broad guidelines to help the clinician choose the most appropriate modality and mode of applying that modality.[1] It is patient driven, rather than specific-modality driven. The modality is not the focus; it is part of an overall rehabilitation plan.

This approach begins with a through evaluation of the injury, establishing long-, medium-, and short-term goals and then selecting modalities and application parameters that will accomplish those specific goals. As the patient progresses, the application is altered to reflect the changing patient needs. Because no two patients or conditions are identical, the skilled clinician can use several tools (modalities) to reach particular treatment goals. The clinician who understands and employs critical thinking adapts to various situations. He alters the application parameters to best meet patient needs and to address the cause of the injury or condition. The critical thinker approach is more flexible than the cookbook approach because it empowers the clinician to speculate and ask, "I wonder what might happen if I try this modality in this situation?" (Fig. 2.2).

STANDARD YET FLEXIBLE OPERATING PROCEDURES

Standard operating procedures (SOPs) are specific guidelines and protocols for performing a specific task. Having SOPs is a form of quality control. A knowledgeable person, or team of people, develops SOPs for all staff to follow when performing the task. For example, your favorite fast food will be the same in Moab, Utah, as it is in New York City because it was prepared by people using the same standard operating procedures. Having SOPs for complex tasks promotes consistency. They help you remember the specific steps and ensure that all essential elements are performed.

Using SOPs for therapeutic modality operation can have some disadvantages. They may lead to cookbook ap-

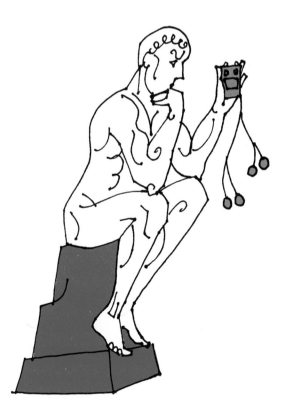

FIGURE 2.2. A critically thinking clinician is always seeking more efficient ways of treating patients.

plications, and the task of learning SOPs for each of the dozens of modalities can be daunting and confusing, especially for modalities that you use infrequently.

The five-step approach outlined in this chapter is a framework for therapeutic modality application.[1] It is not as rigid as typical SOPs because it does not dictate all the specifics of each modality application—it is not a cookbook. We call it a *framework* because it contains all the essential elements. A clinician thinks critically, then adds the specifics of each modality to the general framework. Using the same framework for each modality is a quality control measure because it ensures that all essential elements are included. Using the same five-step procedure for all modalities minimizes the amount of information you need to learn for each modality, thus adding another element of quality control. Remember that this framework is a general outline. Specific information will be presented in subsequent chapters for a variety of modalities.

The Five-Step Application Procedure

The application of all therapeutic modalities should follow a standard procedure to ensure that all essential elements occur and to prevent rogue applications (Fig. 2.3). Although there is a wide range of therapeutic modalities, each one can follow a general application process. Our **five-step application procedure** eliminates the need to learn SOPs for each modality.[1] After learning the five-step framework, you can plug in specifics for each therapeutic modality. By learning and applying this system, you will be more organized and effective in delivering therapeutic modality treatments.

STEP 1: FOUNDATION

A. Definition. A description of the modality and the basics of how it operates (Fig. 2.4).
B. Effects. The physiological and/or pathological changes the modality evokes, both locally and systemically (throughout the body).
C. Advantages. The benefits of the modality that make it more effective in treating injuries than other modalities.
D. Disadvantages. The possible negative effects the modality might cause as well as the benefits that might be lost from using this modality over another.
E. Indications. Situations in which the modality should be used or for which it is a suitable treatment or remedy for the condition.
F. Contraindications. Situations in which the modality should not be used—that is, situations in which it may do more harm than good.
G. Precautions. Situations that could cause harm if the clinician is not careful—for example, failure to move

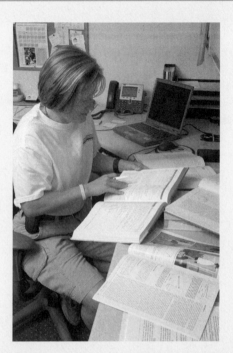

FIGURE 2.4. Before a therapeutic modality can be properly applied, you must have foundational knowledge about the modality and how specific types of injuries respond to the various ways of applying it.

the soundhead during ultrasound treatment could damage tissue or cause extreme pain.

MODALITY MYTH

THERE ARE RELATIVE AND ABSOLUTE CONTRAINDICATIONS

Some clinicians inappropriately use the terms *absolute contraindication* and *relative contraindication* to refer to contraindications and precautions, respectively. The term *absolute contraindication* is redundant. *Contraindication* means "do not use," so it is already absolute. The term *relative contraindication* contradicts itself. It is impossible to "relatively" not use a modality. Use the more precise terms, contraindication and precaution.

STEP 2: PREAPPLICATION TASKS

A. Selecting the proper modality
    1. Determine the pathological and physiological changes associated with the injury by doing the following:
        a. Evaluate (or reevaluate) the injury or problem.
        b. Review the patient's response to any previous treatment (Fig. 2.5).

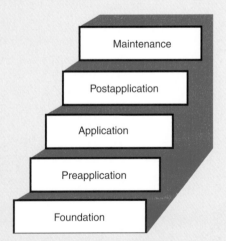

Maintenance

Postapplication

Application

Preapplication

Foundation

FIGURE 2.3. The five-step application procedure is a standardized framework for applying any therapeutic modality. It is rigid enough for quality control, yet flexible enough to allow the clinician to use modalities in the context of a critical thinking approach to rehabilitation.

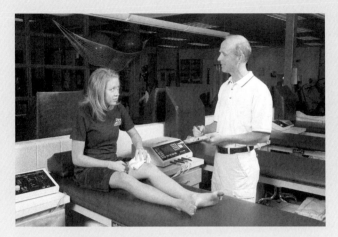

FIGURE 2.5. Patient interaction is an essential preapplication task. Detailed questions about how the patient responded to previous treatments help you decide whether to continue with the present modality or to select another one. Explaining the purpose, the expected outcome, the body's physiological response, and what the patient should feel help prepare the patient psychologically for the treatment.

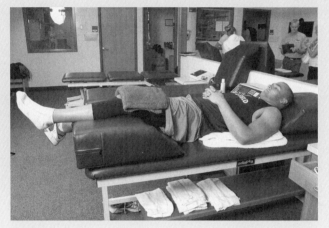

FIGURE 2.6. Pillows and bolsters are helpful in positioning a patient for treatment. You can never have too many pillows and bolsters in an athletic training clinic.

2. Establish the objectives (goals) of the therapy.
3. Match your therapeutic goal with a modality that will help you achieve that goal; consider the effects, advantages, disadvantages, indications, contraindications, and precautions of all the possible modalities you could use to reach your goals.
4. Make sure the modality is not contraindicated for the injury or condition in question.

B. Preparing the patient psychologically. This step entails more than just good bedside manners. As we will discuss in Chapter 7, there is a strong connection between emotions and physiological responses. The patient's psychological state modifies tissue responses to the therapy.
1. Explain the purpose and expected outcome of the procedure.
2. Describe the body's basic physiological response to the treatment, if the patient is interested.
3. Explain what the patient should expect to feel—for example, tingling, pins and needles, or gentle warmth.
4. Demonstrate the procedure on yourself if the patient is apprehensive.
5. Warn the patient about precautions.

C. Preparing the patient physically
1. Remove clothing as necessary.
2. Remove bandages, braces, and so on, as necessary.
3. Position the patient in a manner that will be comfortable, yet allow accessibility to the modality. Have an ample supply of pillows or bolsters (supports) to use in positioning the patient (Fig. 2.6).

D. Preparing the equipment
1. Set up the equipment.
2. Check the equipment operation.
3. Perform a safety check.

3 STEP 3: APPLICATION PARAMETERS

A. Procedures
1. Turn on the unit (if necessary).
2. Adjust the output parameters as needed.
3. Check the patient's response and readjust the output as needed.

B. Dosage
C. Length of application
D. Frequency of application
E. Duration of therapy

4 STEP 4: POSTAPPLICATION TASKS

A. Equipment removal; patient cleanup
B. Equipment replacement; area cleanup
C. Instructions to the patient. *Note:* These should be written if they are extensive or complicated.
1. Schedule the next treatment.
2. Instruct the patient about the level of activity and/or self-treatment she should administer before the next formal treatment.
3. Instruct the patient about what she should feel after treatment.

D. Record of treatment, including unique patient responses (Fig. 2.7).

5 STEP 5: MAINTENANCE

A. Regular equipment cleaning
B. Routine maintenance
C. Simple repairs

CLOSING SCENE

Recall from the opening scene, Jennie, a new student, seemed a bit confused that patients with similar injuries were treated with the same method, even though they responded differently to the treatments. She was also overwhelmed by all of the different kinds of therapeutic modalities housed in the clinic. She wondered about the purpose of each modality and the function of each of the knobs, switches, and lights on the devices. She wondered how long it would take her to master the correct use of all of those machines.

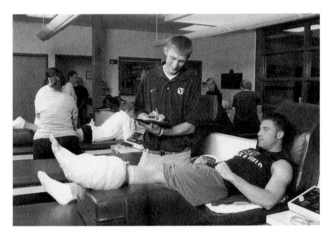

FIGURE 2.7. Properly recording the specifics of the therapeutic modality application, patient response, and instructions to the patient is an often neglected part of the modality application.

Jennie was fortunate to be assigned to work under the direction of a clinical instructor who understood when and why to use modalities. This instructor cautioned her about the flaws of the cookbook approach to treatment. He taught her how to be a critical thinker. This included looking at each patient differently and then determining the appropriate modality to use for each condition. He also taught her the five-step procedure to use when applying modalities. Under his watchful eye, he allowed Jennie to experience what each modality treatment felt like. Within a few months, Jennie understood the functions of each modality and felt confident in using them. As she became more confident, her clinical instructor turned the treatment of some patients over to her. Much to her surprise, the patients got better! Jennie succeeded where others had failed, because she became a clinician skilled in the art of critical thinking.

CHAPTER REFLECTIONS

1. Read and ponder each of the following points. Do you feel you have a clear understanding of each concept? If not, reread the appropriate section of the chapter.
   - Define a standard operating procedure.
   - Explain the cookbook and critical thinker approaches to therapeutic modality application.
   - Discuss the similarities and differences between SOPs and the five-step application procedure.
   - Describe the five-step application procedure, including the sub-elements of each step.
   - Identify the differences between indication, contraindication, and precaution with respect to therapeutic modalities.
   - Explain the importance of each of the following elements in selecting a therapeutic modality: evaluating the patient and injury, therapeutic goals, the physiological effects of the modality on the body, and the advantages of a particular modality over another modality.

2. Write three to five questions for discussion with your class instructor, clinical instructor, classmates, and clinical colleagues.

3. Get together with classmates and quiz each other on the concepts of this chapter. Use the points in exercise 1 and questions you wrote for exercise 2 as a beginning. Explaining concepts out loud to others requires a deeper grasp of the material than feeling you understand it as you read.

CRITICAL THINKING RESPONSE

Critical Thinking 2.1

There are several possible answers:

1. You treat the cause of the injury instead of the symptoms.
2. Your patients get better faster.
3. You know which modality/treatment regimen worked because you tried one or two at a time and there is a cause-and-effect relationship to the outcome.
4. Your patients develop confidence in you.
5. You are able to establish which regimens work and which ones don't.

REFERENCE

1. Knight K, Draper D. Critical thinking and therapeutic modalities. Athl Ther Today 2004;9:28–29.

Injury Record Keeping

OPENING SCENE

Both of us have served as witnesses and consultants in legal cases dealing with the alleged improper use of therapeutic modalities. One such case involved a podiatrist who treated an elderly woman with ultrasound during an office visit after the woman had undergone a bunionectomy. The patient complained that the treatment hurt and asked him to stop. He informed her that she should not feel anything and that the treatment would last for only 10 min. The patient thought the pain and swelling intensified in the days after the treatment. After several weeks of pain, she hired an attorney, who claimed her pain and scarring were excessive and the result of the ultrasound treatment. Were the pain and scarring the result of the surgery or the ultrasound? The patient's treatment records, which described the treatment simply as "ultrasound for 10 min," were inadequate to answer this question The records included only the treatment duration and omitted several important parameters, such as frequency, intensity, ERA, and duty cycle. If the clinician had kept detailed records in this case, he might not be in such a predicament.

The Purpose of Keeping Records

You may think a textbook on health care administration[1,2] is a more appropriate place for a chapter on record keeping. However, maintaining injury and treatment records in an athletic training or physical therapy clinic is essential. You must understand, early in your career, the absolute necessity of keeping accurate records, so we introduce the basics here. You must make record keeping a part of your clinical practice now.

Accurate and detailed **record keeping** is a mandatory part of any athletic training program. Injury records are necessary for the following reasons, in order of importance:

1. *Communication and quality control.* Communicating with other clinicians, the patient, and yourself to increase the quality of care provided to patients.
2. *Legal considerations.* Protecting the clinician in the event of a lawsuit.
3. *Research.* Documenting treatment details to help establish evidence of the effectiveness of the treatment, and/or find newer approaches.
4. *History.* Tracking a patient's injury history.
5. *Traffic patterns.* Monitoring injury and modality use frequency as well as clinic workflow.

COMMUNICATION AND QUALITY CONTROL

By far the most important reason for keeping records is communication—with yourself, with others involved in the treatment, and with the patient. Records enhance the quality of care by preserving details that otherwise might

be forgotten or known only to a single person.

It is impossible for a busy clinician to remember all the details of numerous patients without written records. Periodic review of the records helps a clinician see what progress a patient has made, and may stimulate ideas for improved treatment.

Written records help the various treatment team members understand and discuss the approach, thereby adding continuity to the rehabilitation program (Fig. 3.1). Treatments are often administered by different people, and if the details are not recorded, no one will know what the others are doing. The efforts of each clinician will be isolated rather than being part of a coordinated whole. This often leads to patient confusion, especially if each clinician is giving different advice about self-treatment to

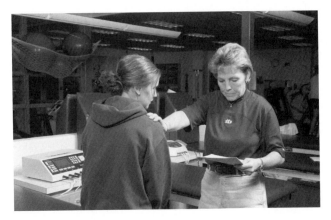

FIGURE 3.1. Clear, concise, and numerous entries on treatment notes help clinicians communicate with each other and thereby provide better care.

supplement the formal regimen. Moreover, the efforts of physicians involved in the rehabilitation program can often be more effective if detailed information about each treatment is communicated to them.

Another way that records help communication is with the patient. Patients frequently express frustration at not recovering from an injury as quickly as expected, and they want to know what else can be done. Although he might claim to be following the prescribed rehabilitation program, the treatment records reveal another story. When confronted with the records, the patient admits to missing some treatments. The problem becomes evident—it is not the program that is wrong; the patient is not following the program. At other times, the program is inadequate and needs to be adjusted. But the adjustments must also be recorded to verify that the patient has faithfully followed the revised program.

LEGAL CONSIDERATIONS

An injury record is a legal document. The value of that document depends on the accuracy and detail of the records. Most lawsuits occur years after the event, usually after any clinician would have forgotten the specific details of any treatment. The statute of limitations is 7 years in most cases, and written records are obviously necessary for providing the details of how a particular patient's injury was treated.

A real court case from 1986 in Illinois illustrates the need for detailed records (KK was a witness). A former high school athlete sued a coach and a cold pack manufacturer for a thermal burn and scarring he claimed resulted from applying a cold pack to his knee overnight. During cross-examination by the defense attorney in the case, the young man was asked a series of questions similar to the following:

>   **DA:** Coach Jones testified that he told you to apply the cold pack for only 30 minutes. Do you contest that?
>   **Athlete:** Yes.
>   **DA:** Are you sure he didn't tell you to apply it for only 30 minutes?
>   **Athlete:** Yes, I am sure, he never told me how long to apply it.
>   **DA:** Have you ever doubted whether or not he told you how long to apply it?
>   **Athlete:** No, I have never doubted it—he did not tell me.
>   **DA:** Did you give a deposition [pretrial testimony] on [date 3 years earlier]?
>   **Athlete:** Yes.
>   **DA:** Will you read the following statement you made during that deposition?

Three years earlier, the patient had testified that he did not think the coach told him how long to apply the cold pack, but he was not sure. Thus his testimony at the trial contradicted his earlier testimony. The jury sided with the coach. Written records help you be consistent in your testimony concerning a lawsuit.

RESEARCH

Research is accomplished by documentation: precise and accurate record keeping. Most clinicians are researchers, whether they realize it or not. Consider the following scenario: A clinician, frustrated with the lack of progress of a patient, tries something new. It seems to work, so she tries it again with other patients and is again satisfied with the results. She then shares the idea with colleagues, who express interest in the concept and ask specific, detailed questions about the cases. The clinician goes back to her treatment records for the details of the case and decides to write a case report. The clinician just conducted a research project. Therapeutic modality use and rehabilitation programs can be improved if clinicians record what they do and then periodically evaluate their records.

HISTORY

The history of an injury is important to all members of the treatment team and to others as well. Because the need for this information sometimes arises months after the injury occurred, accurate and detailed records are critical. Specific details are essential to an insurance company. Claim settlement is often delayed while companies research details. Records also help a patient verify information concerning past injuries. College and professional team recruiters, the military, and some civic and corporate employers often want a patient to report significant sports injuries they have suffered and the extent of their rehabilitation.

TRAFFIC PATTERNS

Injury records provide the only means of establishing daily, weekly, monthly, and yearly traffic patterns in an athletic training clinic. Records can serve as evidence for verifying to the administration the need for additional budget, facilities, and/or staff or the disadvantages of proposed cuts in the clinic's program. Records can also demonstrate increases or decreases in the volume of work handled in the athletic training clinic. If, for example, records show that the use of a particular modality has drastically increased, additional modalities might be authorized.

Using Records and Forms

Several components of athletic training and sports medicine clinics require record keeping. Five types of records are listed in Table 3.1 along with the names of the forms

TABLE 3.1	*Forms Typically Used in an Athletic Training Clinic*
PURPOSE OR TYPE OF RECORD	**SPECIFIC FORM**
Evaluation of injuries	Athletic injury report form
	SOAP notes
Treatment of injuries	Daily treatment log
	Individual treatment sheet
	SOAP note progress
	Daily weight recording form
Referrals to/from others	Medical referral
	Rehabilitation referral
Medical information	Incoming student athlete
	Returning student athlete
Equipment upkeep	Ultrasound calibration
	Electrical stimulator maintenance
	Ground-fault interrupter (GFI) check
	Weight equipment maintenance

that are used at one university for recording that information. (Most clinics have similar forms but probably name them differently.) One of the first things you should do when beginning to work in a new clinic is to familiarize yourself with the various forms and records used in that clinic.

INITIALING ENTRIES ON FORMS

It is important that every entry on recording forms be initialed by the person making the entry. Often one clinician needs more information about a patient than what is on the form. The initials tell the clinician who to go to for additional information.

ELECTRONIC RECORD KEEPING

Not all records need to be kept in paper form. Injury tracking and record-keeping software programs allow records to be computerized (Fig. 3.2). Two popular ones are the Sports Injury Monitoring System (SIMS)[3] and the SportsWare2007[4] injury tracking system. They are designed to document injury and treatment parameters and to improve communication between members of the clinic staff.[1] Two key features of these programs with respect to modality use are daily progress and treatment notes.

Computerized record-keeping programs must be easy to use. They must allow entry on the fly, meaning treatments can be entered as quickly as, or immediately after, they are given. Systems that require clinicians to sit down at the computer in the evening to enter the day's treatment details will result in records that are inaccurate and incomplete.

SOAP NOTES

The **SOAP note** format is a type of problem-oriented medical record.[5,6] SOAP is an acronym for "subjective evaluation, objective evaluation, assessment, and plan."[5]

- *S = subjective.* The subjective evaluation contains information gathered primarily from questioning the patient on his present condition. Patient history and symptoms make up the majority of this information. For example, if a patient presents with ankle pain, saying, "I twisted my ankle and it hurts right here," the subjective evaluation would read, "Lateral ankle pain from twisting ankle."

- *O = objective.* The objective evaluation consists of reproducible information the clinician gathers through tests or evaluative measures. Measurable factors, such

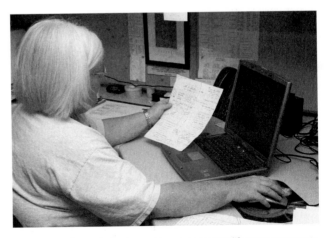

FIGURE 3.2. Computerized record keeping can simplify summary reports.

as laxity during a stress test, girth, volumetric measurements of swelling, and joint range of motion as measured with a goniometer, appear in this portion of the record. The objective evaluation of the patient above might read, "Pain over ATF during palpation and plantar flexion/inversion. Neg malleolar compression test."

- *A = assessment.* The assessment is the clinician's professional judgment or impression of the injury. Continuing with the same example, this section would read "Moderate inversion ankle sprain."
- *P = plan.* The course of action that the clinician and the patient will follow to treat and rehabilitate the injury. Depending on the extent of the injury, this may include an immediate treatment plan and short-term and long-term goals. An immediate treatment plan for this patient with the sprained ankle would read, "Application of an ice pack with an elastic wrap for 30 min repeated every 2 hr." A short-term goal might be, "Cryokinetics to regain full, pain-free ROM and decrease swelling"; a long-term goal might be, "Hot pack to heat the tissues before sport-specific skills and return to competition."

There are three types of SOAP notes:[5]

- **Initial note**, written after the initial assessment (the example just outlined constitutes an initial note)
- **Progress note**, or **interim note**, periodic documentation of the results of the treatment plan
- **Discharge note**, written when treatment is discontinued

CRITICAL THINKING 3.1 *In which of the three types of SOAP notes will most therapeutic modality treatments be recorded?*

SOAP notes record what modalities the clinician uses to manage the patient's rehabilitation program. They are legal documents that protect both the clinician and the patient. SOAP notes are a good way to communicate with others. If a clinician is absent from work or busy treating other patients, her protocol can be easily followed by another practitioner.

SOAP notes provide important information that can be used to determine whether or not a certain modality intervention is working. In cases for which reimbursement might be warranted, clear, concise SOAP notes might make the difference between being paid for modality use or not.

Progress Notes

Progress notes include updates or additional information regarding the patient's status since the most recent note was written (Fig. 3.3).[5] The following is an example of how progress notes could be written with respect to therapeutic modality use for the patient with the ankle sprain introduced earlier.

- *S = subjective.* The progress note after 3 days might read, "The pain has decreased by 50%."
- *O = objective.* Tests and measures are updated or added to the information reported in the last progress note. For example, "Ankle girth has decreased by 1 cm and PF has increased by 5°."
- *A = assessment.* This is typically included in the progress note only if the diagnosis has changed.
- *P = plan.* This includes progress toward short-term or long-term goals and addresses why these goals have been met or why they haven't been met. The progress note after 1 week might read, "Cryokinetics has resulted in pain-free ROM and decreased swelling."

Progress notes *do not* substitute for daily treatment logs. Every treatment should be recorded in both the facility's daily treatment log and in the individual patient's injury record. Progress notes are not intended to be used for every treatment.

Discharge Notes

A discharge SOAP note is written at the time the therapy is discontinued, after a final examination and evaluation are performed. A discharge note addresses the results of the final examination and evaluation, the outcomes and goals achieved, a summary of the interventions, and the final disposition of the patient.[5]

Blackfoot State University
Injury Evaluation

Patient: *Likialiki, Moafua*   Date: *19 Oct. 2005*   Status: (new) ongoing recurring

AT: *D. Draper*   Sport: *football*

Subjective: *Stepped in hole on practice field, can't walk*

Objective: *2+ pain over ATF on palpation & wt bearing*
80% ROM-PF & inv, normal ROM ever & DF

Assessment: *2° ATF Sp*

Plan of treatment: *RICES today, cryokinetics tomorrow*
X-ray

FIGURE 3.3. A typical progress SOAP note form.

CLOSING SCENE

We opened this chapter with an example of how improper record keeping leaves a clinician vulnerable to lawsuits. We could have related the details of any of seven cases when attorneys representing one of our former patients requested our treatment records to review as part of their investigation of a potential lawsuit. No lawsuit was filed, in part because we had good records.

Far more important than protecting us from a few potential lawsuits, our injury records have increased the quality of our care. We have always worked in very busy athletic training clinics, with huge patient loads and numerous clinicians. Our records have been indispensable as we have treated patients using a critical thinking approach.

CHAPTER REFLECTIONS

1. Read and ponder each of the following points. Do you feel you have a clear understanding of each concept? If not, reread the appropriate section of the chapter.
   - Name the five reasons for keeping treatment records, and discuss why each one is important.
   - Discuss the five specific types of records that each athletic training clinic should maintain and name the specific records at your institution that are examples of each type.
   - Explain why it is important to initial each entry in an injury record.
   - Describe the elements of a SOAP note and discuss the type of information that is contained in each section.
   - Explain the similarity and differences between initial, progress, interim, and discharge SOAP notes.

2. Write three to five questions for discussion with your class instructor, clinical instructor, classmates, and clinical colleagues.

3. Get together with classmates and quiz each other on the concepts of this chapter. Use the points in exercise 1 and questions you wrote for exercise 2 as a beginning. Explaining concepts out loud to others requires a deeper grasp of the material than feeling you understand it as you read.

CRITICAL THINKING RESPONSE

Critical Thinking 3.1

Most therapeutic modality treatments are recorded in a progress (interim) note.

REFERENCES

1. Ray RR. Management Strategies in Athletic Training. 3rd ed. Champaign, IL: Human Kinetics, 2005.
2. Rankin JM, Ingersoll CD. Athletic Training Management: Concepts and Application. 3rd ed. New York: McGraw Hill, 2006.
3. Powell N. Med Sports Systems; Sports Injury Information Systems. Available at: www.flantech.net/sims_features.html. Accessed May 2007.
4. Computer Sports Medicine, Inc. CSMi Medical Solutions. Available at: www.csmisolutions.com. Accessed August 2005.
5. Kettenbach G. Writing S.O.A.P. Notes. 3rd ed. Philadelphia: Davis, 2004.
6. Anderson MK, Hall SJ, Martin M. Foundations of Athletic Training. 3rd ed. Baltimore: Lippincott Williams & Wilkins, 2004.

Review Questions

Chapter 1

1. Which of the following modalities is both mechanical and thermal?
   a. massage
   b. traction
   c. electrical stimulation
   d. ultrasound
   e. hot pack

2. Which of the following modalities is both mechanical and cryotherapy?
   a. ice massage
   b. cool whirlpool
   c. vapocoolant spray
   d. ice slush
   e. traction

3. The principle that the body responds to a given demand with a specific and predictable adaptation is known as the _____ principle.
   a. overload
   b. SAID
   c. specificity
   d. RICES
   e. progressive resistive

4. Which of the following is not among the 10 core goals of rehabilitation?
   a. confidence
   b. structural integrity
   c. pain-free joints and muscles
   d. joint flexibility
   e. muscular strength

5. Which of the following is not a good way to stay current with the latest research in therapeutic modalities?
   a. Read the *Journal of Athletic Training* and *Journal of Orthopaedic and Sports Physical Therapy*.
   b. Attend seminars that deal with topics on modalities.
   c. Attend seminars for emergency medical technicians.
   d. Visit poster sessions at seminars geared toward modalities.
   e. Use PubMed and explore other online databases and search engines.

Chapter 2

1. What is the main weakness of a clinician who follows the cookbook approach when using therapeutic modalities?
   a. He is a technician.
   b. He is not a critical thinker.
   c. He treats the symptoms of the injury, not the cause.
   d. He doesn't build trust with his patient.
   e. He takes too many shortcuts.

2. What is the main strength of a clinician who follows the critical thinker approach when using therapeutic modalities?
   a. She is not a technician.
   b. She is guided by standard operating procedures.
   c. She builds trust with her patients.
   d. She treats the cause of the injury, not just the symptoms.
   e. She gets results.

3. The five-step framework for applying therapeutic modalities accomplishes all the following except _____.
   a. ensuring that all essential elements occur during application
   b. helping prevent rogue applications
   c. ensuring that each therapeutic modality is applied the same each time
   d. assisting in the use of SOPs
   e. eliminating the need to learn separate SOPs for each modality

4. Which of the following is not one of the five steps of the five-step application procedure?
   a. application parameters
   b. recording treatments
   c. preapplication tasks
   d. postapplication tasks
   e. foundation

Chapter 3

1. What is the most important reason for keeping records?
   a. preventing lawsuits
   b. research
   c. establishing traffic patterns for future modality use
   d. knowing injury history
   e. keeping communication lines open

2. Which of the following contributes to quality control?
   a. preventing lawsuits
   b. research
   c. establishing traffic patterns for future modality use
   d. knowing injury history
   e. keeping communication lines open

3. Information gathered primarily by questioning the patient is what part of the SOAP note?
   a. history
   b. subjective
   c. objective
   d. assessment
   e. plan

4. The clinician's professional judgment or impression of the injury is what part of the SOAP note?
   a. subjective
   b. diagnosis
   c. objective
   d. assessment
   e. plan

5. The choice to use thermotherapy or cryotherapy would be recorded in what part of the SOAP note?
   a. subjective
   b. objective
   c. analysis
   d. plan
   e. none of the above

6. Which of the following is not a type of SOAP note?
   a. progress note
   b. permanent note
   c. interim note
   d. initial note
   e. discharge note

ORTHOPEDIC INJURY, IMMEDIATE CARE, AND HEALING

The basis of using therapeutic modalities is understanding the injury you are trying to treat and the body's response to that injury. The first topic of Part II is an indepth look at inflammation, the pathophysiological changes that occur after injury. The second topic, immediate care—how you respond right away to the injury—involves the use of modalities that are often more important than anything you do in the subsequent weeks to resolve the problem. The third topic is the healing process and how you can influence it.

Many professionals will think the order of these chapters is odd. Indeed, every other text we have seen places healing immediately after inflammation, and often these topics are discussed in the same chapter. For most of our careers, we taught the concepts of inflammation and healing sequentially. We experimented with the current order a few years ago in an effort to strengthen our presentation of immediate care. It worked so well we haven't even considered going back to our former ordering.

The sequence used here is true to the time course of events. Immediate care procedures should be initiated long before healing begins; and indeed, the earlier they are begun, the more effective they are and the quicker healing is initiated. Although from a pathophysiological standpoint healing follows inflammation, from a chronological and injury management standpoint, healing comes after immediate care. Therefore, our immediate care chapter belongs where it is.

Most of Part II is foundational material. The exception is the last part of Chapter 5, in which we include specific application parameters for immediate care, including cryotherapy. Our treatment of cryotherapy in Chapter 5 is deliberately incomplete because in this part of the book, we are concerned only with immediate care. Chapters 13 and 14 deal with additional uses of cryotherapy during later stages of rehabilitation.

Chapter 5 contains a good deal of content about cryotherapy. Indeed some may feel it is excessive. Our intent is to debunk the vast amount of misinformation about cryotherapy that much of the medical community commonly accepts as true. We choose to acknowledge the existence of these ideas and to discuss why they are wrong, rather than to ignore them. We hope to reduce their influence on how clinicians manage acute orthopedic injury and thereby improve patient care.

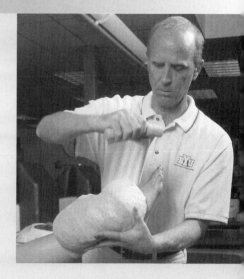

Part II consists of three chapters:

Tissue Response to Injury: Inflammation, Swelling, and Edema

A basketball player grabs a rebound and lands on another player's foot, twists her ankle, and falls to the floor. Rachel, an athletic trainer, rushes to the player's aid, performs a quick evaluation, and assists her off the court. After a thorough evaluation, Rachel determines that the player has a second-degree inversion ankle sprain. The game is over for her. Rachel applies an ice pack, a compression wrap, and a splint; then she helps the player onto the bench and elevates her ankle. Is all of that necessary? Why?

The Inflammatory Response

Injury to the body results in anatomical, physiological, pathological, and psychological changes. Such changes must be addressed in the course of caring for and rehabilitating a patient after an injury. This chapter focuses primarily on the pathological and physiological changes that are part of the inflammatory response. Psychological factors will be discussed in Chapter 7.

Inflammation, also known as the *inflammatory response*, is the local response of the body to an injury or irritant. It occurs at the tissue level and has a dual function (Fig. 4.1):

- To defend the body against foreign substances
- To dispose of dead and dying tissue so repair, the regeneration of viable tissue, can take place

Some authors consider repair to be part of the inflammatory response,[1] whereas others consider these to be separate processes.[2] Still others divide the two processes into three phases.[3,4] Regardless, inflammation and repair are defined by a series of overlapping but sequential events. We treat them as two separate processes to explain each more clearly. Inflammation is the subject of this chapter and repair is the subject of Chapter 6. Thinking of them as one, two, or three processes, however, has no bearing on understanding the events that occur from the time the injury occurs until it is healed.

CARDINAL SIGNS

There are five cardinal, or primary, signs of inflammation, which are often referred to by their Latin names:

- *Rubor:* redness
- *Calor:* heat
- *Edema:* swelling
- *Dolor:* pain
- *Funca laesa:* functional loss

Each of these signs will occur to some degree when tissue is injured and the body responds with inflammation. You may argue that a splinter in the finger will not cause loss of function. It may not prevent the patient from running; but cells in the finger have been damaged, will die, and must be replaced. So there is some loss of function. Also, a splinter in the finger may prevent a baseball pitcher from throwing his best curveball. The primary signs of inflammation always occur in response to an injury, but their magnitude and effect on a person's activity depend on the extent of the injury, where it occurred, and the nature of the activity.

COMMON MISCONCEPTIONS

Many think that inflammation is something bad that should be eliminated; but inflammation is, in fact, good and necessary. Without inflammation, there would be no healing. This misconception persists in part because the signs of inflammation are often mistaken for the inflammatory response itself. Minimizing the *signs* of inflammation, such as swelling and pain, is beneficial, whereas eliminating inflammation will actually prolong the process of healing instead of shortening it.

Another misconception is that the terms *swelling, edema,* and *inflammation* are synonyms for the same phenomenon. Swelling and edema occur during inflammation, but inflammation is a much more complex process (Fig. 4.2). Edema and swelling are not the same. Edema causes swelling, but swelling can occur from other sources: All edema causes swelling, but not all swelling is caused by edema.

SEQUENTIAL, INTERRELATED, OVERLAPPING EVENTS

Inflammation consists of a series of eight sequential, interrelated, and overlapping events:

1. The primary injury
2. Ultrastructural changes
3. Chemical mediation

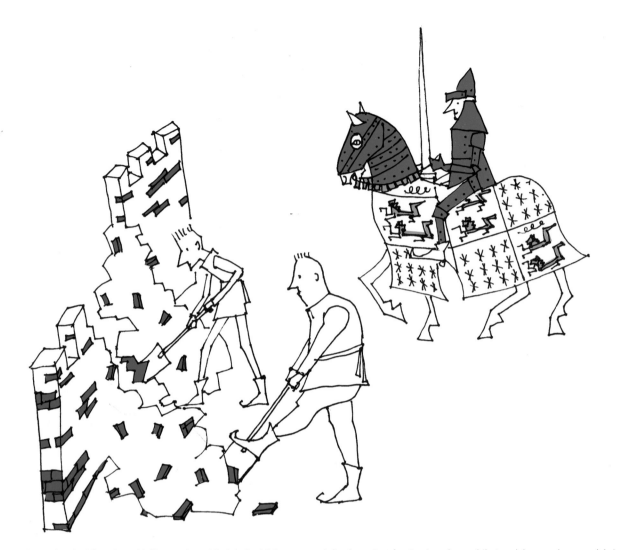

FIGURE 4.1. The dual function of inflammation. A knight in shining armor defends against foreign invaders, while two laborers clean up debris so the "injured" wall can be rebuilt.

4. Hemodynamic changes
5. Metabolic changes
6. Permeability changes
7. Leukocyte migration
8. Phagocytosis

These eight events occur in the order listed, but they can also occur simultaneously at different places within the injured tissue, because they progress at different rates in different parts of the tissue. A helpful analogy is the construction of a highway. The area is first surveyed. Then bridges and culverts are built, hills are leveled, depressions are filled, the roadbed is graded, concrete or asphalt is laid, shoulders are graded, lines are painted, and signs are put up. Bulldozers would not go out before the area is surveyed, nor would lines be painted before the as-

phalt is laid. If the project is many miles long, however, the asphalt may go down at the beginning at the same time bridges are being built toward the end, in sequential, overlapping events, just as in the inflammatory response.

Those who consider inflammation and repair as one process with three phases consider the eight inflammatory events as one phase and divide repair into two phases (discussed in Chapter 6).

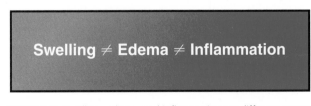

Swelling ≠ Edema ≠ Inflammation

FIGURE 4.2. Swelling, edema, and inflammation are different events.

The Primary Injury

Inflammation is initiated by an injury, an occurrence that impairs the structure or function of tissue and thereby alters the cell's ability to carry out its normal homeostatic mechanisms.[2] This initial tissue disruption is known as **primary injury**. Most **orthopedic injuries**, such as sprains, strains, fractures, and contusions, occur when excessive physical force (stress or strain) causes musculoskeletal structures to fail. There are two types of **trauma**:

- **Macrotrauma**, also called *impact injury* or *contact injury,* is caused by a large insult and results in immediate tissue disruption. Macrotrauma is classified as an *acute injury.*
- **Microtrauma**, also known as *overuse, cyclic loading,* or *friction injury,*[2] is caused by small or low-grade stress that wears away the tissue over time. Microtrauma is classified as *chronic injury.*

Although orthopedic injuries are traumatic, there are many other types of injury, each of which results in the same basic inflammatory response. Additional causes of injury include the following:

- Physical agents (force, burns, radiation)
- Metabolic processes (ischemia and hypoxia)
- Biologic agents (bacteria, viruses, parasites)
- Chemical agents (acids, gases, organic solvents, endogenous chemicals*)

Regardless of the cause of the injury, the same series of responses occurs in the body, although the magnitude of specific reactions vary according to the causative agent. Sometimes the individual may not be aware that an injury has occurred, nor will there be visible signs of the inflammatory process. Nevertheless, each of the inflammation events will occur, even in response to the simplest of injuries.

MODALITY MYTH

TRAUMA IS FORCE

The word *trauma* is sometimes thought of as the force that causes injuries. This is incorrect. Trauma is the injury that results from physical force, not the force itself.

---

*Endogenous chemicals are normal secretions in abnormal locations (such as those that cause gout) or in increased quantity in a normal location (such as those that cause stomach ulcers).

Ultrastructural Changes

Ultrastructural changes refer to the breaking down and eventual disruption of the cellular membrane and its **organelles**, specialized structures within tissue cells. The cell's contents spill out into the **extracellular spaces** (the spaces between cells) and the cell dies.[5] With traumatic injuries, ultrastructural changes occur as a direct result of the primary injury and indirectly as a result of metabolic and/or chemical injury. (Secondary injury will be discussed in more detail later in this chapter.) Secondary injury occurs in cells adjacent to those that undergo primary injury.

Chemical Mediation

Chemical mediators, such as *histamine, bradykinin,* and *cytokines,* are activated by ultrastructural changes; they signal the rest of the body that cells have been damaged, thereby mobilizing the body's resources to respond. They modify and regulate the rest of the inflammatory response, neutralizing the cause of the injury, and start to remove the cellular debris so that repair can take place. Chemical mediators are somewhat like police officers; they come to the site of accidents and direct events until the accident is cleaned up.

Hemodynamic Changes

Hemodynamic changes mobilize and transport defense components of the blood to the injury site and secure their passage through vessel walls into the tissue. These changes occur in blood vessels within the injured area that did not undergo primary injury as well as in vessels on the periphery of the injury.

In response to an injury, arteries dilate and blood flow increases. At the same time, many previously inactive capillaries and venules open, thereby expanding the total blood flow to the area (Fig. 4.3). However, rate of flow through individual vessels is slowed. The slowing of blood flow lets **leukocytes**, white blood cells, fall out of the bloodstream and move to the blood vessel margins (Fig. 4.4a). After tumbling along the margins for a while, the leukocytes stick to the **endothelium** (vessel wall) and/or to other leukocytes (Figs. 4.4b and 4.5). Thus the endothelium becomes paved with leukocytes. Eventually, the leukocytes will pass through gaps in the endothelium and move through the tissue to the injury (Fig. 4.4c–g).

Metabolic Changes

Normal cellular functioning (the cell membrane and organelles) requires energy in the form of **adenosine triphosphate (ATP)**, which is usually supplied by aerobic (oxy-

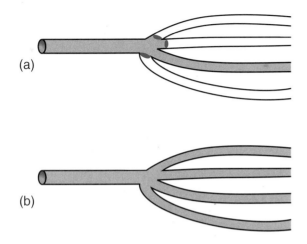

FIGURE 4.3. Hemodynamic changes. **(a)** Inactive vessels **(b)** open after injury to flood the area with blood and decrease the rate of blood flow in individual vessels. These steps allow leukocytes to move from the center of the vessel to the walls and to slow down.

gen-using) metabolism.[7] When a cell is deprived of oxygen, a state known as **hypoxia**, it switches to anaerobic metabolism, or glycolysis, to satisfy its energy requirements. **Glycolysis**, the conversion of glucose to lactic acid when insufficient oxygen is available, is not long lasting, however, and continued hypoxia leads to a steady decrease in energy production. Cell membrane functions slow down as the energy necessary to maintain them decreases. Particularly important is the reduced activity of the sodium pump, a membrane process that maintains the concentration of intracellular sodium at low levels (Fig. 4.6).

The cell membrane is porous to sodium ions (Na^+), so sodium passively diffuses across the membrane if the concentration of sodium between the inside and the outside of the cell is unequal. The cell needs a low internal sodium content to function properly, so the sodium pump actively moves sodium out of the cell. Because this is an active process, it requires energy to function. If sufficient energy is not available, the sodium pump's activity slows or stops, and the sodium concentration within the cell and/or its organelles increases. This causes increased amounts of water to pass into the cell, and the cell begins to swell. Excessive swelling causes the cell to burst and die.

Prolonged anaerobic metabolism also leads to intracellular acidosis, and the buildup of acid within the cell further impairs membrane integrity. Cellular organelles called **lysosomes** contain enzymes that digest foreign matter trapped within the cell. If lysosome membranes rupture from acidosis or from a failure of the sodium pump, their contents will begin attacking and digesting other cellular components, including the cell membrane.

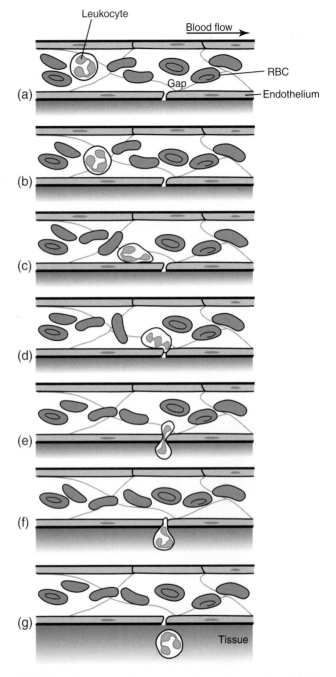

FIGURE 4.4. Hemodynamic changes and leukocyte migration. **(a)** The leukocyte moves to the margin of the blood vessel. It then (b) sticks to the endothelium (pavementing), **(c)** moves over the endothelium surface, **(d)** finds an endothelial gap, **(e)** passes through the gap, and **(f)** leaves the vessel. **(g)** The leukocyte moves about in the tissue. *RBC,* red blood cell.

Permeability Changes

Both histamine and bradykinin increase the permeability of small blood vessels (the same ones involved in hemodynamic changes). The endothelial cells contract or round up, thereby pulling away from each other, creating sizable gaps through which leukocytes move out of the blood vessel into the extracellular spaces (see Fig. 4.4e). Even though the

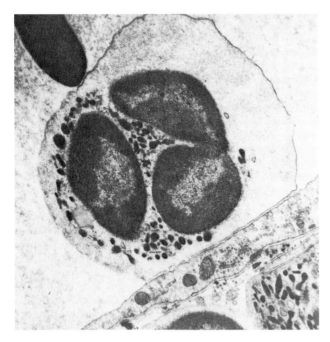

FIGURE 4.5. Electron micrograph of a leukocyte sticking to a blood vessel wall. It will move until it finds a gap in the vessel wall through which it can pass. (Reprinted from McLeod;[6] used with permission from Pfizer Inc.)

gaps are large compared to their normal state, the cells have to work to escape (Fig. 4.7; see also Fig. 4.4e).

Although the purpose of increased permeability is to let leukocytes move to the injury site, it also allows great amounts of protein-rich fluid to escape. The result is increased viscosity of the blood, sometimes to the extent that enough cells are packed in the vessel to block circulation.

Leukocyte Migration

Once the leukocytes have passed to the outside of the vascular wall, **leukocyte migration** to the injury site occurs (see Fig. 4.4g). Leukocyte migration happens in a concentration-limited fashion, meaning that the number of leukocytes is highest at sites where the greatest tissue damage has occurred and is lowest where there is little or no tissue damage. Concentration-limited leukocyte migration is a response to the concentration of chemical mediators in the area; the strongest concentration is at the site of the most damage.

Two types of leukocytes that play a primary role in trauma-induced inflammation are neutrophils and macrophages (Fig. 4.8). Smaller, faster, and more numerous than macrophages, **neutrophils** arrive at the injury site first and provide a temporary first line of defense. They are short lived (~7 hr) and do not reproduce. When they die, they release chemical mediators that attract macrophages to clean up the cellular debris, thus increasing the concentration of chemical mediators released by the cells.

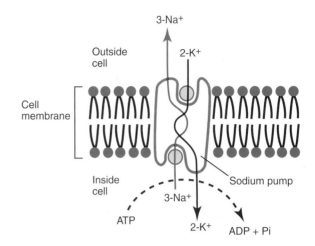

FIGURE 4.6. The sodium pump actively moves sodium ions (Na^+) out of the cell and lesser amounts of potassium ions (K^+) into the cell. The energy necessary to drive this process is supplied by breaking down adenosine triphosphate (*ATP*) into adenosine diphosphate (*ADP*) and free phosphate (*Pi*). (Adapted with permission from Guyton.[7])

The main function of neutrophils is to form a first line of defense against bacterial infections.[8] They contain highly toxic substances that destroy microorganisms and in the process may destroy other neutrophils and/or cause collateral damage to adjacent healthy cells and tissues.[8,9] Regulatory mechanisms, however, reduce or prevent the neutrophils from damaging healthy cells,[9–12] although the extent of their regulation is uncertain.

Macrophages live for months and can reproduce, thereby providing a long-lasting second line of defense.

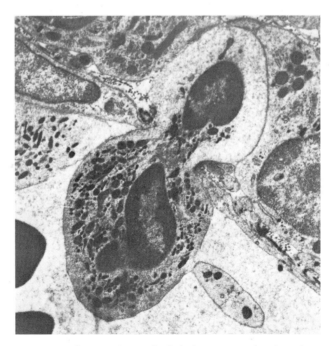

FIGURE 4.7. Electron micrograph of a leukocyte squeezing through an endothelial gap from the vessel into the tissue. Note the platelet (lower right) and a portion of another leukocyte (upper left) adhering to it. (Reprinted from McLeod;[6] used with permission from Pfizer Inc.)

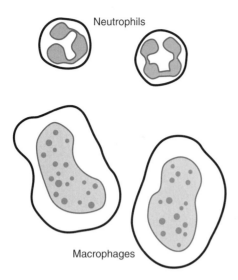

Neutrophils

Macrophages

FIGURE 4.8. Neutrophils and macrophages are the most common leukocytes. Because neutrophils are smaller, they migrate out of the blood vessels first. But they soon die, adding to the cellular debris cleaned up by the macrophages.

Their main function is cleaning up cellular debris. In addition, they release chemical mediators that prolong the inflammatory response and thus aid in healing.

Phagocytosis

The process of digesting cellular debris and other foreign material into pieces small enough to be removed from the injury site via lymph vessels is known as **phagocytosis**. As leukocytes arrive at the injury site, they begin digesting debris and any foreign material that is present, such as bacteria (Fig. 4.9a). The leukocyte engulfs a bacterium or cell particle in its membrane, and lysosomes (cells filled with digestive enzymes) move it (Fig. 4.9b). The membrane encloses the particle, forming a sac called a **phagosome**, which moves to the interior of the cell where it unites with one or more lysosomes to become a **phagolysosome** (Fig. 4.9c). The lysosome contents spill into the phagosome and begin digesting its contents without coming into contact with other essential cellular structures (Fig. 4.9d). This way the cell uses the lysosome's powerful enzymes to digest foreign material or debris without causing its own destruction. The digested contents of the phagolysosome are expelled from the cell as free protein (not part of a structure).

RECURRING AND CHRONIC INFLAMMATION

The phrase *chronic inflammation* is sometimes confusing because it is used to describe events after two very different processes: recurring acute inflammation and microtrauma. **Recurring inflammation** refers to reinitiated acute inflammation before the previous episode of acute inflammation has finished. This occurs when a patient be-

comes overly aggressive and returns to vigorous activity too quickly. Each time acute inflammation is reinitiated before the previous episode is completed, it takes less of an insult to begin the inflammatory response again. An insult that normally would not cause an injury can perpetuate recurring inflammation. Avoid using the term *chronic inflammation* to refer to recurring acute inflammation.

Chronic inflammation begins in a slow, often unnoticed manner; it tends to persist for several weeks, months, or years and has a vague and indefinite termination. It occurs when the inflammatory response is unable to eliminate the cause of the injury (such as with repeated overuse) and restore normal function.[1] The specific mechanisms, however, that cause this condition to become chronic are not known.[2] Macrophages proliferate and release chemical mediators that attract additional macrophages. As more macrophages accumulate, it takes less stress or overuse to keep the process going. Thus activity that normally is nontraumatic becomes a traumatic inflammatory stimulus.

The suffix *-itis* designates conditions with chronic inflammation, such as bursitis (inflammation of the bursae) and tendinitis (inflammation of the tendons). Although these conditions result from microtrauma, not all of them involve an inflammatory response.[14] Cases of clinically diagnosed Achilles tendinitis[14,15] and patellar tendinitis have been reported in which there was no evidence of inflammation. One explanation is that microtrauma can cause significant structural disruption; and microvascular damage can occur, causing pain and other clinical symptoms, before the classic inflammatory response is activated.[2]

An Orthopedic Injury Model

What happens when a muscle is pulled or an ankle is sprained? Although it is correct to answer that the injury evokes the inflammatory response, such a view is somewhat simplistic. Furthermore, an overly simplistic approach is to apply ice to every injury without understanding the inflammatory process. Technique must be based on sound theory if it is to be developed and improved. Before discussing the use of ice, we present a model for understanding the body's response to injury in detail.

 CRITICAL THINKING 4.1 *What is a model, and why are models useful?*

The generalized model presented here describes the processes that occur after an acute trauma. This injury model includes an area of tissue composed of cells, blood vessels, and nerves. Figure 4.10 shows the normal prein-

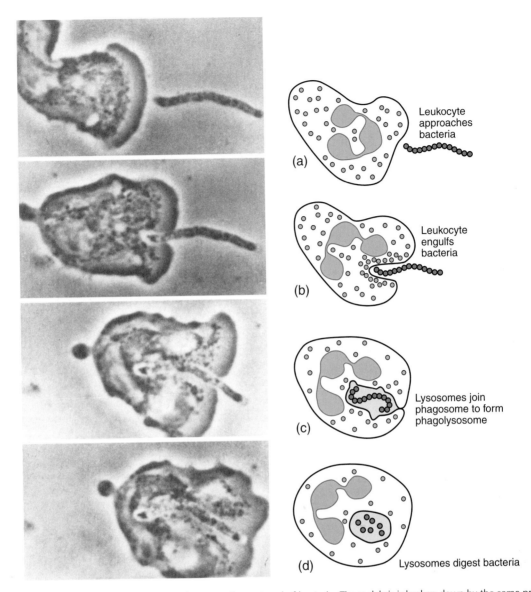

FIGURE 4.9. Phagocytosis. A human neutrophil is phagocytosing a strand of bacteria. Tissue debris is broken down by the same process. (Adapted from Ryan and Majno;[13] used with permission from Pfizer Inc.)

jury tissue. When an injury occurs, whether it's a sprain or strain caused by a stretching force or a contusion caused by direct compression, immediate ultrastructural changes take place in the muscle and/or connective tissue. Figure 4.11 shows the result of the primary injury on the normal tissue. Nerves and blood vessels might be broken at this time as well. All this damage was directly caused by the traumatic force. The damaged tissue becomes debris, which will be removed from the area before new cells can replace the damaged ones.

The cellular debris releases chemical mediators that signal the body that an injury has occurred. The torn nerves send impulses to the brain that are interpreted as pain. Extravascular hemorrhage results from the broken blood vessels (Fig. 4.12). Swelling occurs from the blood

that flows into the extravascular spaces. This hemorrhaging (bleeding) and swelling are usually short lived, however, owing to the clotting mechanism.

Clotting is a multistage process that results in *fibrin* and *platelets*, both of which are blood components, closing a damaged blood vessel.[16] The fibrin forms into strands, which in turn create a network. The fibrin net captures circulating platelets, resulting in a plug that seals the damaged vessel, sometimes completely blocking circulation (Fig. 4.13).

The hemorrhaged blood and cellular debris from the primary injury are collectively known as a **hematoma**. As the hematoma forms, it exerts pressure on undamaged nerve fibers in the area, causing more pain. In addition to outward responses to pain, such as discomfort and nausea,

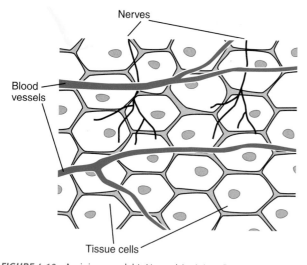

FIGURE 4.10. An injury model I: Normal (uninjured) tissue cells, blood vessels, and nerves.

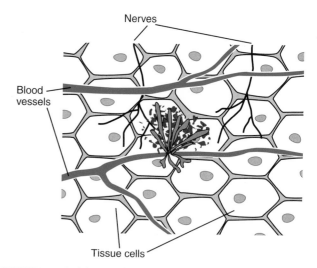

FIGURE 4.12. An injury model III: Hemorrhaging from a ruptured blood vessel into the tissue.

the body responds internally with muscle spasm and inhibition of muscular strength and range of motion. These responses are the body's effort to protect itself by splinting the area, thereby preventing aggravation of the injury.

The body's response to the hematoma is to remove it, and it does so through four of the last five inflammatory events: hemodynamic changes, permeability changes, leukocyte migration, and phagocytosis. These mechanisms take place in the circulatory vessels on the periphery of the injury. Lysosomes in the tissue break down the hematoma, and the resulting pieces of free protein are removed from the area by the lymphatic system. Once the hematoma is resolved, wound healing (repair) can take place (see Chapter 6).

The effects of the inflammatory response are not all positive, however. The combination of slowed blood flow in the vessels on the injury's periphery and a lack of blood flow in the damaged vasculature results in less oxygen delivered to cells near the primary injury. If the inflammatory response is prolonged, metabolic changes will occur in these cells, and they will undergo secondary metabolic injury. Thus the total amount of damaged tissue is increased, and more debris accumulates in the hematoma.

Secondary Injury

The body's response to the traumatized tissue (primary injury) leads to further tissue damage, known as **secondary injury.**[17–20] Many viable cells in the immediate area of, but not damaged by, the primary injury undergo secondary injury as a result of two separate mechanisms: enzymatic action and metabolic deficiency.

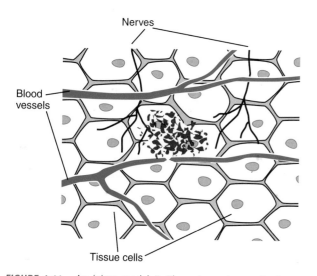

FIGURE 4.11. An injury model II: The primary traumatic damage. Trauma, such as a contusion, causes ultrastructural changes to tissue cells, blood vessels, and nerves. All tissues damaged by the trauma have suffered primary injury. Damage to nerves causes pain.

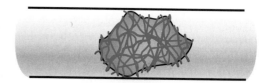

FIGURE 4.13. An injury model IV: Clotting. Strands of fibrin begin forming immediately after the injury to form a fishnet over the damaged vessel. This will later entrap platelets, sealing the lesion, which also plugs the entire vessel.

SECONDARY ENZYMATIC INJURY

When a cell dies (owing to primary injury), its lysosomes release enzymes that digest cellular debris.[2] If these enzymes come into contact with nearby live cells, they start breaking down the membranes of the live cells, leading to additional cellular death; this is known as **secondary enzymatic injury.**[18–20]

A possible second cause of enzymatic injury is the excessive presence and activity of neutrophils.[20] This is speculation, based on the facts that there are many neutrophils in injured tissue and that they have a tendency to cause collateral damage to adjacent healthy cells in response to microorganisms.[8,9] The uncertainty of this theory is twofold:

- We don't know the magnitude of regulatory mechanisms that reduce or prevent the neutrophils from damaging healthy cells.[9,10,12]
- Orthopedic injuries, such as sprains, strains, and contusions, do not involve microorganisms, and the response of neutrophils may be different. Most of our knowledge of the inflammatory response comes from research involving injury caused by substances that remain in the tissue.[21] With trauma, once the primary injury occurs, the cause of the injury is gone.

SECONDARY METABOLIC INJURY

Secondary metabolic injury is caused by three physiological challenges resulting from prolonged local **ischemia**, a deficit of blood to the area. The combination of blood vessel damage by the primary injury and a circulatory slowdown induced by the inflammatory response result in localized ischemia. Ischemia results in hypoxia, inadequate fuel delivery (glucose, fatty acids, etc.), and inadequate waste removal.[22]

All three challenges lead to a deficiency in ATP production:

- Hypoxia results in cells' switching to anaerobic metabolism.
- Aerobic metabolism is cut short because the cellular supply of glucose is limited as a result of reduced blood circulation.
- Aerobic metabolism is further reduced because it is inhibited by waste products such as lactic acid, which are normally removed by the circulation.

In areas where metabolic deficiency is severe enough and long enough, cells die (Fig. 4.14). The resulting debris is added to the hematoma, and the total amount of damaged tissue is increased (Fig. 4.15). A summary of the inflammatory response is presented in Figure 4.16.

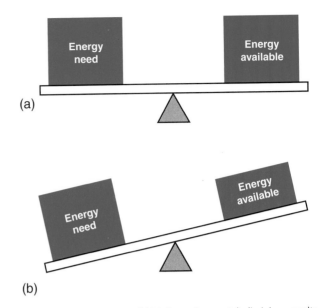

FIGURE 4.14. An injury model V: Secondary metabolic injury results from an imbalance of energy supply and energy consumption in uninjured cells. **(a)** Normal tissue. **(b)** Injured tissue.

MODALITY MYTH

SECONDARY INJURY IS SECONDARY HYPOXIC INJURY

In 1976, the concept of secondary injury was introduced as secondary hypoxic injury to describe tissue damage resulting from a metabolic imbalance resulting from acute traumatic sports injuries.[17] In time, however, it became obvious that there was an enzymatic component to secondary injury[18,19] and that ischemia caused more than just hypoxic challenges to reduced metabolism (as explained in the text).[20] The more inclusive term *secondary metabolic injury* should be used instead of the original term *secondary hypoxic injury*.

Swelling: Hemorrhaging and Edema

Swelling is an increase in tissue volume owing to extra fluid and cellular material in the tissue. Swelling has two sources: direct hemorrhaging into traumatized tissues and edema formation.[23] Initial swelling results from hemorrhaging, and swelling that occurs hours after the injury is from edema.

Whenever blood vessel walls are damaged from an injury, **hemorrhaging** (bleeding) occurs and continues as long as the vessel walls remain open (see Fig. 4.12). Under normal circumstances, clotting begins within 3–5

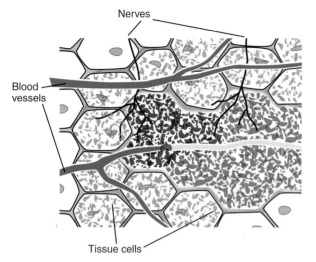

FIGURE 4.15. An injury model V:. A hematoma expands as cellular debris from the secondary injury is added to the debris of the primary injury and hemorrhaging. As the inflammatory process breaks down the cellular debris into free protein, additional secondary injury occurs (see cells at far right).

min after the injury occurs,[24,25] thus sealing the vessel walls and stopping the hemorrhaging.

EDEMA FORMATION

Edema is the accumulation of the fluid portion of blood in the tissues.[26] To understand how edema occurs, it is necessary to first understand normal **fluid dynamics**—the movement of fluid back and forth between capillaries and normal uninjured tissue. If this balanced movement of fluid is upset so that more fluid flows into the tissue than is reabsorbed, the excess fluid is called edema. Thus edema is simply the result of a normal process that is slightly out of balance. The longer it is out of balance, the greater the fluid accumulation and the greater the swelling.

NORMAL FLUID EXCHANGE

In normal tissue, fluid constantly passes between the circulatory system and the extracellular spaces.[7,27] Normally, the fluid that moves out of the capillaries is reabsorbed by the body (Fig. 4.17). The vascular system reabsorbs two-thirds of the fluid directly into the venous end of the capillaries; the lymph vessels reabsorb the remaining third and empties it into the venous system.[28] This fluid movement is caused by differences in fluid pressure between the capillary and the tissue. Edema results when the pressures are upset so that more fluid moves out of the capillary than is reabsorbed.

Two factors make the free movement of fluid possible. First, water molecules diffuse through the capillary walls 80 times more rapidly than blood flows along the capillary.[7] Second, there is a pressure difference between the inside and the outside of the vessels. Known as **capillary filtration pressure**, it is measured as the mathematical

sum of a number of forces known as **Starling forces**.[27] Four components influence filtration pressure according to the following equation:

$$\text{Capillary filtration pressure} = (\text{CHP} + \text{TOP}) - (\text{THP} + \text{COP})$$

where, CHP = capillary hydrostatic pressure; TOP = tissue oncotic pressure; COP = capillary oncotic pressure; THP = tissue hydrostatic pressure.

Hydrostatic pressure is pressure exerted by a column of water; the higher the column of water, the greater the pressure. Swimming provides a practical example of hydrostatic pressure. The deeper you go, the higher the column of water is above you, and the greater the pressure. It is the depth of the water, not the amount of water, that is important. For example, a person 6 ft under water in a swimming pool will experience the same hydrostatic pressure as a person 6 ft under water in the ocean. Hydrostatic pressure is exerted by the water in the blood.

Hydrostatic pressure pushes water. Therefore, **capillary hydrostatic pressure (CHP)** forces fluid out of the capillary and **tissue hydrostatic pressure (THP)** forces fluid back into the capillary.

Oncotic pressure, also called *colloid osmotic pressure*, is pressure resulting from the attraction of fluid by free protein. (It is the similar to osmotic pressure in plants.) Thus **tissue oncotic pressure (TOP)** tends to pull fluid out of the capillary, and **capillary oncotic pressure (COP)** tends to pull fluid back into the capillary.

The net sum of these forces determines which way the fluid travels. At the arteriolar end of the capillary, CHP dominates, and the capillary filtration pressure is positive,[7,27] causing fluid to move out of the capillary and into the tissue. Toward the venular end of the capillary, the pressures that cause fluid to move out decrease and those that cause reabsorption increase; therefore, fluid moves back into the capillary. For instance, CHP averages 23 mm Hg throughout the length of the capillary, but it is much higher at the arteriolar end and much lower at the venular end. If all of the pressures along the length of the capillary are summed and averaged, the net (or overall) average capillary filtration pressure is slightly positive. This explains why one-third of the fluid is not reabsorbed directly into the blood vessel—that which is removed from the area via the lymphatic system. Table 4.1 summarizes capillary filtration pressure components and their effect on fluid exchange between capillaries and tissues.

FLUID EXCHANGE IN INJURED TISSUE

After an acute injury, there are alterations in fluid exchange, and more fluid leaves the circulatory system than is reabsorbed. This fluid accumulates in the tissue, causing edema, and the tissue swells. The driving force of edema accumulation is a change in capillary filtration pressure.

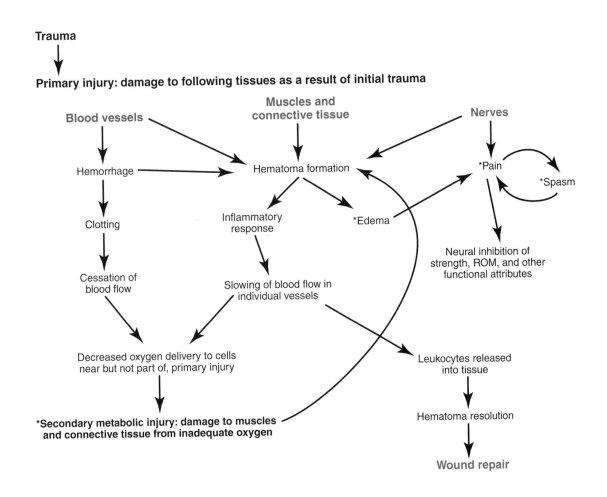

FIGURE 4.16. A summary of the inflammatory response to acute trauma. *, phases of the response that benefit by cold application to the injury; *ROM*, range of motion. See text for details (see also Chapter 5).

Changes in Capillary Filtration Pressure After Injury

With injury there is a change in the average capillary filtration pressure, caused by an increase in TOP.[26] The changes in capillary filtration pressure after an injury are presented in Table 4.2 and Figure 4.18. Because TOP pulls fluid into the tissue, edema and swelling result. Tissue oncotic pressure increases because of increased free protein. As a part of the inflammatory response, tissue debris from primary injury, secondary metabolic injury, and hemorrhaged whole blood is broken down into free protein by macrophages. In addition, some free protein escapes from the circulatory system during the period of hemorrhaging (if a vessel was damaged) or as a result of the increased permeability. The increased tissue free protein upsets the capillary filtration balance, and fluid (edema) builds up in the tissue (Fig. 4.19). The greater the injury, the greater the amount of free protein and eventually edema.

CRITICAL THINKING 4.2 *Because the source of most swelling is excess free protein in the tissue, what must happen to remove the swelling? What effect, if any, does ice have on swelling once it has occurred?*

This process accounts for the delayed nature of most incidences of swelling after acute injury. Both secondary injury and the breakdown of tissue debris by macrophages occur over an extended period of time. Edema, therefore, begins minutes to hours after the injury and continues to develop over many hours. The swelling that occurs immediately after the injury is caused directly by hemorrhaging.

Secondary injury results in increased edema, and increased edema can contribute to increased secondary metabolic injury. Two mechanisms are involved. First, as

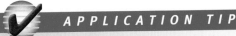

APPLICATION TIP

*USE A COMPRESSION WRAP FOR AN ACUTE INJURY.
Always apply a compression wrap for the first day or so after acute injury, even if the injury appears minor and there is no swelling. Swelling is often delayed. Once it occurs, you cannot turn back the clock. And there is no harm in wearing a compression bandage overnight in situations in which swelling would not occur. It is better to be safe than sorry.*

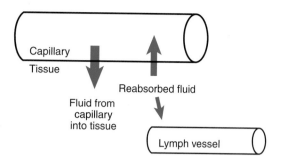

FIGURE 4.17. Normal fluid exchange. Fluid moves constantly between the circulatory system and the body tissue. See text for details.

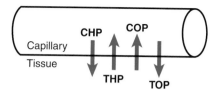

FIGURE 4.18. The influence of the four Starling forces on fluid movement between the capillary and tissue. *Arrows,* the direction of fluid movement (the labels indicate the action). Hydrostatic forces (capillary hydrostatic pressure [*CHP*] and tissue hydrostatic pressure [*THP*]) push fluids, whereas oncotic pressures (capillary oncotic pressure [*COP*] and tissue oncotic pressure [*TOP*]) attract fluid.

edema develops, the distance between the blood vessel and the tissue cells increases, making it harder for oxygen and other nutrients to diffuse from the circulatory system to the target tissue. Second, edema fluid can compress the blood vessel, reducing circulation to the area.

If swelling is from edema, why does the area turn black and blue? Although some discoloration results from oxidized blood, much of the discoloration in muscle may be the result of oxidized **myoglobin**, an oxygen-transporting and storage protein in muscle cells, from damaged musculature.

THE EFFECT OF COLD ON SWELLING

Cold packs are usually applied after clotting has occurred and, therefore, have no effect on hemorrhaging. Once edema has developed, cold applications cannot decrease it. But cold can limit or reduce edema development, if applied soon after the injury. As cold decreases secondary metabolic injury, the amount of free protein in the tissues will be decreased. Thus there will be less tissue oncotic pressure (the major factor for edema). This is covered in more detail in Chapter 5.

REDUCING SECONDARY INJURY AND EDEMA WITH RICES

Both secondary injury and edema can be reduced if appropriate comprehensive measures are initiated quickly after the injury–within minutes, not hours or days. Although cold is the cornerstone of this treatment, it is only part of the necessary therapy. Appropriate immediate care con-

sists of rest, ice (cold), compression, elevation, and stabilization (RICES). Each of these measures is discussed in detail in Chapter 5, including both the theoretical background and the step-by-step application.

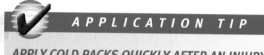

APPLICATION TIP

APPLY COLD PACKS QUICKLY AFTER AN INJURY. The faster you apply the ice, the sooner metabolism will slow down. Thus you protect more tissue from secondary metabolic injury and have less total tissue damage. Do not, however, forgo a thorough evaluation of the injury in order to apply an ice pack.[5] This is the golden period for evaluation: the time when you will be able to gain the most information about the injury.

After injury, the body attempts to protect the injured area by **muscle guarding**, an involuntary process of splinting the injury by inducing a low-grade **muscle spasm** of antagonistic muscle groups. The effectiveness of injury evaluation decreases dramatically once muscle guarding has set in.

MODALITY MYTH

ICE IS USED TO REDUCE INFLAMMATION

Many people think the purpose of ice is to decrease inflammation. But inflammation is necessary to prepare the body for healing. Healing cannot take place until much of the cellular debris is removed from the area. So decreasing inflammation is not helpful. This misconception is the result of confusing inflammation with swelling. The purpose of ice is to minimize swelling. The less swelling, the quicker the injury can be healed (see Chapter 5).

Another misconception concerning ice is that it should be used until the swelling is gone. Ice is effective for preventing swelling (i.e., during the 12–24 hr after injury) but not for removing swelling. Swelling reduction occurs as free protein is removed from the area.

TABLE 4.1	*Normal Capillary Filtration Pressure*
CAPILLARY FILTRATION PRESSURE COMPONENT	**NORMAL AVERAGE PRESSURE (MM HG)***
Capillary hydrostatic	+23
Tissue oncotic	+10
Tissue hydrostatic	−1 to 4
Capillary oncotic	−25
*Net (overall)**	−4 to 7

*If pressure is positive, fluid moves from the capillary into the tissue. If pressure is negative, it moves from the tissue into the capillary.

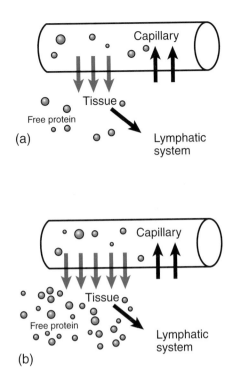

FIGURE 4.19. **(a)** Normal fluid movement. Two-thirds of the fluid exiting the capillary is reabsorbed into the capillary; the other third returns to the circulation via the lymphatic system. **(b)** Edema results when more fluid moves out of the capillary than is reabsorbed, owing to the progressive buildup of excess free protein during hemorrhaging and phagocytosis.

TABLE 4.2	*Changes in Capillary Filtration Pressure Components After Injury*	
CAPILLARY FILTRATION PRESSURE COMPONENT	**NORMAL AVERAGE PRESSURE (MM HG)***	**CHANGE IN PRESSURE OWING TO INJURY**
Capillary hydrostatic	+23	↑
Tissue oncotic	+10	↑
Tissue hydrostatic	−1 to 4	↑
Capillary oncotic	−25	↑
Net (overall)*	−4 to 7	↑

*If pressure is positive, fluid moves from the capillary into the tissue. If pressure is negative, it moves from the tissue into the capillary.

CLOSING SCENE

You now understand that Rachel's actions in treating the injured basketball player were both appropriate and necessary. Inflammation is the body's response to any injury. Its purpose is to protect the body against invasion by foreign bodies and to prepare the injured tissue for repair. The ice pack Rachel put on the patient's injured ankle did nothing for the primary injury, but it did minimize the secondary injury by decreasing both enzymatic and metabolic changes in the tissue. Some swelling resulted from hemorrhaging, although the bleeding was stopped quickly by clotting. Some additional swelling occurred from an increase in free protein and oncotic pressure in the tissue. Much more swelling would have occurred if Rachel had not acted quickly to apply ice, compression, and elevation.

CHAPTER REFLECTIONS

1. Read and ponder each of the following points. Do you feel you have a clear understanding of each concept? If not, reread the appropriate section of the chapter.
   • Describe the inflammatory response, its purpose, its cardinal signs, and the eight inflammatory events. Relate each one to a typical orthopedic injury.
   • Define trauma and its relationship to physical force.
   • Differentiate between macrotrauma and microtrauma.
   • Define metabolic changes, ischemia, and hypoxia. What is their relationship to secondary injury?
   • Explain the function of the sodium pump and its role in inflammation.
   • What is chronic inflammation?
   • Differentiate between primary and secondary injury. What are their causes? How should you manage each one?
   • Explain phagocytosis and the role of neutrophils and macrophages in this process.
   • Explain the common misconceptions about recurring acute inflammation.
   • Define swelling, and differentiate between hemorrhaging and edema.
   • What is capillary filtration pressure? Explain the forces that contribute to capillary filtration pressure and how they are altered after acute orthopedic injury.
   • Describe the difference between preventing and removing swelling. Explain the role of cold in the two processes.
2. Write three to five questions for discussion with your class instructor, clinical instructor, classmates, and clinical colleagues.
3. Get together with classmates and quiz each other on the concepts of this chapter. Use the points in exercise 1 and questions you wrote for exercise 2 as a beginning. Explaining concepts out loud to others requires a deeper grasp of the material than feeling you understand it as you read.

CRITICAL THINKING RESPONSE

Critical Thinking 4.1

A model is a description or an analogy that helps demonstrate or visualize something (such as an atom) that cannot be directly observed; it can also be a simplified description of a complex entity or process. The orthopedic injury model presented in this chapter fits both descriptions because the response to orthopedic injury cannot be directly observed; the physiological and pathological processes are far beyond the scope of this text. By presenting this complex process as a model, we give you a general idea of what happens after an orthopedic injury, so you can understand why and how ice is used to treat injuries.

Critical Thinking 4.2

To reduce or remove swelling, you must remove its source, the free protein. If the fluid is removed without removing the excess free protein, it will just form again. Ice has no effect on removing the free protein; free protein must be removed by stimulating the lymphatic system.

REFERENCES

1. Ferkel RD, Karzel RP, Del Pizzo W, et al. Arthroscopic treatment of anterolateral impingement of the ankle. Am J Sports Med 1991;19:440–446.
2. Leadbetter WB. An introduction to sports-induced soft-tissue inflammation. In: Leadbetter WB, Buckwalter JA, Gordon SL, eds. Sports-Induced Inflammation. Chicago: American Academy of Orthopaedic Surgeons, 1990.
3. Anderson MK, Hall SJ, Martin M. Foundations of Athletic Training. 3rd ed. Baltimore: Lippincott Williams, & Wilkins, 2004.
4. Prentice WE. Arnheim's Principles of Athletic Training. 12th ed. St. Louis: McGraw-Hill, 2006.
5. Fisher BD, Baracos VE, Shnitka TK, et al. Ultrastructural events following acute muscle trauma. Med Sci Sports Exerc 1990;22:185–193.
6. McLeod I. Inflammation. Kalamazoo, MI: Upjohn, 1973.
7. Guyton AC, Hall JE. Textbook of Medical Physiology. 11th ed. Philadelphia: Saunders, 2006.
8. Jones P. Neutrophil. Available at: www.mult-sclerosis.org/neutrophil.html. Accessed January 2006.
9. Mathison RD, Befus AD, Davison JS, Woodman RC. Modulation of neutrophil function by the tripeptide feG. BMC Immunol 2003;4:3.
10. Nkemdirim M, Kubera M, Mathison R. Modulation of neutrophil activity by submandibular gland peptide-T (SGP-T). Pol J Pharmacol 1998;50:417–424.

11. Fujishima S, Aikawa N. Neutrophil-mediated tissue injury and its modulation. Intensive Care Med 1995;21:277–285.
12. Fialho de Araujo A, Oliveira-Filho R, Trezena A, et al. Role of submandibular salivary glands in LPS-induced lung inflammation in rats. Neuroimmunomodulation 2002–2003;10:73–79.
13. Ryan G, Majno G. Inflammation. Kalamazoo, MI: Upjohn, 1977.
14. Clancy WGJ. Tendinitis and plantar fasciitis in runners. In: D'Ambrosia R, Drez DJ, eds. Prevention and Treatment of Running Injuries. Thorofare, NJ: Slack, 1982.
15. Osterman AL, Heppenstall RB, Sapega AA, et al. Muscle ischemia and hypothermia: A bioenergetic study using ^{31}phosphorus nuclear magnetic resonance spectroscopy. J Trauma 1984;24:811–817.
16. Rote N. Inflammation. In: McCance K, Huether S, eds. Pathophysiology: The Biologic Basis for Disease in Adults and Children. 4th ed. St. Louis: Mosby-Elsevier, 2002:197–226.
17. Knight KL. The effects of hypothermia on inflammation and swelling. Athl Train 1976;11:7–10.
18. Knight KL. Cryotherapy in Sport Injury Management. Champaign, IL: Human Kinetics, 1995.
19. Merrick MA, Rankin JM, Andres FA, Hinman CL. A preliminary examination of cryotherapy and secondary injury in skeletal muscle. Med Sci Sports Exerc 1999;31:1516–1521.
20. Merrick MA. Secondary injury after musculoskeletal trauma: A review and update. J Athl Train 2002;37:209–217.
21. Jutte L. The Effects of Acute Blunt Trauma Muscle Injury and local Cryotherapy on Local TNF-a and IL-10 Concentrations. Provo, UT: Exercise Sciences, Brigham Young University, 2005.
22. Majno G, Joris I. Cells, Tissues, and Disease: Principles of General Pathology. 2nd ed. New York: Oxford University Press, 2004.
23. Weisman GB, ed. Mediators of Inflammation. New York: Plenum, 1974.
24. Johnson MG. Potential role of the lymphatic vessel in regulating inflammatory events. Surv Synth Path Res 1983;1:111–119.
25. Mutschler TA, D'Antonio JA, Ferguson GM, et al. Cold therapy reduces blood loss after primary TKA; but pain and swelling are unaffected. Orthop Today 1993;16.
26. Huether S. The cellular environment: Fluids and electrolytes, acids and bases. In: McCance K, Huether S, eds. Pathophysiology: The Biologic Basis for Disease in Adults and Children. 4th ed. St. Louis: Mosby-Elsevier, 2002.
27. Porth CM. Pathophysiology. 7th ed. Baltimore: Lippincott Williams & Wilkins, 2004.
28. Kaempffe FA. Skin surface temperature reduction after cryotherapy to a casted extremity. J Orthop Sports Phys Ther 1989;10:448–450.

5

Immediate Care of Acute Orthopedic Injuries

During a first-aid class, the instructor told Sammy that ice is applied almost universally after sprains, strains, cuts, and bruises. This agreed with what Sammy had observed in an athletic training clinic, and it got him thinking. He realized he had many questions regarding ice: Does it matter when you apply ice after an injury? Does it matter what kind of ice you use? Is it okay to apply an ice pack directly to the skin, or should there be a towel between the skin and the ice bag? How long should ice be applied? Is ice used to reduce swelling or pain or both? Is immediate care just about ice? What about compression, elevation, and rest? During a break, Sammy asked his questions but was disappointed with many of the instructor's answers. "How could such a basic, simple modality be so confusing?" he wondered.

RICES: The Prescription for Immediate Care

In Chapter 4 we discussed the inflammatory response, a series of physiological and pathological changes that occur after an injury. Some of these changes are necessary prerequisites to healing; without them, healing would not occur (see Chapter 6). But some of the changes can lead to further injury and complications that extend the recovery period. Immediate care techniques are designed to limit the unwanted changes, while allowing the necessary changes to occur and thereby facilitate healing and repair.

When applied properly, rest, ice, compression, elevation, and stabilization—known as **RICES**—limit secondary injury, swelling, muscle spasm, pain, and neural inhibition (Fig. 5.1). These efforts result in quicker healing of the injury and thus reduced disability time. Although there seems to be no doubt about using RICES, there is confusion about the pathophysiological response to, and specific protocols for using, these modalities.

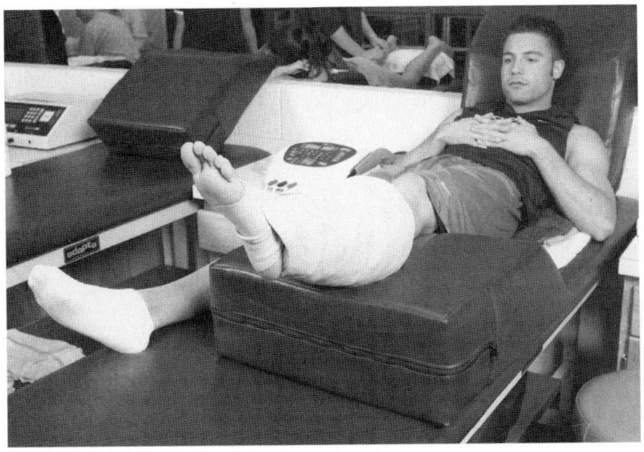

FIGURE 5.1. The immediate care of all acute injuries includes RICES: rest, ice, compression, elevation, and stabilization.

MODALITY MYTH

IMMEDIATE CARE

The following are modality myths about the immediate care of orthopedic injuries:

- Acute care and immediate care are the same.
- Ice decreases swelling.
- The goal of immediate care is to decrease inflammation.
- The purpose of ice is to decrease hemorrhaging.
- Inflammation and swelling are the same.
- Ice should be applied for 20 min during immediate care.
- All injuries should be treated for the same amount of time.

Each of these will be discussed in this chapter.

IMMEDIATE CARE VS. ACUTE CARE

Injuries are usually classified as acute or chronic. **Acute injuries** are of sudden onset, are caused by high-intensity forces, and are of short duration—for example, sprains, strains, and contusions. There are two types of **chronic injuries**: those caused by low-intensity forces of long duration, as in tendinitis and bursitis, and those that are recurring acute injuries, such as a chronic sprained ankle.

The care of acute (and recurring acute) injuries is often divided into three stages: acute (0–4 days), subacute (5–14 days), and postacute (after 14 days). Although this classification is used extensively, there are three problems with it:

- It does not incorporate the concepts of immediate care and emergency care.

- Acute care spans too wide a range of treatments. Treatment given 10 min after the injury is much different from treatment given 3 days after the injury. Acute care therefore must be subdivided.
- Injuries heal at different rates, depending on the type and severity of the injury and the individual patient. Care must be dictated by patient progress, not by specific time frames.

Stages of Acute Injury Care

We suggest the following classification of acute injury care. The general time frames should be considered as points of reference only to help in discussing specific techniques. Actual patient care should be based on patient needs and progress, not on these general time frames.

1. **Acute care**: 0–4 days
   - **Emergency care**: such as cardiopulmonary resuscitation (CPR) or transportation to a hospital, if needed
   - **Immediate care**: 0–12 hr
   - **Transition care**: 12 hr to 4 days
2. **Subacute care**: 4–14 days. An injury in this stage is moving beyond acute but is still "somewhat" or "bordering on" acute.
3. **Postacute care**: after 14 days

ICE, RICE, OR RICES?

The acronym ICE was developed to communicate the combined use of ice, compression, and elevation for treating acute injuries. Most clinicians use RICE because part of the standard practice is for the patient to refrain from activity or to *rest* the injured part. PRICE is used by some because it emphasizes the need to *protect* the injury from further damage. We prefer to use RICES because *stabilizing*, or splinting, the injury lessens pain and neural inhibition in addition to protecting the injury.

RICES is applied to protect the injury from further damage and to decrease or minimize the development of:

- Swelling
- Pain
- Muscle spasm
- Neural inhibition
- Secondary injury

And thus:

- Total injury

What about inflammation? *No!* Review Chapter 4.

Each of the listed elements is important. The majority of professional and public attention, however, has been on controlling swelling through cold application. This is somewhat shortsighted, as we will reveal throughout this chapter.

EVIDENCE FOR THE EFFECTIVENESS OF RICES

Most sports medicine clinicians feel that RICES used immediately postinjury (begun within the first 10–20 min) will control swelling and other negative **sequelae**, or aftereffects, of acute musculoskeletal injuries. Not all agree with this opinion, however. Those who disagree generally cite research in which cold was applied incorrectly.[1,2] Their conclusions should have been that *improperly applied* cold is ineffective, not that cold is ineffective. Others disagree because there is not enough clinical evidence.[3,4]

The few clinical studies on RICES support the effectiveness of the treatment.[5,6] The studies involve hospital patients, so treatment was not initiated as early as typically occurs in athletics. Had treatment been initiated earlier, the results probably would have been even more impressive.

One reason for the lack of clinical studies is that athletic trainers are so convinced of the efficacy of RICES that they cannot in good conscience withhold treatment from athletes who would be assigned to a control group. Athletic trainers have seen the consequences of enough cases of athletes who were not treated properly (because the injury occurred away from campus) to know RICES is necessary. In addition, studies based on patients treated in hospitals and physician's offices do not help because RICES is not applied quickly enough after the injury to be considered immediate care.

TYPES OF INJURIES FOR USING RICES

All acute musculoskeletal injuries should be treated with RICES. In all cases of tissue damage, there is the potential of secondary injury. Failure to treat with RICES will result in greater soft tissue damage and thus delay the final resolution of the injury.

Some authorities advocate RICES for sprains and dislocations, but only ice packs for strains.[7] There is no logic to this recommendation. All acute orthopedic injuries should be treated with RICES.[8]

The Theoretical Basis for RICES

Each element of RICES contributes to the effectiveness of the treatment. None of the elements should be left out. Understanding how the body responds to each element will help you maximize the use of RICES.

REST LIMITS INJURY AGGRAVATION

Rest during immediate care means moving the injured limb as little as possible. The goal is to not aggravate damaged tissue, which could cause further injury[9] and pain, thereby contributing to the pain–spasm–pain cycle. Some define rest during immediate care as "relative rest," meaning decreased activity rather than inactivity.[10] This philosophy is the result of an inadequate definition of immediate care—that is, the idea that immediate care lasts 4–5 days. According to the stages of acute injury care outlined earlier, during immediate care patients should be as inactive as possible. During transition care, patients transition to relative rest, which means protecting the injury but using the rest of the body to prevent deconditioning.

The problem of pain after an injury is not only about the discomfort but about the body's response to the pain. Pain causes the body to shut things down in an attempt to protect itself. It does so by a process called **neural inhibition**, a decrease or absence of normal neuromuscular functions such as strength and range of motion and thus an inhibition of most activity. Often these neural inhibitions continue long after the injury itself has healed,[1] thereby preventing the patient from a full return to normal activity. Resting immediately after an injury (keeping activity below the level where it causes pain) reduces the complications of neural inhibition.

APPLICATION TIP

AVOID PAIN LIKE THE PLAGUE. Two rules of thumb for rehabilitation are "If it hurts, don't do it" and "Work up to the level of pain, but don't go beyond it." The concept of "No pain, no gain" is OK during conditioning exercises but totally wrong during rehabilitation. Pain causes neural inhibition, which prolongs rehabilitation (see Chapter 8). It's not a question of how tough a patient is but how smart he is. Tell the patient to work around the pain, not force his way through it.

The primary rationale for a patient using crutches after a lower-extremity injury is to remove pain. Limping results from pain. Even though a patient may think she can hobble along, doing so invokes pain, which invokes neuromuscular inhibition. The patient should always use crutches until she can walk with a normal gait.

Too little activity may be as detrimental as too much activity. Too little activity results in:

- Delayed healing
- Adhesions
- Muscular atrophy
- Loss of conditioning
- Skills becoming rusty
- Loss of confidence

You must keep your patients as active as possible without causing further problems. Usually this means exercising noninvolved body parts to the maximum and exercising the involved body part to a level just under that which causes pain.

CRITICAL THINKING 5.1 *Why is a three-point gait (walking on both legs, but using the crutches to support the injured leg) more effective than a swing gait (no pressure on the injured leg, it just swings) for a patient who is using crutches 3 days after a moderate ankle sprain?*

ICE LIMITS SECONDARY INJURY

Many think controlling swelling is a major goal of immediate care. Controlling swelling is important, but it is only part of immediate care. Limiting secondary injury and neural inhibition are more important than controlling swelling.

As explained in Chapter 4, swelling is an increase in tissue volume owing to extra fluid and cellular material in the tissue. It results from direct hemorrhaging into traumatized tissues and edema formation. Edema forms when fluid accumulates in the extracellular spaces because of a disruption in the normal fluid exchange between the vascular system and the extracellular spaces; more fluid moves out of the circulatory system than moves back into it. Thus fluid accumulates in the tissues. Cold applications are commonly used to treat swelling.

There are two major theories for why **cryotherapy**, the therapeutic use of cold, should be used for the immediate care of orthopedic injuries: the decreased blood flow theory (or the circulatory theory) and the decreased secondary injury theory.

The Decreased Blood Flow Theory

The traditional theory for immediate care is that cold decreases blood flow.[7,11] The logic of the theory is as follows:

- Cold causes vasoconstriction, which
- Decreases blood flow, and therefore
- Decreases hemorrhaging, and therefore
- Swelling is reduced

Cold does cause vasoconstriction and decreased vascular permeability,[12] compression decreases underlying blood flow,[13,14] and elevation reduces blood pressure.[15] However:

- Cold is rarely applied sooner than 5–10 min after injury. It takes 5–10 min to perform even a cursory evaluation of the injury, transport the patient off the court or field, remove equipment, and then apply RICES.

Often a more comprehensive evaluation of the injury is performed on the sidelines, so the time is extended even longer.

- Once the cold is finally applied, it takes 5–30 min (depending on the depth of the injury) to get significant cooling in the target tissue.
- For most injuries, clotting occurs within minutes after the injury.[16] Thus hemorrhaging ceases long before the blood vessels at the injury site are constricted.
- Therefore the beneficial effects of cold on swelling cannot be attributed to decreased circulation.

Despite the illogical basis of the decreased blood flow theory, many still believe it.[7]

The Decreased Secondary Injury Theory

An alternative theory, proposed in 1976[17] and refined in 1995[18] and 2002,[19] is that cryotherapy has little effect on hemorrhaging; rather it limits the amount of secondary injury and edema.[17] The logic of this theory is twofold. First:

- Without cryotherapy, cells within the injured tissue that escaped ultrastructural damage from the trauma (primary injury) and many cells on the periphery of the primary injury suffer secondary metabolic injury because of inadequate blood flow and oxygen.
- Cryotherapy, however, decreases the metabolic needs of these cells so they require less oxygen. They are put into a state of temporary hibernation.
- These cells are therefore more resistant to the ischemic state caused by the compromised circulation.
- The result is less secondary metabolic injury, so
  - Less total injury
  - Less free protein generated by phagocytosis
  - Less edema

Second:

- Damaged cells release chemicals that attack the tissue and uninjured cells in the vicinity, thus causing secondary enzymatic injury.[18]
- Decreased secondary metabolic injury means there are fewer damaged cells to release these chemicals.

The decreased secondary injury theory is modeled in Figure 5.2. Cryotherapy has no effect on primary traumatic injury nor on the hemorrhaging that occurs before clotting. Nothing can be done about primary injury and hemorrhaging once they have occurred. Early applications of cryotherapy decrease the amount of secondary injury, but they do not totally eliminate it.

The major goal of cryotherapy during immediate care is, therefore, to prevent or minimize secondary injury. With less secondary injury, the total injury is decreased so

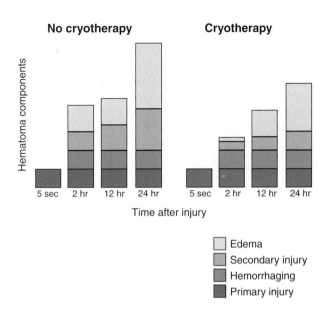

FIGURE 5.2. A model of the effects of immediate cryotherapy on the components of acute orthopedic injury: primary injury, secondary injury, hemorrhaging, and edema. (Adapted with permission from Knight.[17])

there is less damaged tissue to repair. The repair process is much shorter because with less tissue debris to remove, healing begins more quickly. With less total damage, repair runs its course faster.

Cryotherapy and Metabolism

Cryotherapy limits secondary metabolic injury by decreasing tissue metabolism and bringing oxygen demand back into balance with the reduced supply (Fig. 5.3). Damage to blood vessels and the hemodynamic changes of the inflammatory response result in decreased oxygen supply. Cooling reduces cellular energy needs, thereby decreasing the tissue's need for oxygen.[20–23] This same mechanism is used to preserve organs for tissue transplantation; an organ can be removed at one site, packed in a cooler of ice, transported great distances, and safely implanted into another body.[24,25]

There is a direct relationship between tissue temperature and metabolism (Fig. 5.4).[20–22] The greater the cooling, the greater the decrease in metabolism.[*] And the sooner the cold is applied, the more effective it is. Cryotherapy must be applied within minutes after the injury for maximal results.

Heat applications during this period have just the opposite effect. Heat causes an increase in metabolism and therefore increases the oxygen consumption of the tissue. This causes greater secondary metabolic injury and thus more total injury.

---

[*]See Chapter 6 in Knight[18] for more detail.

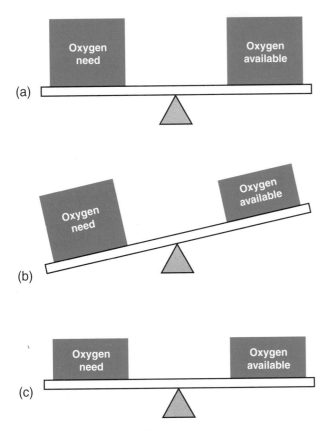

FIGURE 5.3. **(a)** Before injury the oxygen supply and demand were balanced. **(b)** After injury, circulation is decreased and therefore supplies inadequate oxygen to meet the demands. **(c)** Reducing the demand by cooling the tissue reestablishes the balance.

Cryotherapy and Swelling: Decreased Edema, Not Hemorrhage

Cryotherapy reduces edema but has little effect on hemorrhaging. With orthopedic injuries, however, most swelling occurs from edema not hemorrhaging, the exceptions being the immediate "goose egg" and hemarthrosis. A goose egg occurs when a moderate to large vessel near a loose-skinned surface is ruptured. Hemorrhaging occurs immediately into the loose skin, creating a mound of blood. **Hemarthrosis,** the presence of blood in a joint, occurs when the injury involves a joint capsule. Synovial fluid within the capsule prevents total clotting, and blood continues to ooze into the joint.

When Does Edema Occur? When Should Ice Be Applied?

Most edema occurs hours after the injury. The inflammatory process breaks down tissue debris into free protein, which increases tissue oncotic pressure (TOP) and increases capillary filtration pressure (see Chapter 4). Over time, this shift in capillary filtration pressure increases tis-

sue fluid. It is not uncommon for a patient to go to bed a few hours after an acute injury with little swelling and wake up the next morning with significant swelling (edema).

However, it would be misguided to think that the proper time for applying ice is hours after the injury when edema begins forming. The sooner ice is applied—minutes after the injury—the more effective it is.

How Does Ice Decrease Edema?

Cryotherapy cannot decrease TOP, but it can limit the amount of increase by limiting the amount of tissue debris (Table 5.1). This is done in two ways: by decreasing metabolism and by decreasing permeability. Decreased metabolism results in decreased secondary metabolic injury and thus less tissue debris. With less tissue debris, there is less free protein and, therefore, a lower tissue oncotic pressure.

Increased permeability of the blood vessel wall is a necessary part of the normal inflammatory response. In addition to allowing leukocytes to pass through the vessel wall and into the extracellular spaces, permeability lets great amounts of protein-rich fluid escape. This additional protein contributes to increased TOP and increased edema.

Thus cryotherapy, when used immediately after the injury, limits not only the extent of the injury but also the amount of edema that develops as a consequence of the injury. But once secondary injury has occurred, cryotherapy will have no effect on edema or swelling.

COMPRESSION CONTROLS EDEMA

Compression increases pressure outside the capillaries, which, although not a Starling force, decreases capillary filtration pressure and thus helps control edema formation (see Table 5.1). External force pressure—compression—is most beneficial once edema begins occurring and will be effective as long as edema is present. Because it is unknown when edema begins developing, compression should be applied within minutes after the injury and be continued until edema is resolved.

Compression has no effect on normal fluid exchange. An analogy with a balloon will help explain this concept.[18] When the balloon is filled with water, it expands. If the opening of the balloon is not held tightly, the elasticity in the balloon will force the water out. If, however, the balloon is first filled with rocks, the water will occupy spaces between the rocks (Fig. 5.5). As long as just enough water is added to fill the spaces between the rocks, it will not be forced from the balloon—the rocks overcome the balloon's elasticity. Squeezing the balloon (or putting an elastic bandage around it) will similarly have no effect on the water. As more water is added, however,

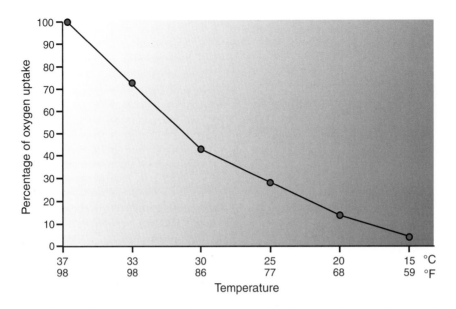

FIGURE 5.4. The relationship between tissue temperature and oxygen consumption. The cooler the tissue, the lower its metabolism. (Adapted with permission from Blair.[21])

and the balloon expands (swells) beyond the rocks, pressure is exerted on the water by the elasticity of the balloon. An elastic bandage around this "swollen" balloon would increase the external force. Also, if the elastic bandage were placed around the balloon before the extra water is added, it would be much harder (i.e., take more force) to add the extra water. The same is true with the human body. An elastic bandage around a normal ankle will have no effect on fluid exchange, but it will tend to retard and/or cause reabsorption of swelling.

While constant compression is essential during immediate care when the goal is to prevent edema, intermittent compression is most effective when the goal is to remove edema (Table 5.2). Intermittent compression stimulates the lymphatic system, which is the route through which tissue debris is removed from the tissue. (Intermittent compression is discussed in more detail later in the chapter.)

Compression also enhances the cooling effect of ice packs, probably by compressing superficial blood vessels and thereby reducing the amount of heat they deliver to the tissue (Fig. 5.6).[14]

ELEVATION CONTROLS EDEMA

Elevation decreases capillary hydrostatic pressure (CHP) and therefore decreases the major factor (in a noninjured state) in forcing fluid out of the capillaries (see Table 5.1). Elevation also decreases tissue hydrostatic pressure (THP), but this has little consequence because THP is small and thus has a minimal effect on fluid filtration.

As discussed in Chapter 4, hydrostatic pressure is caused by the weight of water.[26] The more water above a particular point, the greater the hydrostatic pressure at that point. Capillary hydrostatic pressure is greater when a body part is in a dependent position than when it is elevated because there is more water above.[15,27]

TABLE 5.1	*The Effect of RICES on Capillary Filtration Pressure Components After Acute Injury*				
CAPILLARY FILTRATION PRESSURE COMPONENT	**NORMAL AVERAGE PRESSURE (MM HG)***	**CHANGE IN PRESSURE FROM**			
		Injury	**Ice**	**Compression**	**Elevation**
Capillary hydrostatic	+23				↑
Tissue oncotic	+10	↑	Less ↑		
Tissue hydrostatic	−1 to 4	↑			
Capillary oncotic	−25				
External	0			↓	
Net (overall)†	−4 to 7	↑	↑	↑	↑

**If pressure is positive, fluid moves into the tissue. If pressure is negative, fluid moves out of the tissue.*
†*The net change in pressure owing to the application of ice, compression, and elevation illustrates the additive effect as each one is incorporated into the treatment.*

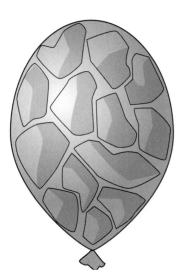

FIGURE 5.5. Rocks in a balloon illustrate how compression on uninjured tissue has no effect on tissue volume. The rocks give the balloon structure (as bones and muscles do for tissue) and therefore prevent it from collapsing under external compression.

STABILIZATION LIMITS NEURAL INHIBITION

The goal of **stabilization** is to support the injured limb so that surrounding muscles can relax. This reduces both pain and neural inhibition. Stabilization should not be confused with compression or rest; its purpose is quite different. It is true that stabilization may provide compression and may force the injured body part to rest, but these are only secondary effects.

Muscle guarding is an unwanted response to injury. The body attempts to protect the traumatized tissue from further injury by causing muscles to spasm and thus splint the joints surrounding the injury. But muscle spasm also causes pain, which causes more muscle spasm, which causes more pain, and so on. Thus a pain–spasm–pain cycle is perpetuated. Early stabilization lets the muscles relax, thereby easing the cycle. There are numerous braces and splints that can be used for stabilization (Fig. 5.7).

> **CRITICAL THINKING 5.2** *Early in the chapter, we stated that focusing the majority of attention concerning RICES on controlling swelling through cryotherapy is somewhat shortsighted. Give a reason for agreeing with this statement and a reason for disagreeing with it.*

The Physics and Physiology of Cryotherapy

When ice is applied to the body it cools the structure it is applied to. Although it sounds pure and simple, there are many factors that determine the amount of cooling. First, we must define *cold*. **Cold** is not a physical substance; it is merely the absence of **heat**, which is the kinetic energy of atoms and molecules. The state of being cold is relative. Consider, for example, that in the northern tier of the United States in October, after a hot summer, when the temperature gets down to 40°F (4.4°C), you feel cold and want to put on a jacket. In March, however, after a cold winter, when the temperature gets up to 40°F (4.4°C), you feel warm and want to take off your jacket.

THE PHYSIOLOGY OF HEAT TRANSFER

During cooling, heat is transferred from the body tissues to the cold modality through a process known as conduction. **Conduction** is the exchange of energy (heat) between two substances that are in contact with each other. Heat moves from the body of higher energy to the body of lower energy, causing the warmer body to cool and the cooler body to warm until they reach equilibrium.[28]

Rate of Conduction

The rate of heat conduction, and therefore the rate of tissue temperature decrease, depends on the interaction of many factors (a list follows). These same principles apply to superficial heating modalities (discussed in Chapter 11) when heat is added to the body:

- *The temperature differential between the body and the cold modality.*[29,30] Heat will conduct more quickly from 95°F (35°C) tissue into a 50°F (10°C) cold pack than it will into a 77°F (25°C) cold pack.
- *The regeneration of body heat and/or modality cooling.*[30] As the tissue gives up heat to the modality, some lost tissue heat is replaced by heat from circulating blood and conduction from surrounding tissues. Simultaneously, the heat given up to the cold modality either is held by the modality, which therefore increases its temperature, or is removed from the modality (e.g., as with a cryomatic

TABLE 5.2	Swelling Management with Cold and Compression	
MODALITY	**CONTROL/LIMIT SWELLING**	**REMOVE SWELLING**
Cold, intermittent (39–50 min)	X	
Compression, continuous	X	
Compression, intermittent		X

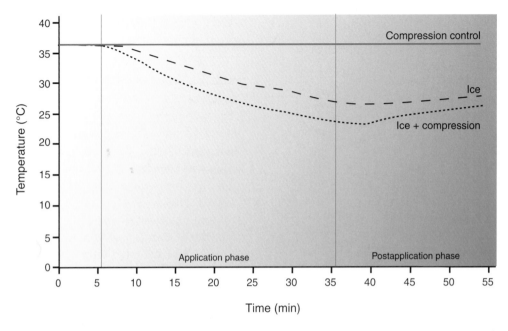

FIGURE 5.6. Compression exerted by an elastic wrap over a crushed ice pack causes a greater tissue temperature reduction than application of the ice pack alone.

unit), which maintains its lowered temperature. Both reheating the body and recooling the modality affect the temperature differential.

- *The heat storage capacity of the cold modality* (explained in the next section). Various modalities can accept differing amounts of heat before they begin warming. Thus a modality that can accept greater amounts of heat will maintain a greater temperature differential between the modality and the tissue. If two cold packs are

identical except for their size, the larger one will have a greater heat storage capacity.

- *The size of the cold modality.* The larger the cold pack, the more heat it can accept.
- *The amount of tissue in contact with the cold pack.* The greater the contact area, the more heat will be extracted from the body and thus more cooling. This is why immersing the forearm in 50°F (10°C) water will cool it to the same degree as a 32°F (0°C) cold pack (Fig. 5.8).

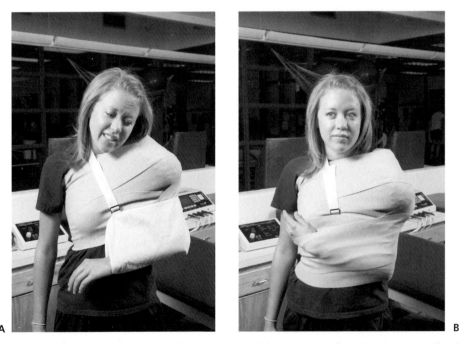

FIGURE 5.7. Stabilization is essential during immediate care. **(a)** Muscles around the injury normally go into spasm to splint the injury, resulting in great pain, even when compression or a sling is used. **(b)** Stabilization allows the muscles to relax, thus breaking the pain–spasm–pain cycle.

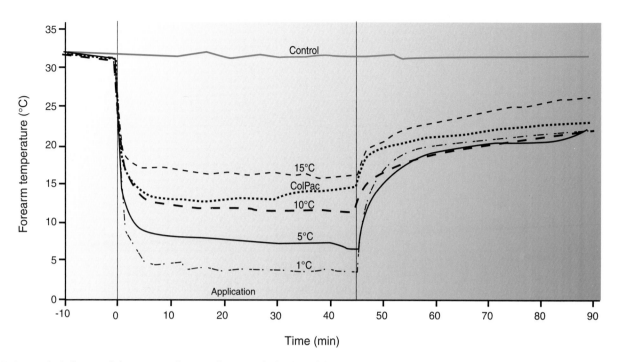

FIGURE 5.8. The influence of the amount of contact between the body and the cold modality on cooling. Note the similarity in tissue temperature during the application of a 32°F (0°C) cold pack and immersion in 50°F (10°C) water. (Adapted with permission from Knight et al.[31])

If other things are equal, a large cold pack will cool a body part more than a smaller one because it covers a larger area of the body and therefore extracts heat from a larger area.

- *The length of application.*[30] The longer the application of the cold modality, the more time for energy to be exchanged and thus more heat removal from the body.
- *Individual variability.* People react differently to cold applications.

An analysis of each of these factors in every type of cold application is beyond the scope of this book. You can evaluate the relative contribution of each factor to the cold modalities of your choice.

Heat Capacity of Modalities

The amount of heat that the same sizes and shapes of various cold modalities can accept depends on their specific heat, their latent heat of fusion, and whether they undergo a phase change.[28] **Specific heat** is the amount of heat energy required to raise 1 kg of a substance 1°C.[32] Therefore, the greater a substance's specific heat, the more heat energy it can withdraw. Water has a very large specific heat, greater than most substances, so it is excellent for cold packs.

Phase change refers to the change from one state (solid or liquid or gas) to another without a change in chemical composition or temperature.[28] Of particular interest here is the phase change from ice to water. The **latent heat of fusion** is the amount of energy needed to convert a sub-stance from its solid state to its liquid state—that is, to undergo a phase change. It takes tremendous amounts of heat energy to change ice at 32°F (0°C) to water at 32°F (0°C).

For example, a 1 kg ice pack would extract 85 kcal of heat from the body if left until the ice melted and warmed to 41°F (5°C). A gel pack of the same mass would extract only 22 kcal by the time it warmed to the same temperature, about 25% as much (Fig. 5.9; Box 5.1 lists specific calculations). This is one of the advantages of crushed ice over gel packs for cooling the body. Crushed ice packs freeze solid and therefore can absorb more heat than gel packs, which do not freeze solid.

TEMPERATURE CHANGES RESULTING FROM CRYOTHERAPY

The beneficial effects of cryotherapy are related to tissue temperature changes. The magnitude and rate of these changes, and of rewarming after application, vary according to the depth of the tissue and the rate of conduction.

Surface Temperature

Cold applications cause an immediate and rapid decline in the temperature of the surface to which the cold is applied, as heat is conducted from the body to the cold modality (see Fig. 5.8). The rate of cooling steadily slows until the surface temperature eventually plateaus a few degrees above the temperature of the modality.[33–37] After application, there is an immediate sharp temperature increase, like the initial decrease but of lesser magnitude,

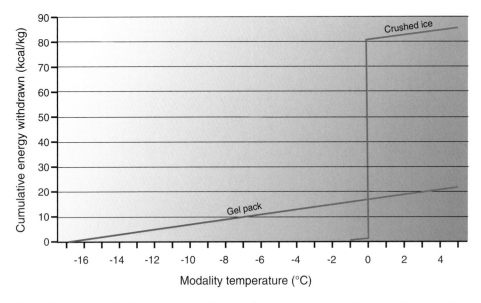

FIGURE 5.9. Crushed ice packs are more effective than gel packs because they undergo a phase change, which results in more heat being withdrawn from the body.

followed by a gradual and prolonged return toward preapplication temperature.

The type of cold modality affects the magnitude of the difference between the modality temperature and the plateaued tissue temperature and whether the tissue temperature begins to rise before the modality is removed. For instance, compare the temperature curves for the ColPac to the 34°F (1°C) and 50°F (10°C) water baths in Figure 5.8. Although the ColPac was initially colder than the 34°F (1°C) water bath, it does not have the capacity to cool the forearm as much as the 34°F (1°C) water bath. In fact, it appears much like the 50°F (10°C) water bath during the first 15 min or so of application. After 15 min, the arm temperature treated with ColPacs began to increase, while the arm temperature in the 50°F (10°C) water bath continued to decrease slightly.

The degree of cooling, but not the rate of cooling, is affected by previous activity (Fig. 5.10).[37,38] Stationary bike riding at a moderate intensity (enough to increase the heart rate to 60–80% of the subject's heart rate range) resulted in an increase of 3.6°F (2°C) in the ankle[37,38] and thigh[37] before, during, and after ice pack application.

Cooling during repeated applications is not consistent. The degree of cooling during a second application depends on the length of the first application, the time between treatments,[37] and the activity of the patient between the two applications.[37,39] The following are principles based on our research on the intermittent application of cold:[37,39]

- Mild activity, such as walking on crutches and showering, causes more rapid rewarming. Therefore, cold should be reapplied immediately after these activities.

- Protocols with cooling to rewarming ratios of 1:2 (i.e., 30:60 min) and less resulted in lower temperatures during the second application–rewarming cycle. If additional reapplication has an additional cooling effect, this may result in tissue damage.

A compression wrap over an ice pack causes a greater decrease in temperature during application and less of an increase after the application of an ice pack in both surface and deep temperatures (see Fig. 5.6).[14]

Tissue Temperature

The response of deep tissue to surface cooling depends on the depth and type of the tissue.[40,41] The reaction of subcutaneous (just below the skin) tissues is the same as that of the skin but decreased in magnitude;[42–44] temperature initially decreases sharply, followed by a more gradual decrease, until it eventually plateaus (Fig. 5.11). Like skin temperature, subcutaneous tissue temperature immediately begins to increase after the application.

Deeper tissue temperatures, on the other hand, do not begin decreasing until minutes after the cold application (see Figs. 5.6 and 5.11).[40,41,45] They then decrease more gradually and to a lesser magnitude than subcutaneous temperature.[40,46,47] Both the delayed response and decreased magnitude of temperature changes in the deeper tissue are the result of the time it takes for heat to exchange between various layers of molecules in the tissue (see Chapter 13).

After cold application, deep tissue temperature continues to decrease (see Figs. 5.6 and 5.11).[41,45,46] The length of the decrease depends on the depth of the tissue[40]—for example, after 5 min of ice massage to the calf, tempera-

BOX 5.1 *LATENT HEAT OF FUSION: COOLING CAPACITY OF AN ICE PACK AND A GEL PACK*

The example given here illustrates the difference in heat energy extracted from tissue during applications of a crushed ice pack and a cold pack (a four-fold difference in this example). For purposes of the illustration, assume the following:

- Both packs weigh 1 kg.
- Both packs are applied to the same surface.
- Both packs are applied until they withdraw enough heat to warm to 41°F (5°C).
- The crushed ice came from a free-standing ice machine, which stored it at 30°F (−1°C).
- The gel pack was stored in a freezer unit at 1°F (−17°C).

Constants required for the equations:[32]

- Heat of fusion of ice (*L*) = 80 cal/g
- Heating ice (*Q*) = 0.5 cal/g
- Heating water (*Q*) = 1 cal/g

Computing the energy associated with the heat withdrawn from the respective modalities requires a single step for the gel pack and three steps for the ice pack (degrees Celsius is the standard convention for these calculations):

Gel Pack

1. Heat water 22°C (from −17°C to 5°C)

   Q = 1 kg × 1 cal per g water/°C × 22°C = 22,000 cal or 22 kcal

Ice Pack

1. Heat ice 1°C (from −1°C to 0°C)

   Q = 1 kg ice × 0.5 cal per g water/°C × 1°C = 500 cal or 0.5 kcal

2. Heat of fusion (ice to water at 0°C).

   Q = 1 kg ice × 80 cal/g = 80,000 cal or 80 kcal

3. Heat water 5°C (from 0°C to 5°C)

   Q = 1 kg ice × 1 cal per g water/°C × 5°C = 5,000 cal or = kcal

   Total = 0.5 + 80 + 5 = 85.5 kcal

Thus the energy differential is 85.5 kcal for the ice pack and 22 kcal for the gel pack: 85.5 ÷ 22 = 3.886. This means that the total energy available for cooling is 3.9 times greater with an ice pack than with a gel pack of equal size and shape.

tures decreased for an additional 2.5 min at 1.0 cm deep, 10 min at 2.0 cm deep, 30 min at 3.0 cm deep, and 50 min at 4.0 cm deep.[40]

The magnitude of the temperature change in deep tissues (at all levels) depends on the magnitude of cold application (the amount of heat removed from the body). This relationship can be seen in the data of Waylonis,[40] who reported that skin temperature was basically the same after 5 min and 10 min of ice massage, but the temperature at 4.0 cm decreased more than twice as much after the 10 min ice massage. This difference in deep tissue temperature reflects a greater conduction owing to the longer application of ice. Some researchers have misinterpreted the effects of ice massage by considering tissue temperature change during application rather than after application.[48]

Adipose tissue insulates deeper tissues and thus decreases the effect of cooling on them.[49,50] Changes in deep tissue temperature correlate with the amount of adipose tissue over the biceps brachii muscle[48] and the thigh muscles[51] when cold is applied to the skin over these muscles and to the percentage of fat of the entire body when application and measurement involve the lower leg.[52]

Intra-Articular Temperature

Intra-articular temperature, or temperature within a joint, resembles that in other tissues—the temperature seems to be a function of the magnitude of heat lost. For instance:

- Cold immersion results in a greater temperature decrease than crushed ice packs (~38°F [21°C] vs. 7.2°F [4°C] in 15 min) and ethyl chloride spray (4.5°F [2.5°C] in 15–30 min).[53]
- Intra-articular temperatures decrease more than adjacent muscle: 4.5°F (2.5°C) vs. 3.6°F (2.0°C), 1.9 cm intramuscularly with 15–30 min ethyl chloride spray[45] and 33°F (18.4°C), 31°F (17.4°C), and 30°F (16.4°C) in the knee joint, adjacent muscle, and adjacent subcutaneous tissue, respectively, as a result of cold packs (43–50°F [6–10°C]) applied for 1 hr.[54]
- Like other deep tissues, the minimum temperature is reached after the ice pack is removed.[53,55]
- The longer the application, the greater the decrease in temperature.[53] For instance, ice packs applied for 5, 15, and 30 min resulted in decreases of 0.6°F (2°C), 7.2°F (4°C), and 11.9°F (6.5°C), respectively.
- Rewarming after cold applications is delayed for hours;[55–57] 215 min after a 30 min application of a frozen gel pack (−23°C) applied over a thin towel to the knees of 10 young healthy bulls.[56] And 150 min after a 30 min crushed ice pack application to 42 human knees, the intra-articular knee temperature was still depressed 8°F (4.5°C).[55]

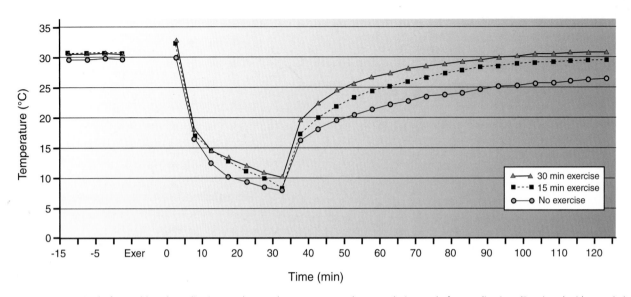

FIGURE 5.10. Exercise before cold pack application moderates the temperature decrease during and after application. (Reprinted with permission from Mancuso and Knight.[38])

Rewarming After Cryotherapy

Rewarming after cryotherapy is a function of three factors:

- The activity level before cryotherapy
- The amount of heat removed from the body during application (i.e., magnitude and duration of cold exposure)
- The amount of heat available to rewarm the area, which is a function of circulation, environmental temperature, and activity

The fingers rewarm much more quickly than the ankle,[34,36] forearm,[36] calf,[46] and interarticular knee.[55,56] Fingers rewarm in 15–20 min, whereas the other body parts take >3 hr (Fig. 5.12). Presumably this is owing to the increased circulation in the fingers.

Deep tissue rewarming is not as straightforward as is surface temperature rewarming. It varies according to the depth of the tissue. Tissues that are more superficial (up to ~2 cm deep) begin rewarming immediately after the cold is removed.[40,52] Deeper tissues continue to decrease.[40,46,58] The longer the cold is applied and the deeper the tissue, the slower the rewarming after application.

Activity during rewarming increases the rate of rewarming.[37] Even mild activity, like walking on crutches and standing in a shower for 20 min, significantly increases the rate of rewarming.

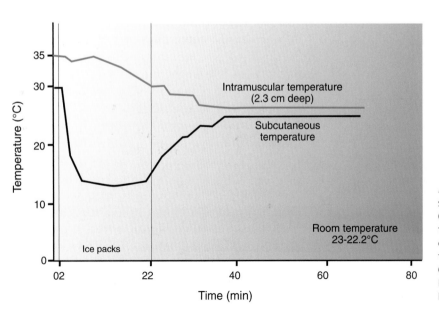

FIGURE 5.11. Subcutaneous temperature responds much like surface tissue temperature (compare with Fig. 5.8). Deep temperature, on the other hand, decreases much more slowly, continues to decrease after application, and returns to preapplication levels much more slowly. (Adapted with permission from Hartviksen.[58] Reproduced with permission from the BMJ Publishing Group)

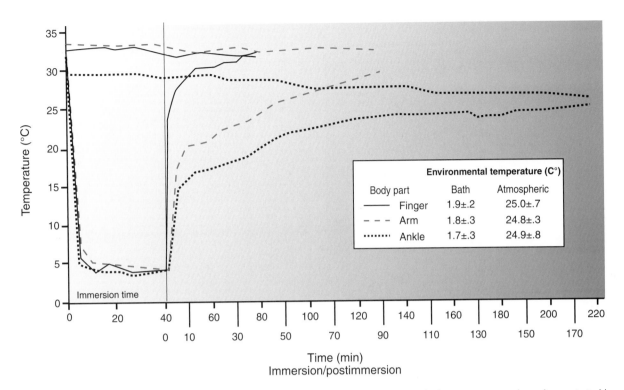

FIGURE 5.12. Fingers rewarm quickly after the removal of a cold pack. Most other body parts take hours to rewarm, here demonstrated by arm and ankle temperatures. (Reprinted with permission from Knight and Elam.[36])

Rewarming after a second application is generally the same as after the first application, as long as the ratio of application time to interval between applications is >2:1 and the application times and the activity level during rewarming are the same.[37]

Cryotherapy Application Principles

Does it matter how you apply cold? Absolutely! The cold modality chosen and how it is applied result in great differences in tissue cooling. Understanding the factors that affect tissue cooling will help you make proper decisions.

Various protocols have been suggested for applying cold during immediate care. In one review of the recommended length, frequency of application, and duration of therapy of >30 published protocols, there were only two instances in which two recommendations were the same.[59] The following discussion will help solve some of the confusion.

FACTORS THAT AFFECT TISSUE COOLING

Numerous factors influence tissue cooling during cold pack application. Some of these were discussed above, including the following:

- The temperature differential between the body and the cold modality
- The regeneration of body heat and/or modality cooling

- The heat storage capacity of the cold modality
- The size of the cold modality (the larger the cold pack, the more cooling)
- The amount of tissue in contact with the cold pack (the greater the area of contact with the cold modality, the more cooling)
- The length of application (the longer the application, the more cooling and the slower the rewarming)
- Individual variability
- Heat capacity of modalities

Other factors that influence tissue cooling and guidelines for application are types of cold packs, application directly to the skin rather than over a towel or elastic wrap, length of application, rate of intermittent application, and the duration of therapy (number of treatments).

TYPES OF COLD PACKS

The four main types of **cold packs** are crushed ice packs, gel packs, artificial ice packs, and crushable chemical packs (Fig. 5.13).

Crushed Ice Pack

A **crushed ice pack** is crushed ice, typically from an ice machine, in a plastic or cloth bag. Ice packs are typically 30°F (−1°C) to 32°F (0°C) when applied to the body. They are the most effective type of cold modality because they undergo a phase change and therefore extract great

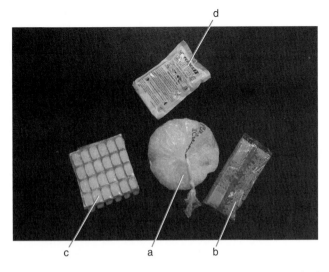

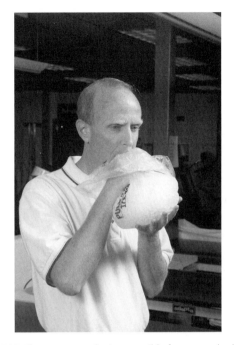

FIGURE 5.13. The four most common types of cold packs: (*a*) crushed ice pack, (*b*) gel pack (cold pack), (*c*) artificial ice pack (with sheets of ice visible on top), and (*d*) crushable chemical pack.

FIGURE 5.14. Remove as much air as possible from a crushed ice pack by sucking it out. Twist the end of the bag before removing it from your face, and then quickly tie the end in a knot.

amounts of heat from the body (see Fig. 5.9). Yet they are not so cold that they cause frostbite, unless applied for hours.

Crushed ice packs are also excellent for on-the-field use. They can be prepared before a practice or event, placed in an insulated cooler, and used hours later. Without a phase change, other types of cold packs are not nearly as effective.

Crushed ice packs are not effective for home use. They cool to about 1°F (−17°C) in a home freezer; if applied directly to the skin they will cause tissue damage. They also become solid when frozen in a home freezer, so they do not conform to irregular body surfaces.

You can make an ice pack by placing 1.5–2.5 lb (0.7–1.2 kg) of crushed or cubed ice in a plastic bag. Suck out as much air as possible from the bag, and tie the end in a knot (Fig. 5.14).

Gel Pack

A **gel pack** is a reusable type of cold pack. It consists of water mixed with an antifreeze, such as alcohol, and a gel substance, in a vinyl pouch. The alcohol keeps the water from freezing solid, and the gel gives it body so the water does not slosh around in the pack. They are cooled in a freezer to about 1°F (−17°C).

Gel packs are not as effective as crushed ice, and they are much more dangerous. The water does not freeze, so they do not go through a phase change when applied. Thus they do not withdraw as much heat from the body. But because they are cooled to ~1°F (~17°C), they might cause frostbite if applied directly to the skin (Fig. 5.15). Applying a barrier to protect the skin from the extreme temperature further decreases their cooling effectiveness.

Artificial Ice Pack

An **artificial ice pack** is a pouch made of vinyl sheets 1 × 1.5 in. (3 × 4 cm). The pouch is filled with water and enclosed in a nylon covering (see Fig. 5.13). The vinyl is meant to keep fruit and vegetables cool during interstate shipping and is cut from large sheets. Artificial ice packs are frozen in a freezer at ~1°F (~17°C), but the nylon covering insulates them so the application temperature is close to 32°F (0°C). Artificial ice packs are not as flexible

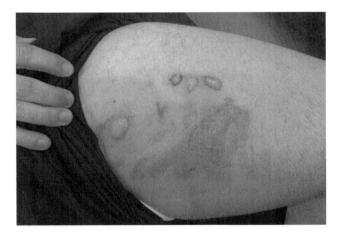

FIGURE 5.15. Frozen gel packs can cause severe skin damage if applied directly to the skin. This individual took a frozen gel pack from our laboratory without permission and applied it directly to his skin (thigh) for 90 min to treat radiating pain. Blisters began forming that evening and continued to grow until 2 days later, when this photograph was taken. The skin healed without scarring but was still mildly sensitive to touch 20 months later.

as gel packs, but they are much more flexible than re-frozen crushed ice packs. Because of their nylon covering, artificial ice packs are not as effective in cooling tissue as is crushed ice, but they are more effective in cooling than a gel pack because they undergo a phase change. They are preferred for home use because they can be safely applied after cooling in a kitchen freezer, are flexible, and go through a phase change as they warm.

Crushable Chemical Pack

A **crushable chemical pack** consists of a thin-walled vinyl pouch of a liquid packaged within a stronger, larger vinyl pouch of dry crystals. When squeezed with sufficient force, the smaller pouch is broken, leaking its fluid into the larger, outer pouch. The fluid and crystals combine in a chemical reaction that cools the fluid. Crushable chemical packs are not recommended because they neither get the body cold enough nor last long enough to be used in place of crushed ice.[60] There also is a danger of chemical burns if the contents of such a pack leak onto the skin. Crushable chemical cold packs should be used only as a last resort.

APPLICATION DIRECTLY TO THE SKIN

In general, crushed ice packs are applied directly to the patient's skin (Fig. 5.16).[61,62] A towel or elastic wrap between the ice pack and the body insulates against the full effect of the cold, thereby making the treatment less effective.[60,63–65] If used for <60 min, most cold packs do not

cause frostbite. Frozen gel packs are an exception, however, and should not be applied directly on the skin. Their temperature may be many degrees below zero and could cause frostbite.

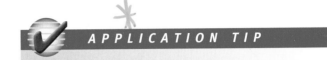

APPLICATION TIP

KNOW WHEN NOT TO APPLY COLD PACKS DIRECTLY TO THE SKIN. Some types of cold packs are too cold to be applied directly to the skin because they will damage the skin. These include frozen gel packs and crushed ice packs using ice frozen in a refrigerator or freezer. Most crushed ice packs are made from ice from an ice machine, which stores the ice just below freezing (30°F or −1°C). But ice from a freezer and gel packs are in the range of −2°F to −5°F (−16°C to −19°C). This is much too cold for the skin and often results in tissue damage.

Placing a towel or elastic wrap between the skin and the cold pack, as many recommend,[7,66] insulates the skin against the cold, decreasing the effectiveness of the cold pack (Fig. 5.17).[60,61–65] Using wet [7,67] or frozen[68] elastic wraps between the skin and the cold pack is preferable to using dry ones, but not as beneficial as application directly to the skin.[61–65]

Most first-aid texts recommend against applying ice packs directly to the skin.[7,69] This is beginning to change,

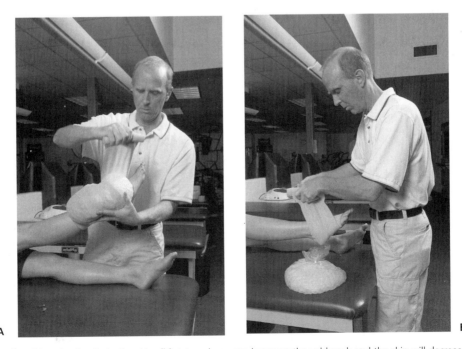

FIGURE 5.16. (a) Apply cold packs directly to the skin. **(b)** A towel or wrap between the cold pack and the skin will decrease the effectiveness of cooling.

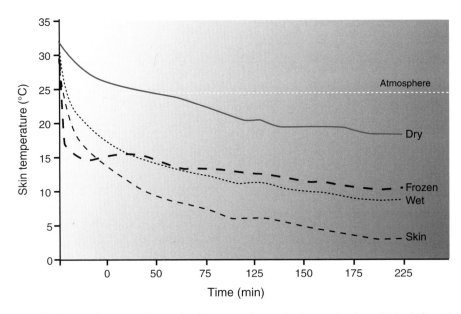

FIGURE 5.17. Applying a crushed ice pack over two layers of a dry, wet, or frozen elastic wrap insulates the body from the cold pack. The most effective cooling occurs when the cold pack is applied directly to the skin. (Reprinted with permission from Urban.[64])

however.[70] The newest text from the American Academy of Orthopaedic Surgeons and the American Academy of Emergency Physicians recommends applying crushed ice packs directly to the skin.[70]

Mirkin[62] claimed that ice packs directly on the skin were safe because living tissue will not freeze until its temperature drops below 25°F (−4.3°C); because an ice pack is 32°F (0°C), it is incapable of causing frostbite. Although his estimate of the freezing temperature of skin was probably low by 3–5°F (2–3°C),[18] he was correct in stating that ice packs can be applied safely to the skin as long as they are not left on >60 min. Long-term application can lead to tissue damage.[71]

We can find no reference to frostbite occurring as a result of a short-term (<60 min) cold application in the literature, nor have we observed frostbite in >30 years of clinical experience applying ice packs directly to the skin of patients for up to 45 min at a time[18] (see also Chapter 14).

LENGTH OF APPLICATION

Ice packs should be applied intermittently. Continuous application is both unnecessary and potentially dangerous. Frostbite can occur with continuous application,[71] and most areas of the body rewarm quite slowly after ice pack application.[35,36,72] The beneficial effects of cold application, therefore, remain after the cold packs are removed. Tissue temperature remains low after removing the cold modality, so tissue metabolism remains depressed. The body part can be kept cool by applying an ice pack for 30–45 min every 2 hr (every hour if the patient is active between applications, such as showering or walking on crutches).

MODALITY MYTH

USING INVALID LENGTHS OF INTERMITTENT COLD APPLICATION

Many clinicians apply ice packs for inappropriate lengths of time, believing their applications are effective. Many applications are less than optimal. Application times for ice packs vary from 6 min to continuously for 24–48 hr.[59] A period of 6 min is much too short to be of any value, and 24 hr is dangerous. The wide variety of application lengths may result from an inadequate theoretical basis for using cryotherapy during immediate procedures.

Most clinicians recommend intermittent applications, even though their reasons for doing so vary.

- Some believe cold-induced vasodilation (CIVD) will increase blood flow to the area if they apply cold for longer than 10–12 min.[73–76] Chu and Lutt[77] felt that initial cold applications should last at least 20 min so the body part could pass through a 3–5 min period of vasodilation and be in a second period of vasoconstriction. CIVD does not occur (see Chapter 13), so this logic is incorrect.
- Some fear frostbite[71,73,78] or nerve palsy[79] if they apply cold for too long, which most define as 15–30 min. The concept is true, but the time frame is much too short. Applications of up to 60 min (for fleshy tissues) are safe.
- Boland[61] believed the application of ice packs for longer than 20–30 min was too painful and should not be done. Ice packs applied for this length are not overly

painful. Ice immersion can be painful, but immersion is not recommended for immediate care.

There is no direct research on how the length of application affects the amount of tissue damage or subsequent resolution of the injury. The rate of rewarming after application, however, indicates that cold packs should be applied for at least 30 min during immediate care.[59] As Figure 5.18 indicates, ankle rewarming after 30, 45, and 60 min ice pack application is significantly slower than after 10 and 20 min ice applications. Thus metabolism remains lowered during the time between intermittent ice pack applications.

The area of the body also affects the length of application. The ankle and forearm temperatures remain depressed for hours after application, whereas the finger rewarms within minutes (see Fig. 5.12).[34,36] The knee reacts like the ankle and forearm. Thick muscular tissues, such as the thigh, require longer to cool than bony areas, such as the ankle,[33,37] and rewarm more quickly.

Deeper tissues cool more slowly than superficial tissues (see Fig. 5.11). The deeper the injury is, the longer the cold pack application. There are few data on which to base specifics. A good guideline is to treat moderately fleshy muscle pulls for 45 min and more fleshy injuries, such as the calf and thigh, for up to 60 min.

The length of cold applications should be adjusted according to the patient's skinfold thickness. The amount of adipose tissue (skinfold thickness) influences cooling.[49,50] In one study, scientists measured how long it took to decrease the intramuscular (anterior thigh, 1 cm below adi-

pose) temperature by 44.6°F (7°C). It took ~8 min in tissue with 0–10 mm skinfold vs. ~59 min in tissue with 31–40 mm skinfold thickness.

RATE OF INTERMITTENT APPLICATION

The question of how long ice packs should be applied involves not just the initial application, but the repeated applications and the time between the applications.

The activity level of the patient determines how quickly subsequent applications should be administered. Generally after the first application, patients will shower and go home. Cold packs should be reapplied immediately. If the patient is inactive, however, applications of more than 30 min every 2 hr will cause a progressive decrease in the temperature of the ankle.[37]

Because reapplication is usually done by the patient or family or friends, **compliance** is a factor. The more complicated the treatment regimen, the less likely it will be followed. Recommendations such as "30 min on and 1 hr off" require too much thinking. A simplified recommendation, which is consistent with the variable application times for various tissues and the data from ankle reapplication,[37,39] is to apply ice packs every 2 hr, rounded to the nearest whole hour (e.g., 2:00, 4:00, 6:00 or 1:00, 3:00, 5:00).

DURATION OF THERAPY

Duration, as used here, refers to the calendar or the length of time that intermittent 30 min applications of cold packs should be continued. How long should RICES continue? There are no available data to indicate an optimal dura-

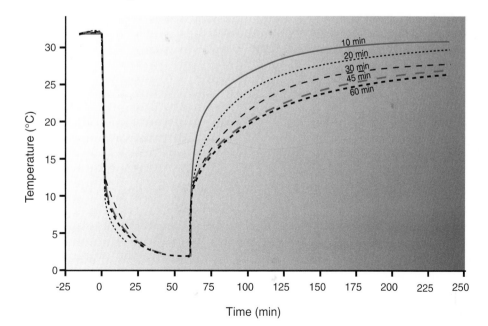

FIGURE 5.18. Ankle cooling and rewarming during and after crushed ice pack applications of 10, 20, 30, 45, and 60 min. The quicker rewarming after 10 and 20 min applications indicates that cold packs should be applied for at least 30 min during immediate care. (Reprinted with permission from Mlynarczyk.[59])

tion. Most clinicians recommend applications for 12–72 hr or until the tendency for swelling has passed.[59] One consideration is the severity of the injury. Immediate care procedures can be terminated earlier when treating a mild injury than when treating a severe injury. Another consideration is the therapy chosen for subacute care. It is possible to transition from immediate care to subacute rehabilitation procedures earlier when using a cryotherapeutic technique for rehabilitation than when using a thermotherapeutic technique. But a definitive answer to the question of the optimal duration of cold applications during immediate care awaits further research.

Two examples of cryotherapy techniques for subacute care are cryokinetics and cryostretch. Both combine cryotherapy with exercise. **Cryokinetics** consists of alternating cold application and active exercise for rehabilitating acute joint sprains. **Cryostretch** consists of alternating cold application, passive stretch, and resistive muscle contraction for rehabilitating acute muscle strains (see Chapter 13).

For first-degree injuries, transition to one of the these cryotherapy techniques after the initial RICES treatment (30 min after the injury) is advisable. For second-degree injuries, continuing RICES treatments until bedtime and until the patient has been evaluated (and possibly via x-ray) the next day is the recommendation. The question is moot for most third-degree injuries, because they generally are treated with surgery and/or immobilization until beyond the acute phase.

PREVENTING SWELLING VS. REDUCING OR REMOVING IT

Cold is effective in preventing or limiting swelling, but it is of little or no value in removing swelling after it has occurred (see Table 5.2). The cause of edema after traumatic injury is excess free protein in the tissue. As explained earlier, cold limits secondary injury. With less total injury, there is less tissue debris, less free protein in the tissue, and less edema. Once swelling has occurred, however, it can be removed only by removing the free protein from the extracellular spaces. As long as free protein remains in the tissue spaces, TOP will be abnormally high, thereby retaining excess fluid in the tissue. The only way to permanently remove edema is to remove the excess free protein.

Protein debris is much too large to be absorbed into the circulatory system. It is removed via the lymphatic system, and such removal requires intermittent compression. The lymphatic system consists of vessels that begin in the tissue and run proximally to the large veins. They have no built-in pumping force, such as the heart, to cause fluid flow. They depend primarily on external compression to force fluid flow (Fig. 5.19). A series of one-way valves al-

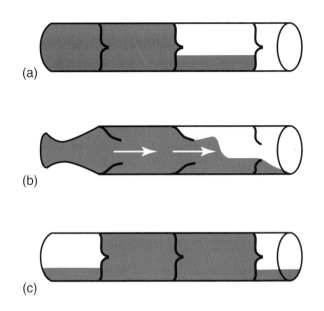

FIGURE 5.19. **(a)** Lymph vessels contain a series of one-way valves. **(b)** Pressure on the vessel forces fluid to flow proximally. **(c)** Release of the pressure creates a vacuum in empty sections of the vessel, which draws lymph into the vessel from surrounding tissue. Ongoing flow occurs from intermittent compression (repeated compression and release).

lows fluid to flow proximally, but prevents backwash. External compression on the vessel forces the valves open and the fluid to move proximally. When the compression is released the valves close, preventing fluid from returning distally. This leaves a vacuum at the distal end of the lymph vessel. This vacuum pulls edema (fluid and free protein) into the vessel.[26] Subsequent compression then forces lymph distally, and the process continues.

Intermittent external force from massage, compression, or lymphedema devices such as the Jobst pump, or the muscle pump, during active exercise stimulates lymph flow.[80,81] Neither heat nor cold applications promote lymph flow. They can be helpful, however, in facilitating one of the other modalities. For instance, with cryokinetics, ice applications decrease pain so that active exercise can begin sooner and be more vigorous. Thus cold application, which has no effect by itself, can facilitate active exercise, which in turn compresses lymph vessels and stimulates lymph flow. (Specific techniques for removing swelling by stimulating lymph flow are presented in Chapter 13.)

Misunderstanding the difference between preventing or limiting swelling and removing it after it has occurred leads many clinicians to use cold applications to "treat" swelling, an effort that is both ineffective and delays proper therapy. An example of this misunderstanding is demonstrated by research on the effects of cold during immediate care that includes patients who were not treated until 12–36 hr after their injury.[6,82] Further, this research included reduction in edema as one of the outcome variables. If a patient's treatment is not initiated within an hour or so of the injury, she is not receiving immediate care.

Intermittent vs. Continuous Cold and Compression

Cold is always applied intermittently. Applications longer than 60 min are unnecessary and potentially dangerous. Compression is applied either intermittently or continuously, depending on the therapeutic goals (see Table 5.2). Preventing swelling during RICES requires continuous application, whereas removing swelling during transitional or subacute care require intermittent compression to stimulate lymphatic drainage.

Compression Application Principles

There are three key considerations for applying compression during RICES: what to apply, where to apply it in relation to cold, and how to apply it.

RICES COMPRESSION DEVICES

Elastic wraps are preferred during RICES. When combined with ice packs, they provide more combined cold and compression than other devices (Table 5.3).[83] Despite its popularity and ease of application, plastic wrap should not be used during RICES (Fig. 5.20). It does not provide either the compression or the cooling of an elastic wrap. Although the ice packs under the plastic wrap and elastic wraps are the same, the greater compression exerted by the elastic wrap assists in providing greater cooling (see earlier discussion).

A Cryo Cuff is used as a cold/compression device, but it should not be used as an alternative for elastic wraps with ice. Dura*Kold should be used strictly as a cold modality because little compression is given by this device.

APPLYING ELASTIC WRAPS OVER ICE PACKS

Elastic wraps should be applied over ice packs, as explained earlier, to maximize tissue cooling (see Fig. 5.17). Some clinicians argue against this, claiming that it compromises compression. Compression is not compromised, however; compression over the anterior talofibular liga-

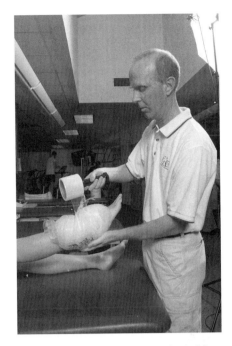

FIGURE 5.20. Plastic wraps are convenient for holding on ice packs, but they do not provide either the compression or the cooling effect of elastic wraps.

ment is the same whether the elastic wrap is under or over the ice pack, as long as the ice pack is tied so that it maintains a constant volume.[33,84]

STRETCHING ELASTIC WRAPS

We recommend that an elastic wrap be stretched to about 75% of its capacity as it is applied. There is no scientific basis for this recommendation, but it is the naturally selected, or intuitive, stretch that students and professionals apply.[33]

CONTRAINDICATIONS AND PRECAUTIONS TO CRYOTHERAPY

Inappropriate use of cryotherapy can cause excessive pain and tissue damage. These fit into three broad categories: cryotherapy that is too cold or applied too long,[85] cryotherapy applied with excessive compression, and applications to patients who suffer from conditions that cause abnormal responses to the cold.[86] These are discussed in general in this section and specific contraindica-

TABLE 5.3	*Temperature and Compression on the Ankle by Various Techniques*	
MODALITY	**AVERAGE 30 MIN TEMPERATURE (°C)**	**AVERAGE 30 MIN PRESSURE (MM)**
Cryo Cuff	13.9 ± 1.8	39.8 ± 6.2
Dura*Kold	14.1 ± 4.1	6.0 ± 2.0
Elastic wrap + ice	7.1 ± 4.8	50.7 ± 21.0
Flexi-Wrap + ice	9.8 ± 5.3	28.6 ± 13.7

tions and precautions are listed in the application section later in the chapter.

There is neither a specific temperature nor a length of application that causes tissue damage. It is the combination of the two that is dangerous.[87] For example, exposure to $-9°F$ ($-4°C$) for <1 min is safe,[88] yet exposure to $45°F$ ($7°C$) for 7 days resulted in gangrene. Intermittent ice water immersion ($32°F$ or $0°C$) for 20–30 min is common during rehabilitation of acute ankle sprains. Yet near continuous immersion for 36–72 hr has caused loss of part of the foot.[71,85] Gel packs (which are frozen to about $1°F$, or $-17°C$) should never be applied directly to the skin (see Fig. 5.15). Ice water immersion and crushed ice packs should be applied to the skin, but not for longer than 1 hr.

Elastic wraps applied over a cold pack can be problematic if applied too tightly, especially in thin people and to body parts where the major nerves are superficial, such as the elbow or knee. Do not apply the wrap too tightly. Cases of temporary **nerve palsy** (local paralysis) from cryotherapy have been reported, but analysis reveals that the combination of an elastic wrap and cold pack probably caused the palsy, not the cryotherapy alone.[18] The incidence of such cases is extremely small compared to the numbers of cryotherapy treatments given, so the risk is minimal.

The most common conditions that cause an abnormal response to cryotherapy include Raynaud disease, cold hypersensitivity, and urticaria. **Raynaud disease** is a circulatory disorder caused by cold or emotion, in which the hands, and less commonly the feet, become discolored and painful. Even mild cold exposure, such as reaching into a refrigerator, causes vascular spasm and extreme pain. Patients with these diseases generally know they have them and will refuse cold application. **Cold hypersensitivity** is a condition manifested by severe pain during cryotherapy.

Cold applications can cause urticaria (hives), in some people.[18] A temporary allergic reaction, **urticaria** is characterized by **wheals**—slightly raised, rounded, or flat-topped areas of skin—usually accompanied by burning or intense itching. It is also caused by exercise, eating certain foods, or from taking certain medicines.

Our experience is that patients with cold urticaria consider it more of a nuisance than a cause for concern. It manifests in patients who have used cold packs previously, often for a number of years. It usually is more intense in the beginning and becomes less severe if the patient continues to receive cold treatments. Our policy is to discuss the situation with patients after the first occurrence and let them decide whether to continue cryotherapy. Most feel the advantages of the cryotherapy outweigh the nuisance of the urticaria, especially as the urticaria decreases in severity over time. Calamine also helps some patients.[89]

Be aware that problems could arise if caution is not exercised when using cryotherapy in the following situations:

- Cardiac disorder
- Compromised local circulation

Electrical Stimulation During Immediate Care

Some clinicians advocate electrical stimulation for the immediate care of orthopedic injuries.[90] We do not recommend this technique at present, for reasons that will become apparent. There have been two schools of thought concerning this issue (see Chapter 9):

- The mistaken belief that high-volt pulsed current stimulation causes vasoconstriction and therefore limits swelling.[91]
- The belief under investigation that sensory-level high-volt pulsed stimulation limits edema development.

THE VASOCONSTRICTION THEORY

The belief that high-volt pulsed current stimulation causes vasoconstriction grew out of early marketing efforts by manufacturers who presented the devices as galvanic simulators. Because galvanic currents are thought to cause vasoconstriction, presumably these units would do so.[91] They are pulsed monophasic, but not galvanic, so they do not cause vasoconstriction. Also, even if they were vasoconstrictive, the goal of immediate care is to decrease secondary injury, not blood flow.

Another problem is that you sacrifice the full benefits of RICES with this technique. Many apply it by immersing the limb in a tub of ice water and inserting one of the electrodes into the bath. This sacrifices elevation. You also have to sacrifice either compression or some cooling. If you apply an elastic bandage to the limb for compression, the bandage will insulate the limb so you have less cooling. On the other hand, to get full cooling you have to sacrifice compression.

Applying electrical stimulation under the traditional RICES does not solve the problem. The thick rubber electrode will insulate the tissue from the cooling of the ice pack.

THE EDEMA-LIMITING THEORY

Limiting edema development by sensory-level high-volt pulsed current stimulation is based on extensive research on small laboratory animals.[90,92–102] The hind limbs of these animals were injured, and the animals were suspended in a sling with the traumatized limbs in a dependent position.[93] The traumatized limbs were immersed in a beaker of water, into which an electrode was placed.

Although research has clearly demonstrated that edema is curbed with high-volt pulsed stimulation, applying this concept is difficult. One problem is that it cannot be used in conjunction with RICES, as scientists suggest doing.[93] Their research suggests that near-continuous treatment is needed throughout the acute inflammatory response.[90,91] A single 30 min treatment decreases edema for 4 hr but does not significantly decrease long-term edema formation.[65,79,87–89] In addition, the animal model involved no compression or elevation.

Another concern is that the research has not been tested against RICES. Therefore, we do not know whether edema retardation is more, less, or the same as that provided by RICES. Scientists have compared electrical stimulation with cold,[92–94] but the protocols used fail to answer the question. The cold water immersion was at a temperature of 55°F (~13°C), which is not as cold as an ice pack. Also, the electrical stimulation and control were applied with room temperature water (75°F, or 23°C), which is ~15°F cooler than tissue, and so the control was actually a mild form of cryotherapy.

We recommend against using electrical stimulation in place of RICES for immediate care. It may have a place if it is used between ice applications and in conjunction with compression and elevation. Further research will, no doubt, clarify how electrical stimulation can augment RICES.

Application of RICES

STEP 1. FOUNDATION

A. Definition. Procedures used immediately after an acute orthopedic injury to limit the negative sequelae of the injury

B. Effects
1. Resting the injured structure minimizes aggravating the injury.
2. Ice cools the tissue, thereby minimizing secondary injury. There is less total injured tissue, less tissue debris, less free protein from phagocytosis of the tissue debris, and less edema. It also limits pain and muscle spasm.
3. Compression helps contain edema and increases the cooling effect of ice.
4. Elevation helps lessen the increase in capillary filtration pressure.
5. Stabilization reduces muscle guarding and pain.

C. Advantages. Less total tissue damage and edema

D. Disadvantages. None, if applied correctly

E. Indications. Acute orthopedic or soft tissue injury

F. Contraindications
1. Do not apply cryotherapy directly to the skin for >1 hr continuously; it can cause frostbite.
2. Do not apply cold packs that have been chilled in a freezer directly to the skin (see Fig. 5.15).
3. Do not apply a compression bandage over a chilled gel pack; it can cause frostbite.
4. Do not apply cryotherapy of any type to patients who have any of the following conditions:
    a. Raynaud disease or any other vasospastic disease
    b. Cold hypersensitivity, manifested by severe pain
    c. Cardiac disorder
    d. Compromised local circulation

G. Precautions
1. The longer you wait after injury, the less effective it is.
2. Unyielding compression: Despite your best efforts, edema may develop. If the edema is excessive, and the compression is unyielding, the pressure may damage tissue in a manner similar to a *compartment syndrome*, as can occur in the lower leg.
3. Be extremely cautious when using cryotherapy for treating patients who:
    a. Have certain rheumatoid conditions
    b. Are paralyzed or in a coma
    c. Have coronary artery disease
    d. Have certain hypertensive diseases

4. Be very careful when applying an elastic wrap over a cold pack, especially in thin people and to body parts for which the major nerves are superficial, such as the elbow or knee.
5. Be aware that cold applications can cause urticaria (hives) in some people.

STEP 2: PREAPPLICATION TASKS

A. Selecting the proper modality
1. Evaluate the injury or problem to:
    a. Rule out life-threatening situations; if one exists, initiate an emergency action plan.
    b. Collect data about the injury. Once muscle guarding develops, the information you obtain from palpation and stress tests will be decreased.
    c. Perform the evaluation thoroughly but quickly.
2. Check for possible contraindications to cold.

B. Preparing the patient psychologically
1. Explain the procedure.
2. Warn about precautions.
3. Reassure the patient; pain and frustration from the injury are usually quite disconcerting.

C. Preparing the patient physically
1. Remove clothing as necessary.
2. Remove bandages, braces, and so on, as necessary.
3. Position the patient in a manner that will be comfortable and allow the injury to be elevated.

D. Preparing the equipment
1. Make an appropriately sized ice pack.
    a. Place crushed ice in a plastic bag. The bag must be big enough so the finished pack will extend 2–3 in. (5–8 cm) beyond the borders of the injury. (Some injuries may require two ice packs.)
    b. Remove as much air as possible from the bag (see Fig. 5.14).
    c. Tie the end of the bag in a knot.
2. Get appropriately sized (width) elastic wrap(s).
    a. For most situations, a 6 in. (15 cm) width is adequate. Never use one <4 in. (10 cm) for immediate care. Smaller wraps don't adequately cover the area and have a greater tendency to roll up and become a tourniquet.
    b. Double-length or multiple wraps are necessary for applications to the knee, thigh, abdomen, chest, and shoulder.
    c. Get a splint or sling.

STEP 3: APPLICATION PARAMETERS

A. Procedures
1. Apply the ice pack so it is centered over the middle of the injury.
   a. Apply directly to the skin.
   b. Shape to the general contour of the body part.
2. Apply the elastic wrap(s) around the ice pack and body part to hold the ice pack in place and to apply compression.
   a. The wrap must extend 2–3 in. (5–8 cm) beyond the borders of the ice pack.
   b. Stretch the wrap to about 75% of its capacity during application.
   c. Secure the end of the wrap with clips or tape, or by tucking it under itself.
3. Check the patient every 5 min to see if the wrap is too tight. Also at this time, shake the ice pack to break up the thermal gradient.
4. Apply a splint, sling, or brace to stabilize the injured body part. The goal is to allow muscles surrounding the joint to relax. (See Fig. 5.7.)
5. Elevate the limb or situate the patient so that the injury is elevated about 6 in. (15 cm) above the heart.

B. Dosage. Use enough ice so that the ice pack(s) and elastic wrap extend 2–3 in. (5–8 cm) beyond the borders of the injury.

C. Length of application
1. Cold, 20–60 min, depending on the injury and the skin-fold thickness of the patient. In general:
   a. 20 min for finger
   b. 30 min for ankle or arm
   c. 45 min for thigh
   d. Add 5 min for each millimeter of skin-fold >1 mm.
2. Rest, compression, elevation, and stabilization continuously. Reapply the elastic wrap and stabilization after removing the ice pack.

D. Frequency of application
1. Begin application 5–10 min after the injury; immediately after the injury evaluation.
2. Second ice application should be 30–60 min later; after the patient has showered and gone home.
3. Apply compression, elevation, rest, and stabilization constantly.
4. Subsequent applications every 2 hr until bedtime. Tell the patient not to stay up into the night just to apply RICES.

E. Duration of therapy
1. Most first-degree injuries: 30–45 min (a single treatment).
2. Second-degree and third-degree injuries: 12–24 hr, if followed by a transitional cryotherapy technique, such as cryokinetics or cryostretch.

STEP 4: POSTAPPLICATION TASKS

A. Equipment replacement; area cleanup
B. Instructions in writing to the patient (Fig. 5.21). These include the following:
1. Time of appointment for the next day (morning if possible).
2. Resting the injury—that is, not stressing the body part to the point of causing pain. Use a sling or crutches as necessary.
3. Specific times for reapplication of the ice pack.
4. *Caution:* Do not reapply more or less frequently than the written instructions specify.
5. Phone number to call if pain or swelling becomes excessive.
C. Record of treatment, including unique patient responses

STEP 5: MAINTENANCE

A. Routine maintenance. Keep the ice machine in good repair, and replace elastic wraps as they deteriorate.

The Use of Crutches

Any patient who is unable to walk without a limp should be on crutches. Crutches make it possible for an injured person to walk properly by using the arms to substitute for, or supplement, leg power. Failure to use crutches will result in the following complications:

• Delayed healing. A person limps because the body weight aggravates the injury and causes pain. Neural inhibition results, thereby prolonging the rehabilitation process.
• Compensating muscle problems. The abnormal gait produced by limping causes muscles and other soft tissue surrounding the hip, knee, and/or ankle or the uninjured limb to shorten and tighten. Sometimes the resulting tightness will persist long after the original injury has healed.

Both of these complications can be minimized by the proper use of crutches. Correct crutch use requires the proper fitting of the crutches, selecting the appropriate crutch walking gait, instructing the patient to walk properly with the selected gait, observing the patient practicing the gait, and periodic reevaluation of the patient to ensure that he is using the crutches properly.

Extended Immediate Care Procedures
University of Moab Sports Medicine

Your activities during the next 12-72 hours are critical to the resolution of your injury. Failure to follow the following procedures may delay your return to full sport participation by as much as two weeks. Help us to help you by doing the following:

Before leaving the Athletic Training Clinic make sure you have:

_____ Had an initial 30- to 45-minute application of ice, compression, and elevation.

_____ Had a second evaluation of the injury.

_____ Showered.

_____ Had an elastic wrap applied to the injured area.

_____ Been fitted for a sling (if shoulder or arm injury) or crutches (if lower extremity injury).

_____ Received instructions in proper use of the sling or crutches (if fitted with them).

After you return to your dorm/apartment/home:

1. Apply an ice or cold pack to the injury for __40__ minutes at the times circled below. To do this, remove the elastic wrap, put the ice pack directly over the injury, and reapply elastic wrap. The wrap should be snug, but not real tight (remove about 3/4 of the stretch).

    1:00   2:00   3:00   │4:00│   5:00   │6:00│   7:00   │8:00│   9:00   │10:00│   11:00   │12:00│

2. After each __40__ minute ice-pack application, remove the ice pack and **reapply** the elastic wrap (snugly, as above). Following the last ice-pack application, wear the elastic wrap through the night until you return for treatment tomorrow.

3. Keep the injured part above the level of your heart as much as possible (constantly if possible) until you go to bed tonight.

4. Tomorrow, report to:

    The Student Health Center at _____ am/pm

    The Athletic Training Clinic at __10__ am/pm

    _____ at _____ am/pm

    _____ at _____ am/pm

5. AT: _____*k.knight*_____

6. If you have problems that you feel need immediate attention, call me at __555-1896__

FIGURE 5.21. Giving written instructions to the patient after the initial RICES treatment increases patient compliance.

PROPER CRUTCH FITTING

Fitting the crutches to the patient is essential to proper use. First, adjust the length of the crutches so that there are 2–3 in. (4.4–6.6 cm) between the axillae and the axillary pads (Fig. 5.22). This adjustment is usually made by removing the two wing nuts and then the two screws near the bottom of the crutches. (Aluminum crutches have a push-button adjustment.) A preliminary adjustment can be made with the patient lying, but the wing nuts should not be tightened until the adjustment has been confirmed with the patient standing.

Second, adjust the handpiece so that the elbow is flexed to ~30°, and the wrist is in a comfortable weight-bearing position (Fig. 5.22). If the position is correct, the patient should lift herself slightly off the floor when pushing down and extending her arms. This adjustment is made by removing the wing nut and screw through the handpiece.

MODALITY MYTH

CRUTCHES GO IN THE ARMPIT

A common misconception is that crutches should fit into the axillae (armpits) so that the shoulders bear the body weight. This is wrong! The weight of the body must be supported almost entirely by the hands; the remainder is supported by the upper lateral chest wall. Carrying the weight of the body in the axillae can cause contusion or concussion to the nerves of the brachial plexus, resulting in **crutch palsy,** a temporary or permanent loss of either sensation or the ability to move or control movement.

SELECTING THE PROPER GAIT

Selecting the appropriate crutch walking gait depends on how much weight the injured limb can take. Although there are a number of crutch walking gaits, two are most applicable to lower extremity trauma patients: the non-weight-bearing gait and the partial-weight-bearing gait. The **non-weight-bearing gait,** also known as the *swing-through gait,* is used when the objective is to completely remove weight from one leg or foot (Fig. 5.23a). The injured limb is lifted and the patient walks alternatively on the good leg and the two crutches. This gait should not be used any longer than necessary, though, because it

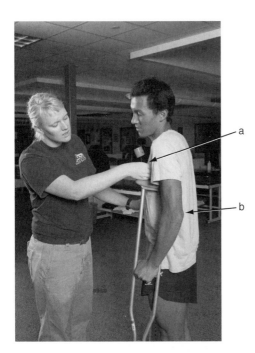

FIGURE 5.22. Crutches are properly fitted when **(a)** there are 2–3 in. (4.4–6.6 cm) between the axilla and axillary pad of the crutch, and **(b)** the elbow is bent ~30°.

can cause the same hip and knee tightness as caused by limping.

The preferred gait for patients with acute orthopedic trauma is the **partial-weight-bearing gait,** also called the *three-point gait* (Fig. 5.23b). The patient walks as with a normal gait, except for using the crutches to remove just enough weight from the injured limb to eliminate pain and limping. Weight borne by the injured leg will vary from light toe touching to almost full body weight. As the patient's injury heals, more weight is taken by the foot, and less by the hands and crutches.

WALKING INSTRUCTIONS

Instructing the patient in the selected gait is merely telling him when to move the crutches.

- "Think of the crutches as part of your injured limb."
- For the partial-weight-bearing gait: "The two crutches are in contact with the ground simultaneously with the injured limb. As you move the injured limb forward, move both the crutches forward also."
- For the non-weight-bearing gait: "Your body weight is totally supported by the uninjured leg while both crutches are placed 12–24 inches in front of your feet. Then transfer your weight to the crutches as you lift your body and swing through to a point 12–23 inches in front of the crutches."

Walking up and down stairs requires special training, because swinging may cause a loss of balance. The following instructions apply no matter which gait the patient uses on level ground:

- For going downstairs: "Begin by lowering the crutches down a step, follow with the injured leg, and then lower the hips down between the crutches. The uninjured leg is brought down last."
- For going upstairs: "The uninjured leg is lifted first, followed by the injured leg, and then the crutches."
- "The phrase 'The good go up to heaven, the bad go down to hell' may help you remember which foot or leg goes first when walking upstairs and downstairs."

The patient should also be instructed not to use a single crutch. With a single crutch, the patient will not stand up straight when walking, and the leaning will cause tightness in the lower back, hip, or knee. Although minimal, the tightness will affect postinjury activities and make the patient susceptible to further injury.

OBSERVING THE PATIENT PRACTICING THE GAIT

Watch the patient walk around until you are satisfied that she has mastered the technique. Going up and down some stairs is part of the practice that should be observed.

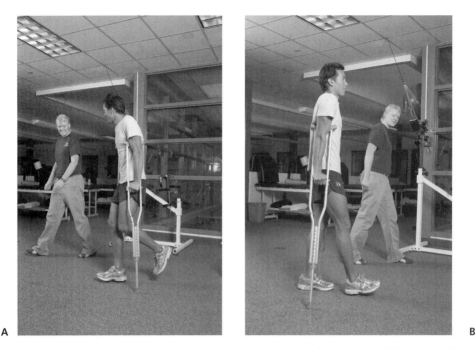

A   B

FIGURE 5.23. The purpose of crutch walking is to remove weight from the injured limb or foot. It can be **(a)** total, as with the non-weight-bearing or swing-through gait, or **(b)** partial, as with the partial-weight-bearing or three-point gait.

PERIODIC REEVALUATION

Periodic reevaluation of the patient should be done so that he will not subconsciously develop a deviant gait pattern that will result in problems after the crutches are no longer needed. This is best done when the patient is unaware that he is being watched. The important thing is for you to make sure that he is walking with as near to a normal gait as possible.

Medicated Ice for Abrasions

Athletes often suffer skin abrasions. An abrasion can become a complicated injury if not handled properly. Proper management includes the standard injury first aid of ice, compression, and elevation to limit pain, swelling, and secondary injury and managing potential bacterial contamination.[103]

Neither of the two most popular treatments for abrasions is comprehensive. One treats the injury like a sprain or strain with RICES and ignores the possibility of infection. The other treats the open wound by cleaning it and applying an antiseptic and sterile wound dressing, but ignores the possibility of secondary injury and swelling. MacLeod[103] suggested combining cryotherapy with an antiseptic by applying ice massage to abrasions with medicated ice cups (Fig. 5.24).

A medicated ice cup is sometimes referred to as a medicated Popsicle. The povidone-iodine in the ice, like all antiseptics, discourages the formation and propagation of bacteria. The indications, contraindications, and precautions for the povidone-iodine and lidocaine are provided with each medicine.

Ice also acts as an analgesic. Using medicated ice composed of 2% lidocaine produces an even greater analgesic effect, which is necessary when brushing or picking dirt and debris out of an open wound. The decrease in pain from the ice and lidocaine also leads to a slowing of the pain–spasm–pain cycle, which helps enhance muscle function around the injury. It is easy to avoid wound infection when the injury is treated early and properly.

PREPARING A MEDICATED ICE CUP

The following materials and medicines are needed to make medicated ice cups:

- Four 2-oz disposable cups
- Plastic stir sticks
- 2% lidocaine
- 10% povidone-iodine
- Distilled or boiled water

Here are the steps:

1. Mix 3 oz of povidone-iodine, 1 oz of lidocaine, and 3 oz of water.
2. Pour the mixture into the four cups.
3. Secure a stir stick vertically in the center of each cup with adhesive tape.

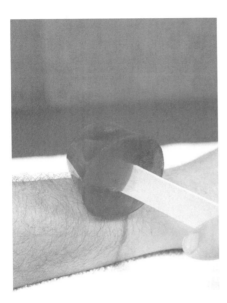

FIGURE 5.24. Ice massage with a medicated ice cup treats abrasions with antiseptic and cryotherapy.

HOW TO APPLY MEDICATED ICE

Here are the steps for applying ice massage to an abrasion using medicated ice cups. Do this as soon as possible after the injury:

1. Seek the advice and approval of a physician before applying medicated ice.
2. Hold the stir stick and roll the ice back and forth along the lacerated skin for about 10 min. As the ice melts, the medicines will flow into the damaged region and produce analgesic and antiseptic effects.
4. Débride the area (remove foreign materials) with gentle sweep with a moist gauze pad, picking out foreign material with tweezers.
5. Treat and protect the injured area as you would any open wound, emphasizing sterility.
6. Apply, or instruct the patient to apply, an ice pack for 20–30 min each hour until bedtime and apply compression constantly (except when applying or taking off the ice pack) for the first 24–72 hr after the injury.

4. Freeze overnight.
5. Clearly label the cups.
6. Isolate the medicated ice cups from other ice cups in the freezer so they are not accidentally used for general ice massage (this wouldn't cause problems, but it would be a waste of resources).

CLOSING SCENE

If Sammy would have read this chapter, he would have realized that there is a lot more to ice application than filling a bag full of ice and putting it on the injury. Among other things, he would have learned the advantages and disadvantages of several types of ice application. He would have learned that applying an ice pack directly to the skin is not only safe but preferred because it provides better cooling than placing a towel between the skin and the ice bag. He would know how long ice should be applied in various circumstances.

CHAPTER REFLECTIONS

1. Read and ponder each of the following points. Do you feel you have a clear understanding of each concept? If not, reread the appropriate section of the chapter.
   • What is immediate care, and when would you use it?
   • List seven modality myths about the immediate care of orthopedic injuries. For each one, briefly state the myth and the truth.

   • Are the terms *immediate care* and *acute care* synonymous? Why or why not?
   • List the stages of acute injury care. Generally when does each occur?
   • What is meant by general time frames for the stages of acute injury care?
   • What does the mnemonic RICES stand for? Briefly

describe each element and say why and when each one is most effective.

- What is swelling, and why and when does it occur?
- Explain what is meant by this statement: Cold during immediate care is more than swelling control.
- What are the two most prominent theories about why cryotherapy is used during immediate care? State the major elements of each theory, and their strengths and weakness.
- What is cold? How is cold transferred from a cold pack to the body?
- Briefly discuss each of the seven factors that influence the rate of heat conduction from the body to a cold pack.
- What is meant by the latent heat of fusion? What role does it play in RICES?
- What is a phase change? How does it apply to cryotherapy?
- Briefly explain the temperature response to cold pack application. Consider surface, tissue, intra-articular, and rewarming after application.
- Briefly discuss each of the four major types of cold packs.
- Should ice be applied directly to the skin? Why or why not?
- What is meant by the depth of target tissue, and how does this apply to RICES?
- What effect does skin-fold thickness have on RICES?
- What is the basis for stretching an elastic wrap to 75% of its capacity when applying it?
- What is the difference between preventing and removing swelling?

- Explain the difference between continuous and intermittent compression. How is each is used?
- Briefly explain the use of crutches during acute orthopedic injury care. Say why and how you would use them.
- What is a medicated ice cup? Why and how is it used?
- Briefly review the five-step process for RICES application.

2. Write three to five questions for discussion with your class instructor, clinical instructor, classmates, and clinical colleagues.

3. Get together with classmates and quiz each other on the concepts of this chapter. Use the points in exercise 1 and questions you wrote for exercise 2 as a beginning. Explaining concepts out loud to others requires a deeper grasp of the material than feeling you understand it as you read.

4. Once you feel you understand the principles of application of RICES and crutch walking, practice applying RICES using the five-step approach with a classmate or clinical colleague. Also, fit crutches to a classmate or clinical colleague and instruct her in properly using them. Alternate applying the modalities to each other. When it is being applied to you, listen and observe carefully to determine whether your classmate is using proper application. Consult your notes when the modality is applied to you and for the first few times you apply the modality to another person. Continue practicing the application until you can do so without using your notes.

CRITICAL THINKING RESPONSES

Critical Thinking 5.1

The swing gait removes all weight from the injured limb, whereas with the three-point or walking gait, the patient uses the crutches to take enough weight off the injured limb that he can walk with a normal gait. As the injury heals, the crutches support less and less weight. It is a matter of total rest (undesirable) vs. relative rest (desirable). One case aggravates the injury and the other helps resolve it.

Critical Thinking 5.2

Agree: Cold application is the only element of RICES that limits additional injury. Thus, in a sense, it is a preventive measure. It also reduces pain and swelling (edema).

Disagree: Focusing attention on ice application might cause you to think rest, compression, elevation, and stabilization are not that important. This could potentially result in your not using these additional elements, which would be a big mistake. Each of these elements contributes to controlling the injury sequelae.

REFERENCES

1. Matsen FA III, Questad K, Matsen AL. The effect of local cooling on postfracture swelling. A controlled study. Clin Orthop 1975; 109:201–206.
2. Sloan JP, Hain R, Pownall R. Clinical benefits of early cold therapy in accident and emergency following ankle sprain. Arch Emerg Med 1989;6:1–6.
3. Bleakley C, McDonough S, MacAuley D. The use of ice in the treatment of acute soft-tissue injury. Am J Sports Med 2004;32:251–261.
4. Hubbard TJ, Aronson SL, Denegar CR. Does cryotherapy hasten return to participation? A systematic review. J Athl Train 2004;39: 88–94.
5. Basur RL, Shephard E, Mouzas GL. A cooling method in the treatment of ankle sprains. Practitioner 976;216:708–711.
6. Hocutt JE Jr, Jaffe R, Rylander CR, Beebe JK. Cryotherapy in ankle sprains. Am J Sports Med 1982;10:316–319.
7. Karren KJ, Hafen BQ, Limmer D, Mitstovich JJ. First Aid for Colleges and Universities. 8th ed. New York: Pearson, Benjamin Cummings, 2004.
8. Altizer L. Strains and sprains. Orthop Nurs 2003;22:404–411.
9. Bergfeld J, Halpern B. Sports Medicine: Functional Management of Ankle Injuries. Kansas City: American Academy of Family Physicians, 1991.
10. Garrett WE Jr. Muscle strain injuries: Clinical and basic aspects. Med Sci Sports Exerc 1990;22:436–443.
11. Bennett D. Water at 67 degrees to 69 degrees Fahrenheit to control hemorrhage and swelling encountered in athletic injuries. J Natl Athl Train Assoc 1961;1f:12-14.
12. Schwartz D, Kaplin KL, Schwartz SI. Hemostasis, surgical bleeding, and transfusion. In: Brunicardi FC, Andersen DK, Billiar TR, et al., eds. Schwartz's Principles of Surgery. 8th ed. New York: McGraw-Hill, 2005.
13. Holloway GA Jr., Daly CH, Kennedy D, Chimoskey J. Effects of external pressure loading on human skin blood flow measured by 133Xe clearance. J Appl Physiol 1976;40:597–600.
14. Merrick MA, Knight KL, Ingersoll CD, Potteiger J. The effects of cold and compression on tissue temperatures at various depths. J Athl Train 1993;28:236–245.
15. Hargens AR. Fluid shifts in vascular and extravascular spaces during and after simulated weightlessness. Med Sci Sports Exerc 1982; 15:421–427.
16. Kozin F, Cochrane CC. The contact activation system of plasma: Biology and pathophysiology. In: Gallin JI, Snyderman R, eds. Inflammation: Basic Principles and Clinical Correlates. 3rd ed. Baltimore: Lippincott Williams & Wilkins, 1999.
17. Knight KL. The effects of hypothermia on inflammation and swelling. Athl Train 1976;11:7–10.
18. Knight KL. Cryotherapy in Sport Injury Management. Champaign, IL: Human Kinetics, 1995.
19. Merrick MA. Secondary injury after musculoskeletal trauma: A review and update. J Athl Train 2002;37:209–217.
20. Seiyama A, Shiga T, Maeda N. Temperature effect on oxygenation and metabolism of perfused rat hindlimb muscle. Adv Exp Med Biol 1990;277:541–547.
21. Blair E. Clinical Hypothermia. New York: McGraw-Hill, 1964.
22. Abramson DI, Kahn A, Rejal H, et al. Relationship between a range of tissue temperature and local oxygen uptake in the human forearm. Lab Clin Med 1957;50:789.
23. Hagerdal M, Harp J, Nilsson L, Siesjo BK. The effect of induced hypothermia upon oxygen consumption in the rat brain. J Neurochem 1975;24:311–316.
24. Rosenfeldt FL. Myocardial preservation 1987: What is the state of the art? Aust N Z J Surg 1987;57:349–353.

25. Shapiro ML, Dunn DL. Transplantation. In: Brunicardi FC, Andersen DK, Billiar TR, et al., eds. Schwartz's Principles of Surgery. 8th ed. New York: McGraw-Hill, 2005.
26. Guyton AC, Hall JE. Textbook of Medical Physiology. 10th ed. Philadelphia: Saunders, 2000.
27. Levick JR, Michel CC. The effects of position and skin temperature on the capillary pressures in the fingers and toes. J Physiol 1978; 274:97–109.
28. Serway RA, Faughn JS, Vuille C. College Physics. 7th ed. Belmont, CA: Thomson-Brooks/Cole, 2006.
29. Fisher D, Solomon S. Therapeutic Heat and Cold. 2nd ed. Baltimore: Waverly, 1965.
30. Barcroft H, Edholm OG. The effect of temperature on blood flow and deep temperature in the human forearm. J Physiol 1943;102: 5–20.
31. Knight KL, Bryan KS, Halvorsen JM. Circulatory changes in the forearm during and after cold pack application and immersion in 1 degree C, 5 degrees C, and 15 degrees C water [Abstract]. Int J Sports Med 1981;1:2.
32. Lide DR. CRC Handbook of Chemistry and Physics. 86th ed. Boca Raton, FL: Chemical Rubber Co., 2005.
33. Varpalotai MA, Knight KL. Pressures exerted by elastic wraps applied by beginning vs advanced student athletic trainers to the ankle vs the thigh with vs without an ice pack. Athl Train 1991;26: 246–250.
34. Knight KL, Aquino J, Johannes SM, Urban CD. A re-examination of Lewis' cold-induced vasodilatation—In the finger and ankle. Athl Train 1980;15:248–250.
35. Knight K, Carmody LW. Rewarming of the ankle and forearm following 30 minutes of ice water immersion. Chattanooga, TN: NATA Annual Meeting, 1984.
36. Knight KL, Elam JE. Rewarming of the ankle, forearm, and finger after cryotherapy: Further re-examination of Lewis' cold-induced vasodilatation. J Can Athl Ther Ass 1981;8:15–17.
37. Palmer J, Knight K. Ankle and thigh skin surface temperature changes with repeated ice pack application. J Athl Train 1996;31: 319–323.
38. Mancuso DL, Knight KL. Effects of prior physical activity on skin surface temperature response of the ankle during and after a 30 minute ice pack application. J Athl Train 1992;27:242–249.
39. Post JB. Ankle skin temperature changes with a repeated ice pack application. Master's thesis, Indiana State University, Terre Haute, 1991.
40. Waylonis GW. The physiologic effects of ice massage. Arch Phys Med Rehabil 1967;48:37–42.
41. Enwemeka CS, Allen C, Avila P, et al. Soft tissue thermodynamics before, during, and after cold pack therapy. Med Sci Sports Exerc 2002;34:45–50.
42. Johannes SM. Temperature response during the warming phase of cryokinetics. Master's thesis, Indiana State University, Terre Haute, 1979.
43. Abramson DI, Chu LSW, Tuck S, et al. Effect of tissue temperature and blood flow on motor nerve conduction velocity. JAMA 1966; 198:1082–1088.
44. Halar EM, DeLisa JA, Brozovich FV. Nerve conduction velocity: Relationship of skin, subcutaneous intramuscular temperatures. Arch Phys Med Rehabil 1980;61:199–203.
45. Borken N, Bierman W. Temperature changes produced by spraying with ethyl chloride. Arch Phys Med Rehabil 1955;36:288–290.
46. Petajan JH, Watts N. Effects of cooling on the triceps surae reflex. J Am Phys Med 1962;41:240–251.
47. Ochs S, Smith C. Low temperature slowing and cold-block of fast axoplasmic transport in mammalian nerves in vitro. J Neurobiol 1975;6:85–102.

48. Lowdon BJ, Moore RJ. Determinants and nature of intramuscular temperature changes during cold therapy. Am J Phys Med 1975;54:223–233.

49. Otte JW, Merrick MA, Ingersoll CD, Cordova ML. Subcutaneous adipose tissue thickness alters cooling time during cryotherapy. Arch Phys Med Rehabil 2002;83:1501–1505.

50. Myrer WJ, Myrer KA, Measom GJ, et al. Muscle temperature is affected by overlying adipose when cryotherapy is administered. J Athl Train 2001;36:32–36.

51. Lehmann JF, DeLateur BJ. Diathermy and superficial heat, laser, and cold therapy. In: Kottke FJ, Lehman JF, eds. Krusen's Handbook of Physical Medicine and Rehabilitation. Philadelphia: Saunders, 1990.

52. Johnson DJ, Moore S, Moore J, Oliver RA. Effect of cold submersion on intramuscular temperature of the gastrocnemius muscle. Phys Ther 1979;59:1238–1242.

53. Bocobo C, Fast A, Kingery W, Kaplan M. The effect of ice on intra-articular temperature in the knee of the dog. Am J Phys Med 1991;70:181–185.

54. Wakim KG, Porter AN, Krusen FH. Influence of physical agents and of certain drugs on intra-articular temperature. Arch Phys Med Rehabil 1951;32:714–721.

55. McMaster W, Liddle S, Waugh T. Laboratory cryotherapy influence on posttraumatic limb edema. Clin Orthop Relat Res 1980;150:283–287.

56. Kern H, Fessl L, Trnavsky G, Hertz H. Kryotherapie: Das verlahten der gelenkstemperatur unter eisapplikation: Grundlage fur die praktishe anwendung. Wein Klin Wochenschr 1984;22:832–837.

57. Kim YH, Baek SS, Choi KS, et al. The effect of cold air application on intra-articular and skin temperatures in the knee. Yonsei Med J 2002;43:621–626.

58. Hartviksen K. Ice Therapy in spasticity. Acta Neurol Scand 1962;38:79–84.

59. Mlynarczyk JH. Skin temperature changes in the ankle during and after ice pack application of 10, 20, 30, 45, and 60 minutes. Master's thesis, Indiana State University, Terre Haute, 1984.

60. Bernards SA, Knight KL, Jutte LS. Surface and intramuscular temperature changes during ice and chemical cold pack application with and without a barrier [Abstract]. J Athl Train 2003;38:S95.

61. Boland AL. Rehabilitation of the injured athlete. In: Strauss RH, ed. Sports Medicine and Physiology. Philadelphia: Saunders, 1979.

62. Mirkin G. Hot and cold: When to apply each to a running injury. Runner. Aug 1980:22–23.

63. Belitsky RB, Odam SJ, Hubley-Kozey C. Evaluation of the effectiveness of wet ice, dry ice, and cryogen packs in reducing skin temperature. Phys Ther 1987;67:1080–1084.

64. Urban CD. Application of ice, compression, and elevation to the lateral aspect of the ankle. Master's thesis, Indiana State University, Terre Haute, 1979.

65. LaVelle BE, Snyder M. Differential conduction of cold through barriers. J Adv Nurs 1985;10:55–61.

66. Prentice WE. Arnheim's Principles of Athletic Training. 12th ed. St. Louis: McGraw-Hill, 2006.

67. Klafs CE, Arnheim DD. Modern Principles of Athletic Training. St. Louis: Mosby, 1977.

68. Wallace L, Knortz K, Esterson P. Immediate care of ankle injuries. J Orthop Sports Phys Ther 1979;1:46–50.

69. National Safety Council. First Aid and CPR Essentials. 98-103 ed. Sudbury, MA: Jones & Bartlett, 1997.

70. Thygerson A, Gulli B, eds. First Aid, CPR and AED. 4th ed. Sudbury, MA: Jones & Bartlett, 2005.

71. Proulx RP. Southern California frostbite. J Am Col Emerg Phys 1976;5:618.

72. Johnson N. The effects of three different ice bath immersion times on numbness (sensation of pressure), surface temperature, and perceived pain. Master's thesis, Brigham Young University, Provo, UT, 2003.

73. Wise D. Application of cold in treating soft tissue injury. Coaching Science Update 1979:53.

74. Hocutt JE Jr. Cryotherapy. Am Fam Physician 1981;23:141–144.

75. DePodesta M. Cryotherapy in rehabilitation. Can Athl Train Assoc J 1979;6:15–16.

76. Ork H. Physical Therapy for Sports. Philadelphia: Saunders, 1982.

77. Chu DA, Lutt CJ. The rationale of ice therapy. J Natl Athl Train Assoc 1969;4:8–9.

78. Hirata I. The Doctor and the Athlete. Philadelphia: Lippincott, 1974.

79. Drez D, Faust DC, Evans JP. Cryotherapy and nerve palsy. Am J Sports Med 1981;9:256–257.

80. Man IOW, Lepar GS, Morrissey MC, Cywinski JK. Effect of neuromuscular electrical stimulation on foot/ankle volume during standing. Med Sci Sports Exerc 2003;35:630–634.

81. Mora S, Zalavras CG, Wang L, Thordarson DB. The role of pulsatile cold compression in edema resolution following ankle fractures: A randomized clinical trial. Foot Ankle Int 2002;23:999–1002.

82. Rucinski TJ, Hooker DN, Prentice WE, et al. The effects of intermittent compression on edema in postacute ankle sprains. J Orthop Sports Phys Ther 1991;14:65–69.

83. Danielson R, Jaeger J, Rippetoe J, et al. Differences in skin surface temperature and pressure during the application of various cold and compression devices. J Athl Train 1997;32:S-76.

84. Duffley H, Knight K. Ankle compression variability using the elastic wrap, elastic wrap with a horseshoe, Edema II boot, and Air-Stirrup brace. Athl Train 1989;24:320–323.

85. Appenzeller H, Ross CT. Utah: Can a student trainer be held to the same standard of care of a physician or surgeon? Sports Courts 1984;5:11–13.

86. Harvey CK. An overview of cold injuries. J Am Podiatr Med Assoc 1992;82:436–438.

87. Keatinge W, Cannon P. Freezing-point of human skin. Lancet 1960;1:11–14.

88. Granberg P. Freezing cold injury. Arctic Med Res 1991;50:76–79.

89. Kendall Demonstration Elementary School Health Services, Gallaudet University. Severe allergic reaction: Hives (uticaria) protocol. Available at: clerccenter.gallaudet.edu/SupportServices/school nurse/hive1b.html. Accessed Jan 2006.

90. Dolan MG, Mendel FC. Clinical application of electrotherapy. Ath Ther Today 2004;9:11–16.

91. Ralston DJ. High voltage galvanic stimulation: Can there be a "state of the art"? Athl Train J Natl Athl Train Assoc 1985;20:291–293.

92. Dolan MG, Thornton RM, Fish DR, Mendel FC. Effects of cold water immersion on edema formation after blunt injury to the hind limbs of rats. J Athl Train 1997;32:233–237.

93. Dolan MG, Mychaskiw AM, Mattacola CG, Mendel FC. Effects of cool-water immersion and high-voltage electric stimulation for 3 continuous hours on acute edema in rats. J Athl Train 2003;38:325–329.

94. Dolan MG, Mychaskiw AM, Mendel FC. Cool-water immersion and high-voltage electric stimulation curb edema formation in rats. J Athl Train 2003;38:225–230.

95. McKeon PO, Dolan MG, Gandolph J, et al. Effects of dependent positioning, cool water immersion and high voltage electrical stimulation on non-traumatized limb volumes. J Athl Train 2003;38(2 suppl):S35.

96. Bettany JA, Fish DR, Mendel FC. Influence of high voltage pulsed direct current on edema formation following impact injury. Phys Ther 1990;70:219–224.

97. Bettany JA, Fish DR, Mendel FC. High-voltage pulsed direct current: Effect on edema formation after hyperflexion injury. Arch Phys Med Rehabil 1990;71:677–681.

98. Fish DR, Mendel FC, Schultz AM, Gottstein-Yerke LM. Effect of anodal high voltage pulsed current on edema formation in frog hind limbs. Phys Ther 1991;71:724–730.

99. Taylor K, Fish DR, Mendel FC, Burton HW. Effect of electrically induced muscle contractions on posttraumatic edema formation in frog hind limbs. Phys Ther 1992;72:127–132.

100. Mendel FC, Fish DR. New perspectives in edema control via electrical stimulation. J Athl Train 1993;28:63.

101. Taylor K, Mendel FC, Fish DR, et al. Effect of high-voltage pulsed current and alternating current on macromolecular leakage in hamster cheek pouch microcirculation. Phys Ther 1997;77:1729–1740.

102. Thornton RM, Mendel FC, Fish DR. Effects of electrical stimulation on edema formation in different strains of rats. Phys Ther 1998;78:386–393.

103. MacLeod J. Treating abrasions with medicated ice. Physician Sportsmed 1985;13(Oct):58.

CHAPTER OUTLINE

Sofia suffered a second-degree medial collateral ligament (MCL) sprain to her knee 2 days ago during basketball practice. She is concerned about her condition and asks you, "Why do I have all of this swelling, and when will it go away? How long until my ligament is healed, and what can I do to ensure that it heals as strongly as possible? When can I begin exercising?"

The Repair of Injured Tissue

Whenever tissue has been damaged during injury, it must be repaired. **Repair** consists of processes that replace dead or damaged cells with healthy ones.[1] Repair follows inflammation, after enough of the cellular debris has been removed to allow the repair processes to begin. Therefore, the bigger the hematoma, the longer it takes for repair to begin.

TYPES OF REPAIR: RECONSTITUTION AND REPLACEMENT

There are two types of repair: reconstitution with the same type of cells as those that were injured and replacement with simpler cells. **Reconstitution** occurs in cells that normally have a high rate of turnover (i.e., skin cells and liver cells). In, *perfect reconstitution,* the cells that were damaged are replaced by identical cells, and there remains no evidence that the injury occurred. In *imperfect reconstitution,* most of the damaged cells are replaced by identical cells, but there is some replacement with connective tissue and thus some scar formation.

Replacement with simpler cells results in scar tissue formation. It occurs in connective tissue, muscle tissue, central nervous system tissue, and in any area where the damage is extensive enough to disrupt the basic cellular framework. This type of repair is also known as *repair by connective tissue,* and it can be either primary union or secondary union. *Primary union* occurs in an area with a small incision, such as a 1/3 in. (1 cm) cut on the chin (Fig. 6.1). It fills and heals rapidly. *Secondary union* occurs when there is a large gap or hole to be filled, such as a 5 in. (13 cm) gaping laceration. Replacement is much slower and leaves a bigger scar.

CRITICAL THINKING 6.1 *Based on the information presented so far in this chapter, why is it important to close lacerations quickly after an injury? Why is it even more important to close them quickly when they are on the face?*

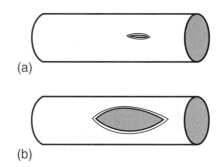

(a)

(b)

FIGURE 6.1. Replacement or repair by connective tissue. **(a)** Primary union occurs when the wound is small and the wound edges are close together. **(b)** Secondary union occurs when there is a large gap or hole to be filled, such as a 5 in. (13 cm) gaping laceration. Replacement is much slower and leaves a bigger scar.

The Phases of Repair

Like the inflammatory response (see Chapter 4), repair is a sequence of events (called phases) that follow one another but that can occur at the same time in different parts of the damaged area.[2] The four phases that constitute the repair process are

- Cellular
- Vascular
- Collagenization
- Contraction and restructuring

THE CELLULAR PHASE

The **cellular phase** of repair is the same as leukocyte migration and phagocytosis in the inflammatory response. Macrophages scavenger the cellular debris. The circulatory and lymphatic systems (mostly lymphatic) drain away the liquified cellular remains, which are mostly small particles of free protein. This is important because the more protein that remains, the bigger the scar that develops.[3]

Lymphatic Drainage and Exercise

The lymphatic system is passive; its vessel walls do not contract, nor is there any pressure to cause fluid to move through it, such as provided by the heart to the venous system. The lymphatic system depends on external force to promote fluid movement—for example, distal to proximal massage or muscular contraction. As a muscle expands in size during contraction, it squeezes the lymph vessels and forces their contents upstream toward their junction with the vascular system (see Fig. 5.19). Thus massage, intermittent compression pumps, or moderate activity during the cellular phase of repair will promote lymphatic drainage and hasten healing.

THE VASCULAR PHASE

The **vascular phase** is a transient phase during which lots of new blood vessels are formed (which later disappear). These vessels are necessary to deliver the great amounts of oxygen and nutrients to the wound area needed for repair. This phase usually takes 4–6 days.

A process known as **capillary budding** is the primary mechanism of the vascular phase of the repair process (Fig. 6.2). Endothelial cells of existing vessels at the edge of the wound begin to divide. The new cells crawl away from, but keep contact with, the existing vessel. New cells push themselves between existing cells, thus forcing the end cells to advance into the wound area.

Adjacent capillary buds migrate toward one another, meet, form together, and create a **capillary arch** (Fig. 6.3). Blood then begins to flow through the arch, and new budding begins from the arch. Soon a network of these arches, or a **capillary arcade**, is formed (Fig. 6.4). The network eventually develops throughout the entire wound area, providing abundant circulation, which is necessary to support collagenization.

Eventually, after collagenization has taken place and the need for abundant circulation has passed, most of the new vessels will atrophy. A few will form into arterioles, some into venules, and some will remain as capillaries.

THE COLLAGENIZATION PHASE

Collagenization is the process of manufacturing and laying down collagen in the wound space. **Collagen**, a fibrous protein found in all types of connective tissue, is the primary solid substance of ligaments, tendons, and scar tissue. It is made by fibroblasts, cells that migrate along strands of fibrin into the wound area; however, these cells do not move far beyond the capillary arcade. They then begin to manufacture fibers of collagen, which extrude haphazardly into the wound space (Fig. 6.5a). Within 4–6 days after the injury, vascularization is maximal, and collagenization is operating at its peak. Most collagen is laid down within 15–20 days after the injury.[4] The wound is not very strong yet; many of the fibers are diagonal or parallel to the wound edges and, therefore, provide little strength. In time, the collagen will realign parallel to the *lines of force*, making the wound strong (Fig. 6.5b). This realignment sometimes takes up to a year, especially if the patient is inactive.

Collagenization requires great amounts of oxygen.[5,6] Oxygen provides energy (through aerobic metabolism) for the fibroblasts and also is an essential building block of collagen. Healing wounds normally do not have all the oxygen that they could use (Fig. 6.6).[6] The amount of collagen accumulated in a wound area and the tensile strength of skin wounds are linearly related to the amount of oxygen available to the healing wound[8] (Fig. 6.7). **Tensile strength** is a measure of the amount of longitudinal stress a wound can withstand before tearing apart. Increasing the percentage of oxygen in the air breathed by injured laboratory rats between days 5 and 15 resulted in greater tensile strength of their wounds.[8]

THE CONTRACTION AND RESTRUCTURING PHASE

The **contraction and restructuring phase** refers to two processes that cause scar tissue to become smaller and

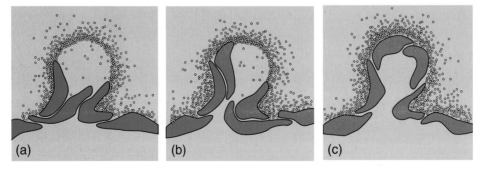

FIGURE 6.2. During capillary budding, new blood vessels are formed as the endothelial cells at a budding site on an existing vessel divide. **(a)** The cells slide past each other into **(b)** positions distal to their place of origin, **(c)** forming a bud.

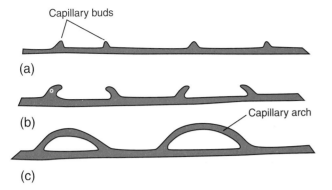

FIGURE 6.3. **(a)** Capillary arches are formed by numerous capillary buds along a vessel. **(b)** Initially, the buds grow randomly into the injured tissue, eventually moving toward each other where **(c)** they join to form a capillary arch. Once the arches form, blood begins flowing through them to supply fibroblasts and oxygen to rebuild the injured tissue.

paler (in light-skinned people). A new scar will appear to be quite red (in a light-skinned person) and mounded or raised above the surrounding tissue. With time, the appearance of the scar changes until it is pale and flat or sunken below the surrounding skin.

Contraction, the first process, is the collapsing of the capillary arcade. Collagen is a relatively inactive tissue; once it is laid down, it does not need much oxygen to satisfy its energy requirements and, therefore, does not need a great deal of circulation. Consequently, much of the capillary arcade collapses and is compressed by the surrounding collagen. This accounts for some of the contraction of the scar. Also, with less blood circulating through the wound, the scar appears paler.

In **restructuring,** the second process, the collagen itself is restructured. The collagen fibers are reorganized from the haphazard way they were laid down to a parallel arrangement (see Fig. 6.5b). This reorganization of fibers

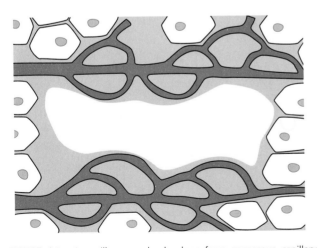

FIGURE 6.4. A capillary arcade develops from numerous capillary arches arising from blood vessels on the periphery of the injured tissue. Most of these new vessels will collapse once the tissue is healed and the need for oxygen drastically decreases.

causes the scar to become more compact, and thus concave. But compactness is not the major reason reorganization occurs.

Collagen fiber reorganization is necessary to give the scar greater strength. Fibers running parallel to the wound edges will not help keep the edges of the wound together. Only fibers connecting the wound edges strengthen the injured tissue.

Collagen restructuring occurs in response to force exerted on the scar. As the body part moves, the scar "senses" the direction of the movement and the collagen fibers line up parallel to the lines of force.[4] Thus active exercise is necessary to the final phase of wound healing, although activity that is too vigorous too early will tear an immature scar.

The Necessity of Exercise

Exercise is necessary during wound healing for two reasons. First, exercise stimulates circulation and thus increases oxygen delivery to the healing tissue. Second, exercise provides the lines of force that are essential for guiding collagen restructuring. Exercise must be controlled, however; too vigorous exercise will disrupt the healing tissue, whereas too little exercise will not provide adequate amounts of oxygen or stress for normal healing to occur. There is a fine line between the amount of exercise that optimizes tissue repair and that which compromises the repair process.

MODALITY **MYTH**

HEALING TISSUE MUST BE RESTED

Some people believe that healing tissue must be rested to prevent tearing the injured tissue. Although it is true that too vigorous exercise is counterproductive, complete rest will actually slow or prevent healing. Moderate, controlled exercise is essential for stimulating collagenization and restructuring of the injured tissue and for maintaining normal nerve function. It also is psychologically beneficial for the patient to be doing something other than waiting for healing to take place.

Healing Modifiers

The body's natural healing process can be facilitated (speeded up) or hindered (slowed down) in many ways. Obviously, your goal is to help the healing process, so you need to eliminate the hindrances and aid the facilitators. The following sections discuss the most common facilitators or modifiers.

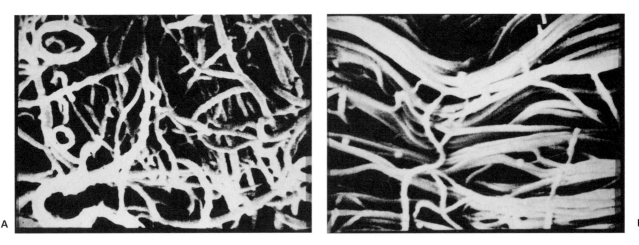

FIGURE 6.5. Electron-micrographs of human collagen. **(a)** New collagen fibers assemble haphazardly at first. **(b)** The same site weeks later after the collagen has realigned in a parallel fashion. Note how the new collagen appears like a plate of cooked spaghetti, while the more mature collagen looks more like uncooked spaghetti right out of the box. (Courtesy of John Bergfeld.)

IMMEDIATE CARE PROCEDURES

The size of the hematoma affects healing time in two ways: the smaller the hematoma is, the quicker repair can begin and the less there is to repair.[2] Can you affect the size of the hematoma? Yes! Aggressively treating the injury as soon after it occurs as possible (within minutes) can have a major influence (see Chapter 5).

CLOSING LACERATIONS QUICKLY

Lacerations must be sutured or treated with Steri-Strips to close the wound gap, thus allowing healing by primary union. For best results, these procedures should be done within 4–6 hr after the wound occurs.

Sutures, Steri-Strips, and Glue

Some surgeons avoid using sutures to close lacerations because implanting sutures into the tissue causes additional tissue injury and invokes additional inflammation as the body tries to destroy the sutures, which constitute a foreign substance. Steri-Strips (Fig. 6.8) or the newly developed tissue glue are less traumatic to the tissue. But they also are not as effective as sutures, especially for athletic injuries, when there are additional stresses on the tissue.

THERAPEUTIC EXERCISE

Therapeutic exercise can either facilitate or hinder healing (see Fig. 1.5). As we discussed earlier, exercise is essential

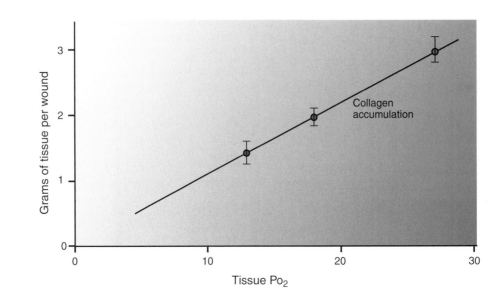

FIGURE 6.6. The need for oxygen in a healing wound is demonstrated by this graph of collagen accumulation and tissue oxygen partial pressure (Po_2). Note the linear relationship between collagen accumulation and Po_2, when Po_2 is less than normal, normal, and higher than normal. (Adapted with permission from Silver.[7])

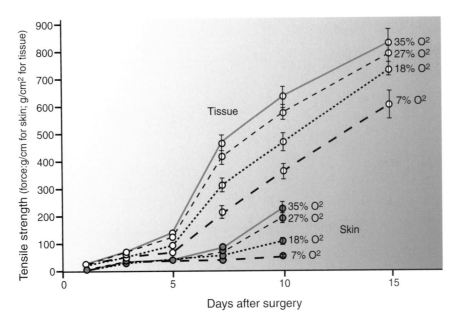

FIGURE 6.7. The effect of changing oxygen supply on wound healing. The more oxygen available, the stronger the wound becomes. (Adapted with permission from Niinikoski.[8] Reproduced with permission from the BMJ Publishing Group.)

to healing—to both stimulate blood flow during collagenization to bring more oxygen to the wound site and to stimulate and guide the reorienting of collagen fibers during the restructuring phase. Lack of exercise will delay healing. On the other hand, too vigorous exercise will tear the healing tissue and thus delay healing.

APPLICATION TIP

KNOW THE RIGHT EXERCISE AMOUNT. *How do you determine how much exercise is enough without going over the line? Remember two principles. First, pain must be avoided during rehabilitation. Pain during an activity tells you the patient is exercising too vigorously. Also, pain on the next day tells you that the previous day's exercise was too vigorous. In either case, reduce the amount of exercise. Second, use progressive resistance exercise. Many patients are reluctant to exercise, thinking exercise will disrupt the healing tissue. Encourage them to begin slow, simple range of motion (ROM) exercises and to progressively increase the complexity.*

THERAPEUTIC MODALITIES

The role of therapeutic modalities is to assist the body in its normal healing process (Table 6.1).[9] Some modalities accomplish this task by stimulating healing. Others pro-

mote lymphatic drainage, which hastens the cellular phase of the repair process. Still others moderate pain, thereby facilitating therapeutic exercise.

PROPER NUTRITION

Many vitamins and trace elements are essential to healing. Although there is no evidence that supplementing with extra amounts of these substances improves or accelerates healing, a lack of them will hinder the process. People who eat a healthy, normal, well-balanced diet do not need to supplement with multiple vitamins.

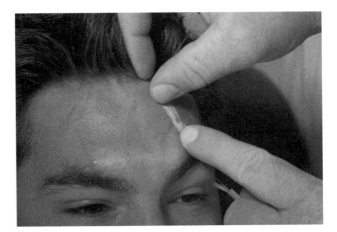

FIGURE 6.8. Steri-Strips are effective in holding small wounds together when there is not too much stress on the tissue.

TABLE 6.1 *The Role of Therapeutic Modalities in Wound Healing*	
THERAPEUTIC GOAL	**MODALITIES**
Stimulate the healing process	Ultrasound Electrical muscle stimulation Hot packs
Promote lymphatic drainage to hasten the cellular phase of the repair process	Massage Cryokinetics Edema pressure devices
Moderate pain, thereby facilitating therapeutic exercise	Cryokinetics Cryostretch Transcutaneous electrical nerve stimulation

CLOSING SCENE

Recall Sofia's questions concerning the healing of her second-degree MCL sprain? You now can give her answers. You tell her of your plan of action to get rid of the swelling. By decreasing the size of the hematoma, healing will take place faster. Then after completing a graded exercise program that is rigorous enough to lay down collagen without tearing it, she will be able to return to activity.

CHAPTER REFLECTIONS

1. Read and ponder each of the following points. Do you feel you have a clear understanding of each concept? If not, reread the appropriate section of the chapter.
   - Define repair and its four phases.
   - Explain the relationship between inflammation and repair.
   - Define the two types of repair and how they differ.
   - Explain why exercise is important during tissue repair and the phases of repair during which it is most beneficial.
   - Explain the difference between a capillary arch and a capillary arcade, and describe the role that each one plays in repair.
   - Explain why a scar is red (in light-skinned people) and mounded at one time and pale and sunken at others.
   - What are modifiers of inflammation? How can they help or hinder repair?

2. Write three to five questions for discussion with your class instructor, clinical instructor, classmates, and clinical colleagues.

3. Get together with classmates and quiz each other on the concepts of this chapter. Use the points in exercise 1 and questions you wrote for exercise 2 as a beginning. Explaining concepts out loud to others requires a deeper grasp of the material than feeling you understand it as you read.

CRITICAL THINKING RESPONSES

Critical Thinking 6.1

The quicker the laceration is closed, the smaller the scar is. The farther apart the wound edges are, the more collagen will be deposited in the space. Minimizing the size of scars is especially important on the face. But there are always some patients who feel scars are a badge of honor. Don't give patients a choice, just patch them up as quickly as possible.

REFERENCES

1. Chettibi S, Ferguson MWJ. Wound repair: an overview. In: Gallin JI, Snyderman R, eds. Inflammation: Basic Principles and Clinical Correlates. 3rd ed. Philadelphia: Lippincott Williams & Wilkins, 1999.

2. Hunt TK, Hopf H, Hussain Z. Physiology of wound healing. Adv Skin Wound Care 2000;13(2 suppl):6–11.

3. Kushner I, Rzewnicki D. Acute phase response. In: Gallin JI, Snyderman R, eds. Inflammation: Basic Principles and Clinical Correlates. 3rd ed. Philadelphia: Lippincott Williams & Wilkins, 1999.

4. Enwemeka CS. Inflammation, cellularity, and fibrillogenesis in regenerating tendon: Implications for tendon rehabilitation. Phys Ther 1989;69:816–825.

5. Niinikoski J. Oxygen and wound healing. Clin Plast Surg 1977;4:361–374.

6. Ehrlich HP, Grislis C, Hunt TK. Metabolic and circulatory contributions to oxygen gradients in wounds. Surgery 1972;72:578–583.

7. Silver IA. The measurement of oxygen tension in healing tissue. Progr Resp Res 1968;3:124–135.

8. Niinikoski J. Effect of oxygen supply on wound healing and formation of experimental granulation tissue. Acta Physiol Scand Suppl 1969;334:1–72.

9. Sussman C, Bates-Jensen B. Wound Care a Collaborative Practice Manual for Physical Therapists and Nurses. 2nd ed. Baltimore: Lippincott Williams & Wilkins, 2001.

Review Questions

Chapter 4

1. A clot is formed by _____ and platelets.
   a. fibrin
   b. collagen
   c. protocollagen
   d. fibroblasts
   e. both b and c

2. Which of the following cleans up most of the tissue debris during the inflammatory response?
   a. polymorph
   b. macrophage
   c. fibrin
   d. fibroblasts
   e. neutrophils

3. Which of the following is *not* a sign of inflammation?
   a. heat
   b. redness
   c. swelling
   d. loss of function
   e. all of the above are signs of inflammation

4. Opening of the endothelial walls of blood vessels and capillaries so that blood cells can move out of the blood vessel occurs during which event of inflammation?
   a. leukocyte migration
   b. metabolic changes
   c. neutrophilic changes
   d. vascular changes
   e. permeability changes

5. A local reaction of the body tissues to any irritant is called _____.
   a. primary injury
   b. secondary injury
   c. pathogenic
   d. inflammation
   e. none of the above

6. Contrast the amount of tissue debris in a wound 24 hr after the injury when ice is applied within 5 min after the injury occurred with the amount of tissue debris when ice is not used at all. If ice is used, the primary injury tissue debris will be _____ and the secondary injury tissue debris will be _____.
   a. less; less
   b. less; more
   c. less; the same
   d. the same; more
   e. the same; less

7. Secondary metabolic injury results from an imbalance between _____.
   a. metabolism and oxygen delivery
   b. metabolism and inflammation
   c. inflammation and oxygen delivery
   d. enzymatic injury and edema
   e. none of the above

Chapter 5

1. Ice, compression, and elevation are indicated for the immediate care of acute injury. What does elevation do that is most beneficial in swelling control?
   a. decreases tissue oncotic pressure
   b. decreases secondary injury
   c. decreases capillary hydrostatic pressure
   d. decreases tissue hydrostatic pressure
   e. decreases external pressure force

2. Which of the following components of capillary filtration pressure is changed the most during the 24 hr after an acute injury as a result of cold pack application immediately after the injury?
   a. capillary hydrostatic
   b. tissue hydrostatic
   c. tissue oncotic   ↓ed metabolism
   d. capillary oncotic
   e. external

3. Swelling _____.
   a. and edema mean the same thing
   b. and inflammation and edema mean the same thing
   c. is a sign of inflammation and edema
   d. is a sign of edema but not of inflammation
   e. none of the above

4. The most important physiological effect of cold applications during the immediate care of acute injuries is _____.
   a. decreased circulation
   b. decreased pain
   c. decreased inflammation
   d. decreased metabolism
   e. decreased tissue elasticity

5. Which of the following should be applied directly to the skin during immediate care procedures?
   a. ice packs Crushed ice pack
   b. cold packs
   c. a wet elastic wrap
   d. a frozen elastic wrap
   e. none of the above

6. During immediate care procedures, compression should be applied to the injury _____.
   a. continuously for 2 hr
   b. continuously until bedtime
   c. for 30 min every 2 hr until bedtime
   d. for 30 min every hour for the first 24 hr
   e. continuously for at least 24 hr

Chapter 6

1. The forming of new blood vessels is known as _____.
   a. collagenization
   b. cascading
   c. capillary budding
   d. arching
   e. both a and c

2. The phase of repair during which fibroblasts manufacture collagen cells is known as the _____ phase.
   a. cellular
   b. vascular

   c. manufacturing
   d. arching
   e. none of the above

3. Fibroblasts usually lay down collagen _____.
   a. parallel to the wound edges
   b. parallel to the bones
   c. parallel to the lines of force
   d. perpendicular to the lines of force
   e. haphazardly

4. The rate of the contraction or restructuring phase of wound repair can be increased by _____.
   a. increasing the oxygen delivery to the wound
   b. using moderate exercise
   c. using vigorous exercise
   d. both a and b
   e. both a and c

5. Oxygen is important during wound healing because it is used _____.
   a. for energy production
   b. as a raw material for collagen production
   c. to promote capillary arcading
   d. to prevent secondary metabolic injury
   e. both a and b

6. Moderate exercise is _____ during wound healing because it _____.
   a. important; stimulates circulation and, therefore, more oxygen is delivered to the wound
   b. important; stresses the tissue and, therefore, guides restructuring
   c. detrimental; stresses the tissue and, therefore, causes reinjury
   d. detrimental; uses up the oxygen so the wound can't heal
   e. both a and b

Understanding Pain and Its Relationship to Injury

Coach Jiminez comes into the high school athletic therapy clinic, where you are interning as a student, to check up on her basketball players before practice. She notices Sofia with hot packs on her knees. "What's wrong?" she asks, "Nothin' coach, it just helps the pain and stiffness go away." She then notices Nikki sitting with her foot in a bucket of ice water. "How's that ankle sprain?" she asks. "It's really improving, I can jog without pain after icing it, Coach. At this rate I'll be practicing in a couple of days." Madison is on a treatment table with an electrical simulator hooked up to her sore elbow. The coach then notices Rachel talking to one of the clinicians about her back. "Is it pain or is it an injury?" Coach Jiminez asks. Then she thinks to herself, "These people sure treat pain in a lot of different ways."

What Is Pain?

Pain is the number one reason an athlete or patient seeks treatment.[1] Everyone knows what pain is, but few can explain it. In fact, some claim that pain has not been adequately defined or objectively measured. Imagine trying to describe the taste of salt to someone who has never tasted it. "Gee, it isn't sweet, and it isn't sour—it's salty." It's very difficult to describe the flavor of salt, but once you've tried it (especially in excess), you know what it tastes like. The same can be said for pain. It is difficult to analyze and evaluate either pain physiology or pain relief.

MODALITY MYTH

PAIN IS A STIMULUS-RESPONSE MECHANISM

Many people incorrectly think that pain is a simple stimulus-response mechanism, that injured tissue stimulates a signal that is sent to the brain where it is interpreted as pain. It also is incorrect to think that the level of pain one feels is a direct result of the amount of tissue damage. Pain and the perception of pain are much more complex than the concept of a simple, rigid, stimulus-response system accounts for. To properly manage pain, you must think of it in a much broader context: as a social, emotional, psychological experience that modulates or modifies the pain-inducing stimulus.

There are several definitions of *pain*. We find this one to be the most useful: **Pain** is an unpleasant sensory and emotional experience associated with actual or potential tissue damage or described in terms of such damage.[2] Most people think of pain in the traditional sense, as a specific response to stimulation by neural input. It is evident now, however, that pain is a multidimensional response to multidimensional stimuli.[3–5]

THE FUNCTION OF PAIN

Pain is both good and bad. Its main purpose is good, but prolonged pain may result in disability, atrophy, circulatory deficiency, and loss of skill (see Chapter 8). Pain plays three main positive roles:

- Pain serves as a warning for withdrawal. For example, when you touch a hot object, pain from the heat causes you to immediately pull your hand away.
- Pain alerts a person that something is wrong. For example, the classic arch pain of plantar fasciitis that someone experiences when first getting out of bed in the morning is a warning sign. If the pain continues to nag the person for several mornings, the pain will prompt him to see a qualified medical professional.
- Pain protects the injured part of the body through muscle guarding (muscle spasm). When a musculoskeletal injury occurs, muscle spasm or guarding usually accompanies the pain. In a sense, the body splints itself to prevent further injury (Fig. 7.1).

A Brief Review of Neuroanatomy and Neurophysiology

This brief review of neuroanatomy and neurophysiology focuses on the terminology necessary for understanding pain and pain relief.

NERVOUS SYSTEM DEFINITIONS: ANATOMY

A. **Central nervous system (CNS):** The brain and spinal cord

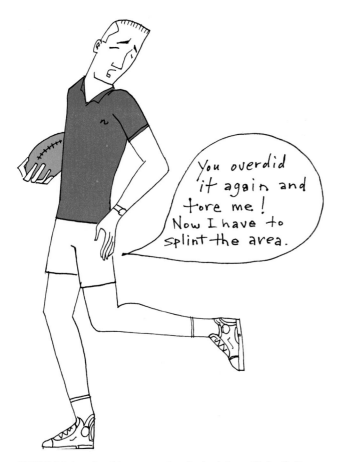

FIGURE 7.1. Imagine this conversation the body has with itself after an injury to a 40-year-old weekend warrior in a backyard game of neighborhood flag football: "All right, you old duff—you overdid it again and tore your hamstring. That will teach ya. I guess I'll send a protective muscle spasm down that leg so you don't damage more muscle fibers."

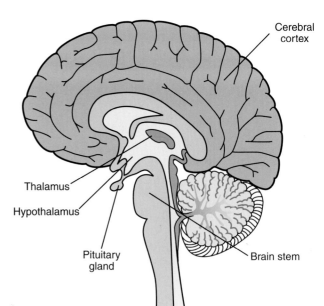

FIGURE 7.2. The brain and brainstem, showing the hypothalamus, thalamus, pituitary, and cerebral cortex.

1. **Hypothalamus:** About the size of a pea, the part of the brain that mainly acts as a central monitoring and control station in a variety of the body's activities. It regulates the functions of the autonomic nervous system and also appears to play a role in mood and motivational states (Fig. 7.2).
2. **Thalamus:** A pair of egg-shaped structures at the top of the brainstem that serves as the main relay center of the brain. Sensations from all the sense organs except the nose are sent to the thalamus, which analyzes the information and relays it on to the higher levels of the brain (cerebral cortex). For example, sensations such as heat, cold, pain, and touch travel along nerves throughout the body to the thalamus, which then sends the signals to the cerebral cortex (Fig. 7.2).
3. **Cerebral cortex:** The outer part of the brain. It has numerous functions; with respect to pain, it coordinates the signals and determines the intensity and location of the pain. The cerebral cortex also initiates descending pain control mechanisms.
4. **Neuron:** The basic functional unit of the nervous system, also called a nerve cell. Its main components are the cell body, dendrites, the axon, and branches that end in axon terminals or twigs (Fig. 7.3). Stimulation of any part of the neuron causes an electrical signal to spread to all parts of the cell.
5. **Nerve fiber:** The axon of a single neuron, or nerve cell, and its multiple dendrites
6. **Nerve:** A bundle of nerve fibers that transmits information via electrical signals among the brain, spinal cord, and other parts of the body
7. **Tract:** A bundle of nerve fibers in the CNS with a common origin, termination, and function. Tracts, also called pathways, can flow in either of two directions:
    a. Descending tracts transmit information from the brain down the spinal cord.
    b. Ascending tracts transmit information up the spinal cord to the brain.
B. **Peripheral nervous system (PNS):** Cranial and spinal nerves
    1. **Sensory nerves:** Nerves that transmit impulses from the periphery of the body to the CNS
    2. **Somatic motor nerves:** Nerves that transmit impulses from the CNS to the periphery of the body and terminate in skeletal muscle. They are controlled voluntarily or through reflex action.
    3. **Autonomic motor nerves:** Nerves that transmit impulses from the CNS to the periphery of the

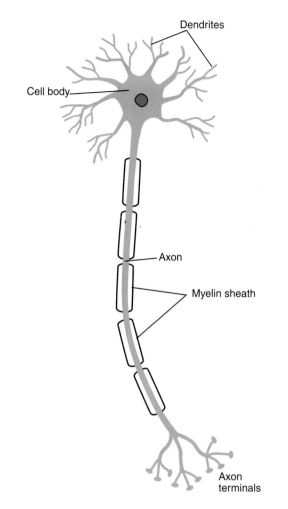

Dendrites

Cell body

Axon

Myelin sheath

Axon terminals

FIGURE 7.3. The main parts of a neuron are dendrites, which receive stimuli from another nerve; the cell body, which receives impulses from the dendrites; the axon, which sends impulses to another location; and branches ending in axon terminals, which release neurotransmitter molecules that either stimulate or inhibit a response in the receiving neuron.

body and terminate in smooth muscle, cardiac muscle, glands, and organs. They are controlled involuntarily.

NERVOUS SYSTEM DEFINITIONS: PHYSIOLOGY

A. **Autonomic nervous system (ANS):** The part of the peripheral nervous system that controls smooth muscle, cardiac muscle, organs, and glands. It is referred to as *self-controlling* because it functions involuntarily and reflexively. The ANS consists of two physiologically and anatomically distinct, mutually antagonistic branches: sympathetic and parasympathetic.

1. **Sympathetic nervous system:** The branch of the ANS that regulates the body's fight-or-flight responses, such as increased heart rate, resulting from stress

2. **Parasympathetic nervous system:** The branch of the ANS that regulates the rest and digest responses, such as decreased heart rate and secretion of digestive enzymes

B. **Somatic nervous system (SNS):** Somatic motor nerves and sensory nerves.

1. **Afferent nerve:** A sensory nerve. It enters the spinal cord via the dorsal horn (Fig. 7.4).

2. **Efferent nerve:** A motor nerve. It exits the spinal cord via the ventral horn.

3. **Dorsal horn:** The posterior portion of the gray matter of the spinal cord, also called the posterior horn. Afferent nerves enter the spinal cord through the dorsal horn.

4. **Ventral horn:** The anterior portion of the gray matter of the spinal cord, also called the anterior horn. Efferent nerves exit the spinal cord through the ventral horn.

5. **Synapse:** The junction between two neurons; the space between the axon terminal of a presynaptic neuron and the cell body or dendrite of a postsynaptic neuron. Impulses can cross the synapse in one direction only.

   a. **Neurotransmitters:** Chemicals that transmit an impulse across a synapse. Neurotransmitter molecules are released by the axon terminals and fit into specific receptors on the cell body or dendrites of the postsynaptic neuron, where they either stimulate or inhibit a response.

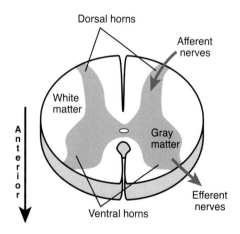

Dorsal horns

Afferent nerves

White matter

Anterior

Gray matter

Efferent nerves

Ventral horns

FIGURE 7.4. The spinal cord consists of thousands of individual nerve fibers. Some fibers are covered with myelin, a white insulating substance that makes areas appear white. In the spinal cord, the white matter is myelinated axons. The gray matter is unmyelinated axons plus neuron cell bodies and dendrites. The pattern of the four areas of unmyelinated fibers makes the gray matter appear to have horns. The dorsal horns are the two horns at the posterior side of the cord. The ventral horns are the two horns at the anterior side. Afferent nerves enter the spinal cord via the dorsal horns and efferent nerves exit the spinal cord via the ventral horns.

b. **Lock and key:** A metaphor for the way neurotransmitters have unique shapes that fit specific receptors on dendrites, like a key fits into a lock (Fig. 7.5). Thus impulses cross a synapse only on the release of the specific neurotransmitter that fits the specific receptor.

6. **Stimulus:** The action of one agent on another (e.g., nerve, muscle) that evokes activity in the receiving structure or agent. The activity does not have to be gross activity; it may be nothing more than a change in permeability in a membrane.

   a. **Noxious stimulus:** A harmful, unhealthy stimulation. Pain is caused by noxious stimuli.

   b. **Threshold:** The minimal point at which a stimulus begins to produce a gross response (psychological or physiological). Individual neurons respond in an all-or-none fashion, so the gross response in a single neuron is the same when the stimulus just barely exceeds a threshold level as it is when the stimulus is many times greater than threshold. Remember, however, that there are many individual neurons with different thresholds within a given area, and a greater stimulus may also evoke a response in adjacent neurons whose threshold is higher. With more nerves responding, the response in the whole tissue is greater.

   c. **Subthreshold stimulus:** Stimulation below the threshold level. It does not evoke a response, but it does cause a change in the electrical activity of the tissue.

7. **Response:** A reaction, such as contraction of a muscle or secretion of a gland, that results from stimulation that exceeds threshold.

8. **Summation:** A process by which subthreshold stimuli add together to evoke a response

   a. **Temporal summation:** Summed over time. This summation occurs when a number of subthreshold stimuli from the same axon are

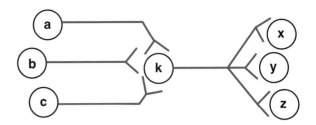

FIGURE 7.6. A simplified model of neural transmission and summation. In reality, there are numerous neurons and thousands of axon terminals and dendrites at each synapse. In this model, neurons *a, b,* and *c* synapse with neuron *k,* which in turn synapses with neurons *x, y,* and *z.* Spatial summation occurs if subthreshold stimuli from a, b, and c all arrive at k simultaneously; if the sum of their individual stimuli (the neurotransmitters) is greater than k's threshold, k will respond and send impulses to x, y, and z.

repeated one after another before the effect of the previous stimulus has dissipated.

   b. **Spatial summation:** Summed over space. This summation occurs when a number of subthreshold stimuli from different axons converge on one cell body simultaneously (Fig. 7.6).

9. **Facilitation:** Enabling a neural response. For instance, during summation, subthreshold stimuli from one neuron make it easier for another neuron to stimulate a postsynaptic neuron by releasing neurotransmitter molecules into the synapse, thereby partially activating the postsynaptic neuron.

10. **Inhibition:** Restraining or repressing a neural response. If, during summation, a presynaptic neuron releases a substance into the synapse that deactivates the neurotransmitter, it will negate the effects of some neurons, thereby preventing impulse transmission or at least making it harder.

11. **Positive feedback:** Activity on a neuron that eventually is returned through a neural network, thereby facilitating further activity on that neuron (Fig. 7.7).

12. **Negative feedback:** Activity on a neuron that eventually is returned through a neural network, thereby inhibiting further activity on that neuron (Fig. 7.7).

Orthopedic Injury Pain

Now that you have been briefed on the anatomy and physiology of the nervous system, let's trace the pathway of pain through your body after an injury (Fig. 7.8). Imagine you are putting the shot and accidentally drop the 8 lb piece of iron on your big toe. The pain signal begins with

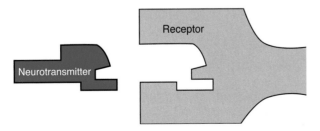

FIGURE 7.5. Lock and key. Neurotransmitters have specific shapes that fit specific receptors, much like a key fitting into a lock. Thus not all neurotransmitters activate all receptors.

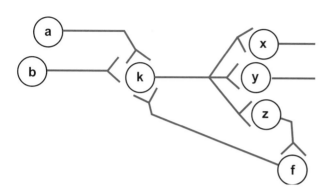

FIGURE 7.7. Positive feedback. Neurons *a* and *b* sum to stimulate neuron *k*, which stimulates neurons *x, y,* and *z*. Neuron *z* stimulates neuron *f*, which then sums with either a or b to stimulate or inhibit k (depending on whether f releases facilitatory or inhibitory neurotransmitters). If f is facilitatory, either a or b can stimulate k by itself, once the initial stimulus begins the feedback loop. Negative feedback occurs if f inhibits k, in which case the sum of neurons a and neuron b would not reach threshold and k would not be stimulated.

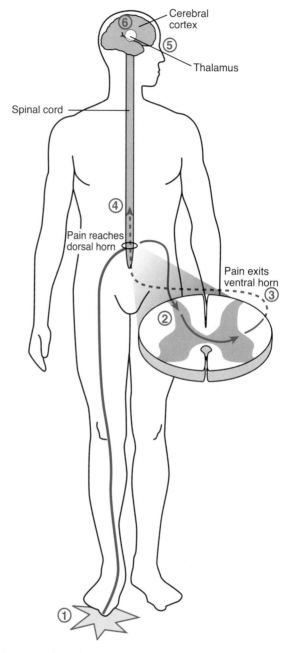

FIGURE 7.8. The pathway that pain travels through the body. The pain signal from (*1*) the injured toe travels as an electrochemical impulse along the nerve up the entire length of the leg. Continuing to (*2,3*) the dorsal and ventral horns of the spinal cord, the signal is then relayed up (*4*) the spinal cord to (*5*) the thalamus and then to (*6*) the cerebral cortex.

the release of potent chemicals stored near nerve endings in your big toe. These chemicals transmit the pain signal from the injured toe as an electrochemical impulse along the nerve, up the entire length of your leg. It continues to the dorsal horn of the spinal cord, a region that runs the length of the spine and receives signals from all over the body.

From there, the signal is relayed up the spinal cord to the thalamus where sensations such as heat, cold, touch, and pain first become noticeable. However, you don't know where the pain is located; you only know that there is pain somewhere in your body.

From the thalamus, the pain signal is relayed to the cerebral cortex, where the exact *location* and *intensity* of the pain are determined. Bystanders might hear you exclaim, "I have pain in my right big toe, and it hurts like heck!" This whole process seems to occur in an instant; the impulse travels from the toe to the brain at an estimated speed of 33 miles per hour![6]

Additional manifestations of this injury could include any or all of the following: jerking your leg, rubbing your toe, shaking your foot, swearing (or wanting to swear), dancing a jig, feeling nauseous, and vomiting. And 6 months later, dropping the shot near the toe could cause all these same responses, even if it did not hit your toe.

NOCICEPTION AND NOCICEPTORS

The ability to feel pain is called **nociception**. It occurs in response to being stimulated by a **nociceptor**, a sensory receptor that responds to pain. Although they are closely related, pain and nociception are not the same.[7] Nociception is a neurophysiological event-specific activity in afferent nerve pathways that conveys information about tissue damage or other painful stimuli to the brain. Pain, on the other hand, is a subjective, emotional experience that results from the modulation of nociception by a host of factors, including heredity, psychosocial experience, prior pain experience, and general life stress. Pain can also occur without a nociceptive stimulus.

Most nociceptors are cutaneous receptors (receptors in the skin), attached to a peripheral nerve.[8] The two most common nociceptors are:

- **Mechanical nociceptors:** Lightly myelinated **A-delta fibers**, activated primarily by strong mechanical displacement of the skin; also called high-threshold mechanoreceptors
- **Polymodal nociceptors:** Unmyelinated **C fibers**, activated by several different types of stimuli, such as heat, mechanical pressure, and inflammatory chemical mediators produced by tissue injury

In addition, nociceptors have been found in every organ and joint capsule of the body.[8] They are stimulated by **endogenous** (internal) chemicals and by mechanical forces. Tables 7.1 and 7.2 show classification systems for peripheral nerves.

COMMON NOXIOUS STIMULI THAT CAUSE PAIN

Various types of stimuli can result in pain. Each of the following stimuli stimulates nociceptors, which are attached to sensory nerves that carry pain signals to the CNS:

- *Mechanical stimulus:* Stimulation caused by pressure put on a nerve, often the result of swelling or muscle spasm, is caused by a mechanical stimulus. This is the most frequent type of noxious stimulus seen in sports medicine
- *Thermal stimulus:* An example of thermal stimulus is stimulation caused by radiant heat, such as the ultraviolet rays of the sun or a burn from touching a hot object.
- *Electrical stimulus:* Touching a hot wire and feeling the buzz from poor grounding of a light socket are examples of mild electrical stimuli.
- *Chemical stimulus:* During the inflammatory response, chemical mediators transmit pain through the body to

alert you that something is wrong (see Chapter 4). One of these chemicals is bradykinin, probably the most painful substance known. Its molecular composition resembles that of snake venom, and just a tiny amount inserted under the skin with a needle can cause excruciating pain.

TYPES OF PAIN

There are several types of pain. Each type is classified according to cause, duration, and intensity.

- **Acute pain** is caused by the activation of nociceptors from external sources (e.g., a contusion or broken bones) or internal sources (e.g., a muscle strain or appendicitis). Acute pain is brief, short term (minutes to days), and often of rapid onset. Many describe acute pain as being of high intensity.
- **Chronic pain** persists beyond the usual course of an acute disease or a reasonable time for an injury to heal (weeks to years). It is also associated with a chronic pathological process that causes continuous pain or in which the pain recurs at intervals for months to years. Often it is pain that is not related to or located at the underlying tissue trauma.

Table 7.3 lists the different effects that acute and chronic pain have on the body.

- **Referred pain** is pain at a site other than the actual location of a trauma. Referred pain tends to be projected outward from the source and distally along the extremities or to the shoulders if the pain is from an injury to an abdominal organ such as the spleen or liver. It is perceived in an area that often seems to have little relation to the pathology. For example, a ruptured spleen will often refer pain to the left shoulder. The site of the referred pain is called a **trigger point**.

TABLE 7.1	*Peripheral Nerve Classification: Letter System*		
TYPE OF FIBER	**DIAMETER (μM)**	**CONDUCTION VELOCITY (M/SEC)**	**GENERAL FUNCTION**
A			
Alpha	13–22	70–120	α-Motor neurons, muscle spindle primary endings, Golgi tendon organs, touch
Beta	8–13	40–70	Touch, kinesthesia, muscle spindle secondary endings
Gamma	4–8	15–40	Touch, pressure, gamma motor neurons
Delta	1–4	5–15	Pain, crude touch, pressure, temperature
B	1–3	3–14	Preganglionic* autonomic
C	0.1–1	0.2–2	Pain, touch, pressure, temperature, postganglionic* autonomic

Preganglionic means from the central nervous system to the ganglia (a group of nerves outside the central nervous system). Postganglionic means from the ganglia to the periphery.

Adapted with permission from Mann.[9]

TABLE 7.2	*Peripheral Nerve Classification: Roman Numeral System*		
TYPE OF FIBER	**DIAMETER (µM)**	**CONDUCTION VELOCITY (M/SEC)**	**GENERAL FUNCTION**
Ia	12–20	70–120	Muscle spindle primary endings
Ib	11–19	66–114	Golgi tendon organs
II	5–12	20–50	Touch, kinesthesia, muscle spindle secondary endings
III	1–5	4–20	Pain, crude touch, pressure, temperature
IV	0.1–2	0.2–3	Pain, touch, pressure, temperature

Adapted with permission from Mann.[9]

- **Radiating pain** originates from an irritated nerve root and travels along that particular nerve's **dermatome** (area of skin innervated by a particular nerve). (An understanding of radiating pain is essential for proper electrode placement when administering electrotherapy; see Chapter 10.)

APPLICATION TIP

CHRONIC PAIN IS MORE DIFFICULT TO TREAT THAN ACUTE PAIN. *Chronic pain is much more difficult to treat because it often involves more social, emotional, psychological input than acute pain does. As such, chronic pain can be perpetuated with much less tissue damage. It is important to manage acute pain aggressively so that it doesn't become chronic pain.*

Theories About Pain

Many theories have been proposed to explain responses to noxious (painful) stimuli. Each has adequately explained the knowledge about pain at the time of its inception. But as additional knowledge about pain has been gained, each theory has been proven to be inadequate, and a newer theory is developed that is consistent with all pain knowledge. Because aspects of each major theory carry forward and are part of newer theories, we present the main ideas of the most important theories.

THE SPECIFICITY THEORY OF PAIN

The specificity theory stated that when specific nociceptors in the periphery of the body are stimulated, the impulse is carried to the brain via nerve pathways, resulting in pain.[10] Specific receptors are a physiological fact, but the direct connection between stimulation of the receptors and pain is a weakness of the theory. This theory cannot explain **phantom limb pain**, why people react differ-

TABLE 7.3	*The Effects of Acute and Chronic Pain on the Body*	
DESCRIPTOR	**ACUTE PAIN**	**CHRONIC PAIN**
Biological function	Warning	None
Time frame	<1 month	>1 month
Nerve fiber transmission	A-δ	C fiber
Patient localization	Well localized and defined	Poorly localized
Psychological and environmental influences	Minor role	Prominent role
Verbal descriptors	Sensory (shooting, hot, sharp)	Emotional or motivational
Most frequent affective problem	Anxiety	Abnormal illness or behavior
Symptoms and dysfunction	Present, easily identifiable	Absent or can't identify
Drug intake	None to appropriate use	Misuse and addiction
Physical activity	Diminished with gradual return	Diminished to absent
Social activity	Diminished with gradual return	Diminished to absent
Probability of divorce	Same as average norms	High
Suicide attempt or consideration	No	Yes

Adapted with permission from Mann.[9]

ently to pain, or how people and animals can be trained to react favorably to noxious stimuli (e.g., Pavlov's dogs).

THE PATTERN THEORY OF PAIN

The pattern theory was developed as a reaction against the specificity theory; it denies the existence of pain receptors and suggests that pain occurs when the rate and pattern of sensory input exceeds a threshold.[10] According to this theory, the intensity of nociceptive stimulation evokes a pattern of impulses in nonspecific receptors that is interpreted by the brain as pain. Moreover, a slowly conducting nerve fiber system carries pain, and normally this system (and thus pain) is inhibited by a rapidly conducting nerve fiber system. In pathological conditions, the intensity of stimulation in the slow system becomes much greater, dominates over the fast system, and results in pain.

There are two main problems with the pattern theory. It is too general, and it does not account for the physiological evidence for the high degree of receptor-nerve specialization. For example, when the eyes (a sensory receptor) are stimulated, they send impulses to the brain via the optic nerve.

THE GATE CONTROL THEORY OF PAIN

Proposed in 1965 by Melzack and Wall,[10] the gate control theory integrates the specificity and pattern theories. Operating at the spinal level, the **gate control theory of pain** proposes a gating mechanism, located in the dorsal horn of the spinal cord, that allows only one sensation at a time to pass through to the brain (Fig. 7.9). Pain and other sensory stimuli travel along both large-diameter and small-diameter nerve fibers. They converge at the **T cell**, which is the gate. The T cell determines which impulse will continue up or down the spinal cord and subsequently to other parts of the body (the action system), where various actions will be invoked.

Sharp, stinging pain travels along large fibers, whereas dull, aching pain travels along small fibers. Other sensations travel along both fiber types. Strong sensory stimulation can control pain by closing the gate to pain, as the gate (the T cell) opens to allow the other sensory stimuli to pass through to the action system.

Another aspect of the gate control theory is an inhibitory mechanism located in the **substantia gelatinosa (SG)** in the dorsal horn of the spinal cord. The SG sends inhibitory neurons to the T cell; it is always active, constantly providing background inhibition to the T cell (this is one reason people react differently to the same noxious stimuli). The SG receives stimuli from both large and small fibers; but the stimuli are different, so the two types

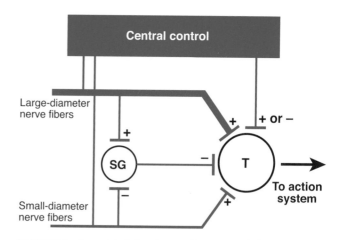

FIGURE 7.9. A model of the three main aspects of the gate control theory of pain. First, both large-diameter and small-diameter afferent nerve fibers facilitate the T cell, which transmits the signal to the action system. Second, a group of cells in the substantia gelatinosa (SG) of the dorsal horn constantly sends inhibitory signals to the T cell. SG cells are facilitated by large sensory nerves and inhibited by small sensory nerves. Third, central control, located in the brain, can either facilitate (+) or inhibit (−) T cell transmission. Central control receives signals from both large and small fibers.

of fibers have different effects on the SG. Large-fiber stimulation facilitates the SG, thus increasing its effects on the T cell (increases its inhibition). Small-fiber stimulation inhibits the SG, thereby decreasing its effects on the T cell (decreases its background inhibition).

The gate control theory also proposes the concept of *central control*, which influences the gating mechanism and therefore the action system. The idea is that pain centers in the brain collect and integrate information from multiple sources, such as memory, vision, smell, and hearing as well as the large-fiber and small-fiber nociceptive and other sensory information. Based on the integrated information, central control can either inhibit or facilitate the T cell, thereby intensifying or decreasing the response to pain. (Central control is discussed in more detail later in this chapter.)

The gate control theory led to the development and use of **transcutaneous electrical nerve simulators (TENS)** (Fig. 7.10). In turn, responses to TENS revealed several problems with the gate control theory of pain:

- Migraine headache is often relieved by TENS application to the temples. But because the temples are not anatomically related to the spinal column, there is no gating mechanism.

- The gate control theory indicates that you must stimulate the exact dermatome serving the site of pain. However, sometimes the placing of electrodes several dermatome levels above or below the pain site is effective in relieving pain.

- There seems to be a memory associated with chronic pain. Sometimes pain is reduced several hours or days

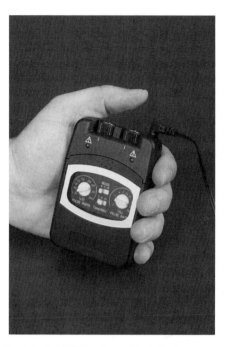

FIGURE 7.10. A typical TENS unit, used to help decrease or change a person's awareness of pain.

after TENS application, rather than during application when the gate should be active.

- Some people are born without the ability to perceive pain, yet they have an overabundance of nociceptors.

Does this mean the gate control theory is wrong and should be discarded? No! Even though some of the details are inaccurate, the concept is solid. Like other major theories in science, the gate control theory contains a key conceptual idea that has a powerful effect on pain research, pain theory, and health care. Many of the basic tenets of the gate control theory remain part of today's established pain theories. As one scholar noted concerning the gate control theory, "ideas need to be fruitful, they do not have to be right."[11] Following are the three major contributions of the gate control theory:

- The dorsal horns are not merely passive transmission stations but sites where the dynamic activities of inhibition, excitation, and modulation occur.
- Pain cannot be explained by peripheral factors alone.
- The brain is an active system that filters, selects, and modulates multiple inputs.

Another deficiency of the gate control theory is that it does not explain the influence of drugs on moderating pain. This is understandable because the bulk of drug information has been discovered since the gate control theory was proposed in 1965. Nevertheless, this deficiency had to be remedied.

OTHER PAIN THEORIES

Numerous theories have been proposed to explain pain since the partial collapse of the gate control theory, the majority of which include the influence of drugs. The most promising and comprehensive is the neuromatrix theory. Details of this theory are given later in the chapter; first we discuss the effects of drugs on pain relief.

Drugs and Pain Relief

To understand current pain control theories, you need to understand how drugs block pain. **Morphine** blocks pain by filling receptors (the locks) so that the neurotransmitters (the keys) cannot occupy those sites (see Fig. 7.5). Thus pain signals cannot cross the synapse, and therefore there is no pain. Scientists discovered **naloxone**, a morphine antidote. It reverses the effect of morphine by bonding with the morphine so that morphine cannot block the neurotransmitter.

Naloxone also reverses electrically induced pain relief in rats and acupuncture pain relief in humans. This finding led scientists to hypothesize that pain relief may be related to a morphine-like substance produced in the body. In 1975, three teams of scientists discovered what we now know are two different substances:

- **Enkephalin** (Greek for "in the head"), discovered in Scotland, is similar in molecular structure to morphine and has similar analgesic properties. Found in the brain, spinal cord, and gastrointestinal (GI) tract, enkephalin has a half-life of only a few seconds, which means it operates at the spinal cord level rather than circulating through the body. Enkephalin is thought to block the gate by interfering with A-delta and C fiber signal transmission to T cells. It is released through somewhat painful sensory stimuli—that is, high-intensity **noxious TENS** or accupressure.
- **Endorphin**, another morphine-like molecule, was discovered simultaneously by two teams of scientists working independently in the United States. (The name is from the words *endogenous* and *morphine*). Produced in the pituitary gland at the base of the brain, endorphin is circulated throughout the body (its half-life is 4 hr). Endorphin exists in several forms, the most active being β-endorphin. It acts in several different areas of the CNS (including the dorsal horn). It inhibits pain signal transmission and decreases the amount of chemical irritants present in the CNS. Modalities that might release endorphins are acupuncture, neuroprobe, high-intensity **low-frequency motor TENS**, and intense exercise.

These discoveries initially caused much speculation.[12] Perhaps people especially sensitive to pain have a deficiency of enkephalin or endorphin receptors. Perhaps the placebo effect occurs because of increased enkephalin and endorphin in the body.

Two additional substances are known to be involved in pain relief:

- **Serotonin:** A biochemical messenger and regulator, found primarily in the CNS, GI tract, and blood platelets.[12] It mediates several physiological functions, including neurotransmission. Serotonin influences pain perception via a descending tract system (brain to spinal cord) that inhibits signals from peripheral nociceptors.
- **Dopamine:** A neurotransmitter in the **extrapyramidal system** of the brain, important in regulating movement. It is also used by the body to synthesize **norepinephrine** and **epinephrine**, major neurotransmitters. It affects brain processes that control movement, emotional response, and the ability to experience pleasure and pain.[14,15]

OPIOIDS: ENDOGENOUS OPIATES

An *opioid* is a synthetic **opiate**, a substance that numbs or decreases pain.[16] In reference to pain control, the term is used to denote the body's naturally occurring endogenous painkillers, such as enkephalin, endorphin, serotonin, and dopamine. Opioids operate in different parts of the nervous system, are thousands of times stronger than morphine, and are effective for varying lengths of time.

Postgate Pain Theories

Many theories were proposed as alternatives to the gate control theory of pain. The three most prominent ones are briefly described in this section.

THE DESCENDING ENDOGENOUS OPIATE THEORY OF PAIN

One theory suggests that a **descending endogenous opiate system (DEOS)** operates at supraspinal levels (i.e., cortical and subcortical areas) and that the spinal gate originates from above—from supraspinal areas that contain opioid-secreting neurons. Fig. 7.11 details the gate control system and the opiate system of pain modulation from using TENS therapy.

THE CENTRAL CONTROL TRIGGER THEORY

The **central control trigger theory** is a modification of the gate control theory. It involves the original gating mechanism plus an additional central inhibitory mechanism. The former modulates the T cell neurons as originally proposed (i.e., central control) and the latter acts via endorphin and enkephalin. Thus there are at least two different mechanisms of pain control and descending tracts.

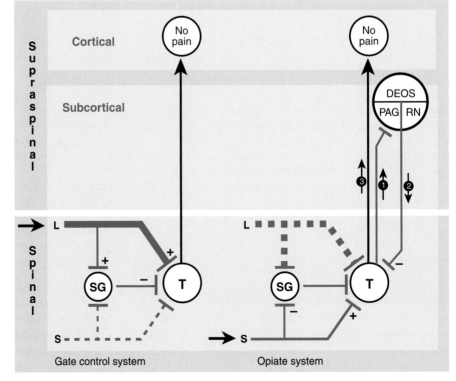

FIGURE 7.11. TENS therapy modulates pain in at least two different ways: by a gating mechanism at the spinal level and through a negative-feedback loop involving spinal levels and the descending endogenous opiate system (*DEOS*). *L*, large fibers; → *L*, preferential electrical stimulation of large-diameter sensory fibers; *PAG*, periaqueductal gray matter; *RN*, raphe nucleus; *S*, small fibers; → *S*, preferential electrical stimulation of small-diameter sensory fibers; *SG*, substantia gelatinosa; *T*, pain-transmitting cells; +, excitatory synapse; −, inhibitory synapse; ↑1, ↓2, negative-feedback loop; ↑3, pathway to the brain. (Adapted with permission from Belanger.[17])

CRITICAL THINKING 7.1 *TENS research substanti-ated the central control trigger theory.[12] A group of 20 patients who achieved TENS pain relief were put into two treatment groups of 10 patients each. One group received TENS over conventional sites, the other group over acupuncture sites. After 3 months of successful pain relief, both groups were given naloxone. The naloxone reversed the pain relief in 6 out of 10 patients in the acupuncture group. Why do you think this happened?*

THE NEUROMATRIX THEORY OF PAIN

The **neuromatrix theory of pain** states that pain is a multidimensional experience produced by characteristic patterns of nerve impulses generated by a widely distributed neural network in the brain.[5,18,19] The basis of this neuromatrix is largely determined by heredity, and it includes psychosocial factors, prior pain experience, cognitive and emotional events, and general life stress. Thus pain is a "biopsychosocial" event,[20] resulting from multidimensional inputs. The response to pain is similarly complex and multidimensional and is unique to each individual.

The neuromatrix theory is the most comprehensive theory since the gate control theory and is now the dominant theory of pain.[11,21]

Pain Management

The process of managing pain is complex, and it must be tailored to each patient. What works with one patient may not work with another. And what worked with a patient one time may not work later for the same patient with a similar injury. Following are some principles on which to base your pain management strategies. Specific techniques are discussed in Chapter 8.

CENTRAL CONTROL

The concept of central control is key to pain management. **Central control** is a concept that previous experiences, emotional influences, sensory perception, and other factors influence the response of the brain to nociceptors and thus the perception of pain. Central control collects and stores information related to pain and mediates the body's response to noxious stimuli. Previous experiences and other sensory input influence pain via central control. Two examples illustrate the idea:

1. The response of an individual (usually a child) to an injury is generally minimal until she notices blood, at which point she responds directly. The noxious stimulus from the injury site was the same before she saw blood, yet the sight of blood—sensory input to central control via the optic nerve—altered the response to the noxious stimulus.

2. One of our former athletes, a moderately successful wrestler, was plagued with minor nicks and scrapes during his early college career. Two years later, after being a two-time All-American and a world medalist, he paid very little attention to these injuries. When asked about the change, he replied that he'd discovered that the difference between a good athlete and a world-class athlete is how each one handles pain and adversity. He still got the minor nicks and scrapes but had learned to ignore them. In other words, minor injuries that were painful early in his career did not cause pain in his later career because of conscious, rational thought (central control).

We are not suggesting that a patient should rationalize away pain or ignore it. Our point is that central control can greatly influence the perception and management of pain.

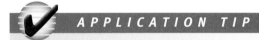
APPLICATION TIP

MANIPULATE THE PLACEBO EFFECT. The concept of central control helps explain how the placebo effect can be so powerful in eliminating pain and why the attitude and approach of the clinician can have such an important effect on a patient's response to an injury. A cheerful, positive approach by the clinician and the patient can change not only the patient's perception of pain but the healing process as well. A negative, defeatist attitude can have the opposite effect. Use this powerful tool to enhance the effects of other treatments.

THE MULTIDIMENSIONAL NATURE OF PAIN PERCEPTION

Pain is multidimensional, meaning that there is more to the perception of pain than the neural impulse from the noxious stimulus. Melzack and Torgerson[3] summarized four dimensions of pain: sensory, affective, evaluative, and miscellaneous.

- *Sensory* refers to the nature of the noxious stimulus or actual sensation of pain—that is, the conduction of impulses from peripheral sense organs to reflex (spinal) or higher centers. It is what you feel, the source of the pain. Words patients use to describe the sensory dimension of pain include *throbbing, stabbing, sharp, stinging, aching,* and *splitting.*

- *Affective* refers to the emotional or autonomic response to the pain stimulus, such as crying or being anxious or depressed owing to painful experiences. It is influenced by mental state, personality type, goals, desires, and the expectations of the patient. *Tiring, sickening, frightening,* and *cruel* are words often used to describe the affective dimension of pain.

- *Evaluative* refers to the conscious thought processes concerning the pain stimulus. A patient compares a noxious stimulus with past experiences and assigns a meaning to the experience. For example, an athlete who sprains her ankle will compare her present pain to the pain she experienced from previous ankle sprains. She will then subjectively judge the overall intensity of the pain. Words that describe the evaluative dimension of pain include *mild, intense,* and *excruciating.*
- *Miscellaneous* is a combination of the other three dimensions. Descriptive words include *cold, numb, tight, nagging,* and *penetrating.*

THE VARIABILITY OF PAIN TOLERANCE

The response to pain differs from person to person. Sometimes the affective dimension of pain overrides the sensory dimension, giving rise to variations in pain tolerance. For example, a separated shoulder might be very painful to a businessman who fell while playing tennis. The recreational athlete may not be used to this level of pain or the fact that the pain will limit his opportunity to relieve some stress via recreation. Yet professional football players have continued to play with this identical injury because the importance of winning the game (the affective dimension) blocks out the pain. It is, therefore, difficult to analyze and evaluate pain physiology, pain tolerance, and pain relief because each one varies so much from person to person. It is often hard to describe the pain you are experiencing to someone else. Pain is whatever the person experiencing it says it is.

APPLICATION TIP

TREAT THE EFFECTS OF PAIN AS WELL AS THE CAUSE OF THE PAIN. It is not enough to treat only tissue damage or the cause of the pain. The social, emotional, and psychological effects of an injury often persist long after the injured tissue has been healed. These factors, if not addressed, can become the source of additional pain and can prevent the patient from realizing her full physical potential. Treating the social, emotional, and psychological effects of an injury helps maximize the mind–body connection.

CRITICAL THINKING 7.2 *The pain experience differs from individual to individual and is influenced by anxiety, distress, and the degree of suffering it causes. One example of this variability occurred during the Battle of Anzio in World War II.[21] The soldiers who fought in this fierce battle suffered broken bones and severe cuts and bruises. The people of the village of Anzio suffered nearly identical wounds, yet the soldiers needed far less morphine than the civilians. Why did the soldiers need fewer painkilling drugs?*

THREE LEVELS OF PAIN CONTROL

Three levels for controlling pain have been described, based on the current theories of pain:

- *Level I: ascending influence pain control.* Pain relief induced by a gating mechanism occurs during the application of modalities such as traditional sensory TENS, massage, and cryotherapy. This is traditional gate control pain relief.
- *Level II: descending influence pain control.* Pain relief modulated by transmissions from higher brain centers, such as the **raphe nucleus** to the dorsal horn of the spinal cord, triggers the release of enkephalin and serotonin to modulate pain. This descending tract is stimulated by noxious stimuli transmitted to the **periaqueductal gray (PAG)** matter in the brain. This model provides a possible explanation for pain relief induced by somewhat painful stimulation of afferent nerves (C fibers), such as acupressure or noxious TENS (delivered at a high intensity and frequency, like the neuroprobe).
- *Level III: β-endorphin-mediated pain control.* Prolonged stimulation of afferent nerves (A-delta fibers) triggers the release of β-endorphin by the pituitary gland from connections between the hypothalamus and the raphe nucleus. Because β-endorphin has a long half-life, this provides long-term stimulation of descending tracts. This model provides a possible explanation for pain relief from modalities such as electroacupuncture and low-frequency motor TENS.

CRITICAL THINKING 7.3 *Conrad, a certified athletic trainer, was covering a youth soccer tournament as part of his clinic's outreach program. A 10-year-old boy came up to Conrad complaining of stomach pain. Conrad asked what the boy had for breakfast and how long ago he had eaten, then determined that the pain wasn't related to diet. He then asked the boy if he had been kicked in the stomach. The boy said, "Yes." Conrad palpated the boy's upper left abdominal quadrant and found that it was rigid. Conrad then asked the boy if he had pain anywhere else, and the boy said, "my left shoulder." Conrad immediately called an ambulance. Why?*

CLOSING SCENE

Recall from the chapter opening scene that you are gaining some clinical experience at a high school. Each day before basketball practice, one of Coach Jiminez's players applies hot packs to her knees to help relieve the pain and stiffness. Other athletes use electrical stimulation or ice to decrease the pain. Why are there so many different treatment therapies for pain reduction? After reading this chapter, you can describe several pain theories and why external stimuli—such as heat, cold, electricity, and manual pressure—stimulate special nerve fibers that help override the pain message.

CHAPTER REFLECTIONS

1. Read and ponder each of the following points. Do you feel you have a clear understanding of each concept? If not, reread the appropriate section of the chapter.
   - Define pain.
   - Discuss the functions of pain.
   - Discuss the four dimensions of pain.
   - How is pain a friend to the patient and clinician? How is it a foe?
   - Discuss the difference between acute and chronic pain.
   - What is the difference between radiating and referred pain?
   - Describe the major points of the specificity and pattern theories of pain

   - Discuss the gate control theory of pain, and four reasons it is inadequate.
   - Discuss the body's internal pain suppressors.
   - Discuss central control and say how you might apply this concept in managing a patient's pain.
   - What is the neuromatrix theory of pain?

2. Write three to five questions for discussion with your class instructor, clinical instructor, classmates, and clinical colleagues.

3. Get together with classmates and quiz each other on the concepts of this chapter. Use the points in exercise 1 and questions you wrote for exercise 2 as a beginning. Explaining concepts out loud to others requires a deeper grasp of the material than feeling you understand it as you read.

CRITICAL THINKING RESPONSES

Critical Thinking 7.1

Because naloxone is a morphine inhibitor, it must have inhibited endorphin release, indicating that endorphins and/or enkephalins were involved in the pain relief. In the conventional group, naloxone had no effect, indicating that the pain was relieved by something other than endorphin or enkephalin—that is, the gating mechanism. This research indicates that there are two different kinds of TENS analgesia and at least two different mechanisms of pain control.

Critical Thinking 7.2

The citizens of Anzio needed more morphine than the soldiers because of the mental stress associated with the battle. Anzio residents also lost homes, jobs, and even loved ones. Although the soldiers didn't lose their homes, they got to go home because of their injuries. The presumed reason the soldiers needed less morphine than the residents of Anzio for identical injuries (now known as the *Anzio effect*) was that the wounds to the residents were a source of anxiety, whereas these same wounds to the soldiers meant a return to their families.

Critical Thinking 7.3

Let's review the symptoms. The boy got kicked in the stomach, had stomach pain, and had pain in the left shoulder. These symptoms are consistent with a ruptured spleen. He was exhibiting referred pain to the left shoulder (Kehr sign). This is a true story. When the ambulance arrived at the emergency room, the young man was taken into the x-ray department where it was determined that he did indeed have a ruptured spleen. The physician took the boy into surgery and removed the spleen. Because of Conrad's knowledge of referred pain patterns, the boy's life was saved.

REFERENCES

1. Turk DC, Melzack R. The measurement of pain and the assessment of people experiencing pain. In: Turk DC, Melzack R, eds. Handbook of Pain Assessment. 2nd ed. New York: Guilford, 2001.
2. Merskey H, Bogduk N. IASP Task Force on Taxonomy. 2nd ed. Seattle: International Association for the Study of Pain, 1994.
3. Melzack R, Torgerson W. On the language of pain. Anesthesiology 1971;34:50.
4. Bond M, Simpson K. Pain: Its Nature and Treatment. New York: Churchill Livingstone, 2006.
5. Melzack R. Pain and the neuromatrix in the brain. J Dent Edu 2001:1378–1382.
6. Silverstein A, Silverstein V. World of the Brain. New York: Morrow, 1986.
7. Charlton JEe. Core Curriculum for Professional Education in Pain. Seattle: International Association for the Study of Pain, 2005.
8. Zimmerman M. Basic physiology of pain perception. In: Lautenbacher S, Fillingim RB, eds. Pathophysiology of Pain Perception. New York: Plenum, 2004.
9. Mann MD. The Nervous System in Action. Available at: www.unmc.edu/Physiology/Mann/index.html. Accessed Mar 2006.
10. Melzack R, Wall PD. Pain mechanisms: A new theory. Science 1965;150:971–979.
11. Nathan PW. The gate-control theory of pain. A critical review. Brain 1976;99:123–158.
12. Svacina L. Pain Control #10. Longmont, CO: Staodynamics, 1977.
13. National Library of Medicine. Medical Subject Headings. Available at: www.nlm.nih.gov/mesh/2003/MBrowser.html. Accessed Apr 2007.
14. Gear RW, Aley KO, Levine JD. Pain-induced analgesia mediated by mesolimbic reward circuits. J Neurosci 1999;19:7175–7181.
15. Wickelgren I. Neuroscience: Getting the brain's attention. Science 1997;278:35–37.
16. Stedman's Electronic Medical Dictionary. Ver. 7. Baltimore: Lippincott Williams & Wilkins, 2006.
17. Belanger AY. Evidence-Based Guide to Therapeutic Physical Agents. Baltimore: Lippincott Williams & Wilkins, 2002.
18. Melzack R. From the gate to the neuromatrix. Pain 1999;suppl 6:S121–126.
19. Melzack R, Coderre TJ, Katz J, Vaccarino AL. Central neuroplasticity and pathological pain. Ann N Y Acad Sci 2001;933:157–174.
20. Gatchel RJ. Clinical Essentials of Pain Management. Washington, DC: American Psychological Association, 2005.
21. Beecher HK. Pain in men wounded in battle. Ann Surg 1946;123: 96–105.

Relieving Orthopedic Injury Pain

You are an athletic training student assigned to the rugby team. A player twists his ankle and limps over to you. The question is, Is it pain or is it injury? Coach Jones wonders whether the distress that caused his athlete to stop practicing is the result of torn tissue or simply all in the athlete's head. It's a legitimate question, you think to yourself. Torn tissue could be aggravated by practicing. But if the distress is only in the athlete's head, he could suck it up or gut it out and continue preparing for the big game. Coach Jones consults with your clinical supervisor to determine whether to let the young man have his pain attended to or to insist that the athlete return to practice.

The Philosophy and Principles of Pain Relief

Drugs, psychological techniques, surgical procedures, and physical therapy have all been used with varying degrees of success for pain relief, but no single method has been consistently successful.[1] This is probably because pain is multidimensional (see Chapter 7) and clinicians sometimes concentrate on a single aspect of the pain. The clinicians we have known who have been the most successful in alleviating pain are directed by a core philosophy. Principles are more important to them than tools. Their therapy is truly an art. The following are the principles that guide these pain control artists.

IGNORE OR LISTEN TO PAIN?

Athletic success requires sacrifice, including ignoring discomfort while meeting a difficult challenge—to push beyond the previous best effort (Fig. 8.1). At times an athlete must ignore the pain and persist in spite of it, especially pain associated with exertion nearing personal limits. But what about pain associated with injury? Some types of injury pain are just an irritant and must be ignored (Box 8.1). Other types will cause neural inhibitions that decrease neuromuscular functioning (range of motion, strength, agility, etc.). Persistent painful activity can enhance neural inhibition to such an extent that a permanent physiological block sometimes results. In this case, ignoring pain will prove detrimental to the athlete and result in chronic irritation and temporary loss of skill.

PAIN: DEMANDING DISCIPLINARIAN OR BENEVOLENT BENEFACTOR?

Is pain pay back for indiscriminately or accidentally pushing your body beyond its limits, thus acting as a demand-

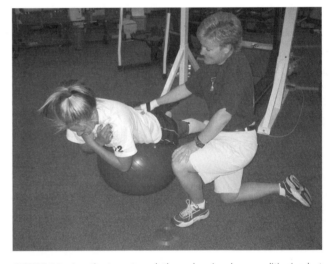

FIGURE 8.1. A patient must work through pain when conditioning but must avoid pain during rehabilitation. Pain during rehabilitation exercises causes neural inhibition, which decreases flexibility, strength, and other physical activity.

ing disciplinarian? Or is pain a protective mechanism to keep you from causing further damage, acting as a benevolent benefactor? Either or both.

The body often mishandles pain. It has a great memory for what it wants to do, but not for why it is doing it.[2,3] Thus pain often persists long after the cause of the pain is resolved. It's that annoying relative who you thought was coming to visit for a few days but who stayed much longer than anticipated. You must respect pain—use it to guide you—but be tough on it when necessary so that it does not take on a life of its own.

NO PAIN, NO GAIN?

When it comes to conditioning, "no pain, no gain" is absolutely right. But this adage does not apply to rehabilitation. During rehabilitation, the mantra is twofold:

- Ignore the pain equals no brain.
- Pandering to pain propagates pain.

Together these statements explain how to both respect pain and be tough on it during rehabilitation. To ignore pain is not smart because it often leads to more pain and disability. On the other hand, if you eliminate all activity to avoid causing any pain, the pain will take on a life of its own, meaning that it will take much less stimulus than normal to evoke a pain response (even minor aches and pains will seem worse than they are).

DEHNE'S SPINAL ADAPTATION SYNDROME

The **spinal adaptation syndrome** is a theory based on a 20-year study of sprains by Ernst Dehne (Box 8.2).[2–5] The logic of the theory is summarized as follows:

- Afferent nociceptive impulses arising from traumatized tissues or tissue in the process of repair alter the integration of central nervous system (CNS) excitation at the spinal cord level.
- These alterations result in decreased response to volitional stimuli and increased response to otherwise subliminal peripheral stresses, resulting in involuntary muscle action.
- The altered muscle response through the mediation of vasomotor reaction (dilation or constriction of blood vessels) determines the local chemical environment that produces the process of repair.
- The process of repair is a highly sensitive state. It responds adversely to additional stress and favorably to the reestablishment of central control.
- The spinal adaptation syndrome seems to operate in all conditions connected with inflammation or repair. Covering such a broad spectrum, it is not specific to any one condition. It appears that all tissue in the process of repair has an extremely sensitive nociceptive potential and reacts violently to all additional stress as well as to stress that would be subliminal in the normal

BOX 8.2 *DEHNE: AN ORTHOPEDIC VISIONARY*

Ernst Dehne[2–5] is often considered the father of modern orthopedic rehabilitation. Although he is relatively unknown, his observations and revolutionary thinking set the stage for the great advances in rehabilitation during the past 30 years. His ideas seemed way out in the 1950s and 1960s, but they are now standard thinking; although few clinicians are aware of how Dehne has influenced their practices.

Dehne was a German orthopedic surgeon who in the 1930s recognized that the standard practice of long-term cast immobilization (often up to 16 weeks) after orthopedic injury and surgery was detrimental to full recovery.[6,7] Through the years, his idea of less immobilization and quicker active use of orthopedically injured limbs grew, even without the support of the mainstream medical community. Markey[8] who served a residency under Dehne, tells of Dehne's frustration with the lack of cooperation by the nursing staff. They were reluctant to follow the surgeon's orders to get the patients out of bed and walking immediately after surgery. It was so bad that Dehne would sometimes pound on a desk, an empty hospital bed, or a table with a baseball bat as he urged the staff to follow his orders.

Although Grant[9] and Hayden[10] do not mention Dehne in their classic papers on cryokinetics (see Chapter 13), they worked one floor below him at Brook Army Hospital in San Antonio, Texas, and treated many of his patients. Their experiment with ice and early active exercise grew, no doubt, from

state. The competitive influence of volitional impulses tends to inhibit and eventually to terminate the nociceptive interference at the spinal cord level.

In short, the theory holds that nociceptive impulses from traumatized tissue inhibit motor functions and tissue repair but that voluntary activity can reestablish central control and prevent this inhibition. In other words, prolonged inactivity after an injury will lead to neural inhibition that could become permanent.

RESETTING CENTRAL CONTROL DURING REHABILITATION

Removing the pain sensation after injury is not enough; you must also get rid of the effects of the pain—that is, reset the system (reset central control). Consider the following analogy.

A plane at Chicago's O'Hare International Airport has a tire blow out during takeoff. Parts of the plane break off as it skids along, leaving the runway littered with debris and luggage. The runway is shut down while crews remove the damaged plane and debris. Within 6 hr the runway is cleaned and can be put back into service (*the pain is removed*).

All is not back to normal, however; thousands of passengers are stranded in the terminal because their flights were canceled. Tens of thousands of additional passengers are stranded in airports around the world because their flights to Chicago were canceled or delayed. Business meetings have to be rescheduled; sports and cultural activities must also be rescheduled because teams, performers, and support personnel didn't arrive on time; hotel reservations for thousands of travelers must be changed; and hundreds of other reservations and activities also have to be changed. It may take weeks or months to get things back to normal—that is, to fix the effects of the blown-out tire in Chicago (*reset central control*).

The concept of resetting central control must be part of the therapy for dealing with pain and injury. Immobilization and injury can cause a physiological block that can become permanent if not handled properly. You must get the whole orchestra playing in unison. If the flutes and violas are just half a beat off, they create discord and noise rather than great, soothing music. The following example from one of our athletes illustrates this principle.

A gymnast suffered an eversion ankle sprain. Weeks after the injury he was pain free while walking and had good muscular strength but could not stick a dismount because of excruciating pain. He had been an All-American the year before and was extremely frustrated. Everything else was normal. He was referred to one of us (KK) for consultation. After reviewing the case and evaluating the injury, we decided to begin a series of graded skill activities to reset central control. Although he was an all-arounder, we concentrated on vaulting, his best event, as follows:

- Approach the pommel horse at 50% speed and jump on the horse into a sitting position.
- Run at 75% speed, straddle the horse, and land on the other side without a flip.
- Repeat the previous step at 90% speed.
- Approach at 90% speed, do a simple flip over the horse, and land on the mat.
- Approach at 90% speed and perform the easiest vault that would score points.

He performed each of these events pain free; and as you might expect, with a bigger grin after each one. We told him to do nothing else but to return that evening (the team had a meet), go through normal warmups, and then perform the same series of activities just before the vault competition. Again there was no pain during any of the jumps and vaults. He competed without pain and scored a 9.2. The following Monday and thereafter, he practiced all events without pain or disability.

This example illustrates both the effects of the spinal adaptation syndrome and the need to reset central control after injury. Make these concepts part of your pain and injury management.

The Placebo Effect and Pain Relief

Derived from the Latin for "I shall please," **placebo** is a medically inactive substance given as a medicine for its suggestive effect or to satisfy the patient's demand for medicine. It is most often thought of as a mock intervention (such as a sugar pill instead of aspirin) that brings about a desired response (pain relief). Patients think they are receiving an actual dose of medicine when they are not, and the psychological effects of their expectations of benefit are responsible for the result.[11] For example, 35% of postoperative patients, people with diabetes, and those suffering chronic headache obtain relief as a result of placebos.[12] In a multicenter study of patients with ulcers, 76% of sufferers treated with Tagamet obtained relief, but 63% of sufferers treated with a placebo obtained relief.[13]

The benefits or effects of placebos occur in response to many types of interventions in addition to taking medically inactive substances.[12] This concept is known as the **placebo effect**—a measurable, observable, or felt improvement in health not attributable to treatment. Psychological factors, particularly the clinician's and the patient's expectations of pain relief, contain powerful therapeutic value in their own right, in addition to the effects of the procedure itself.[14,15] Additional mechanisms, such as learning or conditioned reflex,[16] cognitive modulation,[17] and neurotransmitter reaction,[18] result in a placebo effect. All of these mechanisms fit into the concept of central control (see Chapter 7).

On the negative side, one reason quackery abounds is because of the placebo effect. So-called snake oil salesmen convince their clients that they have a powerful medicine, when in reality the medicine is inert. Another disadvantage relates to research. Sometimes patients will get better as a result of chance or belief in the intervention. That's why good research often requires a large number of subjects, to help separate those who get better because of the placebo effect from those who get better from the intervention being studied.

The placebo effect is a powerful, dynamic, robust, and widespread phenomenon.[19] It is not a nontreatment. Brain mapping with advanced MRI scanners indicate that activity in pain-sensitive brain regions is altered by placebos.[20] A placebo does not interfere with the body's ability to sense pain but instead affects how the brain modulates its interpretation of the body's signals.[20,21] Thus a person's state of mind and previous experiences have a strong effect on descending tract pain control. Clinicians should take advantage of the placebo effect when treating patients (Box 8.3).

PSYCHOLOGICAL ASPECTS AND A POSITIVE ATTITUDE

Psychological and emotional influences surrounding an injury can have a great effect on pain treatments and patient response. For example, if a starting senior guard on the basketball team suffers an anterior cruciate ligament (ACL) sprain, the emotional aspect of this injury—causing him to miss the rest of his college career—will make the immediate pain almost unbearable. If, however, the same injury happened to a third-string sophomore, the emotional impact is likely to be less, and thus the pain will probably be less traumatic.

Another important aspect to consider is attitude. If the patient is negative toward treatment and rehabilitation, the body's healing processes will not work as well. Having a positive attitude toward treatment and rehabilitation helps the body respond to the treatment more favorably (Box 8.4).

Sources of Orthopedic Injury Pain

Orthopedic injury pain results from the stimulation of nociceptors located throughout the body (see Chapter 7). Nociceptors send pain signals to the spinal cord; they are stimulated by the following:

- Injured tissue (mediator release)
- Edema pressure
- Stretching injured tissue

BOX 8.3 *PLACEBO: THE PSYCHOLOGY OF REHABILITATION*

We do not condone the use of unproven treatments to unsuspecting patients; we are advocating the use of highly researched or proven treatments to believing patients. When the clinician and patient both believe in the treatment, there is a high probability of a successful outcome.

It is important that you study the literature and draw your own conclusions about what therapeutic modality treatments work best in given situations. Educate your patients about the modality you are using. Explain how it works and what benefits they should expect to derive from the treatment. It's difficult to determine how much of a patient's response to treatment is owing to the modality and how much is owing to the placebo effect. But one thing is certain—if you have a negative attitude toward your treatment intervention, your patients will lose faith in you, and the powerful mind–body response will be lost.

BOX 8.4 *FINDING THE SILVER LINING IN THE STORM CLOUDS*

In 1991, when I (DD) was the head athletic trainer at a small midwestern university, one of my second-string football players tore his ACL. It was midway through the season of the athlete's senior year, so to him it was the end of his playing career. He was taking the diagnosis quite hard. Knowing that he wanted to be a physical therapist, I said, "You have just suffered what many consider a terrible injury. Can you think of anything positive that might come out of this?"

He responded, "Doc, how could anything about this injury be positive?"

I reminded him that he would be entering physical therapy (PT) school the next fall and that his upcoming surgery, followed by a major rehabilitation process, would prepare him for his subsequent education and career. By going through this process himself, he would experience firsthand what it's like to be a patient recovering from a major injury. He would gain a greater appreciation for pain control, rehabilitation, and modality use. I asked, "How many of your classmates in PT school will have had such an injury and then been involved in the rehabilitation of that injury?"

"Few, I guess," he responded.

"Don't you see how this little bump in the road, your torn ACL, can actually serve as a springboard toward your chosen profession?"

He then started to get the big picture. His attitude changed from being the sad, injured kid to the future therapist excited to learn firsthand what rehabilitation is like.

• Otherwise normal activity in a tissue that is sensitized from disuse after injury

Direct vs. Indirect Pain Relief

There are two main approaches to treating orthopedic injury pain: direct and indirect. The indirect method focuses on removing the cause of pain. For example, if a basketball player with an ankle sprain is experiencing pain from the pressure of edema on nociceptors, using an intermittent compression pump and elevation will reduce the swelling in this area and thus relieve the pain.

The direct method of pain relief addresses the pain itself. The application of transcutaneous electrical nerve stimulation (TENS) to a sprained ankle to gate the pain or release endogenous opiates is an example of direct pain relief.

USING A VARIETY OF TECHNIQUES

It is important to have a variety of pain relief methods at your disposal. Just as all patients do not respond to pain in the same way, not all patients respond to treatments in the same manner. If a technique isn't working after three or four treatments, try something else. Change methods when necessary; sometimes the body adapts to the treatment method and the method becomes ineffective. Here are two examples:

• Some athletes are sensitive to cold and so cryokinetics is not possible (see Chapter 13). TENS can be used instead to facilitate exercise.[22]
• A football wide receiver suffered from a moderate-plus quadriceps contusion. Although he initially responded well to cryostretch treatments (see Chapter 13), after 2 or 3 days, the cold no longer facilitated therapeutic exercise. The athletic trainer then switched his treatment to TENS and exercise. The athlete continued to progress for another couple of days and then plateaued. He was then treated with analgesic balm and therapeutic exercise for 2 days, and then went back to the cryostretch. The player continued the rotation through the three techniques for pain relief as the athletic trainer continued the therapeutic exercise until the athlete was able to perform pain free.

Tools for Relieving Pain

A variety of techniques are available to relieve pain. Differences in injury and in patient response dictate the therapeutic approach, so clinicians need to be skilled in using a number of techniques. It's essential to remember that the tool is not as important as the philosophy of the approach.

THERAPEUTIC EXERCISE

Low-level, controlled therapeutic exercise decreases edema-induced pain by stimulating lymph flow, thereby reducing the pressure on nociceptors. Isometric contractions interspersed with static stretching relieve pain by reducing muscle spasm (see Chapter 13).

Immobilization, therapeutic modalities, and therapeutic exercise are all techniques used to decrease pain (Fig. 8.2). Therapeutic exercise should be relatively pain free. It is acceptable if the activity is mildly uncomfortable, but serious discomfort is a warning from the body that something is wrong. Therapeutic exercise or activity during rehabilitation should not evoke the same type of pain that was experienced when the injury occurred.

COUNTERIRRITANTS

Counterirritants are substances that irritate the skin when applied; causing mild skin inflammation. The irritation closes the gate on mild pain in muscles, joints, or internal organs. In essence, the counterirritant causes the brain to switch its attention from the mild pain to the counterirritant. Counterirritation is perhaps one of the oldest[23] and simplest methods of pain relief. Examples are as follows:

• Ethyl chloride spray
• Hot water bottle
• Ice packs
• Vibration
• Tactile stimulation (pressure)
• Neuromuscular electrical stimulation (NMES)

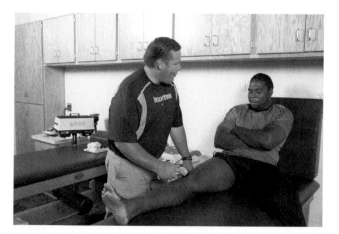

FIGURE 8.2. Therapeutic modalities modulate pain so that patients can begin therapeutic exercise.

- Static electricity
- Analgesic balms

The use of most of these counterirritants is straightforward. Analgesic balms are an exception. Claims of their effects are often misstated, and the products are sometimes misused. Therefore we will discuss them in more detail.

Analgesic Balms

Analgesic balms make up most of the counterirritants used by the public (e.g., sports cream, Ben-Gay, Icy Hot, Flexall) An **analgesic balm** is an externally applied drug that has a topical analgesic, anesthetic, or anti-itching effect by depressing cutaneous sensory receptors or has a topical counterirritant effect by stimulating cutaneous sensory receptors.

There are several over-the-counter (OTC) analgesic lotions, creams, and patches that patients can use to reduce aches and pains. The active ingredient in most of these topical analgesics is menthol, methyl salicylate, or capsaicin, used singly or in combination with one or both of the others.

Menthol is an alcohol obtained from oil of peppermint and derived from the mint plant. Menthol is classified as an irritant that produces a cooling sensation when used at 1.25–16%. Menthol is included in analgesic balms to provide a sensation of cold, although some patients describe a cool burning sensation. The amount of menthol in many OTC topical analgesics ranges from 1% to 16%.

Methyl salicylate is wintergreen oil, produced synthetically or from the distilled leaves of sweet birch. Methyl salicylate is classified as an irritant that produces redness when used at 10–60%. It is included in analgesic balms to provide a sensation of heat. For methyl salicylate to be classified as an active ingredient, it needs to make up 10–60% of the product. **Capsaicin**, a derivative of the hot pepper (chili) plant, is an irritant included in analgesic balms to provide a sensation of heat.

Scientists have studied the effects of topical analgesics in reducing pain associated with delayed-onset muscle soreness.[24] Pain perception was measured with a visual analog scale 48 hr after eccentric exercise. Subjects were then divided into three groups: placebo, menthol/methyl salicylate, and capsaicin. The treatments were applied over the most painful area for 5 min and then removed. Subjects in the menthol/methyl salicylate group experienced a significant reduction in pain compared to the other two groups.

Using an animal model, scientists reported that administration of menthol (1.9%) to the skin surface of contracting muscles decreased autonomic responses to static muscle contractions.[25] This effect was independent of higher brain processing and strongly suggests that menthol application to the skin has analgesic effects on pain signals located in the muscle.

Scientists who have performed research on products that contain either menthol or methyl salicylate as an active ingredient have reported that these products produce no significant increase in muscle or skin temperature.[26] How do these products provide the sensations of heat or cold, and how do they relieve pain?

The mechanism by which menthol works has not been well understood until recently.[24,27] It seems that some of the same receptors in the skin that respond to cold stimuli (temperatures between 46°F and 86°F [8°C and 30°C]) also respond to menthol.[24] Because the same receptor is stimulated by both cold and menthol, patients might notice a sensation of cooling, or burning cold, after the menthol application.[24] These sensations, in turn, may reduce the amount of pain patients experience.[28]

The fact that these products don't increase or decrease the temperature does not mean that they are ineffective. They may help reduce pain in two ways. First, because these chemicals (menthol or methyl salicylate) stimulate the cutaneous sensory receptors, pain signals may be altered at the dorsal horn of the spinal cord. Second, the action of massaging the analgesic cream into the area and the stimulating effects of the counterirritant may increase large-diameter afferent nerve input. Indeed, topically applied external analgesics appear to provide some benefit for pain relief. In fact, the American College of Rheumatology supports these agents as primary therapy for disorders such as osteoarthritis of the knee and promote their use before relying on nonsteroidal anti-inflammatory drugs (NSAIDs).[29]

THERMOTHERAPY

Pain reduction is probably the most frequent indication for the use of heat in a therapeutic setting.[30] Topical heat is effective for reducing pain associated with rheumatoid arthritis,[31,32] adhesive capsulitis[33] and neck and back **trigger point pain**[34] (a hypersensitive area or site in muscle or connective tissue, usually associated with myofascial pain syndromes). Experimental research on patients with low-back pain has demonstrated that topical heat provided greater pain relief and resulted in lower disability for 24 hr after thermotherapy application, compared to no treatment.[35] Similar effects were also shown in the treatment of trapezius myalgia with low-level topical heat.[36] Heat's pain-relieving qualities are related to its ability to increase local blood flow,[37–39] promote the relaxation of soft tissue,[38–40] and reduce muscle spasm.[41–42]

Erasala et al.[39] used Doppler ultrasound to demonstrate increased blood flow in the trapezius muscle after topical thermotherapy. This increased blood flow is thought to "wash away" chemical irritants such as bradykinin. In addition to increased blood flow, heating is also believed to cause a counterirritant effect through the stimulation of cutaneous nerves, specifically **thermoreceptors**, sensory receptors that respond to heat or cold.[38] As a result of thermoreceptor activity, both sedation and relaxation are facilitated, which often leads to pain modulation.[30,38] Although the mechanisms underlying these phenomena are not completely understood, both the gate control theory and a decrease in the response rates of specific nerves (axons of γ-motor neurons) that supply muscles have been proposed as possible mechanisms for the decreased pain and muscle relaxation that occurs with the application of thermotherapy.[30,38,44]

Finally, as a muscle spasm is relaxed, pressure on nociceptors is lessened, thereby leading to a reduction in pain, called reduction of the pain–spasm–pain cycle. Thermo-therapy is discussed in detail in Chapters 11 and 12.

ELECTROTHERAPY

Various forms of electrical nerve stimulation devices provide pain relief for several conditions, including osteoarthritis,[45,46] low-back pain,[47,48] neck pain,[49] and postoperative orthopedic surgery pain.[50–52] Electrical stimulating currents are thought to reduce pain in three ways:

- By reducing muscle spasm, hence relaxing the muscle
- By releasing endogenous opiates at pain receptor sites
- By stimulating the nonpainful nerves, thus modulating the pain

Electrotherapy is discussed in Chapter 10.

CRYOTHERAPY

Cold is a powerful pain-relieving modality. It is perhaps the most effective modality available, certainly more effective than heat applications in relieving pain during acute care.[53] Heat, however, appears to be superior in decreasing dull pain that is common the day after extreme exertion or toward the end of subacute care. Here are two guidelines:[54]

- Treat specific acute injuries with cryotherapy but general aches and pain with a warm whirlpool or hot tub.
- In a subacute injury, if pain prevents normal range of motion (ROM) or gait, use ice to facilitate exercise; if ROM and gait are normal, use heat applications to relieve the dull aches.

Cryotherapy: Powerful Pain Medicine

In the 1940s, Allen et al.[55,56] used cold applications (ice packs and immersion for 1–5 hr) as the only analgesic for limb amputation. Cold applied to the leg can prevent tooth pain resulting from the electrical stimulation of teeth fillings and laser-evoked pain.[12,19] Postoperative medication and complications are minimized after orthopedic surgery when cold is applied.[57]

Cryotherapy is also effective in minimizing chronic pain induced by repetitive strain. Baseball pitchers who immersed their arms in ice water after a simulated game were more accurate and could throw with greater velocity in a subsequent game 3–4 days later.[58,59]

The most common use of cold with acute orthopedic injury is to modulate the pain of sprains, strains, and contusions to facilitate therapeutic exercise (Fig. 8.3).[9,10,60–63] The discovery of this technique, known as cryokinetics, in the mid-1960s dramatically changed the approach to the rehabilitation of these injuries. These concepts are discussed in greater detail in Chapters 13 and 14.

Pain Resulting from Cold Immersion

Immersion in a slush bucket, with the water temperature near 34°F (1°C) is very painful during the first few ses-

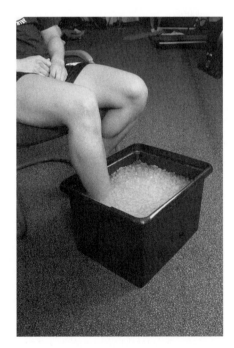

FIGURE 8.3. Cryokinetics, the alternating of cold application and therapeutic exercise, is a powerful technique that combines the pain-modulating effects of both cold and controlled, progressive therapeutic exercise.

sions. For this reason, some clinicians avoid using certain cryotherapy techniques. But patients quickly adapt to cold pain and find that faster recovery more than compensates for the initial pain.

Monitoring and Assessing Pain Relief During Rehabilitation

Pain must be monitored throughout the rehabilitation process. As discussed in Chapter 1, pain during an activity indicates the activity is too strenuous or complex; residual pain, or pain the next day, indicates that the previous day's activity was too strenuous. Activities that result in pain during rehabilitation will hinder the rehabilitation process by inducing neural inhibition.

Because pain tolerance varies from person to person and the perception of pain is subjective, pain itself is difficult to measure, and pain relief is hard to quantify. The best assessment tools are questionnaires and scales that quantify a person's subjective evaluation of the pain. Most instruments measure a single quality of pain, such as intensity. One scale, the McGill Pain Questionnaire, measures multiple qualities of pain. These are the most common pain assessment instruments:

- Number scale
- Verbal rating scale
- Visual analog scale
- Graphic rating scale
- McGill Pain Questionnaire

THE NUMBER SCALE

Number scales are used to measure pain intensity. They consist of a range of numbers (such as 0–10) and descriptors associated with some or all of the numbers (Fig. 8.4). Patients are instructed to select the number that best describes their pain. For example, 0 means no pain, and 10 means pain so severe that the patient feels a need to go to the hospital.

THE VERBAL RATING SCALE

Verbal rating scales consist of a group of descriptors but no numbers. For example, patients may be asked to rate their pain as absent, mild, moderate, or severe or their pain relief as none, slight, moderate, or good. Verbal rating scales are thought to be insensitive to slight changes.[65,66]

THE VISUAL ANALOG SCALE

The **visual analog scale (VAS)** consists of a line of specific length, usually 100 mm (4 in.), with contrasting descriptors at each end of the line. Descriptors may indicate any quality of pain, such as "no pain" and "severe pain," "annoying" and "unbearable," "dull" and "sharp" (Fig. 8.5). There are no numbers displayed on the line. The patient simply makes a vertical slash on the line where she feels her pain is. The clinician then measures from the left side of the scale to the slash to assess the pain. The measurement (in millimeters) is then converted to a percentage. The VAS is thought to represent a robust, sensitive, and reproducible measure of pain.[66–68]

Circle the word and/or number that best describes the intensity of your pain:

0	Nothing at all
0.5	Very, very weak (just noticeable)
1	Very weak
2	Weak (light)
3	Moderate
4	Somewhat strong
5	Strong (heavy)
6	
7	Very strong
8	
9	
10	Very, very strong (almost maximal)
	Maximal

FIGURE 8.4. A number scale for quantifying pain. (Adapted with permission from Borg.[64])

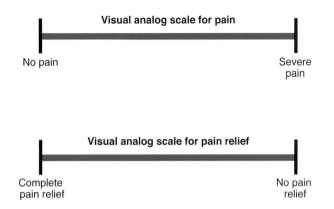

FIGURE 8.5. A visual analog scale for assessing pain. The patient makes a vertical slash on a 100 mm line where she feels her pain is.

One area of contention concerning the VAS is whether to allow patients to see previous results when assessing subsequent pain. For example, if you wanted to assess the effectiveness of a single treatment or a course of treatments, you would measure pain before and after treatment. Knowledge of the first measurement will influence the subsequent measurement. A purist would say the two measurements must be independent. Yet the subjective nature of assessing pain almost demands that assessing change be done from the perspective of the initial assessment. We favor the latter.

CRITICAL THINKING 8.1 *You use a TENS unit to treat a patient with elbow pain and want to see how effective your treatment is at relieving pain. What could you use to measure pain relief? How would you know if you were making progress?*

THE GRAPHIC RATING SCALE

The **graphic rating scale** is a horizontal line, similar to the VAS, with anchor points at each end and descriptors spread along the line (Fig. 8.6). It is administered and scored the same as the VAS. Some feel is it a better scale than the VAS because it is more sensitive to intensity,[69] is easier to use,[70] and has greater within- and between-subject reliability.[71]

THE MCGILL PAIN QUESTIONNAIRE

The **McGill Pain Questionnaire** is the most complex of the pain measurement tools. It uses pictures, scales, and words to help patients describe sensory and affective aspects as well as magnitude and changes in their pain. A sample of the questionnaire is presented in Figure 8.7.

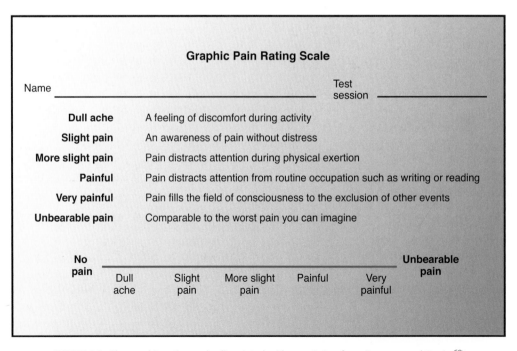

FIGURE 8.6. The graphic rating scale. (Reprinted with permission from Denegar and Perrin.[69])

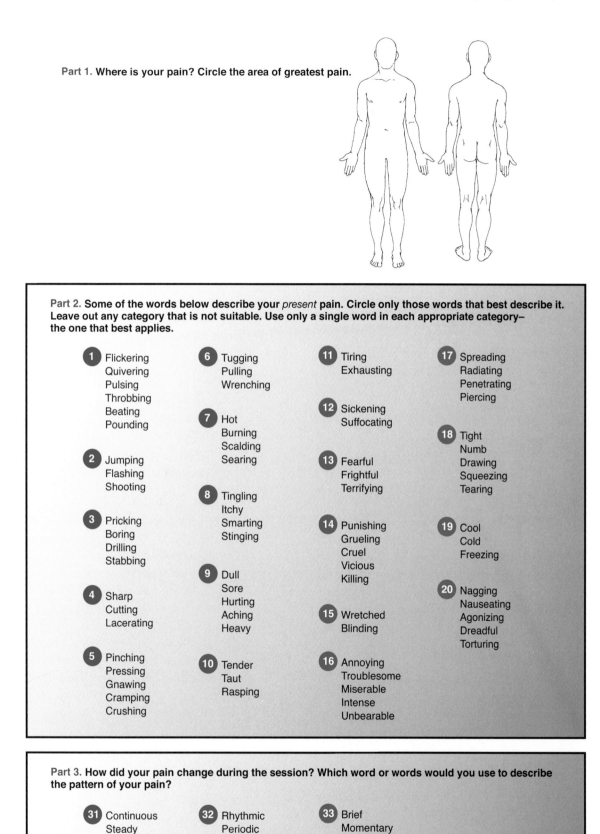

Part 1. Where is your pain? Circle the area of greatest pain.

Part 2. Some of the words below describe your *present* **pain. Circle only those words that best describe it. Leave out any category that is not suitable. Use only a single word in each appropriate category–the one that best applies.**

1. Flickering
   Quivering
   Pulsing
   Throbbing
   Beating
   Pounding

2. Jumping
   Flashing
   Shooting

3. Pricking
   Boring
   Drilling
   Stabbing

4. Sharp
   Cutting
   Lacerating

5. Pinching
   Pressing
   Gnawing
   Cramping
   Crushing

6. Tugging
   Pulling
   Wrenching

7. Hot
   Burning
   Scalding
   Searing

8. Tingling
   Itchy
   Smarting
   Stinging

9. Dull
   Sore
   Hurting
   Aching
   Heavy

10. Tender
    Taut
    Rasping

11. Tiring
    Exhausting

12. Sickening
    Suffocating

13. Fearful
    Frightful
    Terrifying

14. Punishing
    Grueling
    Cruel
    Vicious
    Killing

15. Wretched
    Blinding

16. Annoying
    Troublesome
    Miserable
    Intense
    Unbearable

17. Spreading
    Radiating
    Penetrating
    Piercing

18. Tight
    Numb
    Drawing
    Squeezing
    Tearing

19. Cool
    Cold
    Freezing

20. Nagging
    Nauseating
    Agonizing
    Dreadful
    Torturing

Part 3. How did your pain change during the session? Which word or words would you use to describe the pattern of your pain?

31. Continuous
    Steady
    Constant

32. Rhythmic
    Periodic
    Intermittent

33. Brief
    Momentary
    Transient

FIGURE 8.7. The McGill Pain Questionnaire. (Adapted with permission from Melzack.[71])

CLOSING SCENE

Recall from the chapter opening scene, that you are an athletic training student assigned to the rugby team. A player twists his ankle and limps over to the staff AT, obviously in pain. His coach asks if the player actually has an injury that would sideline him or if the young man can play through the pain. The staff AT informs Coach Jones that she will evaluate the ankle to determine the extent of the injury. You are to use a pain assessment scale to determine the extent of the pain and then recommend when the athlete will be able to return to practice.

CHAPTER REFLECTIONS

1. Read and ponder each of the following points. Do you feel you have a clear understanding of each concept? If not, reread the appropriate section of the chapter.
   - Discuss the relative effectiveness of drugs, psychological techniques, surgical procedures, and physical therapy for pain control.
   - Why is it important to develop a philosophy about pain and pain relief?
   - Discuss each of the following principles of pain relief, including how each contributes to your philosophy of pain control:
     - Conditioning vs. rehabilitation
     - Pain: demanding disciplinarian or benevolent benefactor?
     - No pain, no gain
     - Dehne's spinal adaptation syndrome
     - Resetting central control during rehabilitation
   - Give an example of the application of each of the previous pain relief principles when treating patients.
   - What is the placebo effect?
   - What effect does a positive attitude have on pain control?
   - Name four sources of orthopedic injury pain and briefly discuss the mechanism of each one.
   - Differentiate between direct and indirect pain relief.
   - Discuss the use of each of the following tools for relieving pain:
     - Therapeutic exercise
     - Counterirritants
     - Thermotherapy
     - Electrotherapy
     - Cryotherapy
   - Discuss the concept of assessing pain and quantifying pain relief.
   - Discuss the advantages and disadvantages of the following pain scales: number scale, verbal rating scale, visual analog scale, graphic rating scale, McGill Pain Questionnaire.

2. Write three to five questions for discussion with your class instructor, clinical instructor, classmates, and clinical colleagues.

3. Get together with classmates and quiz each other on the concepts of this chapter. Use the points in exercise 1 and questions you wrote for exercise 2 as a beginning. Explaining concepts out loud to others requires a deeper grasp of the material than feeling you understand it as you read.

CRITICAL THINKING RESPONSE

Critical Thinking 8.1

You can use the visual analog scale to measure pain relief. You know if you are making progress by subtracting the current treatment's score from the previous treatment's score. For example, before your treatment, the patient made a mark on the line at 66 mm from the left anchor point. After the treatment, she makes a mark 22 mm from the left anchor point.

$$66 - 22 = 44$$

This reveals a 67% reduction in pain.

REFERENCES

1. Svacina L. Pain Control #10. Longmont, CO: Staodynamics, 1977.
2. Dehne E. The spinal adaption syndrome (a theory based on the study of sprains). Clin Orthop 1955;5:211–220.
3. Dehne E, Torp RP. Treatment of joint injuries by immediate mobilization. Based upon the spinal adaptation concept. Clin Orthop 1971;77:218–232.
4. Dehne E. The rationale of early functional loading in the healing of fractures. Clin Orthop Relat Res 1979;146:18–27.
5. Dehne E. The rationale of early functional loading in the healing of fractures: A comprehensive gate control concept of repair. Clin Orthop Relat Res 1980;146:18–27.
6. Dehne E. Beurteilung und Behandlung der Verletzungen desBandapparates am Knie unter Zugrundelegung einer mechanistischen oder einer physiologischen Betrachtungsweise [Physiological consideration in treatment of tears of ligaments of the knee]. Arch Orthop Unfallchir 1938;39:319.
7. Dehne E. Ein Fall von unvollstandiger Luxation des Talus als Folge wiederholter Verletzungen im oberen Sprunggelenk [Subluxation of the ankle]. Zentralbl Chir 1933;60:688.
8. Markey KL. Personal communication with KK, 1985.
9. Grant AE. Massage with ice (cryokinetics) in the treatment of painful conditions of the musculoskeletal system. Arch Phys Med Rehabil 1964;44:233–238.
10. Hayden CA. Cryokinetics in an early treatment program. J Am Phys Ther Assoc 1964;44:990–993.
11. Charlton JE. Core curriculum for professional education in pain. Seattle: International Association for the Study of Pain, 2005.
12. Wall PD. The placebo and the placebo response. In: Wall PD, Melzack R, eds. Textbook of Pain. Edinburgh, UK: Churchill Livingstone, 2003.
13. Kirsch I, Sapirstein G. Listening to Prozac but hearing placebo: A meta-analysis of antidepressant medication. Prev Treat [serial online]. 1998;Item 2A.
14. Kirsch I. Specifying nonspecifics: Psychological mechanisms of placebo effects. In: Harrington A, ed. The Placebo Effect: An Interdisciplinary Exploration. Cambridge, MA: Harvard University Press, 1999.
15. Voudouris N, Peck C, Coleman G. The role of conditioning and expectancy in the placebo response. Pain 1990;43:121–128.
16. Montgomery C, Kirsch I. Classical conditioning and the placebo effect. Pain 1997;72:107–113.
17. Villemure C, Bushnell M. Cognitive modulation of pain: How do attention and emotion influence pain processing. Pain 2002;95:195–199.
18. Amanzio M, Benedetti F. Neuropharmacological dissection of placebo analgesia: Expectation-activated opioid systems versus conditioning-activated subsystems. J Neurosci 1999;19:484–494.
19. Gustafson D. Categorizing pain. In: Aydede M, ed. Pain: New Essays on Its Nature and the Methodology of Its Study. Cambridge, MA: MIT Press; 2005:219–241.
20. Wager T, Rilling J, Smith E, et al. Placebo-induced changes in FMRI in the anticipation and experience of pain. Science 2004;303:1162–1167.
21. Wager TD, Nitschke JB. Placebo effects in the brain: Linking mental and physiological processes. Brain Behav Immun 2005;19:281–282.
22. Peppard A, Riegler H. Ankle reconditioning with TNS. Phys Sportsmed 1980;8:105–106.
23. Gammon GD, Starr I. Studies on the relief of pain by counterirritation. J Clin Invest 1941;20:13–20.
24. McKemy D, Neuhausser W, Julius D. Identification of a cold receptor reveals a general role for TRP channels in thermosensation. Nature 2002;416:52–57.
25. Ragan BG. Menthol based analgesic balm attenuates the pressor response evoked by muscle afferents. J Athl Train 2003;38:S34.
26. Draper D, Trowbridge C, Wells A, Egget D. The ThermaCare HeatWrap increases paraspinal muscle temperature greater than the IcyHot Patch and the Mentholatum Patch. J Athl Train 2003;38:S45.
27. Zucker C. A cool ion channel. Nature 2002;416:17–18.
28. Hill J, Sumida K. Acute effect of two topical counterirritant creams on pain induced by delayed-onset muscle soreness. J Sport Rehabil 2002;11:202–208.
29. Kuritzky L. Topical analgesics: Are they underused? Hosp Pract 1997;15:131–132.
30. Bell GW, Prentice WE. Infrared modalities (therapeutic heat and cold). In: Prentice WE, ed. Therapeutic Modalities in Sports Medicine. St. Louis: Mosby College, 1998.
31. Hawkes J, Care G, Dixon JS, et al. Comparison of three physiotherapy regimens for hands with rheumatoid arthritis. Br Med J (Clin Res Ed) 1985;291(6501):1016.
32. Ayling J, Marks R. Efficacy of paraffin wax baths for rheumatoid arthritic hands. Physiotherapy 2000;86:190–201.
33. Miller MD, Wirth MA, Rockwood CA Jr. Thawing the frozen shoulder: The "patient" patient. Orthopedics 1996;19:849–853.
34. McCray RE, Patton NJ. Pain relief at trigger points: Comparison of moist heat and shortwave diathermy. J Orthop Sports Phys Ther 1984;5:175–178.
35. Steiner D, Erasala GN, Hengehold DA, et al. Continuous low-level heat therapy for acute muscular low back pain. Paper presented at the 19th annual scientific meeting of the American Pain Society, Atlanta, GA, 2000.
36. Steiner D, Erasala GN, Hengehold DA, Goodale MB. Continuous low-level heat therapy for trapezius myalgia. Paper presented at the 19th annual scientific meeting of the American Pain Society, Atlanta, GA, 2000.
37. Abramson DI, Mitchell RE, Tuck S, et al. Changes in blood flow, oxygen uptake and tissue temperatures produced by the topical application of wet heat. Arch Phys Med Rehabil 1961;42:305–318.
38. Belanger AY. Evidence-Based Guide to Therapeutic Physical Agents. Baltimore: Lippincott Williams & Wilkins, 2002.
39. Erasala GN, Rubin JM, Tuthill TA, et al. The effect of topical heat treatment on trapezius muscle blood flow using power Doppler ultrasound. Paper presented at the meetings of the American Physical Therapy Association, 2001, Anaheim, CA.
40. Lehmann JF, Masock AJ, Warren CG, Koblanski JN. Effect of therapeutic temperatures on tendon extensibility. Arch Phys Med Rehabil 1970;51:481–487.
41. Cordray YM, Krusen EM. Use of hydrocollator packs in the treatment of neck and shoulder pains. Arch Phys Med Rehabil 1959;40:105–108.
42. Fountain FP, Gersten JW, Sengir O. Decrease in muscle spasm produced by ultrasound, hot packs, and infrared radiation. Arch Phys Med Rehabil 1960;41:293–298.
43. Lehmann J, DeLateur BJ. Therapeutic heat. In: Lehman J, ed. Therapeutic Heat and Cold. 4th ed. Baltimore: Williams &d Wilkins, 1990.
44. Lehmann JF, Brunner GD, Stow RW. Pain threshold measurements after therapeutic application of ultrasound, microwaves and infrared. Arch Phys Med Rehabil 1958;39:560–565.
45. Taylor AG, West BA, Simon B, et al. How effective is TENS for acute pain? Am J Nurs 1983;83:1171–1174.
46. Zizic TM, Hoffman KC, Holt PA, et al. The treatment of osteoarthritis of the knee with pulsed electrical stimulation. J Rheumatol 1995;22:1757–1761.
47. Melzack R, Vetere P, Finch L. Transcutaneous electrical nerve stimulation for low back pain. A comparison of TENS and massage for pain and range of motion. Phys Ther 1983;63:489-493.
48. Cheing GL, Hui-Chan CW. Transcutaneous electrical nerve stimulation: Nonparallel antinociceptive effects on chronic clinical pain and acute experimental pain. Arch Phys Med Rehabil 1999;80:305–312.

49. Nordemar R, Thorner C. Treatment of acute cervical pain—A comparative group study. Pain 1981;10:93–101.

50. Arvidsson J, Eriksson E. Postoperative TENS pain relief after knee surgery: Objective evaluation. Orthopedics 1986;9:1346–1351.

51. Jensen JE, Conn RR, Hazelrigg G, Hewett JE. The use of transcutaneous neural stimulation and isokinetic testing in arthroscopic knee surgery. Am J Sports Med 1985;13:27–33.

52. Cornell PE, Lopez AL, Malofsky H. Pain reduction with transcutaneous electrical nerve stimulation after foot surgery. J Foot Surg 1984;23:326–333.

53. Chapman CE. Can the use of physical modalities for pain control be rationalized by the research evidence? Can J Physiol Pharmacol 1991;69:704–712.

54. Knight KL. Cryotherapy in Sport Injury Management. Champaign, IL: Human Kinetics, 1995.

55. Allen FM. Reduced temperature in surgery, I: Surgery of limbs. Am J Surg 1941;52:225–237.

56. Crossman LW, Ruggiero WF, Hurley V, Allen FM. Reduced temperature in surgery, II: Amputation for peripheral vascular disease. Arch Surg 1942;44:139–156.

57. Schaubel HJ. The local use of ice after orthopedic procedures. Am J Surg 1946;72:711–714.

58. Carbajal FJ, Nelson DO. The effect of cold pack application on the recovery from pitching a baseball. Athl J 1967;47:8–11,85–86.

59. Kato D. Effect of static stretch and ice immersion on pitching performance after induced muscle performance. Master's thesis, Indiana State University, Terre Haute, 1985.

60. Juvenal JP. Cryokinetics, a new concept in the treatment of injuries. Scholast Coach 1966;35:40–42.

61. Hocutt JE Jr, Jaffe R, Rylander CR, Beebe JK. Cryotherapy in ankle sprains. Am J Sports Med 1982;10:316–319.

62. Behnke RS, Blackwell HJ, Nicolette RL, Moore RJ. Ice therapy. Paper presented at the meetings of the National Athletic Trainers' Association, June 1967.

63. Moore RJ, Nicolette RL, Behnke RS. The therapeutic use of cold (cryotherapy) in the care of athletic injuries. J Natl Athl Train Assoc 1967;2:6.

64. Borg GA. Psychophysical bases of perceived exertion. Med Sci Sports Exerc 1982;14:377–381.

65. Ohnhaus E, Adler R. Methodological problems in the measurement of pain: A comparison between the verbal rating scale and the visual analogue scale. Pain 1975;1:379.

66. Huskisson E. Pain Measurement and Assessment. New York: Raven, 1983.

67. Scott J, Huskisson E. Vertical and horizontal analogue scales. Ann Rheum Dis 1979;38:560.

68. Carlsson AM. Assessment of chronic pain. I. Aspects of the reliability and validity of the visual analogue scale. Pain 1983;16:87–101.

69. Denegar CR, Perrin DH. Effect of transcutaneous electrical nerve stimulation, cold, and a combination treatment on pain, decreased range of motion, and strength loss associated with delayed onset muscle soreness. J Athl Train 1992;27:200–206.

70. Jensen MP, Karoly P, Braver S. The measurement of clinical pain intensity: A comparison of six methods. Pain 1986;27:117–126.

71. Melzack R. The McGill Pain Questionnaire: Major properties and scoring methods. Pain 1975;1:277–299.

Review Questions

Chapter 7

1. Which theory about pain by Melzack and Wall proposes a mechanism, located in the dorsal horn of the spinal cord, that allows only one sensation at a time to pass through to the brain?
   a. central control
   b. gate control
   c. endogenous opiate
   d. pattern
   e. specificity

2. Pain that is brief, short term, and often of rapid onset and high intensity is called _____.
   a. chronic pain
   b. acute pain
   c. radiating pain
   d. referred pain
   e. phantom pain

3. Pain that persists a month beyond the usual course of an acute disease or a reasonable time for an injury to heal (also described as continuous pain) or that recurs at intervals for months to years is known as

   _____.
   a. chronic pain
   b. acute pain
   c. radiating pain
   d. referred pain
   e. phantom pain

4. Pain that is felt at a site other than the actual location of a trauma, that tends to be projected outward from the torso and distally along the extremities, and that is perceived in an area that often seems to have little relation to the pathology is known as

   _____.
   a. chronic pain
   b. acute pain
   c. radiating pain
   d. referred pain
   e. secondary pain

5. A pain theory that considers previous experiences, emotional influences, sensory perception, and other factors as influencing the transmission of the pain messages and thus the perception of pain is called

   _____.
   a. central control
   b. gate control
   c. endogenous opiate
   d. pattern
   e. specificity

6. In what part of the body is the pain gate located?
   a. cerebral cortex
   b. brainstem
   c. ventral horn
   d. substantia gelatinosa
   e. none of the above

7. What are the voluntarily controlled nerves that transmit impulses from the central nervous system (CNS) to the periphery of the body and terminate in skeletal muscle?
   a. somatic motor nerves
   b. autonomic motor nerves
   c. somatic sensory nerves
   d. autonomic sensory nerves
   e. all of the above

8. The body's naturally occurring painkillers are referred to as _____.
   a. endogenous opiates
   b. T cells
   c. nociceptors
   d. dopamines
   e. morphine

9. Which of the following is not an endogenous opiate?
   a. enkephalin
   b. endorphin
   c. serotonin
   d. bradykinin
   e. none of the above

Chapter 8

1. Which pain assessment tool is a scale that consists of no numbers but is a 100 mm line with contrasting descriptors, such as "no pain" and "severe pain," on the anchor points at the ends of the line.
   a. number scale
   b. verbal rating scale
   c. visual analog scale
   d. graphic rating scale
   e. McGill Pain Questionnaire

2. Which pain measurement tool uses pictures, scales, and words to help patients describe sensory and affective aspects as well as magnitude and changes in their pain?
   a. number scale
   b. verbal rating scale
   c. visual analog scale
   d. graphic rating scale
   e. McGill Pain Questionnaire

3. A medicinally inactive substance or mock intervention given to a patient to bring about a desired response and satisfy the patient's demand for medicine is known as _____.
   a. a counterirritant
   b. a placebo
   c. an irritant
   d. central control
   e. a sugar pill

4. Which of the following is false with respect to exercise and pain?
   a. Therapeutic exercise should be relatively pain free. T
   b. It is acceptable if the exercise is moderately uncomfortable as long as swelling does not increase.
   c. Therapeutic exercise or activity during rehabilitation should not evoke the same type of pain that was experienced when the injury occurred. T
   d. Pain during an activity indicates the activity is too strenuous or complex. T
   e. Sharp pain after an activity indicates the activity is too strenuous or complex. T

5. Activities that result in pain during rehabilitation will hinder the rehabilitation process by inducing _____.
   a. neural inhibition
   b. the spinal adaptation syndrome
   c. central control
   d. proprioceptors
   e. swelling

6. Electrical stimulating currents are thought to reduce pain by all of the following except by _____.
   a. reducing muscle spasm, hence relaxing the muscle
   b. releasing endogenous opiates at pain receptor sites
   c. releasing morphine-like drugs from the thalamus
   d. stimulating the nonpainful nerves
   e. modulating neural inhibition

7. The most common use of cold with acute orthopedic injury is to modulate the pain of sprains, strains, and contusions to facilitate _____.
   a. reduction of swelling
   b. healing
   c. therapeutic exercise
   d. reduction of spasm
   e. endorphin release

ELECTROTHERAPY

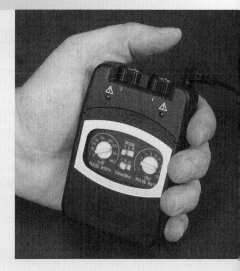

For most students and many clinicians, understanding electricity and how to use it therapeutically is difficult, partly because in many cases their background in chemistry and physics (the basis of electricity) is not as strong as their background in anatomy and physiology. In addition, not all clinicians and manufacturers of electrotherapy devices use the same vocabulary to explain how various electrotherapy devices work.

Chapter 9 is a review of the basic science of electricity. We review basic chemistry and physics and then discuss the principles and characteristics of electricity that are necessary for understanding electrotherapy. We then discuss various current characteristics: how these characteristics are manipulated to produce different output forms and how the output form is transmitted from the device to the patient. Last, we present general principles of electrotherapy application for achieving various therapeutic goals. In Chapter 10 we present specific application techniques for achieving the most common electrotherapeutic goals.

Principles of Electricity for Electrotherapy

BOX 9

OPENING SCENE

While visiting his uncle's dairy farm, a young city boy was invited to play a game of tag with some neighboring farm children. As he chased the other children, he noticed they took the long way around a wire fence through a gate and out across a field. Sensing an opportunity to take a shortcut and catch up, he grabbed hold of the wire fence to pull it down low enough to step across it. Whap! He felt a jolt as he touched the wire and quickly let go. The other kids heard his painful cry and began laughing and joking about the city slicker who thought he could outsmart them. You see, the boy's uncle had installed an electric fence around the field to keep the cows contained. The boy learned a few things about electricity that day, and he learned to respect it.

A Common Language

The therapeutic value of electrical currents is centuries old. Your great-grandparents could have purchased an "electrical stimulator" from their Sears, Roebuck catalog or from one of many other vendors.[1] But the claims of its efficacy were so outlandish that the use of electrical modalities waned. The discovery of silicon resistors and microcircuits during space exploration led to the introduction of high-volt and Russian current stimulators in the 1980s, and a rebirth of the modality occurred.

Many types of electrical stimulators followed. To be competitive, manufacturers developed variations, with a plethora of electrical current characteristics, and they used arbitrary terms to differentiate these characteristics.[1] In an effort to sell their products, the manufacturers made unfounded claims about effectiveness. The combination of the variety of electrical current characteristics and the inconsistent terminology for describing them led to confusion. It seemed as though each manufacturer spoke a different language.

In 1990, the Section on Electrophysiology of the American Physical Therapy Association published a common language for electrotherapy. The use of these common terms by educators, clinicians, and manufacturers has helped minimize confusion.

Clinicians must understand and use a common language for two important reasons. First, they need to be able to use electrical stimulation intelligently. Decision-making professionals must understand *why* as well as how to use electrical stimulation so they can provide the most benefit to patients. Second, they need to be capable of intelligently discussing the features of various electrical stimulation units with sales personnel and thus make informed purchasing decisions when the need arises.

The Basics of Electricity

Numerous definitions of electricity can be found. Here are four definitions, all correct, each one emphasizing a different aspect of electricity:

- A property of certain fundamental particles of all matter that have a force field associated with them, manifested by either an accumulation of, or an absence of, electrons on an atom or body[2]
- A form of energy associated with the existence and interaction of electrical charge, manifested by the accumulation of, or absence of, electrons on an atom or body; exhibits magnetic (electromagnetic), chemical, mechanical (electrokinetic), and thermal properties
- A form of energy that exhibits magnetic, chemical, mechanical, and thermal effects; formed from the interaction of positive (+) and negative (−) charges[3]
- The physical phenomena associated with the existence and interaction of electrical charge, either static charges (electrostatics) or moving streams of charge (current)[4]

STATIC AND CURRENT ELECTRICITY

There are two types of electricity: static and current. **Static electricity** is frictional electricity, created by rubbing two objects together. In the process, one object gains electrons, the other object loses electrons. Examples are rubbing your shoes on carpet, running a comb through dry hair, and rubbing a balloon on hair. Static electricity can be stored in an insulated conductor in which the charges are in a state of tension, ready to flow. The discharge is often a single discharge into the ground or through something else and into the ground. The body of the earth is considered an electrical sink, which means it can accept

the electrons will move back and forth in the metal plates and wire, which by definition is alternating current. As long as the mechanical power keeps the magnet turning, AC current will flow.

An Electrical Motor vs. an Electrical Generator

An electrical motor is conceptually the same as a generator; they consist of the same basic components, but they have opposite processes. A generator converts mechanical power to electrical power, whereas an electrical motor converts electrical power to mechanical power.

Alternating Current Terms

A graph of AC flow versus time appears as a sine wave as the current flows in one direction and then the other (Fig. 9.7). The following elements are essential to understanding the use of electrical currents in therapy:

- **Impulse:** AC flow in a single direction. In Figure 9.7, impulse appears as a half circle (or egg); the portion of the graph representing current flowing from the baseline to the maximum in one direction and back to the baseline. In the example given earlier of generating AC, it represents electron flow during the time the magnet rotates 180°.
- **Cycle:** Two impulses. The portion of the graph representing current flowing from the baseline to the maximum in one direction, back across the baseline to the maximum in the opposite direction, and back to the baseline. In the previous example of generating AC, it represents electron flow during the time the magnet rotates 360°.
- **Frequency:** The rate of passage of crests on a wave form, expressed in cycles per second (cps) or hertz (Hz). Ordinary electricity in the United States is 60 cps; in Europe and parts of Asia it is 50 cps. Low-frequency current is <1,000 cps; high-frequency current is >10,000 cps.

Devices for measuring and regulating electricity are described in Box 9.2.

Output Current Characteristics

Therapeutic medical devices operate on (are powered by) either AC or DC, which is called the input current. The device then sends either pure current (AC or DC) or a modulated (manipulated) pulsed current. The three basic

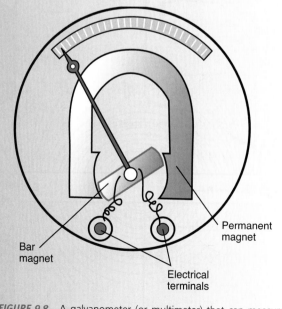

BOX 9.2 *DEVICES FOR MEASURING AND REGULATING ELECTRICITY*

Measurement instruments are based on the electromagnetic effects of current. In the simplest case, they include a permanent magnet and an electromagnet that can rotate. When the electromagnet is charged, the two magnets repel each other, causing the electromagnet to rotate away from the permanent magnet. The amount of repulsion is proportional to the strength of the electromagnet, which is proportional to the amount of current flowing through it. Adding a display and calibrating it creates a measuring device. The generic device is called a **galvanometer** (Fig. 9.8). With additional circuitry, it can be configured to become an **ampmeter** (ampere meter), which measures the flow rate of current (most are actually milliampmeters); a **voltmeter**, which measures voltage; or an **ohmmeter**, which measures resistance to current flow.

FIGURE 9.8. A galvanometer (or multimeter) that can measure amps, volts, or ohms.

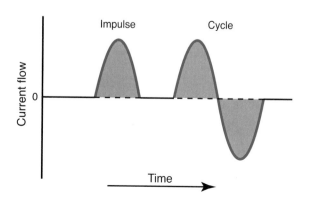

FIGURE 9.7. Impulse and cycle on a graph of current flow vs. time.

forms of output current, in order of increasing complexity, are (see Fig. 9.1):

- *DC:* Continuous flow of electrons in a single direction
- *AC:* Continuous flow of electrons; defined by frequency or cycles per second; can be turned off and on to create bursts
- *Pulsed current:* Interrupted electron flow

The simplest form of pulsed current interruption is turning the switch on and off. The process is much more complicated, however, as the input current is manipulated, regulated, and adjusted in numerous ways to create many different output current forms.

CURRENT MODULATION

Current modulation includes all the manipulating, regulating, and adjusting of the input current to create a variety of specific output wave forms. Most electrotherapy

output is pulsed. A **pulse** is a finite period of charged particle movement, separated from other pulses for a limited time during which no current flows. A pulse consists of one or more **phases**, which is a period of unidirectional charged particle movement (current flow). Characteristics of the most commonly used electrotherapy phases and pulses are explained in Box 9.3.

A second way that input currents are modulated is the timing of the current flow. The basic unit of timing is **phase duration** (sometimes called *pulse width*), the time during which current flows in a single direction. This and other aspects of current timing modulation are explained in Box 9.4.

Amplitude (*intensity, output*) is measured in one of two ways: voltage delivered to the electrodes, or current flowing through the circuit (which includes the body part being treated). Current amplitude modulation is explained in Box 9.5.

BOX 9.3 *PHASE AND PULSE CHARACTERISTICS*

Phase and pulse characteristics are defined by the following:

- **Phase shape:** The shape of an output current after being modulated. The phase shapes that are most commonly used therapeutically are rectangular, spike, triangular, and sawtooth.
- A pulse is characterized by the number of its phases (Fig. 9.9):
  - **Monophasic:** One phase (current flows in one direction only)
  - **Biphasic:** Two phases (current flows in both directions)
  - **Triphasic:** Three phases
  - **Polyphasic:** Many phases
- **Phase charge:** The total electrical charge of a single phase, expressed in coulombs (microcoulombs for NMES). It is the time integral (area under the

curve); the result of both amplitude and duration (Fig. 9.10).
- **Pulse charge:** The amount of electrical charge of a single pulse; the sum of phase charges
- **Pulse symmetry:** The relationship between the shapes of the two phases of a biphasic pulse (Fig. 9.10):
  - **Symmetrical pulse:** A pulse with identical phases
  - **Asymmetrical pulse:** A pulse with different phases
- **Pulse charge balance:** The relationship between the charges of two phases of a biphasic pulse, independent of the symmetry of the phases (Fig. 9.10):
  - **Balanced phase:** A pulse containing equal phase charges
  - **Unbalanced phase:** A pulse containing unequal phase charges
- **AC train:** A continuous repetitive series of pulses at a fixed frequency (or a segment of AC)
- **Burst:** A finite series of pulses (or a finite interval of AC at a specific frequency) flowing for a limited time period, followed by no current flow. Think of it as turning a pulse train or AC on and off (Fig. 9.11).
  - **Burst interval:** The time during which a burst occurs, usually measured in milliseconds
  - **Interburst interval:** The time between bursts, usually measured in milliseconds

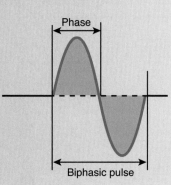

FIGURE 9.9. Two continuous phases form a biphasic pulse.

BOX 9.3 **PHASE AND PULSE CHARACTERISTICS (continued)**

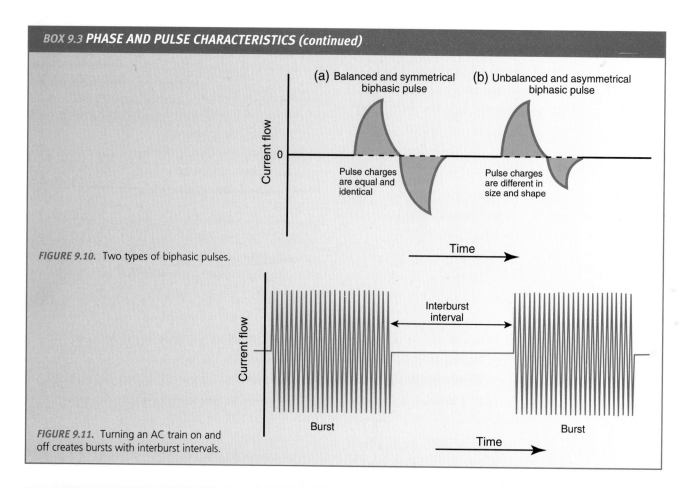

(a) Balanced and symmetrical biphasic pulse

Pulse charges are equal and identical

(b) Unbalanced and asymmetrical biphasic pulse

Pulse charges are different in size and shape

Current flow

Time

FIGURE 9.10. Two types of biphasic pulses.

Current flow

Interburst interval

Burst   Burst

Time

FIGURE 9.11. Turning an AC train on and off creates bursts with interburst intervals.

BOX 9.4 **CURRENT TIMING MODULATION**

Phase duration and the timing of current flow are defined by the following (Fig. 9.12):

- **Rise time:** The time from the beginning of a phase until it reaches maximal amplitude
- **Decay time:** The time from maximal amplitude to the end of a phase
- **Pulse duration** *(pulse width):* The time required for each pulse to complete its cycle, usually reported in microseconds or milliseconds
  - *Short pulse duration:* A pulse that lasts <150 μsec
  - *Long pulse duration:* A pulse that lasts >200 μsec

- **Interpulse interval:** The time between successive pulses
- **Pulse period:** The beginning of the pulse to the beginning of the subsequent pulse; pulse duration plus interpulse interval
- **Pulse rate** *(pulse frequency):* The number of pulses per second (pps; in Hz).
- **Duty cycle:** The percentage of time that current is flowing (pulse duration) over one pulse period. Thus current with an on time of 10 msec and an off time of 40 msec would have a 20% duty cycle.

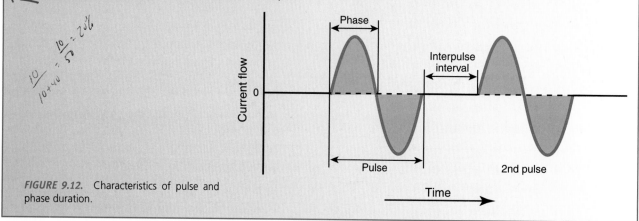

Phase

Interpulse interval

Current flow

Pulse   2nd pulse

Time

FIGURE 9.12. Characteristics of pulse and phase duration.

BOX 9.5 *CURRENT AMPLITUDE MODULATION*

Current amplitude is characterized by the following (Fig. 9.13):

- **Peak current:** The highest magnitude of the pulse
- **Average current:** The average magnitude of a pulse. It is computed in one of two ways: the average current during the pulse or the average current during the period. The second method includes the off time between pulses.
- **Stimulation pattern:** The structure of the pulses used in the current
- **Constant stimulation pattern:** Stimulation in which amplitude of successive pulses (or cycles) is the same
- **Surged stimulation pattern:** Stimulation in which amplitude of successive pulses (or cycles) gradually increase from zero to a maximum preset intensity (Fig. 9.14)
- Surge characteristics
- **Ramp up:** The time during which the intensity of an electrical charge increases
- **Plateau:** The time during which pulses remain at maximum preset intensity
- **Ramp down:** The time during which the intensity of an electrical charge decreases
- **Time on:** The time during which current flows from the beginning to the end of a surge
- **Time off:** The time during which current does not flow; the time between surges

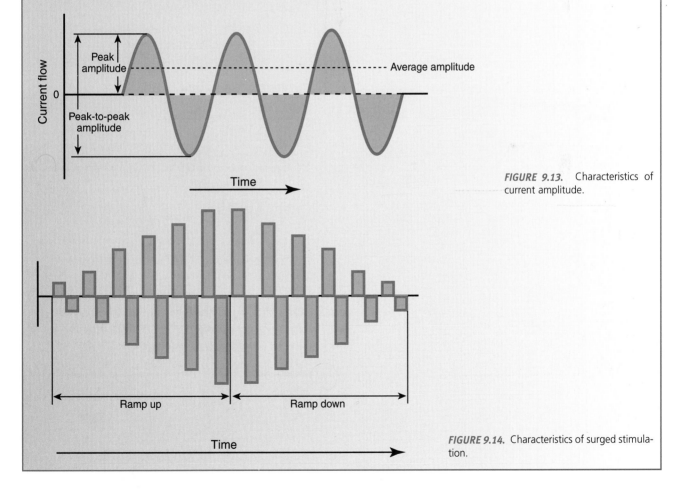

FIGURE 9.13. Characteristics of current amplitude.

FIGURE 9.14. Characteristics of surged stimulation.

A **wave form** is the shape of an electrical current, created when the current is graphed with amplitude on the vertical axis and time on the horizontal axis. The modulation of DC and AC produces a variety of output forms. The most commonly used therapeutic wave forms are described in Box 9.6. Originally, electrical simulators output a single wave form. Manufactures vigorously argued the merits of their specific wave form, claiming it was superior to the others. In time, however, as technology advanced, manufacturers began to develop generators that could output a variety of wave forms.

BOX 9.6 COMMONLY USED WAVE FORMS

Following are nine frequently used electrotherapy wave forms with their descriptions:

1. **Direct (galvanic) wave form:** Pure DC, used for iontophoresis

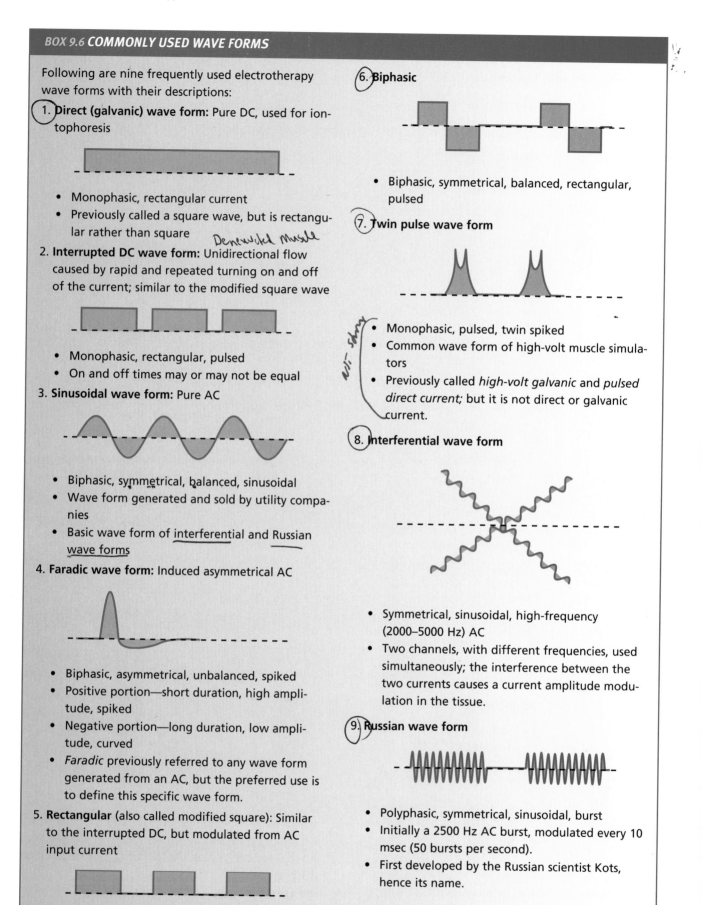

- Monophasic, rectangular current
- Previously called a square wave, but is rectangular rather than square *Denervated Muscle*

2. **Interrupted DC wave form:** Unidirectional flow caused by rapid and repeated turning on and off of the current; similar to the modified square wave

- Monophasic, rectangular, pulsed
- On and off times may or may not be equal

3. **Sinusoidal wave form:** Pure AC

- Biphasic, symmetrical, balanced, sinusoidal
- Wave form generated and sold by utility companies
- Basic wave form of <u>interferential</u> and <u>Russian</u> wave forms

4. **Faradic wave form:** Induced asymmetrical AC

- Biphasic, asymmetrical, unbalanced, spiked
- Positive portion—short duration, high amplitude, spiked
- Negative portion—long duration, low amplitude, curved
- *Faradic* previously referred to any wave form generated from an AC, but the preferred use is to define this specific wave form.

5. **Rectangular** (also called modified square): Similar to the interrupted DC, but modulated from AC input current

- Monophasic, rectangular, pulsed

6. **Biphasic**

- Biphasic, symmetrical, balanced, rectangular, pulsed

7. **Twin pulse wave form**

- Monophasic, pulsed, twin spiked
- Common wave form of high-volt muscle simulators
- Previously called *high-volt galvanic* and *pulsed direct current;* but it is not direct or galvanic current.

8. **Interferential wave form**

- Symmetrical, sinusoidal, high-frequency (2000–5000 Hz) AC
- Two channels, with different frequencies, used simultaneously; the interference between the two currents causes a current amplitude modulation in the tissue.

9. **Russian wave form**

- Polyphasic, symmetrical, sinusoidal, burst
- Initially a 2500 Hz AC burst, modulated every 10 msec (50 bursts per second).
- First developed by the Russian scientist Kots, hence its name.

Tissue Responses to Electrical Stimulation

Therapeutic electrical applications cause four types of responses in the tissue: thermal, chemical, magnetic, and kinetic. Thermal effects will be discussed in Chapter 16. Aspects of the other three are presented in this section.

CHEMICAL EFFECTS

The chemical effect of electrical stimulation involves driving ions of medication into the body. When a direct electrical current is passed through the solution, the ions wander or move:

- Positively charged ions move to the negative pole, the cathode.
- Negatively charged ions move to the positive pole, the anode.

This effect is illustrated by two classic, simple experiments performed by LeDuc in the 1890s.[5]

LeDuc's Experiments

In his first experiment, LeDuc cut a hole in a potato and filled it with a potassium iodine solution, which was partially dissociated into positive potassium ions and negative iodine ions (Fig. 9.15). He then stuck wires into either end of the potato and attached them to a battery. As the DC passed through the potato, the ions were attracted to the two poles: the positive potassium ion to the negative pole and the negative iodine ion to the positive pole.

In LeDuc's second experiment, he placed two rabbits in series in an electrical circuit so that the current passed through both animals. This experiment is described in Figure 9.16.

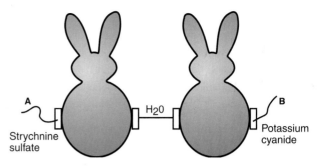

FIGURE 9.16. The chemical effects of electrical stimulation: LeDuc's rabbit experiment. Two rabbits are placed in series in an electrical circuit, with an electrode soaked in a strychnine sulfate solution attached to one rabbit and an electrode soaked in potassium cyanide attached to the other. The electrodes attached to the wire between the rabbits were soaked in plain water (H_2O). The battery was attached so that electrode A was negative and electrode B was positive, and the current passed through the rabbits without harming them. When the battery was reversed, both rabbits died, the first from strychnine poisoning and the second from cyanide poisoning. The positive A pole repelled the positive strychnine and caused it to enter the first rabbit. The negative B pole repelled the negative cyanide and caused it to enter the second rabbit.

LeDuc's two experiments clearly illustrated that direct current can drive ionized molecules into the skin. This concept is the basis of iontophoresis (discussed later in this chapter).

Requirements for Ion Migration

Continuous monophasic DC electron flow is necessary for ion migration. The process is moving electrons against gradient, so if the electron flow is discontinuous, the electrons will diffuse back to their starting position during the "no flow" time. It is like pushing a car up a hill; if you push for a while and then rest, the car will roll back down to the starting position.

In the 1980s there was a misconception that high-volt twin-pulsed simulators created a chemical effect.[6,7] In fact, they were once called "high-volt galvanic simulators." They do produce a monophasic wave form; but they are pulsed, so they do not produce the continuous electron flow necessary to cause a chemical effect.

Iontophoresis

Iontophoresis is the application of a mild direct electrical current (DC) for transporting negatively or positively charged ions from a drug solution into a patient's skin and underlying tissues.[8–10] It requires long-term flow (5–10 min) of a pure DC. The medication must ionize in solution and be placed under the appropriate electrode so that the active ion is driven into the tissue.

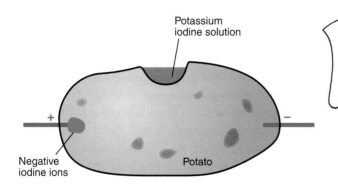

FIGURE 9.15. The chemical effects of electrical stimulation: LeDuc's potato experiment. As a direct current was passed through a potato containing a small pool of potassium iodine solution, negative iodine ions migrated to the end of the potato with the positive pole. Analysis was easy. The iodine interacted with the starch near the positive pole to form blue starch iodine, visible with the naked eye.

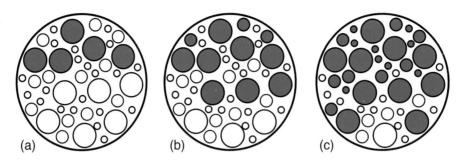

FIGURE 9.19. The influence of nerve size and depth on nerve excitability. *Solid circles,* stimulated neurons. **(a)** A current that is just strong enough to reach threshold will stimulate only the largest and most superficial fibers of a mixed nerve. **(b)** A more intense current will also stimulate medium-size superficial fibers and large fibers in the middle of the nerve bundle. **(c)** A still larger current will also stimulate small superficial fibers, medium-size fibers in the middle, and large fibers deep in the nerve.

Current Density

Current density is a measure of the quantity of charged ions moving through a particular cross-sectional area of an electrode and the skin beneath the electrode (Fig. 9.20). For example, a current of a 500 mA applied through a 25 cm^2 electrode would have a current density of 20 mA/cm^2. If the electrodes through which the current flows are of equal size, the current density will be equal. If one of the electrodes is bigger than the other, it will have less current density.

> **CRITICAL THINKING 9.5** (a) *If the current density under a 2 cm × 2 cm electrode is 80 mA/cm^2, what would the current density be under its paired electrode, which is 8 cm × 8 cm? (b) What would it be under a paired electrode that was 2 cm × 2 cm?*

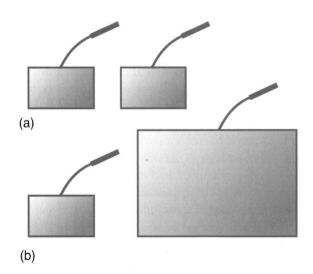

FIGURE 9.20. Current density is a measure of the quantity of charged ions moving through a particular cross-sectional area of an electrode. **(a)** If the electrodes through which the current flows are of equal size, the current density underneath the electrodes will be equal. **(b)** If one of the electrodes is bigger than the other, the bigger electrode will have less current density.

Interaction of Current Amplitude and Pulse Duration

Current strength is a product of its amplitude and pulse duration (Fig. 9.21). Thus average current (and fiber recruitment) can be increased by increasing either current amplitude or pulse duration (as long as the other remains constant). This relationship also explains why a low-volt simulator can cause greater muscle contraction than a high-volt simulator. Although voltage is five times greater in the high-volt simulator, its pulse duration is much shorter, so the average current is lower.

Frequency of Stimulation

Frequency of stimulation has no effect on the stimulation threshold of individual muscle fibers; however, the force of whole muscle contraction and muscle fatigue increase. As the frequency of stimulation increases, muscle fibers don't have time to relax between stimuli (action potentials), so the contraction becomes steady, as opposed to a series of individual twitches. This is known as a **tetanic contraction**, and the point at which it begins is known as **tetany**. Tetany occurs when the stimulation

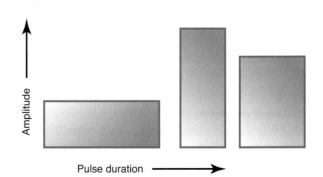

FIGURE 9.21. Current strength is the product of its amplitude and pulse duration. For example, each of the three wave forms shown here (graphs of current amplitude by pulse duration) has the same current strength.

frequency exceeds 20–30 pps, depending on the type of muscle fiber.

Electrode Orientation

Muscle conducts electricity four times better longitudinally than transversely.[4] Therefore, electrodes should be applied parallel to muscle fibers rather than perpendicular to them.

Motor Point

The **motor point** is the place where a given amount of current will elicit the greatest muscular contraction. It is the point where the motor nerve enters the muscle, usually located at the beginning of the muscle belly. The clinician should be aware of the following:

- Motor points are located by trial and error, by looking for a good sharp muscle contraction while moving the electrode over the muscle.
- Charts can help identify motor points, but there is a certain amount of anatomical variation in location.
- Motor point should not be confused with trigger point. A trigger point is a localized area of the body that is extremely sensitive to palpation, electrical stimulation, and ultrasound.

ELECTRODES

Electrodes are devices attached to the terminals of a generator or electrical stimulator unit through which current enters and leaves the body. Electrodes come in a variety of sizes, shapes, and materials and are named according to their function. The three most popular electrode systems over the years have been the following:

- *Metal-sponge electrodes:* A thin metal plate attaches to the wire from the terminal. A wet sponge is placed between the metal plate and the skin to increase the conductivity between the two. These are held in place with a flexible rubber belt or a sand bag.
- *Carbon- or silicon-impregnated rubber electrodes with sponge, paper towel or conductive gel interface:* Carbon or silicon is added to the rubber, which is an insulator, so that it becomes a conductor. A wet sponge, a wet paper towel, or conductive gel is placed between the rubber plate and the skin to increase the conductivity between the two. These are held in place with a flexible rubber belt or a sand bag.
- *Adhesive backed carbon- or silicon-impregnated rubber electrodes:* Adhesive is used in place of the sponge or paper towel and rubber belt or sand bag. These are quicker and easier to apply but more expensive than other systems. They were intended to be single-use,

disposable electrodes, but most people reuse them 8–10 times, until the adhesive loses its stickiness.

Recently, companies have begun to distribute inexpensive single-use electrodes (Fig. 9.22). These electrodes resemble a sticker or roll of stamps. You simply remove the electrode from the backing and stick it on the treatment site. After the treatment, the electrode is removed and thrown into a trash receptacle. Manufactures claim these electrodes deliver current to the body as effectively as adhesive reusable electrodes.

Physical Characteristics

The shape of an electrode is not important. Most of them are round, square, or rectangular. However, the size and the material that electrodes are made of are significant.

- *Size:* The size of the electrode and its placement determine the number of motor units that are stimulated. A small electrode placed over a single muscle will stimulate only that muscle, whereas a larger electrode can stimulate a number of muscles. The size of electrodes also has a bearing on the current density under the electrode. The smaller the electrode is, the greater the current density will be, as long as the current output is the same.
- *Material:* The conductivity of the material will affect the amount of current flow. Carbon- or silicon-impregnated rubber electrodes seem to have better conductivity than do metal-sponge electrodes, but their useful life is limited. The carbon or silicon will leach out with use, reducing the electrode's conductivity.

Cross-Contamination of Reusable Electrodes

Self-adhesive electrodes should be reused only on the same patient. If used on different patients it may transfer

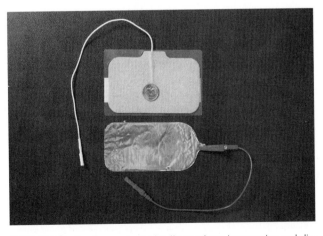

FIGURE 9.22. Single-use electrodes (*bottom*) are inexpensive and discarded after each use. Note: The dime on the multiple-use electrode shows size.

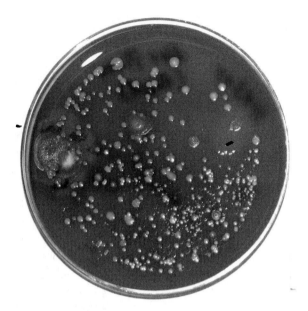

FIGURE 9.23. Bacterial culture from an electrode that had been applied on multiple patients. Notice the several colonies of bacteria growing on the electrode. (Courtesy of Alex Pinto.)

bacteria from one patient to the next. Figure 9.23 shows a culture dish with several colonies of bacteria on it. This culture was taken from a randomly selected electrode in a sports medicine and physical therapy clinic. It is important that the area to be treated be cleaned before treatment and that electrodes are not used on several patients; these measures help prevent the cross-contamination and the spread of germs among patients. Plus there is no risk of cross-contamination with single-use, self-adhesive electrodes because they are discarded after use.

Electrode Function

An electrode's function—what happens to the tissues under it when stimulated—depends on its relative size in relation to its paired electrode. Electrodes are classified as active or dispersive:

• **Active electrode**: An electrode under which the current density is great enough to elicit the desired response (Fig. 9.24)

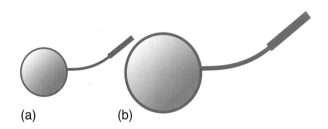

(a)   (b)

FIGURE 9.24. Electrodes may be active or dispersive, depending on their size relative to the opposite electrode of their pair. **(a)** An active electrode is always much smaller than **(b)** a dispersive electrode and therefore has a greater current density.

• **Dispersive electrode** *(indifferent electrode)*: An electrode under which the current density is not great enough to elicit the desired response. An electrode is dispersive when it is much larger than the electrode(s) from the opposite terminal. It is used to complete the circuit and usually is applied to a location remote to the area being treated.

Placement Techniques

There are three basic techniques for placing electrodes (Fig. 9.25). These techniques facilitate different responses by the tissues under them:

• **Bipolar technique:** Electrodes from the two terminals are of equal size, resulting in essentially equal current density under them. (There will be some difference in current density if there is a difference in tissue resistance under the two electrodes.) Both electrodes are, therefore, active. The electrodes are

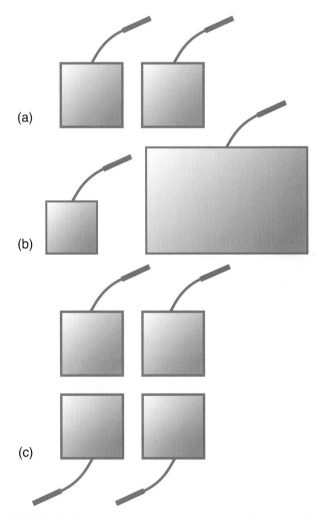

(a)

(b)

(c)

FIGURE 9.25. Three electrode placement techniques: **(a)** bipolar, with a pair of equal size electrodes; **(b)** unipolar, with a pair of unequal size electrodes; and **(c)** quadripolar with four electrodes of equal size.

both applied to the treatment area, in relative proximity to each other.

- **Unipolar technique:** Electrodes from the two terminals are of unequal size, thus creating active and dispersive electrodes. There may be multiple active electrodes, all coming from the same generator terminal, as long as their aggregate size is less than the dispersive electrode. The active electrode(s) is (are) applied to the treatment area and the dispersive electrode is applied to a remote location.
- **Quadripolar technique:** Four electrodes of equal size are used, a pair from each of two channels. Generally they crisscross the target tissue. The most popular use of this technique is with interferential stimulation, by which two currents of different frequencies are applied.

Polarity

Polarity is the positive or negative voltage on the active electrode compared to the voltage on the dispersive electrode. This should not be confused with unipolar and bipolar placement techniques. Polarity applies only when a unipolar placement technique is used. Polarity appears to affect the excitability of nerves, but some people respond better to negative polarity and others to positive polarity.

Therapeutic Uses of Electrical Stimulation

There are five types of tissue responses to electrical stimulation, four of which are evoked by therapeutic stimula-

tion (Table 9.2). The five types of responses are:

- **Ion migration:** Ions move through the tissue in response to continuous DC stimulation.
- **Sensory twitch:** Repetitions of brief isolated sensory ticks in response to moderate-amplitude, low-frequency pulsed stimulation. This response is not used therapeutically.
- **Fused response:** A sustained sensory response that feels like pins and needles, in response to moderate-amplitude, high-frequency pulsed or AC stimulation.
- **Twitch contraction:** Repetitions of isolated brief muscular contraction followed by relaxation in response to low-frequency, high-amplitude pulsed stimulation. It occurs in individual muscle fibers or in entire muscle groups.
- **Tetanic contraction:** A sustained muscular contraction in response to repetitive high-frequency, high-amplitude pulsed or AC stimulation of at least 20–30 pps. It occurs in individual muscle fibers or in entire muscle groups.

Specific uses of these types (except sensory twitch) and the applications that invoke them are presented in Chapter 10.

TABLE 9.2	**Tissue Responses to Electrical Stimulation and Types of Stimulators**			
	CURRENT CHARACTERISTICS			
TISSUE RESPONSE	**Amplitude**	**Frequency**	**THERAPEUTIC GOAL**	**WAVE FORM**
DC STIMULATORS				
Ion migration	Moderate	None	Iontophoresis	DC
AC STIMULATORS				
Sensory twitch	Low	Low	None known	All but DC
Sensory fused	Low	High	Pain reduction	Interferential
			Wound healing	Twin pulse
			Edema reduction	Twin pulse
Twitch (pulsed) contraction	Moderate	Low	Muscle reeducation	Biphasic, Russian
			As part of ultrasound for tendinitis	Twin pulse, biphasic, Russian
Tetanic contraction (with surge)	High	High	Strength development	Biphasic, Russian
			Spasm reduction	Biphasic, Russian

CLOSING SCENE

Recall from the chapter opening scene that a young boy got shocked when he touched an electric fence on his uncle's dairy farm. (This is a true story that happened to DD.) After reading this chapter, you now know that the electrical shock would have been increased if the boy were standing in water and would have been absent if he had touched the fence while wearing rubber gloves. You also know that the power of electricity can be harnessed and used to decrease pain or elicit a muscle contraction. Our goal for this chapter was to provide you with a basic understanding of electricity and how it relates to therapeutic modalities, which you will appreciate when you use electrical stimulation clinically.

CHAPTER REFLECTIONS

1. Read and ponder each of the following points. Do you feel you have a clear understanding of each concept? If not, reread the appropriate section of the chapter.
   - Why is there confusion about the therapeutic use of electrical currents?
   - What is meant by a common language in relation to NMES? Why is this concept important for clinicians, scientists, and manufacturers?
   - What is electricity?
   - What is an electrical charge?
   - Differentiate between static and current electricity.
   - Give three examples of why an understanding of chemistry and physics is essential for understanding electricity.
   - Differentiate between AC, DC, and pulsed currents. How is each type of current produced?
   - What is Ohm's law?
   - Explain the relationship between electricity and magnetism.
   - Differentiate between conductor, insulator, semiconductor, and partial conductor.
   - Discuss the following aspects of quantifying electricity: coulomb, voltage, ampere, and ohm.
   - Compare and contrast electrical current and the flow of water. Include the requirements of each.
   - Describe each of the following elements of electrical equipment: generator, terminal, electrical circuit, muscle stimulator, nerve stimulator, circuit breaker, GFI.
   - Discuss how electricity is generated and converted, including the requirements in each case.
   - Compare and contrast an electrical motor and an electrical generator.
   - Define each of the following as they apply to electrical stimulation: impulse, cycle, frequency, pulsed current, current modulation, phase, phase duration, phase shape, pulse, monophasic pulse, biphasic pulse, polyphasic pulse, phase charge, pulse charge, pulse symmetry, pulse charge balance, burst, pulse duration (width), interpulse interval, period, pulse rate, duty cycle, amplitude, peak current, average current.
   - Differentiate between constant and surged stimulation. When would you use each?
   - Define the following: ramp up, plateau, ramp down, time on, time off.
   - What is a wave form? Define the most commonly used electrotherapy wave forms.
   - Describe LeDuc's experiments, and explain their relevance to electrical stimulation.
   - What role do magnetic effects have on tissue rehabilitation?
   - Define each of the following and explain its relevance to NMES: polarized neuron membrane, action potential, and nerve excitability.
   - What is a mixed nerve?
   - Differentiate between A fibers, B fibers, and C fibers, including size, speed, and function.
   - Explain the effect of the following on nerve excitability: nerve size, nerve depth, and tissue resistance.
   - What is current density, and what is its role in NMES?
   - Discuss the relationship between pulse duration, current amplitude, and frequency of stimulation on muscle fiber recruitment.

- Explain the difference between a trigger point and a motor point. Describe the role of each in NMES.
- Discuss the role of electrodes in NMES, including physical dimensions, function, and placement techniques.
- Define and differentiate among the following tissue responses to NMES: chemical, thermal, magnetic, and kinetic.
- Define and differentiate the five basic types of tissue responses to electrical stimulation. Include the characteristics of each response, generator settings necessary to evoke each one, and why each is used.

2. Write three to five questions for discussion with your class instructor, clinical instructor, classmates, and clinical colleagues.
3. Get together with classmates and quiz each other on the concepts of this chapter. Use the points in exercise 1 and questions you wrote for exercise 2 as a beginning. Explaining concepts out loud to others requires a deeper grasp of the material than feeling you understand it as you read.

CRITICAL THINKING RESPONSES

Critical Thinking 9.1

a. 0.005 amp or 5 mA; 100 V/20,000 Ω
b. 0.01 amp or 10 mA; 100 V/10,000 Ω

Critical Thinking 9.2

Increase voltage, and decrease resistance. Yes, cleaning oils from the skin will decrease its resistance and current flow will increase.

Critical Thinking 9.3

The battery generates DC. We know this because electrons flow from one place to another.

Critical Thinking 9.4

When electrode A was negative and electrode B was positive, negative electrode A attracted the positive strychnine and repelled the negative sulfate. At the same time, positive electrode B attracted the negative cyanide and repelled the positive potassium. Thus the current passed through the rabbits but the poisons did not.

When electrode A was positive and electrode B was negative, positive electrode A attracted the negative sulfate and repelled the positive strychnine. Simultaneously negative electrode B attracted the positive potassium and repelled the negative cyanide. Thus, as the current passed through the rabbits, it drove the poisons into them—the strychnine into the first rabbit and the cyanide into the second rabbit.

Critical Thinking 9.5

a. 5 mA/cm^2. The second electrode is 16 times as big; 2 × 2 = 4; 8 × 8 = 64; 64 ÷ 4 = 16. Did you mistakenly think it was 4 times as big? Granted, 8 is four times 2, but we are talking about area here, not linear dimensions.
b. 80 mA/cm^2. The two electrodes are the same size.

REFERENCES

1. Behray J. The Turn of the Century Electrotherapy Museum: Tesla Library. Available at: www.electrotherapymuseum.com/Library/index.htm. Accessed April 2006.
2. Merriam-Webster's Collegiate Dictionary. 11 ed. Springfield, MA: Merriam-Webster, 2003.
3. Tabers Cyclopedic Medical Dictionary. 20th ed. Philadelphia: FA Davis Co, 2004.
4. Benton LA, Baker LL, Bowman BR, Walters RL. Functional Electrical Stimulation: A Practical Clinical Guide. 2nd ed. Downey, CA: Rancho Los Amigos Rehabilitation Engineering Center, Rancho Los Amigos Hospital, 1981.
5. Shriber WJ. A Manual of Electrotherapy. 4th ed. Philadelphia: Lea & Fibiger, 1975.
6. Ralston DJ. High voltage galvanic stimulation: Can there be a "state of the art?" Athl Train 1985;20:291–293.
7. Voight M. Reduction of post traumatic ankle edema with high voltage pulsed galvanic stimulation. Athl Train 1984;19:278–279, 311.
8. Hasson SM, Wible CL, Barnes WS, Williams JH. Dexamethasone iontophoresis: Effect on delayed muscle soreness and muscle function. Can J Sport Sci 1992;17:8–13.
9. Kahn J. Iontophoresis and ultrasound for postsurgical temporomandibular trismus and paresthesia. Phys Ther 1980;60:307–308.
10. Kahn J. Iontophoresis dissected. Biomechanics 1996;3:81–83.
11. Lunt MJ. Magnetic and electric fields produced during pulsed-magnetic-field therapy for non-union of the tibia. Med Biol Eng Comput 1982;20:501–511.
12. Brighton CT, Pollack SR. Treatment of recalcitrant non-union with a capacitively coupled electrical field. A preliminary report. J Bone Joint Surg Am 1985;67:577–585.
13. Guyton A. Textbook of Medical Physiology. Vol. 18. 8th ed. Philadelphia: Saunders, 1991.

Application Procedures: Electrotherapy

Jose, a clinic director, is reviewing the day's treatment forms after an unusually busy day. Patients have come in for the treatment of acute and chronic pain, muscle spasms, and acute and chronic edema and for the prevention of postoperative muscle atrophy. In fact, a soccer player has even been in for treatment of a slow-healing strawberry (abrasion) on her thigh caused by sliding on the turf in a game. Jose noticed that when the staff used electrotherapy for these conditions, they often chose the wrong parameters. He decides it's time for a refresher course on standard operating procedures for electrotherapy modalities.

Electrotherapy Applications: An Overview

There are a variety of electrotherapy devices, each with different current characteristics and resulting in somewhat different responses. The competing claims by various manufacturers has created much confusion. An analogy with vehicles helps cut through this confusion. A subcompact car is excellent for one or two people to commute to work and could serve the needs of a family. A minivan would be a better vehicle for a family but would not be as economical as the subcompact car for commuting. A family with a large yard, lots of trees, a big vegetable garden, and snow mobiles for winter recreation would find a pickup truck very useful. A minivan could tow the snow mobiles and haul fertilizer to and waste from the garden and orchards, but it would not be as effective as a pickup truck.

Electrotherapy modalities are similar to the vehicles. One type of electrotherapy modality might be the best tool for a certain indication and be appropriate for several other purposes, but it might not work as effectively as other electrotherapy modalities. Stated another way, several electrotherapeutic modalities can cause a muscle to contract, but some do it better than others. If you owned just one electrotherapy modality, you would use it to decrease pain, decrease swelling, decrease muscle spasm, increase strength, and increase range of motion. To offer the best care, however, you need to have a variety of electrotherapy modalities and use each one to treat only the conditions for which it is most effective. Modern technology has made it possible to own a variety of devices.

For years, manufacturers argued the merits of the current characteristics of their particular devices. Owing to technological advances and clinical and research results, most of them now produce electrotherapy modalities with multiple current forms. It is not uncommon to see TENS, interferential current, neuromuscular electrical stimulation, high-volt pulsed current, and microcurrent with ultrasound or light therapy included on one machine. Continuing the vehicle analogy, it would be like having push-button controls for converting your vehicle into a subcompact car, a minivan, a pickup truck, or a sports utility vehicle (SUV).

The multicurrent devices strain our vocabulary. What were four to six modalities of 15 years ago are now in a single device. In an effort to avoid confusion, we discuss each of the various current types as separate electrotherapy modalities. As for the other modalities presented in this book, you need to learn the advantages and disadvantages of each individual modality (or current type) so you can choose the best tool to use to reach specific therapeutic goals.

STANDARD OPERATING PROCEDURES

Standard operating procedures (SOPs) for the five most common electrotherapy modalities are presented in this chapter. They are:

- Transcutaneous electrical nerve stimulation for pain relief
- Interferential current therapy for pain relief
- Neuromuscular electrical stimulation for muscle reeducation, preventing disuse atrophy, decreasing muscle spasm, and decreasing edema
- Iontophoresis for transcutaneous drug delivery
- High-volt pulsed current stimulation for wound healing and edema control

Key parameters for these modalities are summarized in Table 10.1.

Think of an SOP as a roadmap. For example, on a road trip, there are several routes you can take to get from one

TABLE 10.1	Key Parameters for Electrotherapy Modalities				
PARAMETER	TENS	IFC THERAPY	NMES	IONTOPHORESIS	HVPC STIMULATION
Current type	AC	Two ACs crisscross, forming one interference current	AC	DC	AC (monophasic)
Wave form	Biphasic	Sine	Russian or biphasic	Rectangular	Twin pulse
Total current flow	1–100 mA	1–100 mA	0–200 mA	1–5 mA	0–500 mA
Frequency	1–150 pps	Carrier: 2500–5000; beat: 0–299 pps	1–200 pps	—	1–120 pps
Pulse width	10–500 msec	NA	20–300 msec	—	13–100 msec
Electrode placement	Directly on pain, dermatome, motor points, trigger points, acupuncture points, nerve root, contiguous, contralateral	Crisscross with area to be stimulated in center of the X	Bipolar on motor point and on belly of muscle	Monopolar with drug delivery electrode on treatment site	Monopolar; active electrode on area to be treated
Primary indications	Acute and chronic pain	Acute and chronic pain; muscle spasm	Disuse atrophy; muscle reeducation; muscle spasm; postacute edema	Acute and chronic pain; inflammation arthritis	Acute and chronic edema; wound healing;

AC, alternating current; DC, direct current; TENS, transcutaneous electrical nerve stimulation.

place to another. But you need to determine which route is the best, most efficient one under certain circumstances. As you read this chapter, think of how you can use electrotherapy modalities to reach your treatment goals. Don't fall into the habit of using SOPs inattentively; it might lead to a dead end.

Transcutaneous Electrical Nerve Stimulation for Pain Relief

Transcutaneous electrical nerve stimulation (TENS) is a modality that uses surface electrodes to deliver a pulsed electrical current through the skin to stimulate nerves for the purpose of controlling and relieving pain (Fig. 10.1). The word *transcutaneous* means through the skin, and *nerve stimulation* refers to the current having enough intensity to depolarize sensory nerves.

A SHORT HISTORY OF TENS

The establishment of TENS for pain relief began in the early 1970s, based mainly on the findings of Canadian psychologist Ronald Melzack and British neuroanatomist Patrick Wall.[1] In 1965, these scientists published their classic paper on the gate control theory of pain (see Chapter 7) and how stimulating afferent nerves could close a gate in the spinal column to pain signals coming

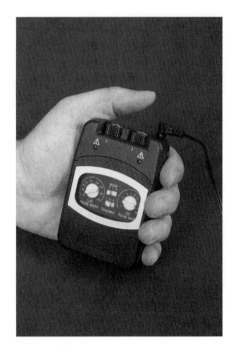

FIGURE 10.1. A portable TENS unit.

from other nerves.[2] Several companies began marketing transcutaneous electrical nerve stimulators. Later Melzack and Wall revised their theory to include how cognition might affect pain.[3,4]

THE PHYSIOLOGICAL EFFECT OF TENS

The physiological effect of TENS is selective depolarization of afferent nerves. Electrodes are placed on the skin, usually at the site of the pain. By adjusting different parameters on a TENS unit, the clinician can change the patient's perception of acute and chronic pain.

TENS MODES

There are three major modes of TENS, each applied by modulating the intensity and beat frequency (adjustable pulses per second):

- **Sensory TENS:** Used to treat acute pain by stimulating large-diameter sensory nerves. The beat frequency is high (80–200 pps), and the intensity is adjusted to the point at which the patient reports a buzzing or tingling. This is conventional or traditional TENS.
- **Motor TENS:** Used to treat chronic pain by stimulating small-diameter afferent nerves. The beat frequency is low (1–5 pps) and the intensity is higher than sensory TENS (to the patient's tolerance). The patient reports some burning, needling sensation, and a slight muscle twitch.
- **Brief-intense TENS:** Used to treat chronic pain before rehabilitation by stimulating C fibers. The beat frequency varies between low and high and changes periodically. The intensity is also higher than sensory TENS (to the patient's tolerance). The patient reports some burning, needling sensation, and twitch and tetanic muscle contractions.

HOW TENS WORKS

There are several theories about how TENS works. Many scientists believe that pain modulation during and after TENS is achieved through either the gate control system or the opiate system (see Chapter 7). The gate control system is typically activated by sensory TENS mode, whereas the opiate system is activated by motor TENS and brief-intense TENS modes.

Evidence supports the opiate system for pain modulation when a particular TENS mode, such as motor or brief-intense TENS is used. When patients whose pain was being relieved by TENS treatment were given naloxone, an inhibitor of exogenous and endogenous opiates, the pain returned rapidly.[4,5]

RESEARCH ON TENS

Because TENS is used primarily for pain management, research in this area is often difficult to perform. Recall from Chapter 7 that pain varies from one person to the next and measuring pain and pain relief is hard to do.

TENS relieves pain associated with osteoarthritis,[6] rheumatoid arthritis,[7] dysmenorrhea,[8,9] and low-back pain.[10,11] Reports of postoperative pain relief with TENS include total knee-replacement surgery,[12,13] shoulder surgery,[14] and other orthopedic conditions.[15–17] To date, the results are still mixed on the effectiveness of TENS to produce analgesia postoperatively. TENS has not been effective in relieving myofascial pain.[18]

 CRITICAL THINKING 10.1 *What is an advantage of using TENS postoperatively?*

MAKING TENS THERAPY MORE EFFECTIVE

To be successful in using TENS, consider the following:

- *Do not treat all your patients the same* (i.e., don't use a blanket protocol for everyone): Patients are not alike; therefore, parameters, electrode placements, and treatment protocols need to be modified to meet the needs of individual patients.
- *Be flexible:* Scientists are unclear regarding which TENS mode is more effective under which conditions. It might be best to start with sensory TENS because it is easily tolerated by the patient. If the patient doesn't respond, progress to either motor TENS or brief-intense TENS.
- *TENS by itself is not a cure for pain:* It can, however, relieve pain long enough to help a patient complete an exercise session or get a good night's sleep.

Now that you have a little background, you are ready for the five-step application procedure for TENS therapy.

Application of TENS

STEP 1: FOUNDATION

A. Definition. TENS is a modality that uses surface electrodes to deliver a pulsed electrical current through the skin to stimulate nerves.

B. Effects
    1. Afferent nerve stimulation
    2. Pain relief
    3. Some motor nerve stimulation (and associated muscular contraction) at higher amplitudes

C. Advantages
    1. Portable; can be used while exercising or at work
    2. Self-treatment
    3. Alternative to cold during cryokinetics
    4. Alternative to painkilling medication

D. Disadvantages
    1. Eliminates pain; does not treat the cause of the pain
    2. May mask more serious problems
    3. Inconclusive research results
    4. Sometimes becomes a cure-all

E. Indications
    1. Pain of peripheral origin
    2. Acute pain
    3. Chronic pain

F. Contraindications
    1. Do not use with a person who has
        a. An implanted pacemaker
        b. A history of heart disease
    2. Do not treat the transthoracic area.
    3. Discontinue use if a skin irritation develops.

G. Precautions
    1. Be cautious when using TENS over an area with:
        a. Impaired sensation
        b. Skin lesions (cuts, abrasions, new skin, recent scar tissue, etc.)
    2. A patient should be cautious when using TENS while driving or operating heavy machinery because reaction time might be hindered.
    3. Remember that a temporary decrease in pain does not mean the cause of the pain has gone (although pain sometimes persists long after its cause has been resolved).
    4. A TENS unit is delicate; instruct the patient to handle it carefully.

STEP 2: PREAPPLICATION TASKS

A. Make sure TENS is the proper modality for this situation.

1. Reevaluate the injury or problem. Make sure you understand the patient's condition.
2. If TENS was applied previously, review the patient's response to the that treatment.
3. Establish (or confirm) treatment goals.
4. Confirm that the objectives of therapy (goals) are compatible with TENS.
5. Make sure TENS is not contraindicated in this situation.

B. Preparing the patient psychologically
    1. Explain the procedure if the patient is being treated for the first time or if the treatment is being changed.
        a. Describe the expected sensation (e.g., pricking pins and needles).
        b. Only a small amount of current will be used.
        c. TENS will not cause electrocution.
        d. It should not be painful; if it is, ask the patient to let you know, then lower the intensity.
    2. Demonstrate the procedure on yourself if the patient seems particularly apprehensive.
    3. Check for and warn the patient about precautions.

C. Preparing the patient physically
    1. Remove clothing, tape, etc. from the electrode contact area. It is not necessary to remove them from the area between the two contact points.
    2. Place the patient in a comfortable position.

D. Preparing the equipment
    1. Make sure the output is at the minimal setting.
    2. Prepare the electrodes.
        a. Attach the electrodes to the leads (cords) and the leads to the TENS unit.
        b. Apply a conducting medium (electrode gel) to the electrode surface (unless self-adhering electrodes are used).
    3. Electrode placement is very important, but most clinicians use trial and error to determine the best placement. The following systems are recommended:
        a. Over acupuncture points
        b. Directly over the pain
        c. Proximal-distal to pain (Fig. 10.2)
        d. Crisscross over the pain (requires a two-channel unit)
        e. Over a motor point
        f. Along a dermatome
    4. Check the equipment and electrode operation.
        a. If nonadhering electrodes are used, place them on the table and cover the electrodes

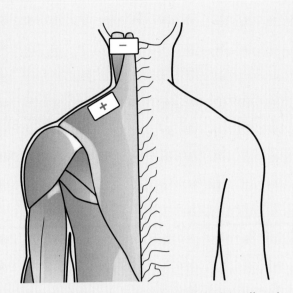

FIGURE 10.2. Electrodes placed distal-proximal of the affected area.

with your hand (Fig. 10.3). Turn up the intensity until current is felt.

   b. Check the connecting leads, especially for loose-fitting electrode tips, if current is absent or reduced.

5. Place the electrodes on the patient's skin.

   a. Electrodes must be firmly attached to the body part, while also allowing movement of the body part (especially if worn during athletic activity or at work).

   b. Good contact is essential but sometimes hard to achieve.

   c. If nonadhering electrodes are used, tape them to the skin and/or wrap with an elastic or Velcro strap.

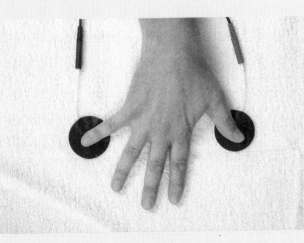

FIGURE 10.3. Testing electrodes to confirm they are functioning properly.

STEP 3: APPLICATION PARAMETERS

A. Procedures. The following are general procedures for TENS. The parameters for treating specific conditions are given in Table 10.2. Also see the manufacturer's manual for specific instructions concerning the modality your clinic uses.

1. Select the pulse width and rate, according to the manufacturer's guidelines.
2. Turn the unit on.
3. Tell the patient you are beginning.
4. Slowly increase the current intensity.

   a. Ask the patient to tell you when he begins to feel pins and needles.

   b. Increase the current until it feels most comfortable to the patient (for sensory TENS).

   c. There should be no muscular contraction (for sensory TENS).

5. Adjust the pulse width and rate; here are two options:

   a. Go through the entire range and select the most comfortable setting.

   b. Use specific settings for specific problems.

     i. For treating acute pain, set a narrow pulse width (75 μsec) with a high pulse rate of 80–200 pps. (Pain relief is almost immediate, but lasts only a few minutes to 1 hr.)

     ii. For treating chronic pain; set a wide pulse width (200 μsec) with a low pulse rate of 1–5 pps (Pain relief may take 30 min, but it may last 6–7 hr.)

6. Show the patient how to increase the intensity and pulse rate. (TENS is often a take-home modality, so it is important that the patient knows how to use it.)

B. Dosage

1. Use the maximal current that is comfortable for the patient.
2. It might be necessary to increase every 10 min as the body adapts to the stimulus.

C. Length of application. Extremely variable, from 30–60 min to hours.

D. Frequency of application. Three or four times a day as needed for pain.

E. Duration of therapy. Use until TENS is no longer effective.

STEP 4: POSTAPPLICATION TASKS

A. Equipment removal; area clean up

1. Turn off the power.
2. Return all controls to off or the minimum setting.

TABLE 10.2	*Key Parameters of TENS Therapy for Various Conditions*		
PARAMETER	**ACUTE PAIN (SENSORY TENS)**	**CHRONIC PAIN (MOTOR TENS)**	**PAIN REDUCTION BEFORE REHABILITATION (BRIEF-INTENSE TENS)**
Pulse duration	60–100 μsec	150–250 μsec	>250 μsec
Pulse rate	80–200 pps	1–5 pps	Variable
Electrode placement	Directly on painful area; nerve root and dermatome	Motor points, trigger points, acupuncture points	Motor points, trigger points, acupuncture points
Output intensity	Pleasant tingling without contraction	To tolerance; burning needling sensation; slight muscle twitch	To tolerance; visible twitch and tetanic muscle contraction
Modulation	Modulated rate	Modulated burst	Modulated amp
Treatment sequence	15–30 min; 1–2 times daily	15–30 min; 1–2 times daily	10–20 min; 1–2 times daily
Onset of relief	<10 min	20–40 min	<15 min
Duration of relief	30 min to 2 hr	6–7 hr	<30 min
Opioid peptide	dynorphin	β-Endorphin	Enkephalin
Fiber activation	A-beta	A-delta and C	A-beta, A-delta, and C

TENS, transcutaneous electrical nerve stimulation.

3. Remove and clean the electrodes.
4. Place the electrodes and TENS unit in proper place, preferably locked up.

B. Instructions to the patient
 1. Schedule the next treatment.
 2. Instruct the patient about the level of activity and/or self-treatment before the next formal treatment.

C. Record of treatment, including unique patient responses

D. Battery recharging (if charging unit is used)

5 STEP 5: MAINTENANCE

A. Batteries
 1. Keep a spare set.
 2. Keep charged (if charging unit is used).

B. Electrodes
 1. Must be kept clean; body oils will accumulate.
 2. Wash the electrodes with warm water and a mild detergent.
 3. Do not wash self-adhering electrodes, as this will cause the adherent and coupling medium to dissolve.
 4. Make sure the wire is firmly attached to the electrode post.

Interferential Current Therapy for Pain Relief

Interferential current (IFC) therapy is the application of two separate medium-frequency sinusoidal currents of different frequencies to the same area.[1,19] The two currents interfere with each other so that their individual effects are increased, diminished, or neutralized (Fig. 10.4). The resulting current is thus different from either of the beginning currents. If you have ever been in a speeding motorboat, you have seen the large wake or waves that are created by the boat. As another boat crosses these waves at a 90° angle, the other boat may fishtail a little, and the mu-

tual action of the bisecting (or interfering) waves causes an agitating, uneven, sometimes bigger wave (Fig. 10.5).

The use of IFC therapy started in Europe in the 1950s and was introduced in the United States and Canada in the early 1980s. This took place about the same time as the publication of several texts on the subject.[20–22] In 1999, it ranked as high as fifth among the most frequently used therapeutic modalities by physical therapists in Ireland[23] and Australia.[24,25]

THE THEORY OF IFC THERAPY

Advocates of IFC therapy claim that you can achieve the stronger physiological effects of low-frequency (<250

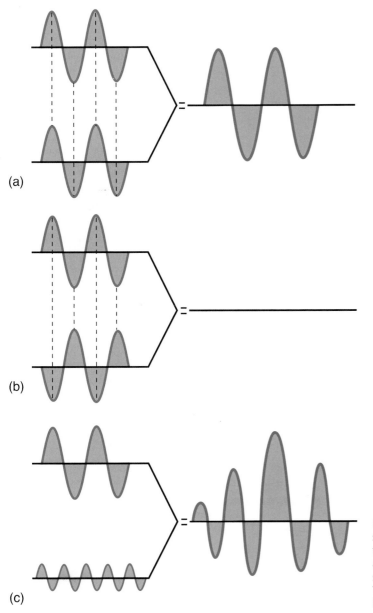

FIGURE 10.4. IFC therapy is based on the concept of two sinusoidal currents (at *left*) interacting with each other to create a third current (at *right*). **(a)** two currents of the same frequency and in phase double the amplitude. **(b)** Two currents of the same frequency and 180° out of phase cancel each other. **(c)** Two currents of differing frequency create a current with varying amplitude.

pps) electrical stimulation of muscle and nerve tissues without the associated painful and unpleasant side effects of such stimulation.[26] They claim that to produce low-frequency effects at sufficient intensity and depth, most patients experience considerable discomfort. This is because the resistance of the skin is inversely proportional to the frequency of the stimulation. The lower the stimulation frequency, the greater the resistance to the passage of the current; thus more discomfort is experienced. The skin impedance at low frequency (50 Hz) is ~3200 Ω; whereas at medium frequency (4000 Hz), it is reduced to ~40 Ω.[26] Thus a medium-frequency current will pass more easily through the skin, requiring less electrical energy input to reach the deeper tissues and giving rise to less discomfort.

We note that this concept is not supported by all scientists, as some believe that medium frequency is no more comfortable to the patient than low frequency.

There is no scientific evidence to support or refute this theory. Our experience with NMES (low-frequency stimulation) indicates that the strength of contraction, rather than pain, is the limiting factor to the amount of current a patient can tolerate. Also, clinicians generally use NMES to produce high-intensity muscle contraction.

USING IFC THERAPY

The main use of IFC is for pain relief, although there are protocols for edema control, muscle reeducation, and bone

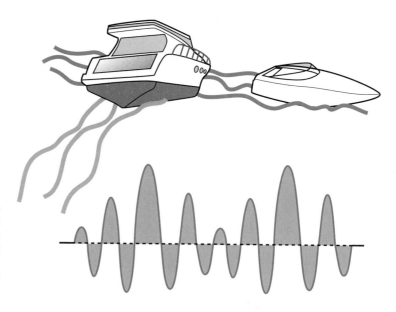

FIGURE 10.5. Interference waves or current. Notice the large waves created by the speeding motorboat. As another boat crosses these waves at a 90° angle, the other boat may fishtail a little; the mutual action of the bisecting (or interfering) waves causes an agitating, uneven, sometimes bigger wave. In essence, this is what happens when electrical currents cross during IFC therapy.

stimulation.[19] Probably its greatest advantages over traditional TENS therapy are its ability to cover a large area and perhaps its ability to penetrate deeper into the tissues.[19]

Two channels (and four electrodes) are used to deliver IFC. One channel has a set frequency, which is called the **carrier frequency**. The other channel has an adjustable frequency, which is used to produce a **beat frequency**, the difference between the two frequencies. For example, if the carrier frequency is 5000 Hz and the second frequency is 5200 Hz, the beat frequency would be 200 Hz.

The four electrodes are applied in a crisscross pattern, so that each channel forms one of the legs of the X. The location where the two currents cross or interfere is called a vector. There are two types of vectors: static and dynamic. A **static vector** does not move, but stays centered where the currents cross. A **dynamic vector** moves throughout the treatment field between the four electrodes. This is done by altering the beat frequency (by changing the second current's frequency), a feature known as sweep or scan. The advantages of the vector pattern are that you can treat both localized pain, with a static vector (Fig. 10.6), and poorly defined pain, with a dynamic vector (Fig. 10.7).

Suppose you want to decrease a patient's poorly localized back pain. Your carrier frequency is 5000 Hz, and you decide to choose a beat frequency (the frequency that can be adjusted) of 100 Hz. After the patient has guesstimated the area of most pain, apply four electrodes on the patient in a crisscross pattern with the pain centered in the middle. Hook up two electrodes to one channel and two electrodes to another. Then slowly turn up the intensity to the point at which the patient feels tingling without contracting of the muscle. One channel will run the current at 5000 Hz, while the other runs it at 5100 Hz.

Because the pain is poorly localized, you can use a dynamic vector (or sweep or scan, depending on the manufacturer's instructions). As the vector moves throughout the back, it stimulates a large area, treating most of the area bracketed by the electrodes (Fig. 10.7).

There is a setting on most machines that have IFC labeled *premodulated*. This is for treating mainly longitudinal areas in which four electrodes can't effectively bracket the treatment area. With this two-pole stimulation, electronic manipulation of the currents results in interference in the machine, not the body.

THE EFFECTIVENESS OF IFC THERAPY

Palmer[27] expressed the opinion that IFC is unlikely to produce physiological and therapeutic effects different from those of a TENS unit. Alon[28] referred to IFC as sim-

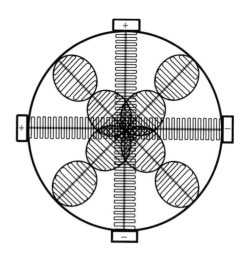

FIGURE 10.6. In IFC therapy, a static vector can be locked on to the area where the pain is easily located. (Adapted with permission from Castel D. International Academy of Physio Therapeutics [clip art].)

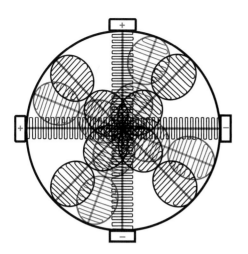

FIGURE 10.7. In IFC therapy, a dynamic vector moves the current throughout a large area to treat pain that is hard to pinpoint. (Adapted with permission from Castel D. International Academy of Physio Therapeutics [clip art].)

ply a different, more expensive, redundant approach to achieving the same effects as other electrical stimulators capable of generating pulsed current wave forms with short pulse duration.

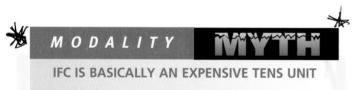

IFC IS BASICALLY AN EXPENSIVE TENS UNIT

It is true that the beat frequency of IFC brings about responses similar to a TENS unit. However, owing to the medium-frequency generator of IFC and less resistance by the skin, IFC can deliver a total current to the tissues of 70–100 mA greater than TENS.[29]

The differences in opinion about the effectiveness of IFC are probably owing to the lack of, and conflicting, clinical research. One group of scientists[30] reported IFC therapy to be effective at increasing blood flow, whereas others failed to show an increase in circulation with IFC.[31–33] IFC therapy was beneficial for osteoarthritic pain in one study[34] while showing little or no benefit in others.[35,36] Chronic post-traumatic edema was reduced owing to the milking of the venous and lymphatic return systems through electrically evoked muscle contractions using IFC.[37]

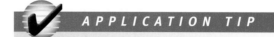

APPLICATION TIP

WHEN PAIN REDUCTION IS DESIRED, USE IFC FOR LARGE, DEEP AREAS AND TENS FOR SMALL, SUPERFICIAL AREAS. The bottom line is that IFC can cover a large area and can stimulate deep tissues. The vector field can be crossed at the joint providing more current density and pain relief to the deeper tissues. TENS is ideal for treating painful conditions, such as trigger points. Most trigger points are superficial and are within the appropriate range to be treated with low-frequency currents (i.e., TENS).

To achieve success in using IFC, review the information earlier in this chapter about how to make TENS treatments more beneficial. Also consider that those who have had success with IFC therapy do the following:[19]

- Correctly position the vector to stimulate the target tissue
- Use the appropriate size and positioning of the electrodes to stimulate the target tissue
- Use the appropriate stimulation parameters (frequency, amplitude) for activation of the correct sensory fiber
- Persevere, if pain relief is not immediately obtained

Application of IFC Therapy

1 STEP 1: **FOUNDATION**

A. Definition. IFC therapy is the interference or super-imposition of at least two separate medium-frequency sinusoidal currents on one another.

B. Effects
  1. Pain relief
  2. Some motor nerve stimulation (and associated muscular contraction) at higher amplitudes
  3. Muscle spasm reduction
  4. Edema control (perhaps)

C. Advantages
  1. Stimulates tissues deeper than can a TENS unit (owing to medium carrier frequency)
  2. Larger coverage area than with TENS because of crisscross pattern of four electrodes surrounding the area of pain
  3. Possibly more comfortable than a TENS unit because of narrow pulse duration and low skin resistance. Medium-frequency currents (IFC) meet with less skin resistance than low-frequency currents (TENS).

D. Disadvantages
  1. Eliminates pain; does not treat the cause of the pain
  2. May mask more serious problems
  3. Few, if any, portable units are available
  4. Sometimes becomes a panacea

E. Indications
  1. Acute pain
  2. Chronic pain
  3. Pain that covers a large area
  4. Muscle spasm (by decreasing pain)

F. Contraindications
  1. Do not use on a person who has
    a. An implanted pacemaker
    b. A history of heart disease
  2. Do not treat the transthoracic area.
  3. Discontinue use if a skin irritation develops.

G. Precautions
  1. Be cautious when using IFC over an area with:
    a. Impaired sensation
    b. Skin lesions (cuts, abrasions, new skin, recent scar tissue, etc.)
  2. A patient should be cautious when using IFC while driving or operating heavy machinery.
  3. Remember that a temporary decrease in pain does not mean the cause of the pain has gone (although pain sometimes persists long after its cause has been resolved).

2 STEP 2: **PREAPPLICATION TASKS**

A. Make sure IFC therapy is the proper modality for this situation.
  1. Reevaluate the injury or problem. Make sure you understand the patient's condition.
  2. If IFC was applied previously, review the patient's response to the that treatment.
  3. Confirm that the objectives of therapy are compatible with IFC.
  4. Make sure IFC is not contraindicated in this situation.

B. Preparing the patient psychologically
  1. Explain the procedure if the patient is being treated for the first time or if the treatment is being changed.
    a. Describe the expected sensation (e.g., pricking pins and needles).
    b. Only a small amount of current will be used.
    c. IFC will not cause electrocution.
    d. It should not be painful; if it is, ask the patient to let you know, then lower the intensity.
  2. Demonstrate the procedure on yourself if the patient seems particularly apprehensive.
  3. Check for, and warn the patient about, precautions.

C. Preparing the patient physically
  1. Remove clothing, tape, etc. from the electrode contact area. It is not necessary to remove them from the area between the two contact points.
  2. Position the patient in a comfortable position, usually sitting or lying.

D. Preparing the equipment
  1. Make sure the output is at the minimal setting.
  2. Prepare the electrodes.
    a. Attach four electrodes to the leads and the leads to the IFC unit.
    b. Apply a conducting medium (electrode gel) to the electrode surface (unless self-adhering electrodes are used).
  3. Check the equipment and electrode operation.
    a. If nonadhering electrodes are used, place them on the table and cover them with your hand. Turn up the intensity until current is felt.
    b. Check the connecting leads, especially for loose-fitting electrode tips, if current is absent or reduced.
  4. Find out where the patient's pain is, and make a small mark on that area with an erasable marker. Bracket the pain with the electrodes.

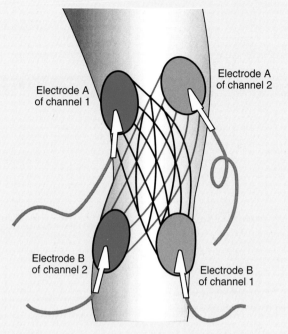

FIGURE 10.8. IFC therapy and crisscrossing over the painful area. Find out where the patient's pain is, and make a small mark on that area with an erasable marker. Bracket the pain with the electrodes.

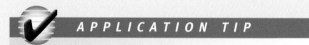

APPLICATION TIP

LOCATE THE CENTER OF PAIN. Imagine a clock on which the pain is at the center of the clock's face. The two electrodes from channel 1 are placed at 9 o'clock and 3 o'clock and two electrodes from channel 2 are placed at 12 o'clock and 6 o'clock. Thus the electrodes crisscross, and the pain is in the center (Fig. 10.8).

5. Place the electrodes on the patient's skin.
   a. Electrodes must be firmly attached to the body part, while also allowing movement of the body part (especially if worn during athletic activity or at work).
   b. Good contact is essential but sometimes hard to achieve
   c. If nonadhering electrodes are used, tape them to the skin and/or wrap with an elastic or Velcro strap.

3 ■ STEP 3: **APPLICATION PARAMETERS**

A. Procedures. The following are general procedures for reducing pain using IFC therapy. The parameters for treating other conditions are given in Table 10.3. Also see the manufacturer's manual for specific instructions concerning the modality your clinic uses.

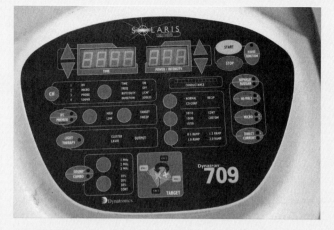

FIGURE 10.9. A typical IFC control panel on a multimodality unit.

1. Turn the unit on.
2. Tell the patient you are beginning.
3. Slowly increase the current intensity (Fig. 10.9).
   a. Ask the patient to tell you when she begins to feel pins and needles.
   b. Increase the current until it feels most comfortable to the patient.
   c. There should be no muscular contraction.
4. Adjust the pulse rate settings for specific problems.
   a. For treating acute pain, use a high pulse rate of 80–200 pps. (Pain relief is almost immediate but lasts only a few minutes to 1 hr.)
   b. For treating chronic pain, use a low pulse rate of 1–5 pps. (Pain relief may take 30 min but may last 6–7 hr.)
   c. Target or vector: For pain that is easily identifiable and pinpointed, use the target or vector buttons to move the spot where the current intersects to the area directly over the pain. For pain that is hard to pinpoint, use the dynamic vector (this will continuously move the intersection of the currents throughout the area, thus treating a larger area of pain).
B. Dosage
   1. Use the maximal current that is comfortable for the patient.
   2. It might be necessary to increase every 10 min as the body adapts to the stimulus.
C. Length of application. 20–30 min
D. Frequency of application. Once or twice daily, as needed for pain (Table 10.3)
E. Duration of therapy. Use until IFC is no longer effective.

4 ■ STEP 4: **POSTAPPLICATION TASKS**

A. Equipment removal; area cleanup
   1. Turn off the power.

TABLE 10.3	Key Parameters of IFC Therapy for Various Conditions					
CONDITION	CARRIER FREQUENCY (HZ)	PULSE RATE (PPS)	ELECTRODE PLACEMENT	OUTPUT INTENSITY	VECTOR	TREATMENT SEQUENCE
Acute pain	4000–5000	80–150	Crisscross painful area; dermatome of involved tissue	Pleasant tingling without contraction	Target (specific pain) or sweep to increase treatment area	10–30 min; 3–4 times daily
Chronic pain	2500	1–10	Crisscross painful area; dermatome of involved tissue	Pleasant tingling with or without mild twitch contraction	Target (specific pain) or sweep to increase treatment area	10–30 min; 1–2 times daily
Muscle spasm	2500	4 pps	Crisscross local trigger points	Moderate visible muscle contraction	Target (specific spasm) or sweep to increase treatment area	10–30 min; 1–2 times daily
Nerve block	4000–5000	Continuous	Over local peripheral nerve(s), innervating the painful area(s)	Pleasant tingling without contraction	Target specific pain	10 min; 1–2 times daily
Bone healing	4000–5000	100	Crisscross the fracture	Pleasant tingling without contraction	Target specific area	10–20 min; daily
Edema control	4000–5000	50	Crisscross the swelling	Strong but comfortable contraction	Sweep to cause pumping action	10–30 min; 3–4 times daily

IFC, interferential current.

2. Return all controls to off or the minimum setting.
3. Remove and clean the electrodes.
4. Place the electrodes, leads, and wraps in the proper place, not on top of the unit.
B. Instructions to the patient
1. Schedule the next treatment.
2. Instruct the patient about the level of activity and/or self-treatment before the next formal treatment.
C. Record of treatment, including unique patient responses
D. Return of the generator cart to the proper place; area cleanup

5 STEP 5: MAINTENANCE

A. Check the fuse in back if the unit will not turn on (also make sure it is plugged in).
B. Electrodes
1. Must be kept clean; body oils will accumulate.
2. Wash the electrodes with warm water and a mild detergent.
3. Do not wash self-adhering electrodes, as this will cause the adherent and couplant to dissolve.
4. Make sure the leads are firmly attached to the electrode post.

CRITICAL THINKING 10.2 *Suppose you want to use IFC with a carrier frequency of 2500 Hz. Your goal is long-lasting pain relief for someone with chronic pain. (a) What would be a good range for your beat frequency? (b) What would be a good range for your carrier frequency?*

CRITICAL THINKING 10.3 *You are treating a patient who has low-back pain. You feel he could benefit from electrical current stimulation for pain control at home, yet your IFC unit is too large. What option do you have?*

CRITICAL THINKING 10.4 *You are treating a patient who has pain in her hip. When you ask her to point to the pain she replies, "It's hard to localize, and seems to move around." Which modality would be best to use under these circumstances and why?*

Neuromuscular Electrical Stimulation

Neuromuscular electrical stimulation (NMES) refers to eliciting a muscle contraction with electrical currents. In orthopedics and rehabilitation, muscle contractions via NMES therapy are indicated for:

- Muscle reeducation—that is, reestablishing or strengthening muscle contraction
- Preventing disuse atrophy
- Decreasing muscle spasm
- Decreasing edema

A BRIEF HISTORY OF NMES

NEMS has been used for decades. It was first combined with ultrasound to provide a sensation so patients would feel they were getting something from the ultrasound treatment. However, it was not used aggressively through the 1950s because of a common belief that faradic (alternating current) stimulation was too painful.

The Russians began using NMES to increase muscle strength in trained athletes during the 1970s. In 1977, the Russian physiologist Yakov Kots[38] made some astounding claims and demonstrations at a meeting of Canadian and Soviet scientists.[1] Kots claimed that the use of his "Russian current" could produce the following:

- Up to 30% more force than a voluntary maximal contraction
- Lasting strength gains of up to 40% in healthy athletes
- No sensory discomfort; *painless* treatment[1]

In 1980, a Canadian company started manufacturing these so-called Russian current stimulators. To date, no North American scientist has been able to duplicate Kots's claims of pain-free current flow during high-level muscle contractions. In fact, most subjects in the studies complained of a great amount of pain as the current amplitude tried to replicate the force of a voluntary muscle contraction.[1] Indeed, NMES increases muscle strength; however, it does not appear to be superior to voluntary training.[39–46]

In the 1970s high-volt pulsed current (HVPC) was introduced. Advocates claimed that it was more comfortable than traditional low-volt stimulation and that it penetrated deeper and, therefore, would result in greater muscle contraction than low-volt modified square wave stim-

ulators. Research, however, proved that it did not result in greater muscle contraction.[47] The interest generated by the Russian and HVPC stimulators turned attention back to low-volt pulsed current stimulators.

NMES FOR MUSCLE REEDUCATION AND PREVENTION OF DISUSE ATROPHY

If a healthy athlete can generate a stronger voluntary muscle contraction than an electrically induced contraction, why use NMES? The answer is simple. Neuromuscular electrical stimulation is used on patients who cannot perform a voluntary muscle contraction. These might be patients for whom peripheral nerve innervation is intact but normal voluntary contraction is weak or limited from muscle atrophy after prolonged immobilization, after surgery, or as a result of pain. Scientists have found NMES not only to be of value in maintaining muscle integrity and combating disuse atrophy but also to be effective in promoting early active range of motion in postsurgical and immobilized limbs.[48–51]

The Effect of NMES on Injured Muscle

When a patient suffers a musculoskeletal injury or undergoes surgery, he often loses the ability to fully contract some muscles. NMES can help restore muscle function; follow this process:

- Hook up the patient to a NMES device.
- By depolarizing α-motor neurons, NMES causes muscles to involuntarily contract.
- After several repeated contractions, the central nervous system (CNS) receives and processes afferent feedback from the muscle.
- This improves the patient's proprioceptive and visual sense of the motions.
- The patient begins to relearn the motions.
- As the patient gets stronger, he needs to isometrically contract his muscles as much as possible during the stimulation.[52]

The use of NMES on a muscle with strength deficits increases a patient's awareness of contractile motions by providing proprioceptive, kinesthetic, and sensory input. Treatment goals focus on assisting with motion and on reeducating a muscle toward normal motion so that an active exercise program can begin as soon as possible.[52] Key parameters for muscle reeducation and the prevention of disuse atrophy are given in Table 10.4.

Avoiding Replacing Strength Training with NMES

It is important that a patient not become too dependent on NMES. Electrical muscle stimulation recruits fibers in the

TABLE 10.4	Key Parameters of NMES for Various Conditions		
PARAMETER (DISUSE ATROPHY)	**POSTACUTE EDEMA**	**MUSCLE SPASM**	**MUSCLE REEDUCATION**
Carrier frequency	5000 Hz	5000 Hz	2500–5000 Hz
Pulse rate	30–50 pps	50–70 pps	50–70 pps
Electrode placement	Bipolar on muscle group proximal to edema	Bipolar on motor points and muscle spasm	Bipolar on motor points and muscle belly for optimal contraction
Output intensity	Visible muscle contraction	Visible muscle contraction	Visible muscle contraction
Duty cycle	5–10 sec on; 5–10 sec off	10 sec on; 10 sec off	10 sec on; 50 sec off; then 10 sec on; 30 sec off, later during rehab
Ramp	Minimum (0.5 sec on; 0.5 sec off) to none	1–2 sec on; 1–2 sec off	2–3 sec on; 2–3 sec off
Patient duty	Elevate part	Try to relax	Contract with on cycle
Treatment sequence	10–20 min; twice daily	10–20 min; daily	20 min daily

NMES, neuromuscular electrical stimulation.

opposite order than a voluntary contraction. For example, when a patient is hooked up to an NMES unit and allows the machine to produce a passive contraction, the large nerve fibers fire first, followed by the smaller fibers. However, when a patient performs an active voluntary contraction, the small fibers fire first, followed by the larger ones. Thus the patient needs to move on to more traditional weight training as soon as possible to develop muscle strength appropriately.

- The order of stimulation of muscle fibers is the reverse of normal; large fibers are stimulated first. In a voluntary contraction, small fibers are stimulated first.

- The exercise is not effortless. It is nonvoluntary but not effortless. The muscle still contracts, using adenosine triphosphate (ATP) and all the other metabolic components and mechanisms.

MODALITY MYTH

EFFORTLESS EXERCISE WITH NMES CREATES WASHBOARD ABDOMINALS

You might have seen some advertisements claiming that muscle stimulation of the abdominal muscles will result in improved muscle tone and strength to this area. This idea is entirely false, for three main reasons:

- Electrical muscle stimulation cannot cause as strong a muscle contraction as a voluntary muscle contraction can. Also, if it were possible to elicit a strong enough contraction with a machine to produce a six-pack, or washboard abdominals, the intensity would have to be turned up so high that it would be unbearable.

NMES FOR DECREASING MUSCLE SPASM

The exact cause and mechanism of a muscle spasm are not clearly defined. By *spasm,* we mean a low-grade contraction or tightness as opposed to a muscle cramp, which is a complete, massive, sudden-onset contraction. A spasm can result from microtrauma, macrotrauma, accumulation of chemical irritants, muscle weakness, and pain. Regardless of the original cause, pain and discomfort lead to more pain and a protective muscle spasm. As the spasm puts pressure on sensitive nerve endings, more pain is produced, causing the vicious pain–spasm–pain cycle.

Avoid being overly concerned with what caused the muscle spasm, because the pain derived from the spasm is the reason the patient is seeing you. The goals of the treatment should be to break the pain–spasm–pain cycle while providing normal range of motion to the area of pain.

Tetanic Contraction Stimulation

The goals of tetanic contraction stimulation are to:[52]

- Increase local circulation
- Remove metabolic wastes
- Mechanically stimulate muscle fibers
- Induce some muscle spasm fatigue

Key parameters for reducing muscle spasm are given in Table 10.4.

NMES FOR DECREASING EDEMA

Neuromuscular electrical stimulation can produce cyclic muscle contractions (twitch contractions) to stimulate lymphatic flow and help remove free protein and edema from the area. If the patient is able, she should contract the muscles being treated during the on phase of each stimulation to help milk out the edema.

Application of NMES

STEP 1: FOUNDATION

A. Definition. NMES is the eliciting of muscle contraction by electrical currents.

B. Effects
   1. Muscle contraction to:
      a. Increase blood flow
      b. Retard atrophy development
      c. Decrease or retard neuromuscular inhibitions
      d. Increase muscle relaxation, decrease spasm
   2. Pain relief, possibly by decreasing muscle spasm

C. Advantages
   1. Can be applied to immobilized body part
   2. Can supplement voluntary muscular contraction

D. Disadvantages. Sometimes becomes a cure-all.

E. Indications
   1. Residual or chronic muscle spasm
   2. Any time normal neuromuscular function is not possible
   3. Muscle strains
   4. During cast immobilization or disuse atrophy
   5. Pain (owing to muscle spasm)

F. Contraindications. Do not use
   1. On a person with a pacemaker
   2. Over the heart or brain
   3. Over recent or nonunion fractures
   4. Over potential malignancies

G. Precautions. Be cautious when using NMES over an area with:
   1. Impaired sensation
   2. Skin lesions (cuts, abrasions, new skin, recent scar tissue, etc.)
   3. Decreased range of motion
   4. Extensive torn tissue

STEP 2: PREAPPLICATION TASKS

A. Make sure NMES is the proper therapy for this situation.
   1. Reevaluate the injury or problem. Make sure you understand the patient's condition.
   2. If NMES was applied previously, review the patient's response to the that treatment.
   3. Confirm that the objectives of therapy are compatible with NMES.
   4. Select or review the electrical current characteristics of your NMES unit.
   5. Make sure NMES is not contraindicated in this situation.

B. Preparing the patient psychologically
   1. Explain the procedure if the patient is being treated for the first time or if the treatment is being changed.
      a. Describe the expected sensation—moderate, prickling pins and needles progressing to strong contraction.
      b. Explain that:
         i. Electricity will cause the muscle to contract (say how much)
         ii. Only a small amount of current will be used
         iii. NMES will not cause electrocution
         iv. NMES should not be painful; if it is, tell the patient to let you know.
   2. Demonstrate the procedure on yourself if the patient seems particularly apprehensive.
   3. Check for, and warn the patient about, precautions.
      a. Inspect the skin for cuts, abrasions, new skin, etc. and make sure it is clean and free from oils.
      b. If the area to be treated has excess hair, it will need to be shaved to ensure electrode conductivity.
      c. Determine that skin sensation is not impaired by lightly taping or rubbing the skin and asking the patient if and where he feels pressure.
      d. Determine that joint range of motion is not impaired by moving the joint though complete range of motion.

C. Preparing the patient physically
   1. Remove clothing, tape, etc. from electrode contact area. It is not necessary to remove them from the area between the two contact points.
   2. Position the patient in a comfortable position.

D. Preparing the equipment
   1. Turn the unit on to warm up (necessary only in older units).
      a. Make sure the output is at minimal setting.
      b. Pulse rate (at least 30 Hz) must be displayed in the output window.
   2. Prepare the electrodes.
      a. Attach the electrodes to the leads and the leads to the generator.
      b. No preparation is needed for self-adhering electrodes.
      c. Prepare carbon-rubber electrodes with the proper medium.

i. Carbon-rubber electrodes require either water or a gel-based couplant.

ii. A gel-based couplant is applied directly to the electrode and is placed between the skin and the electrode.

iii. When water is used as a couplant, it is applied to a small sponge that is placed between the skin and the electrode. In that case, wet the sponge; remove excess water but do not squeeze dry.

3. Check the equipment and electrode operation.

   a. If nonadhering electrodes are used, place them on the table and span them with your hand. Turn up the intensity until current is felt.

   b. Check the connecting leads, especially for loose-fitting electrode tips, if current is absent or reduced. Reduce the current to zero before the next step.

4. Firmly attach bipolar electrodes on the patient's skin; place one near the center of the muscle belly and the other on the proximal or distal end of the muscle (Fig. 10.10).

   a. Good contact is essential.

   b. Remove the adhesive backing for self-adhering electrodes.

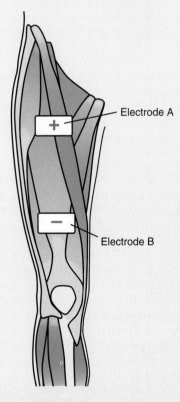

FIGURE 10.10. In NMES therapy, to produce a strong muscle contraction, one electrode is applied to the muscle belly and the other electrode is applied near the distal or the proximal end of the muscle.

Electrode A

Electrode B

c. For nonadhering electrodes, place a wet sponge, or piece of wet paper towel between the electrode and skin and use elastic belts, straps, body weight, sandbags, etc. to hold the electrodes in place.

STEP 3: APPLICATION PARAMETERS

A. Procedures. The following are general procedures for conditions requiring muscle contraction. The parameters for treating specific conditions are given in Table 10.4. Also see the manufacturer's manual for specific instructions concerning the modality your clinic uses. A NMES control panel is shown in Figure 10.11; refer to it as an example of the various switches and knobs on a NMES unit.

1. Set the pulse rate:

   a. <10 pps for twitch contraction, which is used for:

      i. Edema control

      ii. Chronic pain

   b. >30 pps for tetanic contraction, which is used for:

      i. Spasm reduction

      ii. Disuse atrophy

2. Set the duty cycle (amount of time the current will be on, compared to the amount of time the current will be off).

3. Set the timer.

4. Adjust the surge (ramp) controls as necessary. If you are inducing a tetanic contraction, you must use a surge (ramp).

5. Tell the patient that you are beginning the treatment and that she must tell you when it is uncomfortable.

6. Slowly increase the current intensity until the patient responds.

   b. Decrease the intensity slightly.

   c. Intensity must be sufficient to cause muscle contraction.

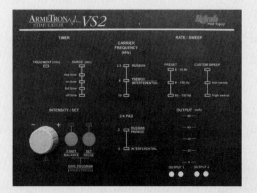

FIGURE 10.11. A typical NMES control panel.

7. Skin resistance may decrease after 5–10 sec and then intensity may be increased.
8. If treating a motor point, move the electrode around to find the motor point.
   a. Look for the area that causes maximal contraction.
   b. Pause 5–10 sec in each area to overcome skin resistance.
9. If the patient complains of discomfort, the following might be the cause:
   a. Too much current (most probable cause).
   b. Insufficient moistening of sponge.
   c. Minor small denuded area (scratches, cuts, abrasions, etc.)
   d. The patient's hypersensitivity
   e. Poor electrode conformity
10. As the patient gets stronger, resistance can be applied during the contraction (Fig. 10.12).

B. Dosage. Use the maximal current that is comfortable for the patient.
C. Length of application
   1. 10–30 min
   2. See individual manufacturer instructions

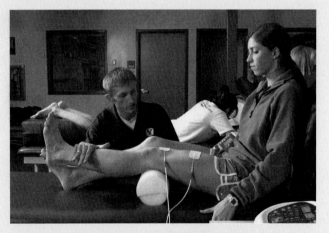

FIGURE 10.12. In NMES therapy, resistance can be applied during the muscle contraction as the patient gets stronger.

D. Frequency of application. As often as twice per day if separated by 3–4 hr
E. Duration of therapy. Continue treatment until the goals have been met, which usually means active exercise is under way.

STEP 4: POSTAPPLICATION TASKS

A. Equipment removal; area cleanup
   1. The timer will stop the current.
   2. Return all controls to off or the minimum setting.
   3. Remove the electrodes.
   4. Place the electrodes and belts in the proper place, not on top of the unit.
B. Instructions to the patient
   1. Schedule the next treatment.
   2. Instruct the patient about the level of activity and/or self-treatment before the next formal treatment.
C. Record of treatment, including unique patient responses
D. Return of the generator cart to the proper place; area cleanup

STEP 5: MAINTENANCE

A. Check the fuse in back if the unit will not turn on (also make sure it is plugged in).
B. Electrodes
   1. Must be kept clean; body oils will accumulate.
   2. Wash sponges or carbon-rubber electrodes with warm water and a mild detergent.
   3. Do not wash self-adhering electrodes, as this will cause the adherent and couplant to dissolve.
   4. Make sure the wire is firmly attached to the electrode post.
   5. The carbon in the electrode will leach out with time. Check the current flow, and assess the need for a new electrode.

CRITICAL THINKING 10.5 *If NMES doesn't provide for as strong a muscle contraction as a voluntary contraction, why do clinicians use it postoperatively?*

Iontophoresis for Transcutaneous Drug Delivery

Iontophoresis is the application of a mild direct current (DC) to drive negatively or positively charged ions of a drug solution into a patient's skin and underlying tissues.[53–55] Most units are small (about the size of a TENS unit); they are portable battery-operated devices of one or two channels (Fig. 10.13).

HOW IONTOPHORESIS WORKS

The underlying principle is that like charges repel each other, so the drug ions are repelled or pushed into the skin and surrounding tissues by direct current. Two electrodes—one to deliver the drug and one larger dispersive electrode—are applied to the patient's skin at least 6 in. (15 cm) apart. The drug delivery electrode can be either

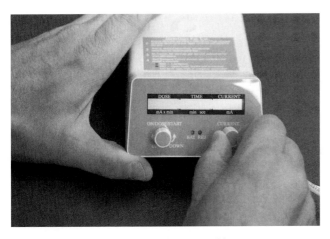

FIGURE 10.13. An iontophoresis unit uses a mild DC to transport negatively or positively charged ions from a drug solution into a patient's skin and underlying tissues.

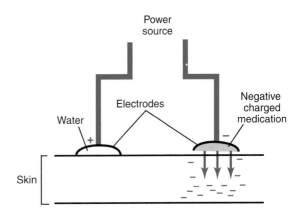

FIGURE 10.14. In iontophoresis, drug ions are repelled or pushed into the skin and surrounding tissues. The positively charged electrode delivers (repels or pushes) positively charged drug ions, or (as shown here) the negatively charged electrode delivers (repels or pushes) negatively charged drug ions.

positively or negatively charged depending on the charge of the ion to be pushed. Ionized medication is placed under the active electrode, and its polarity is selected so that it is same as the drug ion (Fig. 10.14).

When a DC is applied:

- The positively charged electrode delivers (repels or pushes) positively charged drug ions into the skin and surrounding tissues.
- The negatively charged electrode delivers (repels or pushes) negatively charged drug ions into the skin and surrounding tissues.

THE BENEFITS OF IONTOPHORESIS

Iontophoresis has the benefit of delivering medicine, such as anti-inflammatories and painkillers, directly to the area safely without the following disadvantages:

- Painful needle injections
- Risk of infection from nonsterile needle injections
- Systemic effects from taking a pill, such as stomach or intestinal irritation

Patients report a mild tingling or warm sensation during treatment, much like the sensation derived from a TENS unit.

There is an ongoing debate about whether iontophoresis can actually cause ions to penetrate the skin, although research has shown that it delivers medication 6–20 mm below the skin.[56,57] Iontophoresis has been effective in reducing pain and inflammation associated with plantar fasciitis,[58] temporomandibular joint (TMJ) disorders,[59] and epicondylitis[60] when dexamethasone, lidocaine, or sodium salicylate was used. Unfortunately little research exists on how much medicine actually enters the tissues and is delivered to the treatment site.

COMMON DRUG IONS USED IN ORTHOPEDIC MEDICINE

Some of the more common drug ions used for iontophoresis in orthopedic medicine, their polarities, and their function, are:

- *Dexamethasone (negative ion):* Helps reduce inflammation by inhibiting the biosynthesis of prostaglandins and various other inflammatory substances
- *Acetate (negative ion):* Helps dissolve calcium deposits and scar tissue in soft tissues such as muscles and tendons
- *Hydrocortisone (positive ion):* Helps decrease tissue inflammation by inhibiting the biosynthesis of prostaglandins and various other inflammatory substances
- *Lidocaine (positive ion):* Helps decrease local pain by blocking nerve impulse transmission

Before using a needle to inject children, pediatricians use iontophoresis to deliver lidocaine and numb the area. This might sound antiproductive because the child needs to get a shot anyway. But children need to be vaccinated against diseases, and if the area can be anesthetized to lessen the pain of the shot, why not give it a try? It requires at least 10 min of current stimulation before the skin is anesthetized with a 50% concentration of lidocaine.[61]

NEGATIVE EFFECTS OF USING IONTOPHORESIS

Even though iontophoresis is delivered in small doses (<5 mA), skin irritation can occur from using a DC. The skin under the electrodes may turn light red, from the expansion of small blood vessels in the skin. DC can also cause *mast cells*, which synthesize and store histamines, to release histamine, causing small bumps or red dots to appear at either electrode site. Patients sometimes complain of dry skin or itching around the area. Factors that increase skin reactions include:

- *Skin type:* Fair-skinned people show a tendency toward skin irritation.
- *Skin pigmentation:* In darker-skinned patients, the normal reddening is usually less visible than with lighter-skinned people.

Some patients find out that they are sensitive to DC. Typical symptoms of DC sensitivity are redness and hives resembling small white bumps.

To help reduce the risk of skin irritation:

- Use an alcohol scrub on the skin to clean off any oils or dirt before treatment.
- After the treatment, apply a lotion containing aloe vera gel.
- Increase the size of the anode or cathode to decrease current density.
- Increase the spacing between the electrodes to decrease current intensity.

Application of Iontophoresis for Transdermal Drug Delivery

STEP 1: FOUNDATION

A. Definition. Iontophoresis is an active transdermal drug delivery process that delivers drug ions through the skin using a direct current.
B. Effects. Depends on the drug ion being delivered:
  1. Pain relief
  2. Anesthesia
  3. Decreased inflammation
  4. Decrease in size of calcium deposits
C. Advantages
  1. Prevents the pain and skin damage that accompanies needle injection of drug medication
  2. Avoids the accidental needle injection to clinicians
  3. Localized drug delivery; does not have to travel through the entire system (as a pill does)
  4. Avoids the gastrointestinal (GI) side effects of nonsteroidal anti-inflammatory drugs (NSAIDs) and cyclooxygenase 2 (COX-2) inhibitors.
  5. Portable; the patient can travel with it.
D. Disadvantages
  1. Eliminates pain or inflammation; it does not treat the cause of the pain or inflammation.
  2. DC runs a slight risk of electrode burns.
  3. Some believe transdermal drug delivery is not possible.
E. Indications
  1. See Effects.
  2. Delivery of soluble salts and drug ions into the body for medical purposes as an alternative to needle injection or taking a pill.
F. Contraindications
  1. Do not use with a person who has
    a. An implanted pacemaker
    b. Damaged or denuded skin on the treatment area
    c. Drug allergies to medicine to be delivered transdermally
    d. Recent laceration of the treatment area
  2. Do not treat the transcranial area.
  3. Do not treat the orbital region.
G. Precautions. Be cautious when using iontophoresis over an area with:
  1. Impaired sensation
  2. Recent scar tissue
  3. Exposed metal (it is safe to use over implanted surgical metal, screws, plates, etc.)

STEP 2: PREAPPLICATION TASKS

A. Make sure iontophoresis is the proper modality for this situation.
  1. Reevaluate the injury or problem. Make sure you understand the patient's condition.
  2. If the modality was applied previously, review the patient's response to that treatment.
  3. Confirm that the objectives of therapy are compatible with iontophoresis.
  4. Make sure iontophoresis is not contraindicated in this situation.
  5. Above all else, make sure you have a physician's prescription to deliver the medication.
B. Preparing the patient psychologically
  1. Explain the procedure if the patient is being treated for the first time or if the treatment is being changed.
    a. Describe the expected sensation—mild tingling or warm.
    b. Electricity will not cause the muscle to contract.
    c. Only a small amount of current will be used.
    d. Iontophoresis will not cause electrocution.
    e. It should not be painful; if it is, tell the patient to let you know. Decrease the intensity (but the treatment will take a few minutes longer).
  2. Demonstrate the procedure on yourself if the patient seems particularly apprehensive. Do a dry run; do not use any medication or open any electrode packages.
  3. Check for and warn the patient about precautions.
C. Preparing the patient physically
  1. Place the patient in a comfortable position.
  2. Use an alcohol preparation to clean the area where the electrodes are going to be applied.
D. Preparing the equipment
  1. Remove the electrodes from the pouch or container. Make sure both the delivery electrode and the dispersive electrode appear to be in working order.
  2. Prepare the medication. Fill a syringe or marked eyedropper with the appropriate amount of medication typically used for iontophoresis.

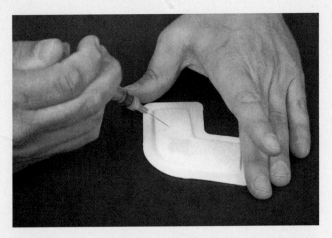

FIGURE 10.15. In iontophoresis, medication that is ionized in solution is placed on the appropriate electrode so that the active ion is driven into the tissue.

3. Prepare the active (drug delivery) electrode:
   a. Remove the backing on the electrode.
   b. Place it on a table and saturate the sponge side of the electrode with the medication (Fig. 10.15). Do not overfill; no medication should seep over onto the adhesive backing.
4. Apply the electrodes:
   a. Remove the backing on the dispersive pad and attach it on a large muscle belly at least 6 in. (15 cm) away from the active electrode site.
   b. Apply the saturated active electrode to the area to which you want the drug ions delivered (Fig. 10.16).
5. Attach the electrodes to the appropriate cords or lead clips. Make sure the leads are connected properly for the polarity of the drug you are delivering (see the manufacturer's manual).

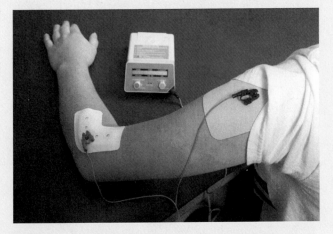

FIGURE 10.16. Electrode application in iontophoresis. See text for details.

STEP 3: APPLICATION PARAMETERS

A. Procedures. The following are general procedures for iontophoresis. See the manufacturer's manual for specific instructions concerning the modality your clinic uses.
   1. Turn the unit on.
   2. Tell the patient you are beginning.
   3. If the unit has an automatic ramp, the current amplitude will slowly increase to maximize the patient's comfort.
   4. If the unit does not have an automatic ramp, you can maximize the patient's comfort by:
      a. Slowly increasing current intensity.
      b. Ask the patient to tell you when he begins to feel mild tingling or warm under the drug delivery electrode.
   5. Adjust the intensity according to the patient's tolerance and dosage. Many electrodes are operational up to a maximum total delivered dose of 80 mA/min when negative polarity is used and 40 mA/min when positive polarity is used.
B. Dosage
   1. Set the unit to deliver the recommended dose of medication (Table 10.5).
C. Length of application. Dose specific; see Table 10.5
D. Frequency of application. Every other day
E. Duration of therapy. Up to 3 weeks

STEP 4: POSTAPPLICATION TASKS

A. Equipment removal; area cleanup
   1. Turn off the power.
   2. Return all controls to off or the minimum setting.
   3. Remove and dispose of the electrodes (the dispersive electrode can be reused, after cleaning).
   4. Place unit in the proper place, preferably locked up.
B. Battery recharging, if necessary
C. Instructions to the patient
   1. Schedule the next treatment.
   2. Instruct the patient about the level of activity and/or self-treatment before the next formal treatment.

TABLE 10.5	*Sample Dose Delivery for Ionotophoresis*	
TOTAL CHARGE	**CURRENT**	**TIME**
40 mA/min	2 mA	20 min
40 mA/min	3 mA	13.5 min
40 mA/min	4 mA	10 min

D. Record of treatment, including unique patient responses
   1. Typical skin reactions that occur from a DC are
      a. Erythema (redness) under one or both electrodes
      b. Small bumps
   2. Neither is of any significance and typically disappear in a few hours.

5 STEP 5: **MAINTENANCE**

A. Batteries
   1. Keep a spare set.
   2. Keep them charged (if a charging unit is used).
B. Electrodes
   1. Keep specific iontophoresis electrode pouches on hand.
   2. Make sure the wire is firmly attached to the electrode post.

CRITICAL THINKING 10.6 *A patient with fair skin received an iontophoresis treatment. The next day she reports to you that the treatment was uncomfortable. You notice redness on the skin where the treatment occurred. What can you do to help prevent this irritation during the next treatment?*

High-Volt Pulsed Current Stimulation for Wound Healing

High-volt pulsed current (HVPC) is a twin-peak, monophasic, pulsed current driven by its characteristically high electromotive force or voltage. High-volt stimulators enable the clinician to use either positive or negative polarity, but because of the low average current and duty cycles, skin injuries caused by changes in skin pH are unlikely.[62] HVPC stimulators are versatile and are used in several treatments, including:

- Wound management
- Edema management
- Muscle reeducation and spasm reduction
- Pain modulation

Its major advantage, however, is promoting wound healing. The other functions are more effectively performed by other types of electrical stimulation.

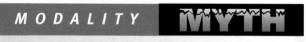

M O D A L I T Y **MYTH**

HVPC IS DANGEROUS

Some people are under the impression that HVPC is dangerous because it uses higher voltages than most electrotherapeutic devices. This is not true; the pulse width is much smaller than other devices, so the average current is less than other devices. Thus amperage is also less.

CHARACTERISTICS OF HIGH-VOLT STIMULATORS

Electrical stimulators that generate <150 V are termed low volt. Electrical stimulators that can generate >150 V are termed high volt. An HVPC stimulator uses 150–500 V. Therefore, the chief characteristics of HVPC are high peak voltages with a low average current. HVPC uses a twin-peak monophasic wave form, resembling a double spike with a fast rise followed by a fast decline (see Box 9.6). Its pulse widths are short, in the microsecond range (65–200 μsec), with pulse rates of 1–200 Hz. Box 10.1 lists the typical features of a HVPC stimulator.

HVPC and Electrode Polarity

Many HVPC stimulators include the option of selecting polarity (either negative or positive). This grew out of an early misconception that HVPC produced galvanic stimulation. Because it does not, we question what changing polarity does. We have observed that uninjured subjects have a definite preference for one or the other when stimulated for a maximal tetanic contraction, although the selection did not

M O D A L I T Y **MYTH**

HVPC STIMULATION CAUSES ION MIGRATION

In the 1980s, there was a misconception that high-volt twin-pulsed simulators created a chemical effect. In fact, they were once called "high-volt galvanic simulators." While it's true that these are monophasic, they are pulsed, so they do not produce the continuous electron flow necessary to cause a chemical effect. Continuous monophasic DC electron flow is required for ion migration. The process is moving electrons against a gradient, so if the electron flow is discontinuous, the electrons will diffuse back to their starting position during the no flow time. It's like pushing a car uphill; if you push for a while and then rest, the car will roll back down to the starting position (see Chapter 9).

BOX 10.1 *TYPICAL FEATURES OF HVPC STIMULATION*

- Current
  - Twin peaked, pulsed unidirectional
  - Each peak 65–200 μsec wide
- Controls
  - Amplitude or amount of current; controlled by output control knob
  - Continuously variable up to 500 V
  - Pulse rate; controlled by pulse rate knob
  - 1–120 pps
  - Surge rate or ramp control
- Technique
  - Can use monopolar or bipolar technique. Monopolar is used for wound healing or when treatment is directed over a large area (edema reduction, acute pain control). Bipolar technique is used for muscle contraction or chronic pain.
- Treatment time
  - 15 min if pulsed or if the patient is going to engage in vigorous activity after treatment.
  - 15–30 min if surge mode is used or the patient is not engaging in vigorous activity.

change the strength of the contraction. We also note that wound repair protocols include the suggestion that polarity be changed every few days.[63,64]

HVPC FOR WOUND MANAGEMENT

Wound management with HVPC involves high-frequency, low-amplitude stimulation, creating a sustained sensory response that many report as pins and needles. Most of the research on HVPC has been done on wound management of pressure sores (ulcers). Results are as follows:

- HVPC has a greater effect in treating pressure ulcers than whirlpool and HVPC treatments combined.[65]
- Pressure ulcers treated with HVPC for 45 min per day, 5 days a week were completely healed within 7.3 weeks. In the same study, ulcers not treated with HVPC increased in size by 29%.[64]
- Scientists reported that pressure ulcers treated with HVPC (200 V; 100 Hz) 1 hr a day for 20 days decreased by 80%, compared to 52% for a control group.[66]

How HVPC Stimulates Wound Repair

Bioelectrical currents exist in the body's vascular and interstitial tissues. Structures such as blood vessel walls, insulating tissue matrix, extracellular fluid, and intravascular plasma are capable of conducting bioelectricity.[67] When tissues are damaged, an electrical potential is created between the injured and the noninjured tissues. The DC potentials of the skin, subcutaneous tissue, and blood vessels may stimulate cellular activity when injured, thereby stimulating tissue regeneration and tissue remodeling. The use of HVPC may speed up healing by promoting the natural healing process, including the development of a difference in potential, referred to as the *injury potential*, between the wound area and the surrounding healthy tissue. The injury potential typically becomes positive 24–48 hr after the injury and becomes negative 8–9 days after the injury. As the wound heals, the difference in potential slowly returns to baseline.[68,69] Therefore, HVPC stimulation can be used to enhance the natural process of tissue recovery and healing.[52]

Many clinicians are under the mistaken notion that HVPC outputs a DC and tissue responses to HVPC are similar to those of DC.[70] There is no question that HVPC stimulates wound healing, and skepticism is probably unfounded. Keep this in mind as you read the next three paragraphs.

Individual cells migrate toward DC electrodes; the direction and speed of migration are influenced by the strength of the field and polarity of the electrodes.[71] Negative polarity increases vascularity and stimulates fibroblastic growth, collagen production, and epidermal cell migration. Negative polarity has also been shown to inhibit bacterial growth. Positive current polarity attracts macrophages and promotes epithelial growth.[72,73]

Most treatments begin with the negative polarity. The negative polarity encourages blood clots to dissolve and increases inflammatory by-products, leading to the healing of damaged tissues.[63] Positive polarity encourages clot formation around the wound and in granulation tissue.[63]

If after a few days of treatment the condition is not improving, switching electrode polarity might help. For example, when Kloth and Feedar[64] used HVPC for would healing of pressure ulcers, they began their study using the positive electrode polarity. When a patient reached a healing plateau, the electrode polarity was switched to the negative side. If a second plateau was reached, electrode polarity was switched again. This technique seemed to be effective for reducing wound size or complete healing. In three animal studies, the best healing results for epithelialization involved using the negative polarity for 3 days and then switching to the positive polarity.[74–76]

HVPC FOR EDEMA MANAGEMENT

HVPC stimulation is used for two purposes in edema management: curbing edema formation and resolving edema once it has formed, although NMES may be a better choice for resolving edema.

Edema is the accumulation of the fluid portion of blood in the tissues (see Chapter 4). To understand how edema accumulates, it is necessary to first understand normal fluid dynamics, the movement of fluid back and forth between capillaries and normal injured tissue. If this balanced movement of fluid is upset so that more fluid flows into the tissue than what is absorbed, the excess fluid is called edema. Thus edema is simply the result of a normal process that is slightly out of balance. The longer it is out of balance, the greater the edema accumulation and the greater the swelling.

Laboratory results are mixed with respect to the effect that HVPC has on edema management. Michlovitz et al.[77] report that there was no difference in edema control when HVPC stimulation was included with the application of ice, compression, and elevation in the treatment of acute ankle sprains. Cosgrove et al.[78] studied the effects of HVPC; symmetrical, biphasic pulsed current; and placebo electrical current on edema reduction after blunt trauma to rats. There were no differences in edema reduction among the groups.

The application of HVPC may be effective in curbing post-traumatic edema for 4 hr, yet long-term edema was not significantly reduced.[79,80] Taylor et al.[81] report that HVPC using either the positive or the negative polarity was effective in decreasing macromolecular leakage from blood vessels in hamster cheek pouches after histamine treatment. Dolan et al.[82] report that 3 hr of HVPC or a combination of HVPC and cold water immersion was effective at curbing edema formation by 50% in rats. Ideally, the treatment should be applied as soon as possible after the injury, and it should be maintained during the entire time that edema is forming.[82]

HVPC is sometimes confused with direct currents and the belief that the negative electrode repels plasma proteins, thus preventing them from moving from the capillary to the extracellular spaces and therefore thwarting edema formation. Because HVPC is not a DC, and because of the short duty cycle (1–2%) of HVPC, it is unlikely that it prevents edema formation this way. The physiological mechanism for curbing edema formation seems centered on the ability of HVPC to decrease the permeability of blood vessels. Reed[83] and Taylor et al.[81] suggest that HVPC decreases the leakiness of the vessels, thereby reducing the number of plasma proteins and amount of fluid that leave the vessels and enter the extracellular spaces.

Based on the results of animal studies, two protocols for curbing edema formation with HVPC have been proposed. The first, called the water-immersion technique,[84] involves HVPC applied with negative polarity, 120 pps , and 90% of visible motor threshold for 30 min every 4 hr (Fig. 10.17). Advocates of this technique advise that application begin as soon as possible after the injury and continue as long as the edema is still forming.

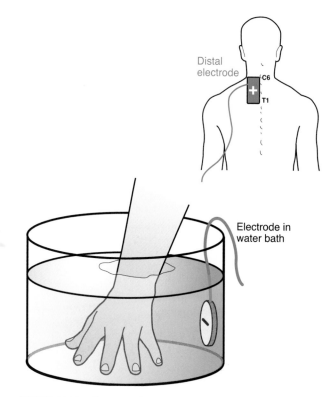

FIGURE 10.17. The water-immersion technique using HVPC.

The second protocol is similar to the first, but it is applied in a near-continuous format along with rest, ice, compression, elevation, stabilization (RICES).[62] It is based on the concept that HVPC is effective only while it is being applied.[82]

Like NMES, HVPC stimulation can be used in a muscle-pumping action to get rid of edema once it has formed. In this case, the intensity is increased until there is a strong muscle contraction. We prefer NMES, however, because it produces stronger muscle contractions.[85] And better still is active exercise, if possible.

HVPC FOR MUSCLE REEDUCATION AND SPASM REDUCTION

Muscle contraction for reeducation involves high-frequency, high-amplitude, surged stimulation that generates a tetanic contraction. HVPC is not as effective as NMES for this purpose because its average current is not as high as low-volt stimulators and therefore does not generate as strong a contraction.[85] We recommend that HVPC be used only if NMES is unavailable.

HVPC FOR PAIN MODULATION

HVPC is ineffective in reducing the pain of delayed-onset muscle soreness.[86,87] However, HVPC stimulation appears to help relieve pain owing to muscle spasm.[88]

Application of HVPC Stimulation

STEP 1: FOUNDATION

A. Definition. HVPC stimulation is the production of a twin-peak monophasic pulsed current driven by a large electromotive force.

B. Effects
1. Wound healing
2. Pain relief
   a. Sensory level (acute pain)
   b. Motor level (chronic pain)
3. Muscle contraction
   a. Disuse atrophy
   b. Spasm reduction
   c. Edema reduction
4. Edema control (maybe)

C. Advantages
1. The only electrical stimulator proven to promote wound healing
2. Can be applied to immobilized body part
3. Highly versatile in function

D. Disadvantages
1. Cannot provide as strong a contraction as low-volt stimulators (NMES)
2. Many units are not portable
3. Sometimes trial and error is needed to determine the appropriate electrode polarity for wound healing

E. Indications
1. Wound lesions (pressure sores, scarring from incisions)
2. Pain
3. Residual or chronic muscle spasm (if a low-volt unit is unavailable)

F. Contraindications
1. Do not use on a person with a pacemaker.
2. Do not use in these locations:
   a. Over the heart or brain
   b. Over the lumbar and abdominal area of pregnant women
   c. Over potential malignancies
   d. Over the anterior cervical area

G. Precautions.
1. Be cautious when using HVPC over an area with:
   a. Impaired sensation
   b. Extensive torn tissue
   c. Hemorrhage
2. Patients with epilepsy should be monitored during treatment.

STEP 2: PREAPPLICATION TASKS

A. Make sure HVPC is the proper therapy for this situation.
1. Reevaluate the injury or problem. Make sure you understand the patient's condition.
2. If HVPC stimulation was used previously, review the patient's response to that treatment.
3. Confirm that the objectives of therapy are compatible with HVPC.
4. Select or review the electrical current characteristics.
5. Make sure HVPC is not contraindicated in this situation.

B. Preparing the patient psychologically
1. Explain the procedure if the patient is being treated for the first time or if the treatment is being changed.
   a. Describe the expected sensation, depending on treatment goals.
      i. Wound repair or acute edema reduction: moderate prickling pins and needles over smaller electrode; little sensation over large dispersive electrode
      ii. Sensory level pain (acute pain reduction): moderate prickling pins and needles
      iii. Conditions requiring muscle contraction: moderate prickling pins and needles progressing to strong contraction
   b. Electricity will cause the muscle to contract or assist the normal healing of the body.
   c. Only a small amount of current will be used
   d. HVPC stimulation will not cause electrocution.
   e. It should not be painful; if it is, ask the patient to let you know.
2. Demonstrate the procedure on yourself if the patient seems particularly apprehensive.
3. Check for and warn the patient about precautions.
   a. Inspect the skin for cuts, abrasions, new skin, etc. and make sure it is clean and free from oils.
   b. If the area to be treated has excess hair, it will need to be shaved to ensure electrode conductivity.

c. Determine whether skin sensation or joint range of motion is impaired. If the patient lacks sensation in the area, she may not be able to determine when the current intensity is painful.

C. Preparing the patient physically

1. Remove clothing, tape, etc. from the electrode contact area. It is not necessary to remove them from the area between the two contact points.

2. Place the patient in a comfortable position.

D. Preparing the equipment

1. Turn the unit on.
   a. Make sure the output is at the minimal setting.
   b. Set the pulse rate.

2. Prepare the electrodes.
   a. Attach the electrodes to the leads and the leads to the generator.
   b. No preparation is needed for self-adhering electrodes.
   c. Prepare carbon-rubber electrodes with the proper medium.
      i. Carbon-rubber electrodes require either water or a gel-based couplant.
      ii. A gel-based couplant is applied directly to the electrode and is placed between the skin and the electrode.
      iii. When water is used as a couplant, it is applied to a small sponge placed between the skin and the electrode. In that case, wet the sponge; remove excess water but do not squeeze dry.

3. Check the equipment and electrode operation.
   a. If nonadhering electrodes are used; place them on the table and span them with your hand. Turn up the intensity until current is felt.
   b. Check the connecting cords, especially for loose-fitting electrode tips, if current is absent or reduced.

4. Firmly attach the electrodes on the patient's skin.
   a. Monopolar: active electrode over the injury and the dispersive electrode over a remote site, such as the back, abdomen, or thigh
   b. Bipolar: proximal and distal to the muscle belly
   c. Good contact is essential
   d. Remove the adhesive backing for self-adhering electrodes
   e. For nonadhering electrodes, place a wet piece of paper towel between the electrode and the skin and use elastic belts, straps, body weight, sandbags, etc. to hold the electrodes in place.

3 | **STEP 3: APPLICATION PARAMETERS**

A. Procedures. The following are general procedures for HVPC stimulation. The parameters for treating specific conditions are given in Table 10.6. Also see the manufacturer's manual for specific instructions concerning the modality your clinic uses.

1. Set the pulse rate.
   a. <15 pps for individual or twitch contractions
   b. >50 pps for moderate to tetanic contractions

2. Set the polarity. Negative over motor point (monopolar).

3. Set the duty cycle.

4. Set the timer.

5. Tell the patient you are beginning the treatment.

6. Slowly increase the current intensity.
   a. Ask the patient to tell you when it is uncomfortable.
   b. Decrease the intensity slightly.
   c. Intensity must be sufficient to cause muscle contraction.

7. Skin resistance will decrease after 5–10 sec, and then the intensity may be increased.

8. If treating a motor point, move the anode electrode probe around to find the motor point.
   a. Look for the area that causes maximal contraction.
   b. Pause 5–10 sec in each area to overcome skin resistance.

TABLE 10.6	**Key Parameters of HVPC Stimulation for Various Conditions**			
CONDITION	**POLARITY**	**PULSE SETTING**	**ELECTRODE PLACEMENT**	**OUTPUT**
Edema control	Negative	120 pps	Under water or large surface	90% of visible motor threshold
Wound management	Negative to attract fibroblasts; positive to attract macrophages	100 pps	Active electrode in wound or adjacent to wound edges	Pins and needles; tingle

HVPC, high-volt pulsed current.

9. If the patient complains of discomfort, the following might be causes:
    a. Too much current
    b. Insufficient moistening of sponge
    c. Minor small denuded area (scratches, cuts, abrasions, etc.)
    d. The patient's hypersensitivity
B. Dosage. Use the maximal current that is comfortable for the patient.
C. Length of application.
    1. 15 min if pulsed or if the patient is going to exercise vigorously after the treatment.
    2. 15–30 min if surge mode is used or the patient is not going to exercise vigorously after the treatment.
    3. See the individual manufacturer's instructions.
D. Frequency of application. As often as three time per day if separated by 3–4 hr.
E. Duration of therapy. Continue treatment until goals have been met.

4 STEP 4: POSTAPPLICATION TASKS

A. Equipment removal; area cleanup
    1. The timer will stop the current.
    2. Return all controls to off or the minimum setting.
    3. Remove the electrodes.

4. Place the electrodes and belts in the proper place, not on top of the unit.
B. Instructions to the patient
    1. Schedule the next treatment
    2. Instruct the patient about the level of activity and/or self-treatment before the next formal treatment.
C. Record of treatment, including unique patient responses.
D. Return of the generator cart to the proper place; area cleanup

5 STEP 5: MAINTENANCE

A. Check the fuse in back if the unit will not turn on (also make sure it is plugged in).
B. Electrodes
    1. Must be kept clean; body oils will accumulate.
    2. Wash sponges or carbon-rubber electrodes with warm water and a mild detergent.
    3. Do not wash self-adhering electrodes, as this will cause the adherent and couplant to dissolve.
    4. Make sure the wire is firmly attached to the electrode post.
    5. The carbon in the electrode will leach out with time. Check the current flow, and assess the need for a new electrode.

Microcurrent Electrical Nerve Stimulation

Microcurrent electrical nerve stimulation (MENS) is the therapeutic use of constant (DC) and pulsed (interrupted) currents in which the stimulus amplitude is in the microamperage (millionth of an ampere) range. Because microcurrents are a major factor in the control of various body functions, it seems reasonable that treatment with MENS would be effective. The evidence does not support the therapeutic use of this modality. Despite the lack of evidence, there are many passionate adherents of MENS therapy.

THE MANY NAMES FOR MENS

The term *microcurrent electrical nerve stimulation* does not accurately describe this modality because the current intensity is too low (<1 mA) to cause nerve depolarization.[89] Perhaps this is why the American Physical Therapy Association labeled it low-intensity direct current (LIDC) in 1990.[90]

Other than MENS, this modality has been referred to as:[91]

- Low-intensity direct current (LIDC)
- Low-voltage pulsed microamperage stimulation
- Biostimulation
- Bioelectric therapy
- Low-intensity electrical stimulation
- Microcurrent

Despite the logic of these other names, most people continue to use MENS, so we will also use this term.

THE THEORY BEHIND MENS

The creation of MENS originated with studies by Becker[69] on animal soft tissue healing and limb regeneration in the 1960s. According to Becker, after injury or disease, injured cells from skin, nerve, and muscle are theorized to posses their own injury currents in the microamperage range that might play a role in healing the injury. Thus if human tissue repair is mediated in part by electrical signals, an electrical current applied to the injury site may enhance the injury process.

For example, neutrophils, macrophages, and fibroblasts (key cells involved in wound healing) carry a positive or negative charge. By applying the anode or cathode over the wound, the microcurrent helps in the galvanic attraction of these cells into the wound, thereby promoting wound healing.[1]

The MENS unit is programmed to produce a specific current intensity so low that often the patient cannot feel the current. Manufacturers of microcurrent devices state that a primary characteristic is its ability to generate a fixed current by adjusting the voltage to account for variations in skin resistance. Some scientists doubt that microamperage current can even penetrate the skin.[92] Regardless, many companies are including MENS on their multimodality machines.

The Effectiveness of MENS

There is no clear-cut research supporting the therapeutic use of MENS. Scientists have found it to have a positive effect in treating:

- Pressure ulcers[93]
- Diabetic ulcers[94]
- TMJ disorders[95]

However, other scientists have reported it to have no effect in treating:

- Pressure ulcers[96]
- TMJ pain[97]
- Delayed-onset muscle soreness[87,98–100]
- Coracoacromial arch pain[101]
- Surgically induced wounds[102]

Most of the instances in which MENS might play a positive role is in wound healing, an area that is typically outside the practice of athletic trainers. Further research is needed to determine whether this modality has a place in treating orthopedic injuries.

For those who wish to use MENS as a modality, follow the manufacturer's directions. It is safe; however, the same precautions that apply to TENS apply to this modality.

CLOSING SCENE

It has now been 2 weeks since the clinic staff took a refresher course on electrotherapy. The staff is showing improved use of electrotherapy, based on observations of treatments and review of the treatment forms. The staff is using the correct modality and optimal parameters to reach treatment goals, and the patients are responding positively to the treatments. Jose is pleased.

CHAPTER REFLECTIONS

1. Read and ponder each of the following points. Do you feel you have a clear understanding of each concept? If not, reread the appropriate section of the chapter.
   - Define TENS.
   - Explain the theoretical basis of TENS therapy.
   - What are the indications and contraindications for using TENS?
   - Describe how a TENS treatment is applied.
   - Define IFC therapy.
   - Explain the theoretical basis of IFC therapy.
   - What are the indications and contraindications for using IFC therapy?
   - Describe how an IFC treatment is applied.
   - Define NMES.
   - Explain the theoretical basis of NMES therapy.
   - What are the indications and contraindications for using NMES?
   - Describe how an NMES treatment is applied.
   - Define iontophoresis.
   - Explain the theoretical basis of iontophoresis therapy.
   - What are the indications and contraindications for using iontophoresis?
   - Describe how an iontophoresis treatment is applied.
   - Define HVPC stimulation.
   - Explain the theoretical basis of how HVPC therapy.
   - What are the indications and contraindications for using HVPC stimulation?
   - Describe how an HVPC treatment is applied.
   - Define MENS.
   - Explain the theoretical basis of MENS therapy.
   - What are the indications and contraindications for using MENS?

2. Write three to five questions for discussion with your class instructor, clinical instructor, classmates, and clinical colleagues.

3. Get together with classmates and quiz each other on the concepts of this chapter. Use the points in exercise 1 and questions you wrote for exercise 2 as a beginning. Explaining concepts out loud to others requires a deeper grasp of the material than feeling you understand it as you read.

4. Once you feel you understand the principles of application of TENS, IFC, NMES, iontophoresis, and HVPC

treatments, practice applying them using the five-step approach with a classmate or clinical colleague. Alternate applying the modalities to each other. When it is being applied to you, listen and observe carefully to determine whether your classmate is using proper application. Consult your notes when the modality is applied to you and for the first few times you apply the modality to another person. Continue practicing the application until you can do so without using your notes.

CRITICAL THINKING RESPONSES

Critical Thinking 10.1

The advantage of using TENS postoperatively is that the patient might require fewer painkilling drugs, thereby negating the possibility for drug dependency.

Critical Thinking 10.2

Settings for long-lasting analgesia:
a. 1–5 Hz or pps
b. 2501–2505 Hz.

Critical Thinking 10.3

Because your IFC unit is too large, loan the athlete a portable TENS unit or have the physician write him a prescription for TENS. (Some insurance companies will pay for a TENS unit.)

Critical Thinking 10.4

Because the patient has hip pain that is hard to localize, the best modality would be IFC because it has a dynamic

vector that can move the current to cover a large area for treating pain that is difficult to pinpoint.

Critical Thinking 10.5

NMES is often used postoperatively because the muscle is often weak and cannot elicit a strong contraction. NMES is used to assist the patient in contracting the affected muscles.

Critical Thinking 10.6

The following will help prevent electrode irritation during an iontophoresis treatment on a fair-skinned patient:

*   Use an alcohol scrub on the skin to clean off any oils or dirt before treatment.
    *   Increase the size of the anode or cathode to decrease current density.
    *   Increase the spacing between electrodes to decrease current intensity.
    *   After the treatment, apply a lotion containing aloe vera gel.

REFERENCES

1. Belanger AY. Evidence-Based Guide to Therapeutic Physical Agents. Baltimore: Lippincott Williams & Wilkins, 2002.
2. Melzack R, Wall PD. Pain mechanisms: A new theory. Science 1965; 150:971–979.
3. Wall PD. The gate control theory of pain mechanisms. A re-examination and re-statement. Brain. 1978;101:1–18.
4. Wall PD. Textbook of Pain. 3rd ed. London: Churchill Livingstone, 1994.
5. Mannheimer JS, Lampe GN. Clinical Transcutaneous Electrical Nerve Stimulation. Philadelphia: Davis, 1984.
6. Fargas-Babjak A, Rooney P, Gerecz E. Randomized trial of Codetron for pain control in osteoarthritis of the hip/knee. Clin J Pain 1989;5: 137–141.
7. Abelson K, Langley GB, Sheppeard H, et al. Transcutaneous electrical nerve stimulation in rheumatoid arthritis. N Z Med J. 1983; 96:156–158.
8. Dawood MY, Ramos J. Transcutaneous electrical nerve stimulation (TENS) for the treatment of primary dysmenorrhea: A randomized crossover comparison with placebo TENS and ibuprofen. Obstet Gynecol 1990;75:656–660.
9. Lundeberg T, Bondesson L, Lundstrom V. Relief of primary dysmenorrhea by transcutaneous electrical nerve stimulation. Acta Obstet Gynecol Scand 1985;64:491–497.
10. Melzack R, Vetere P, Finch L. Transcutaneous electrical nerve stimulation for low back pain. A comparison of TENS and massage for pain and range of motion. Phys Ther 1983;63:489–493.
11. Cheing GL, Hui-Chan CW. Transcutaneous electrical nerve stimulation: Nonparallel antinociceptive effects on chronic clinical pain and acute experimental pain. Arch Phys Med Rehabil 1999;80: 305–312.
12. Walker RH, Morris BA, Angulo DL, et al. Postoperative use of continuous passive motion, transcutaneous electrical nerve stimulation, and continuous cooling pad following total knee arthroplasty. J Arthroplasty 1991;6:151–156.

13. Angulo DL, Colwell CW. Use of postoperative TENS and continuous passive motion following total knee replacement. J Orthop Sports Phys Ther 1990;11:599–604.

14. Morgan B, Jones AR, Mulcahy KA, et al. Transcutaneous electric nerve stimulation (TENS) during distension shoulder arthrography: A controlled trial. Pain 1995;64:265–267.

15. Arvidsson J, Eriksson E. Postoperative TENS pain relief after knee surgery: Objective evaluation. Orthopedics 1986;9:1346–1351.

16. Jensen JE, Conn RR, Hazelrigg G, Hewett JE. The use of transcutaneous neural stimulation and isokinetic testing in arthroscopic knee surgery. Am J Sports Med. 1985;13:27–33.

17. Cornell PE, Lopez AL, Malofsky H. Pain reduction with transcutaneous electrical nerve stimulation after foot surgery. J Foot Surg 1984;23:326–333.

18. Kruger LR, van der Linden WJ, Cleaton-Jones PE. Transcutaneous electrical nerve stimulation in the treatment of myofascial pain dysfunction. S Afr J Surg 1998;36:35–38.

19. Castel D. Electrotherapy and Ultrasound Update. 2nd ed. Reno, NV: International Academy of Physio Therapeutics, 1996.

20. de Domenico G. Basic Guidelines for Interferential Therapy. Sydney, Australia: Theramed Boors, 1981.

21. de Domenico G. New Dimensions in Interferential Therapy. A Theoretical and Clinical Guide. Lindfield: Reid Medical Books, 1987.

22. Savage B. Interferential Therapy. London: Faber & Faber, 1984.

23. Foster NE, Thompson KA, Baxter GD, Allen JM. Management of nonspecific low back pain by physiotherapists in Britain and Ireland. A descriptive questionnaire of current clinical practice. Spine 1999; 24:1332–1342.

24. Lindsay DM, Dearness J, Richardson C, et al. A survey of electromodality usage in private physiotherapy practices. Aust J Physiother 1990;36:249–256.

25. Lindsay DM, Dearness J, McGinley CC. Electrotherapy usage trends in private physiotherapy practice in Alberta. Physiother Can 1995; 47:30–34.

26. Watson T. Electrotherapy on the Web. Available at: www.Electrotherapy.org. Accessed April 2007.

27. Palmer ST, Martin DJ, Steedman WM, Ravey J. Alteration of interferential current and transcutaneous electrical nerve stimulation frequency: Effects on nerve excitation. Arch Phys Med Rehabil 1999;80: 1065–1071.

28. Alon G. Principles of electrical stimulation. In: Nelson RM, Hayes KW, Currier DP, eds. Clinical Electrotherapy. 3rd ed. Stamford, CT: Appleton & Lange, 1999.

29. Kloth LC, Cummings JP, Section on Clinical Electrophysiology and the American Physical Therapy Association. Electrotherapeutic Terminology in Physical Therapy. Alexandria, VA: American Physical Therapy Association, 1990.

30. Noble JG, Henderson G, Cramp AF, Walsh DM, Lowe AS. The effect of interferential therapy upon cutaneous blood flow in humans. Clin Physiol 2000;20:2–7.

31. Nussbaum EL, Rush P, Disenhaus L. The effects of interferential therapy on peripheral blood flow. Physiotherapy 1990;76:803–807.

32. Indergand NJ, Morgan BJ. Effect of interference current on forearm vascular resistance in asymptomatic humans. Phys Ther 1995;75: 306–312.

33. Olson SL, Perez JV, Stacks LN, Walsh MH. The effects of TENS and interferential current on cutaneous blood flow in healthy subjects. Physiother Can 1999;51:27–31.

34. Shafshak TS, el-Sheshai AM, Soltan HE. Personality traits in the mechanisms of interferential therapy for osteoarthritic knee pain. Arch Phys Med Rehabil 1991;72:579–581.

35. Quirk A, Newham RJ, Newham KJ. An evaluation of interferential therapy, shortwave diathermy, and exercise in the treatment of osteoarthrosis of the knee. Physiotherapy 1985;71:55–57.

36. Hurley DA, Minder PM, McDonough SM, et al. Interferential therapy electrode placement technique in acute low back pain: A preliminary investigation. Arch Phys Med Rehabil 2001;82:485–493.

37. Hobler C. Case study: Reduction of chronic posttraumatic knee edema using interferential stimulation. Athl Train 1991;26:364.

38. Kots YM. Electrostimulation. Paper presented at the Canadian-Soviet Exchange Symposium on Electrostimulation of Skeletal Muscles. Concordia University, Montreal, Dec 6–15, 1977.

39. Currier DP, Mann R. Muscular strength development by electrical stimulation in healthy individuals. Phys Ther 1983;63:915–921.

40. Wolf SL, Ariel GB, Saar D, et al. The effect of muscle stimulation during resistive training on performance parameters. Am J Sports Med 1986;14:18–23.

41. Selkowitz DM. Improvement in isometric strength of the quadriceps femoris muscle after training with electrical stimulation. Phys Ther. 1985;65:186–195.

42. Laughman RK, Youdas JW, Garrett TR, Chao EY. Strength changes in the normal quadriceps femoris muscle as a result of electrical stimulation. Phys Ther 1983;63:494–499.

43. McMiken DF, Todd-Smith M, Thompson C. Strengthening of human quadriceps muscles by cutaneous electrical stimulation. Scand J Rehabil Med 1983;15:25–28.

44. Wadey VMR. The effects of daily adjustable progressive resistive exercise and electrical stimulation on strength [master's thesis]. Terre Haute: Indiana State University, Department of Physical Education, 1988.

45. Massey BH, Nelson RC, Sharkey BC, et al. Effects of high frequency electrical stimulation on the size and strength of skeletal muscle. J Sports Med Phys Fitness 1965;5:136–144.

46. Mohr T, Carlson B, Sulentic C, Landry R. Comparison of isometric exercise and high volt galvanic stimulation on quadriceps femoris muscle strength. Phys Ther 1985;65:606–612.

47. Wadey VM, Knight KL. Four week training of quadriceps strength with electrical muscle stimulation and the isotonic DAPRE technique. J Can Athl Ther Assoc 1989;16:14–20.

48. Knight KL. Electrical muscle stimulation during immobilization. Physician Sportsmedi 1980;8:147.

49. Eriksson E, Haggmark T. Comparison of isometric muscle training and electrical stimulation supplementing isometric muscle training in the recovery after major knee ligament surgery. A preliminary report. Am J Sports Med 1979;7:169–171.

50. Godfrey CM, Jayawardena H. Comparison of electro-stimulation and isometric exercise in strengthening the quadriceps muscle. Physiother Can 1979;31:265–267.

51. Gould N, Donnermeyer D, Gammon GG, et al. Transcutaneous muscle stimulation to retard disuse atrophy after open meniscectomy. Clin Orthop 1983:190–197.

52. Hecox B, Mehreteax TA, Weisberg J. Physical Agents. Norwalk, CT: Appleton & Lange, 1994.

53. Hasson SM, Wible CL, Barnes WS, Williams JH. Dexamethasone iontophoresis: Effect on delayed muscle soreness and muscle function. 1992;17(1):8–13.

54. Kahn J. Iontophoresis and ultrasound for postsurgical temporomandibular trismus and paresthesia. Phys Ther 1980;60:307–308.

55. Kahn J. Iontophoresis Dissected. Biomechanics 1996;3:81–83.

56. Hasson SH. Exercise training and dexamethasone iontophoresis in rheumatoid arthritis: A case study. Physiother Can 1991;43:11–29.

57. Glass JM, Stephen RL, Jacobson SC. The quantity and distribution of radiolabeled dexamethasone delivered to tissue by iontophoresis. Int J Dermatol 1980;19:519–525.

58. Gudeman SD, Eisele SA, Heidt RS Jr, et al. Treatment of plantar fasciitis by iontophoresis of 0.4% dexamethasone. A randomized, double-blind, placebo-controlled study. Am J Sports Med 1997;25: 312–316.

59. Schiffman EL, Braun BL, Lindgren BR. Temporomandibular joint iontophoresis: A double-blind randomized clinical trial. J Orofac Pain 1996;10:157–165.

60. Demirtas RN, Oner C. The treatment of lateral epicondylitis by iontophoresis of sodium salicylate and sodium diclofenac. Clin Rehabil 1998;12:23–29.

61. Oshima T, Kashiki K, Toyooka H, et al. Cutaneous iontophoretic application of condensed lidocaine. Can J Anaesth 1994;41:677–679.

62. Dolan MG, Mendel FC. Clinical application of electrotherapy. Athl Ther Today 2004 2004;9:11–16.

63. Feedar JA, Kloth LC, Gentzkow GD. Chronic dermal ulcer healing enhanced with monophasic pulsed electrical stimulation. Phys Ther 1991;71:639–649.

64. Kloth LC, Feedar JA. Acceleration of wound healing with high voltage, monophasic, pulsed current. Physl Ther 1988;68:503–508.

65. Akers TK, Gabrielson AL. The effect of high voltage galvanic stimulation on the rate of healing of decubitus ulcers. Biomed Sci Instrum 1984;20:99–100.

66. Griffin JW, Tooms RE, Mendius RA, et al. Efficacy of high voltage pulsed current for healing of pressure ulcers in patients with spinal cord injury. Phys Ther 1991;71:433–442; discussion 442–434.

67. Nordenstrom BE. Biologically Closed Electric Circuits: Clinical, Experimental and Theoretical Evidence for an Additional Circulatory System. Stockholm: Nordic Medical, 1983.

68. Burr H, Taffel M, Harvey S. An electrometric study of the healing wound in man. Yale J Biol Med 1940;12:483–485.

69. Becker RO, Murray DG. Method of producing cellular dedifferentiation by means of very small electrical current. Trans NY Acad Sci 1967;29:606–615.

70. Ralston DJ. High voltage galvanic stimulation: Can there be a "state of the art"? Athl Train 1985:291–293.

71. Mustoe TA, Pierce GF, Thomason A, et al. Accelerated healing of incisional wounds in rats induced by transforming growth factor-beta. Science 1987;237:1333–1336.

72. Gentzkow GD, Miller KH. Electrical stimulation for dermal wound healing. Clin Podiatr Med Surg 1991;8:827–841.

73. Reich JD, Tarjan PP. Electrical stimulation of skin. Int J Dermatol 1990;29:395–400.

74. Fakhri O, Amin MA. The effect of low-voltage electric therapy on the healing of resistant skin burns. J Burn Care Rehabil 1987;8:15–18.

75. Brown M, McDonnell MK, Menton DN. Electrical stimulation effects on cutaneous wound healing in rabbits. A follow-up study. Phys Ther 1988;68:955–960.

76. Brown M, McDonnell MK, Menton DN. Polarity effects on wound healing using electric stimulation in rabbits. Arch Phys Med Rehabil 1989;70:624–627.

77. Michlovitz S, Smith W, Watkins M. Ice and high voltage pulsed stimulation in treatment of acute lateral ankle sprains. J Orthop Sports Phys Ther 1988;9:301–304.

78. Cosgrove KA, Alon G, Bell SF, et al. The electrical effect of two commonly used clinical stimulators on traumatic edema in rats. Phys Ther 1992;72:227–233.

79. Taylor K, Fish DR, Mendel FC, Burton HW. Effect of electrically induced muscle contractions on posttraumatic edema formation in frog hind limbs. Phys Ther 1992;72:127–132.

80. Mohr TM, Akers TK, Landry RG. Effect of high voltage stimulation on edema reduction in the rat hind limb. Phys Ther 1987;67:1703–1707.

81. Taylor K, Mendel FC, Fish DR, et al. Effect of high-voltage pulsed current and alternating current on macromolecular leakage in hamster cheek pouch microcirculation. Phys Ther 1997;77:1729–1740.

82. Dolan MG, Mychaskiw AM, Mattacola CG, Mendel FC. Effects of Cool-Water immersion and high-voltage electric stimulation for 3 continuous hours on acute edema in rats. J Athl Train 2003;38:325–329.

83. Reed BV. Effect of high voltage pulsed electrical stimulation on microvascular permeability to plasma proteins. A possible mechanism in minimizing edema. Phys Ther 1988;68:491–495.

84. Mendel FC, Fish DR. New perspectives in edema control via electrical stimulation. J Athl Train 1993;28:63.

85. Rauh JG. Comparison of muscular force production as a result of voluntary contraction and three electrical stimulators. Terre Haute, IN: Indiana State University, Physical Education, 1982.

86. Butterfield DL. The effects of high-volt pulsed current electrical stimulation on delayed-onset muscle soreness. J Athl Train 1997;32:15.

87. Wolcot C. A comparison of the effects of high volt and microcurrent stimulation on delayed onset muscle soreness. Phys Ther 1991;71:S117.

88. Morris L, Newton RA. Use of high voltage pulsed galvanic stimulation for patients with levator ani syndrome. Phys Ther 1987;67:1522–1525.

89. Picker RI. Current trends: Low-volt pulsed microamp stimulation, Part 1. Clin Manag 1989;9:10–14.

90. American Physical Therapy Association, Section on Clinical Electrophysiology. Electrotherapeutic Terminology in Physical Therapy. Alexandria, VA, American Physical Therapy Association, 1990.

91. Driban JB. Bone stimulators and microcurrent: clinical bioelectrics. Athl Ther Today 2004;9:22–27.

92. Merrick MA. Unconventional modalities: Microcurrent. Athl Ther Today 1999;4(5):53–54.

93. Wood JM, Evans PE, 3rd, Schallreuter KU, et al. A multicenter study on the use of pulsed low-intensity direct current for healing chronic stage II and stage III decubitus ulcers. Arch Dermatol 1993;129:999–1009.

94. Baker LL, Chambers R, DeMuth SK, Villar F. Effects of electrical stimulation on wound healing in patients with diabetic ulcers. Diabetes Care 1997;20:405–412.

95. Bertolucci LE, Grey T. Clinical comparative study of microcurrent electrical stimulation to mid-laser and placebo treatment in degenerative joint disease of the temporomandibular joint. Craniology 1995;13:116–120.

96. Baker LL, Rubayi S, Villar F, DeMuth SK. Effect of electrical stimulation waveform on healing of ulcers in human beings with spinal cord injury. Wound Repair Regen 1996;4:21–28.

97. Zuim PRJ, Garcia AR, Turcio KHL, Hamata MM. Evaluation of microcurrent electrical nerve stimulation (MENS) effectiveness on muscle pain in temporomandibular disorders patients. J Appl Oral Sci 2006;14:61–66.

98. Allen JD, Mattacola CG, Perrin DH. Effect of microcurrent stimulation on delayed-onset muscle soreness: A double-blind comparison. J Athl Train 1999;34:334–337.

99. Weber MD, Servedio FJ, Woodall WR. The effects of three modalities on delayed onset muscle soreness. J Orthop Sports Phys Ther 1994;20:236–242.

100. Denegar C. The effects of low-volt microamperage on delayed onset muscle soreness. J Sport Rehab 1992;1:95.

101. Sinnreich MJ. Microcurrent electrical nerve stimulation (MENS) and coracoacromial arch pain: The effects after one treatment. Phys Ther 1992;72:S68.

102. Byl NN, McKenzie AL, West JM, et al. Pulsed microamperage stimulation: A controlled study of healing of surgically induced wounds in Yucatan pigs. Phys Ther 1994;74:201–213; discussion 213–218.

Review Questions

Chapter 9

1. What is the resistance found in a 40 V circuit possessing a current flow of 10 A?
    a. 4 Ω
    b. 400 Ω
    c. 0.25 Ω
    d. 30 Ω
    e. 10 Ω

2. Monopolar stimulation involves the use of active and dispersive electrodes. The parameter that determines which pad(s) will be active is the _____.
    a. polarity adjustment
    b. average current
    c. pulse duration
    d. current density
    e. electrode material

3. During NEMS, the A electrode is 10 × 5 in. and electrode B 7 × 7 in. This type of stimulation would be classified as _____.
    a. monopolar
    b. bipolar
    c. quadripolar
    d. polypolar
    e. unipolar

4. The amount of energy required to produce a muscle contraction is _____.
    a. <10 mA
    b. 11–20 mA
    c. >30 mA
    d. 1–15 µA
    e. 15–30 µA

5. Which of the following would provide the most resistance to current flow?
    a. material with many free electrons
    b. material that is short
    c. material of wide cross-sectional size
    d. material of low temperature
    e. both a and d

6. The most common AC wave form is _____.
    a. square
    b. triangular
    c. sine
    d. rectangular
    e. sawtooth

7. To form a closed circuit in the body's tissues, at least one electrode from each of the generator's output leads must _____.
    a. touch the skin
    b. be larger than the other electrode
    c. be saturated in water
    d. be smaller than the other electrode
    e. be made of insulated material

8. What happens when the number of twitch contractions per second rises?
    a. improved lymphatic drainage
    b. relaxation
    c. tetany
    d. pain reduction
    e. all of the above

9. Two equal-size electrodes are placed in the target treatment area and an equal amount of stimulation is felt under each electrode. This is known as _____.
    a. bipolar placement
    b. monopolar placement
    c. quadripolar placement
    d. dual-polar placement
    e. all of the above

10. The large electrode that is used with a unipolar technique is called _____.
    a. alternating
    b. an ampere
    c. the circuit
    d. dispersive
    e. the cathode

11. Any alteration in the magnitude or any variation in the duration of an electrical current is called _____.
    a. frequency
    b. modulation

c. ohm

d. adaptation

e. on–off ratio

12. A unit of measure that indicates the rate at which electrical current is flowing is the _____.

    a. volt

    b. ampere

    c. ohm

    d. watt

    e. joule

Chapter 10

1. Which type of modality uses medium frequency as its carrier frequency?

    a. TENS

    b. MENS

    c. iontophoresis

    d. IFC

    e. HVPC

2. Which type of modality uses a direct current?

    a. TENS

    b. MENS

    c. iontophoresis

    d. IFC

    e. both b and c

3. Which type of modality uses a low-frequency alternating current?

    a. TENS

    b. MENS

    c. iontophoresis

    d. IFC

    e. HVPC

4. Which on–off cycle would be the best for the prevention of atrophy during the early phases of rehabilitation using Russian stimulation?

    a. 10/10

    b. 20/20

    c. 30/10

    d. 10/30

    e. 10/50

5. Which on–off cycle would be the best for reducing a muscle spasm using NMES?

    a. 10/10

    b. 20/20

    c. 30/10

    d. 10/30

    e. 10/50

6. Which type of TENS is used primarily to treat acute pain by stimulating the large-diameter sensory nerves using a frequency of 80–200 pps with the intensity adjusted to the point at which the patient reports a buzzing or tingling?

    a. sensory TENS

    b. motor TENS

    c. brief-intense TENS

    d. opiate TENS

    e. noxious TENS

7. Which type of TENS is used to treat chronic pain by stimulating the small-diameter afferent nerves using a low frequency of 1–5 pps with an intensity that results in a twitch contraction?

    a. sensory TENS

    b. motor TENS

    c. brief-intense TENS

    d. opiate TENS

    e. all of the above

8. Which type of modality uses a twin-peak monophasic pulsed current driven by a large electromotive force?

    a. TENS

    b. MENS

    c. iontophoresis

    d. IFC

    e. HVPC

9. Which of the following modalities is primarily used to modulate pain?

    a. TENS

    b. MENS

    c. IFC

    d. HVPC

    e. a and c

10. Which modality uses DC and pulsed currents with a stimulus amplitude that is imperceptible?

    a. TENS

    b. MENS

    c. iontophoresis

    d. IFC

    e. HVPC

THERAPEUTIC HEAT AND COLD

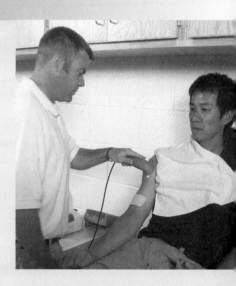

Therapeutic heat and cold form the bulk of the traditional therapeutic modalities. Heat modalities have historically been the workhorse of rehabilitation. For decades, clinicians thought that heat applications increase blood flow, thereby carrying away injury wastes and bringing nutrients to rebuild damaged tissue. This does occur. A more powerful reason for therapeutic heat has emerged, however. It now appears that the primary purpose of heat application is to facilitate therapeutic exercise (specifically stretching) and reduce general soreness.

Cryotherapy has emerged as a powerful rehabilitative tool as well, although many people still think of cold only for immediate care to prevent swelling. Cold facilitates active exercise, especially during the early stages of acute orthopedic injury rehabilitation. Thus therapeutic exercise can begin sooner and progress more quickly.

The chapters in Part V contain a rich smattering of history, because the past forms the foundation of the present and future. You will also find many references to our research. After more than a combined 30 years of clinical experience, 50 years of research, and the pursuit of thousands of clinical questions, we are quite passionate about understanding and explaining the proper application of therapeutic heat and cold. We hope to impart some of this passion to you as you expand your theoretical understanding and practical skills to improve the health of your patients.

Part V begins with Chapter 11 on the principles of heat as it applies to thermotherapy, including what it is and why it is used therapeutically. This foundation is essential for understanding how to properly use therapeutic heat and cold. In addition, advances in the use of these modalities require this foundational knowledge. Much of this chapter is a review of concepts taught in a basic physics class.

Chapter 12 covers the application of numerous superficial heat modalities. The theoretical basis and application of the two most effective deep-heating modalities (ultrasound and diathermy) are presented in Chapters 15 and 16.

In Chapter 13, we discuss the theoretical basis for the use of cryotherapy beyond immediate care and dispel many of the myths concerning its use. We also present a concise list of principles on when to use heat and cold therapeutically. In Chapter 14, we present application techniques for the most common uses of cryotherapy for acute orthopedic injury rehabilitation beyond immediate care.

Principles of Heat for Thermotherapy

You are in the athletic training clinic, taping an athlete's ankle. You overhear Andrew, a staff athletic trainer (AT) talking to a baseball player. Andrew suggests a regimen of heat therapy for the player's chronic case of supraspinatus tendinitis (shoulder). The athlete asks, "What kind of heat treatment? Is there a difference between using a whirlpool, hot pack, and ultrasound? What causes the difference?" How would you answer these questions?

Defining Thermotherapy

Thermotherapy is the therapeutic use of heat: the application of a device or substance with a temperature greater than body temperature, thus causing heat to pass from the thermotherapy device to the body. **Cryotherapy** is the therapeutic use of cold: the application of a device or substance with a temperature less than body temperature, thus causing heat to pass from the body to the cryotherapy device.

Heat is a form of energy produced by the movement of atoms and molecules. All substances with a temperature above *absolute zero* ($-450°F$, $-273°C$) possess heat. Technically, there is no such thing as cold; **cold** is the absence of heat or something that has less heat than one would desire.

Temperature is the measure of an object's ability to spontaneously give up energy. It is used to indicate the level of molecular motion associated with heat.

> **CRITICAL THINKING 11.1** *Let's review an example from Chapter 5. Is it hot or cold? In the fall, if the temperature drops down to 40°F (4.5°C), you think it's cold out and put on a jacket. In the spring, if the temperature gets up to 40°F (4.5°C), you think it's warm out and shed your coat. Why is your perception of the temperature different even though the temperature is the same?*

SUPERFICIAL AND DEEP HEAT

There are two classifications of thermotherapy: superficial and deep. **Superficial thermotherapy** is the application of modalities to the surface of the body that primarily heat the surface tissues (<1 cm) (Table 11.1). We should note, however, that *superficial thermal modalities* will heat tissues deeper than 1 cm, but the amount of heating is not enough to evoke the desired therapeutic effects. Hot packs, whirlpool, and paraffin are examples of superficial thermal modalities. These modalities heat primarily by conduction and infrared radiation.

Deep thermotherapy is the application of modalities that cause a *tissue temperature rise* (TTR) in deeper tissues (3–4 cm). Ultrasound and diathermy are *deep thermal modalities,* and they heat by conversion and radiation. Diathermy radiation has different characteristics from infrared radiation and therefore evokes different physiological effects.

Transferring Heat to and from the Body

Therapeutic heat and therapeutic cold applications use one of three types of heat transfer between the therapeutic modality and the body: conduction, convection, or radiation. Conversion is sometimes considered a type of heat transfer, although this is a misnomer, as discussed later in the chapter. Heat is always transferred from the object of higher temperature to the object of lower temperature.

CONDUCTION

Conduction is heat transfer between two objects of uneven temperatures after coming into contact with each other. In the human body conduction occurs on the cellular level, as hotter, rapidly moving, or vibrating atoms and molecules interact with cooler, neighboring atoms and molecules, transferring some of their energy (heat) to the cooler atoms. Given enough time, the process occurs until the objects reach thermal equilibrium. Examples of modalities that transfer heat by conduction are hot packs, whirlpool, ice packs, and slush buckets. Conduction is the most frequently used method of heat transfer in physical medicine.

A **thermal gradient** always develops when heat is transferred by conduction. This means there is a gradual change in temperature from the interior of one object to the interior of the other object (Fig. 11.1). The slope of the gradient becomes less with time as heat is withdrawn from

TABLE 11.1	Temperature Changes Owing to Application of Various Thermal Modalities					
MODALITY	**PARAMETERS**	**DEPTH (CM)**	**TISSUE**	**DURATION (MIN)**	**TEMPERATURE CHANGE (°C)**	**REFERENCE**
Hot pack		1	Triceps surae	15	3.6	1
		2	Quadriceps	10	0.8	2
		2	Quadriceps	20	2.0	2
		2	Quadriceps	30	3.0	2
		3	Triceps surae	15	0.8	1
Whirlpool	40.6°C	1.5	Triceps surae	20	2.8	3
Contrast therapy	40.6°C/15.6°C	1.5	Triceps surae	20	0.4	3
	41°C/10°C	1.5	Triceps surae	20	0.44	4
Topical heat wrap	Knee wrap	5	Knee joint capsule	120	2.6	5
	Back wrap	1.5	Paraspinals	120	2.7	6
	Back wrap	1.5	Paraspinals	150	1.8	7
	Back wrap	2	Paraspinals	120	1.1	8
	Knee wrap	1.5	Vastus medialis	120	3.2	5
Shortwave diathermy	Pulsed at 48 W	2	Suprailiac fat	20	7.2	9
	Pulsed at 48 W	3	Triceps surae	20	4	10
	Pulsed at 48 W	3	Triceps surae	20	4.6	11
	Pulsed at 48 W	5	Knee capsule	20	3.2	12
Ultrasound, 1 Mz	1 W/cm^2	2.5	Triceps surae	10	2	13
		5	Triceps surae	10	2	13
	1.2 W/cm^2	4	Triceps surae	10	2.5	14
	1.5 W/cm^2	2.5	Triceps surae	10	3	13
		5	Triceps surae	10	3	13
		2.5	Triceps surae	12.5	4	15
		3 and 5	Triceps surae	10	3.2	16
		5	Triceps surae	12.5	3.5	15
		5	Triceps surae	10	4	17
	1.5 W/cm^2 gel	3	Triceps surae	10	4.8	18
	1.5 W/cm^2, water bath	3	Triceps surae	10	2.1	18
	1.5 W/cm^2; 2 ERA	4	Triceps surae	10	3.5	19
	1.5 W/cm^2; 6 ERA	4	Triceps surae	10	1.3	19
	1.5 W/cm^2, ice	3	Triceps surae	15 (ice);10 (US)	0.6	20
		5	Triceps surae	5 (ice);10 (US)	1.8	17
	1.6 W/cm^2; BNR 2.3:1	3	Triceps surae	10	3	21
	1.6 W/cm^2; BNR 2.4:1	3	Triceps surae	9	4.5	21
	1.6 W/cm^2; BNR 7.7:1	3	Triceps surae	8.8	4.2	21

(continued)

TABLE 11.1	*Temperature Changes Owing to Application of Various Thermal Modalities (continued)*					
MODALITY	PARAMETERS	DEPTH (CM)	TISSUE	DURATION (MIN)	TEMPERATURE CHANGE (°C)	REFERENCE
Ultrasound, 3 MHz	0.5 W/cm²	0.8	Triceps surae	10	3	13
		1.6	Triceps surae	10	3	13
	1 W/cm²	1	Fat (triceps)	10	8.4	22
		1	Patellar tendon	4	8.3	23
		0.8	Triceps surae	10	6	13
		1.6	Triceps surae	10	6	13
	1 W/cm², gel	1	Lateral ankle	10	7.7	24
	1 W/cm², gel pad	1	Lateral ankle	10	6.7	24
	1.2 W/cm²	1 and 2.5	Triceps surae	5.5	4.4	25
	1.4 W/cm²	2	Triceps surae	5	3.3	14
	1.5 W/cm²	1.2	Triceps surae	6	5.3	26

BNR, beam nonuniformity ratio; *ERA,* effective radiating area; *US,* ultrasound.

deeper within the warmer object and heat increases deeper in the cooler object. Results from one of our hot pack studies illustrate the thermal gradient in tissue. After a hot pack was applied to the quadriceps for 20 min, temperature had risen 6.5°F (3.6°C) at a depth of 1 cm, but there was only a 1.4°F (0.8°C) increase at 3 cm (see Table 11.1).[1]

Many factors affect the rate of heat conduction between various modalities and the patient. These were discussed in Chapter 5 in relation to cold and are listed below:

- The temperature differential between the body and the modality
- The dissipation of tissue heat and/or modality heating
- The heat storage capacity of the modality
- The size of the modality
- The amount of tissue in contact with the modality
- The length of application
- Individual patient variability

CONVECTION

Convection is the transfer of heat to or from an object by the passage of a fluid or air past its surface. Central heating and cooling of a home or building are examples of heat transfer by convection. Examples of modalities that transfer heat by convection are whirlpool and fluidotherapy. A whirlpool transfers heat by both conduction and convection.

RADIATION

Radiation, also called *radiant energy,* is the transfer of energy in the form of rays, waves, or particles, often from a

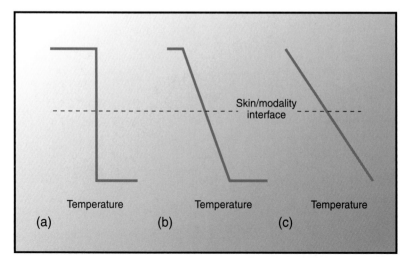

FIGURE 11.1. A thermal gradient develops over time during heat transfer between two objects of different temperatures in contact with each other. *Dotted line,* interface between the two objects; *solid line,* temperatures of the objects in contact. **(a)** Immediately upon contact, **(b)** after the passage of time, **(c)** after the passage of additional time.

central source. All substances with a temperature above absolute zero radiate heat to a substance of lower temperature through infrared rays. The sun heats the Earth, in part by radiation of infrared rays. The heat you feel coming off asphalt pavement on a hot summer day is also caused by infrared radiation. Diathermy, laser, infrared (heat), and ultraviolet lamps are the most common examples of therapeutic modalities that use radiation to transfer heat. Radiation and electromagnetic waves are discussed in greater depth later in the chapter.

CONVERSION

Many consider **conversion**, another type of heat transfer, defining it as a process that occurs when a form of energy other than heat (electricity, chemical, mechanical, etc.) is converted to heat within the body. Although conversion is the process by which deep tissues are heated and is an essential part of thermotherapy, another form of energy—not heat—is transferred from outside into the body. Examples of modalities that heat by conversion are ultrasound and diathermy.

Conversion is the only way of increasing the temperature of deep tissues to therapeutic levels. Both conduction and convection deliver heat to the surface of the body, which is then conducted into the body. But most of the heat is dissipated by the subcutaneous circulation before it can substantially increase the temperature of deeper tissues. The depth of penetration of deep heat depends on the modality and on the physiological and anatomical characteristics of the individual body part.

MODALITY MYTH

HEAT IS NECESSARY FOR REHABILITATION BECAUSE IT INCREASES BLOOD FLOW AND PROMOTES HEALING

Increasing blood flow is beneficial during healing, and local heat applications do increase blood flow. However, therapeutic exercise increases blood flow many times more than heat applications do. Therefore, therapeutic exercise is more important than heat applications during rehabilitation.

The Therapeutic Use of Heat

Traditionally, the primary reason heat was used as a therapeutic agent was to increase blood flow to the injured body part. In the process of carrying away the heat, blood also delivers nutrients to the area and carries metabolites and other waste products away. It is assumed that these latter two functions increase the rate of healing of the injury, although the theory has never been tested. Another argument against the traditional reason for applying thermotherapy is that active exercise increases blood flow much more than therapeutic heat.

Therapeutic heat modalities are indispensable for other reasons, however. They promote relaxation, relieve general soreness, and facilitate connective tissue stretching. Also, you can use therapeutic heat modalities to target increased blood flow to a specific area, such as the knee of a patient that is too sore to warm up on a treadmill.

PHYSIOLOGICAL EFFECTS OF HEAT

A major reason for using therapeutic modalities is to stimulate an increased rate of normal functions. The tissue temperature rise (TTR) caused by thermotherapy results in the following:

- *Increased circulation:* 1.5–2 times normal resting blood flow
- *Increased metabolism:* Beneficial during wound healing but devastating during immediate care because it will increase secondary metabolic injury. Therefore, heat should never be applied until 2–3 days after an acute injury.
- *Increased inflammation:* Increased phagocytosis and wound healing
- *Decreased pain (analgesia):* A general sedative effect that promotes relaxation; effective for general soreness, aches, and pains but not as effective as cold applications in removing acute injury pain. Therefore, it is not as effective as cryotherapy for facilitating active exercise (see Chapter 13).
- *Decreased muscle spasm*
- *Decreased tissue stiffness:* Thermotherapy decreases fluid viscosity, which makes joints and muscles less stiff, and causes the cross-linked fibers in collagen to release, thereby facilitating the elongation of connective tissue (see Fig. 6.6).

✓ APPLICATION TIP

***WHEN TO USE HEAT AND COLD.** Therapeutic heat is most effective in decreasing general soreness and in preparing soft tissues for stretching and joint mobilization. Therapeutic cold is most effective in relieving pain and inhibition in acutely injured soft tissue, thereby facilitating therapeutic exercise.*

HEAT SINKS

Regardless of the cause of local TTR, circulation to the area removes heat and thereby prevents local thermal damage (cooking the tissue). Heat is carried by the blood to **heat sinks**, areas of the body that can accept and dissipate great amounts of heat. The two primary heat sinks in the human body are the lungs and skin. The lungs dissipate heat through respiration, and the skin dissipates heat through perspiration and radiation. As long as the heat sinks dissipate the heat at least as quickly as it is added to the body by the modality, the application is safe. If, however, heat is added to the body faster than it is dissipated, the body part will gradually increase in temperature, and local heat injury can result. This is why it is a contraindication to apply heat to areas of compromised circulation, such as the feet of a patient with diabetes. If the heat application gets too warm, inadequate blood flow to cool the area can result in overheating and associated tissue destruction.

APPLICATION TIP

WHIRLPOOL TEMPERATURE DEPENDS ON HEAT SINKS. *The maximal temperature of a whirlpool is determined by the amount of the body that is immersed in the bath (see Chapter 12). The concept of heat sinks explains why. If only a foot or arm is in the bath, about 5% of the body surface is being heated and about 95% acts as a heat sink (along with the lungs). At the other extreme, if the patient is immersed up to the neck, 95% of the body surface is being heated and 5% acts as a heat sink. In the latter case, a small area must dissipate the large amount of heat being added to the body. Thus the following principle: The more of the body that is in a whirlpool bath, the lower the temperature should be.*

GENERAL HEAT CONTRAINDICATIONS

In most situations, the application of topical heat is safe; however, there are three general heat contraindications, or contraindications to all forms of heat application. In addition, there are specific contraindications to specific thermal modalities. The general contraindications are

- Do not apply any form of heat to an acute injury within the first 48–72 hr of injury. Increased metabolism will cause an increase in secondary metabolic injury if heat is applied too quickly to an acute injury.
- Do not apply any form of heat to an area with compromised circulation. Inadequate blood flow prevents cooling, and the tissue could suffer heat injury.
- Do not apply any form of heat to an area with compromised sensation. The same problem potentially exists

as with compromised circulation. If the body cannot sense the temperature of the heat application, it may not respond with increased circulation to the area.

scored

Radiation and Electromagnetic Waves

Much of this section is a review of principles taught in a basic physics class. This material will help you understand the principles on which ultrasound, diathermy, lasers, infrared lamps, and ultraviolet lamps are based and why they are used therapeutically. This information will keep you from being a knobologist (see Chapter 1). Radiation, radiant energy, electromagnetic waves, and electromagnetic radiation are similar and the terms are often used interchangeably.

Understanding scientific notation and the metric system will help you understand radiation. If you need a review, the basics are in Boxes 11.1 and 11.2, and Critical Thinking 11.2 will test your knowledge.

 CRITICAL THINKING 11.2 *Which is bigger, 23×10^2 or 3×10^3?*

SIMILARITIES AND DIFFERENCES AMONG FORMS OF RADIATION

As mentioned earlier, radiation propagates energy through empty space as **electromagnetic waves**, which take many forms, including heat, light, electricity, x-rays, and cosmic rays (Fig. 11.2). Forms of radiation have the following in common:

BOX 11.1 *SCIENTIFIC NOTATION*

Scientific notation is a way of expressing very large numbers—for example, 6.98×10^4. This expression consists of a coefficient (6.98) multiplied by 10 raised to an exponent (4). To convert this to a more familiar number, multiply the 10 by the number of the exponent: $6.98 \times 10 \times 10 \times 10 \times 10 = 69,800$. A simple way to multiply by 10s is to move the decimal point to the right, adding extra zeroes as needed. If the exponent is negative (10^{-4}), move the decimal point to the left. Here are three more examples:

- $3 \times 10^8 = 300,000,000$
- $1 \times 10^2 = 100$
- $10^3 = 1 \times 10^3 = 1,000$

BOX 11.2 *METRIC SYSTEM ABBREVIATIONS*

ABBREVIATION	MEANING	VALUE
K	kilo	10^3 or 1,000
M	mega	10^6 or 1,000,000
c	centa	10^{-2} or 1/100
m	milli	10^{-3} or 1/1000
μ	micro	10^{-6} or 1/1,000,000
μm	millimicro	10^{-9} or 1/1,000,000,000
n	nano	10^{-9} or 1/1,000,000,000
Å	angstrom	10^{-10} or 1/10,000,000,000

- All are caused by minute particles moving through space.
- All are called electromagnetic waves.
- All travel at the same linear speed in space, which is 186,000 mi./sec or 3×10^8 m/sec.

The various forms of radiation have these main differences:

- Some forms are visible (such as light).
- Some forms are audible (such as radio waves).
- Some forms you can feel (such as electricity and infrared).
- Some forms can pass through you (such as x-rays).
- Each form has different energy.

The differences among various forms of radiation result from their different energy levels, which result from their specific wavelengths and frequencies (see Fig. 11.2).

ELECTROMAGNETIC WAVES

Electromagnetic waves consist of oscillating electric and magnetic fields at right angles to one another and to the propagation direction (Fig. 11.3). Individual electromagnetic waves, although dual in nature, behave as a single wave and are often represented as such. Each has a unique wavelength and frequency.

Wavelength is the distance, expressed in meters or centimeters, of one repetition of the wave (Fig. 11.4). **Frequency** is the rate of passage of crests on the wave form, expressed in cycles per second (cps) or hertz (Hz). Even though all electromagnetic waves are sinusoidal waves with the same linear speed, they travel differently. As one changes, the other one changes proportionally in the opposite direction; as one increases, the other one decreases. This is so because the linear speed is constant. Therefore, wavelength multiplied by frequency will always equal 186,000 mi./sec, or $= 3 \times 10^8$ m/sec. The giant and dwarf analogy presented in Box 11.3 helps explain this principle.

If you know either the wavelength or the frequency, you can compute the other. For example, if a particular electromagnetic wave had a wavelength of 186,000 mi., its frequency would be 1 cps or 1 Hz. If its wavelength was 1 mi., its frequency would be 186,000 Hz.

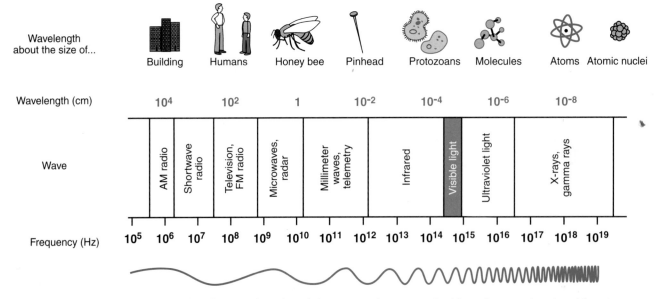

FIGURE 11.2. The electromagnetic spectrum illustrates the variety of electromagnetic waves, each with a unique wavelength and frequency.

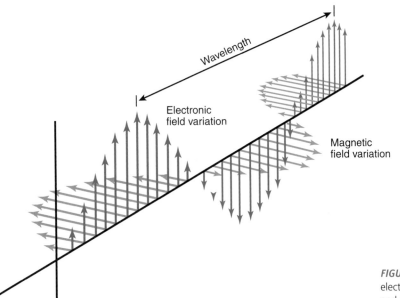

FIGURE 11.3. Electromagnetic waves consist of oscillating electric and magnetic fields at right angles to one another and to the propagation direction.

CRITICAL THINKING 11.3 *(a) If an electromagnetic wave is 6,200 mi. long, what is its frequency? (b) If another wave has a frequency of 2000 Hz, what is its wavelength?*

CLASSIFICATION OF ELECTROMAGNETIC WAVES

Because every electromagnetic wave form has a unique wavelength and unique frequency, waves can be classified according to either wavelength or frequency. There is no convention as to which is used. Some are classified by wavelength, others by frequency, and some by both. Electricity and radio waves are examples of electromagnetic waves that are classified according to frequency. Lasers are classified by wavelength. Diathermy is named for its wavelength (shortwave), but it is classified by its frequency, which sometimes causes confusion (see Chapter 16).

> **BOX 11.3 *THE GIANT AND DWARF ANALOGY***
>
> The relationship between wavelength and frequency is illustrated by an analogy of a foot race between a giant and a dwarf. Imagine that the NBA's tallest center (perhaps 7 ft. 6 in.) and shortest guard (say 5 ft. 4 in.) raced from baseline to baseline on a basketball court. Assume they tie. If the center's stride length is 6 ft., he traveled the distance in 16 strides. If the guard's stride length is only 4 ft., it took him 24 strides to travel the same distance. So it is with electromagnetic waves: The shorter the wavelength, the greater the frequency.

> **A P P L I C A T I O N   T I P**
>
> *THE THERAPEUTIC EFFICACY OF LASERS IS WAVELENGTH SPECIFIC. The body responds differently to electromagnetic waves of different wavelengths, so one laser does not fit all purposes (see Chapter 19). You cannot use your TV remote control to heal orthopedic injuries.*

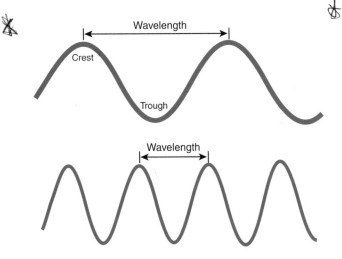

FIGURE 11.4. Two sinusoidal waves with different wavelengths.

PROPERTIES OF ELECTROMAGNETIC WAVES

The two most important properties of electromagnetic waves in relation to therapeutic modalities are their energy and their inertia. Both are a function of the photon, a particle produced by molecular motion.

Photons

A **photon** is the basic unit of radiant energy. The amount of energy in photons is a function of the frequency of the electromagnetic wave that produced it, so photons of a given frequency will always have the same amount of energy. There is no such thing as half a photon of energy; photons of a given frequency always occur in precisely the same-size energy chunks.

Photons do posses differing amounts of energy, however. Because a photon's energy is a function of the frequency of the electromagnetic wave, the greater the frequency (or shorter the wavelength), the more energy it has. Thus x-rays have much greater energy than do radio waves. The energy at lower frequencies is so small that it has no therapeutic value.

Reflection, Refraction, Transmission, Absorption

Photons possess inertia, so they exert pressure on any object or substance they strike. All electromagnetic waves move in a straight line until they come into contact with some other substance. One, or a combination, of four things will then occur (Fig. 11.5):

- **Reflection:** As waves hit the substance, they bounce back; there is no penetration of the substance. The angle of reflection is determined by the angle of the strike.
- **Refraction:** The waves bend as they pass through the substance; an example is light passing through a prism. The amount of bending depends on the frequency of the waves.
- **Transmission:** The wave is transmitted through the substance. Transmission can be complete, such as with γ-rays through a door, or partial, such as x-rays

through an arm. The depth of penetration is a function of the energy of the waves.
- **Absorption:** Partially transmitted waves are absorbed by the tissues and turned into heat.

Thermal Effects of Electromagnetic Waves

All electrical currents cause a rise in temperature in the substance thorough which they flow because of the conversion of electricity to heat. The amount of heat produced is defined by the principles of Joule's law:

- Heat produced is directly proportional to the square of the current strength.
- Heat produced is directly proportional to the resistance of the conductor.
- Heat produced is directly proportional to the duration of the passage of a current.

Two examples are the light bulb and an electrical fuse. In a light bulb, carbon or tungsten filaments are high resistance, so heat is produced as electricity passes through the filament. As current passes through a fuse, the metal rod in the middle heats. If the current is too strong, it heats to the point that the metal rod melts and the circuit is broken.

THE INFLUENCE OF TISSUE RESISTANCE

The tissues of the body possess varying resistances. This should mean that tissues with higher resistance would heat up more, but it's not so. Electricity flows along the path of least resistance.

Applying Radiation

The following laws and principles relate to the application of all forms of radiation:

- **Inverse square law:** $I = 1/d^2$. The intensity (I) of radiation is inversely proportional to the distance squared (d^2). Thus decreasing the distance between the source and the patient will cause a much greater increase in its intensity. For example, decreasing the distance by half increases the intensity fourfold. This is one of the reasons that infrared lamps (Chapter 12) and microwave diathermy (Chapter 16) are dangerous. Moving the source closer to the body greatly intensifies the radiation delivered to the body.
- **Cosine or right-angle law:** The optimum radiation occurs when the source of the radiation is perpendicular

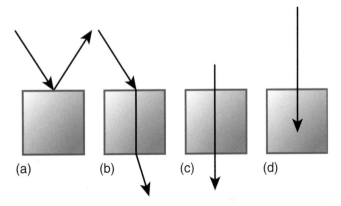

FIGURE 11.5. The possible responses of electromagnetic energy when it comes in contact with matter. *Arrows,* the movement of photons. **(a)** Reflection, **(b)** refraction, **(c)** transmission, and **(d)** absorption. See the text for details.

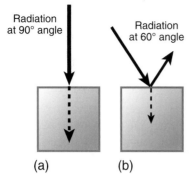

Radiation at 90° angle

Radiation at 60° angle

(a)   (b)

FIGURE 11.6. The effects of the cosine or right-angle law. **(a)** When radiation is at a 90° angle, or perpendicular to the surface, all of it transmits. **(b)** When radiation is applied at a different angle, some of the radiation is reflected.

to the center of the surface of the area to be radiated. When the source is at an angle, some of it is reflected to the side rather than moving into the tissue (Fig. 11.6). The amount of transmission is a function of the angle of application: full effects are achieved at 90°, 86% at 60°, and only 50% when radiation is applied at 30°.

- **Law of Grotthus-Draper:** Waves must be absorbed to be beneficial. Also known as the *principle of photochemical activation* and the *Draper law*, this law was proposed in the nineteenth century to define the effect of photons in stimulating photochemical reactions in a substance.[27] It had nothing to do with heat. However, because not all of the absorbed light brings about chemical action, most of the "excess" absorbed energy is converted into thermal energy. So indirectly the law applies to heat as well. Another interpretation of this law that can reasonably be applied to therapeutic modalities is that there is an inverse relationship between the amount of energy absorption and the depth

of penetration of the energy. Energy that is absorbed by superficial layers is no longer available to deeper-lying tissues. This law explains why the effects of laser and infrared radiation are only superficial.

- **Arndt-Schultz principle:** There is an optimal amount of energy absorption per unit of time that is beneficial. Less than this amount will not cause a reaction, and more than this amount will be detrimental. The old adage "More is better" applies only up to a point as far as therapeutic modalities are concerned.

Acoustic Waves

Acoustic waves (sound, ultrasound) are not electromagnetic waves. They differ from electromagnetic waves in two dramatic ways:

- Acoustic waves transmit best through solids and not at all through a vacuum. Electromagnetic waves transmit best through a vacuum and poorly through solids. Electromagnetic waves are slowed by collisions. Acoustic waves are transmitted by collisions; as density increases, so does transmission. For example, ultrasound will transmit 0.3 mm in the atmosphere, 1.5 mm in soft tissue, and 3.5 mm in cortical bone.
- Acoustic waves do not travel as fast as electromagnetic waves; in fact, they travel much more slowly— a few hundred thousand m/sec (10^5) as opposed to 10^8 m/sec for electromagnetic waves. As in electromagnetic waves, linear speed equals wavelength times frequency.

CRITICAL THINKING 11.4 *Why must the head of an ultrasound unit be in good contact with the body?*

CLOSING SCENE

Recall from the chapter opening scene that Andrew, a staff AT, suggested a regimen of heat therapy for a baseball player's chronic supraspinatus tendinitis. The athlete wondered if there was a difference in the heating effects produced by a whirlpool, hot pack, and ultrasound. You now know that whirlpools and hot packs produce moderate heat in the superficial tissues, whereas ultrasound can generate even greater amounts of heat into the deep tissues. Since the supraspinatus is a fairly deep muscle, located underneath the deltoids, you conclude that ultrasound would be the modality of choice for heating this deep structure.

CHAPTER REFLECTIONS

1. Read and ponder each of the following points. Do you feel you have a clear understanding of each concept? If not, reread the appropriate section of the chapter.
   - What is heat?
   - Explain why heat is used therapeutically.
   - What are the general indications and contraindications to the therapeutic use of heat?
   - Define conduction, convection, radiation, and conversion and describe how they relate to heat transfer.
   - Provide an example of radiant energy.
   - What are some common properties of electromagnetic waves?
   - When is it appropriate to use heat?

2. Write three to five questions for discussion with your class instructor, clinical instructor, classmates, and clinical colleagues.

3. Get together with classmates and quiz each other on the concepts of this chapter. Use the points in exercise 1 and questions you wrote for exercise 2 as a beginning. Explaining concepts out loud to others requires a deeper grasp of the material than feeling you understand it as you read.

CRITICAL THINKING RESPONSES

Critical Thinking 11.1

The sensation of being hot or cold is relative. In the summer you get used to the temperature being hot, so 40°F (4.5°C) is colder than what you are used to and you interpret it as being cold. During the winter the opposite is true. You get used to it being cold, and because 40°F (4.5°C) is hotter that what you have been used to, you interpret it as being warm.

Critical Thinking 11.2

$23 \times 10^2 = 2300$. $3 \times 10^3 = 3000$. So 3×10^3 is bigger than 23×10^2.

Critical Thinking 11.3

Remember that wavelength times frequency equals 186,000 mi./sec. So:

a. Frequency = 30 Hz (186,000 mi./sec ÷ 6,200 mi. = 30 Hz).

b. Wavelength = 93 mi. (186,000 mi./sec ÷ 2,000 Hz = 93 mi.)

Critical Thinking 11.4

Ultrasound is a mechanical wave that cannot be transmitted through air. Therefore, if the transducer is not in complete contact with the skin and coupling agent, the energy will not be transmitted.

REFERENCES

1. Draper DO, Harris ST, Schulthies SS, et al. Hotpack and 1 MHz ultrasound treatments have an additive effect on muscle temperature increase. J Athl Train 1998;33:21–24.
2. Morris AK. Moist Heat Pack Re-Warming Following 10, 20, 30 min Application. Master's thesis, Brigham Young University, 2003.
3. Myrer JW, Draper DO, Durrant E. Contrast therapy and intramuscular temperature in the human leg. J Athl Train 1994;29:318–322.
4. Wertz AS, et al. Intramuscular and subcutaneous temperature changes in the human leg due to contrast therapy. J Athl Train 1997; 32:S33.
5. Mitra A, Draper DO, Hopkins T, Anderson MA. Application of the ThermaCare knee wrap results in significant increases in muscle and intracapsular temperature. J Athl Train 2005;40:S88–S89.
6. Draper DO, Trowbridge CA. Continuous low-level heat therapy: What works, what doesn't. Athl Ther Today 2003;8:46–48.
7. Draper D, Trowbridge CA. The ThermaCare HeatWrap increases skin and paraspinal muscle temperature greater than the CuraHeat Patch. J Athl Train 2004;39:S93.
8. Trowbridge C, Draper DO, Feland JB, Eggett D. The ThermaCare air-activated heat wrap heats paraspinal muscles greater than two menthol-based pain patches. J Orthop Sports Phys Ther 2004;34: 549–558.
9. Draper DO, Castel C. The effect of pulsed shortwave diathermy on temperature elevation in adipose tissue. J Athl Train 1998;33:S70.
10. Draper DO, Knight KL, Fujiwara T, Castel JC. Temperature change in human muscle during and after pulsed short-wave diathermy. J Orthop Sports Phys Ther 1999;29:13–18; discussion 19–22.
11. Garrett CL, Draper DO, Knight KL. Heat distribution in the lower leg from pulsed short-wave diathermy and ultrasound treatments. J Athl Train 2000;35:13–22.
12. Draper DO, Anderson M. An explanation of knee joint intracapsular temperature rise following pulsed shortwave diathermy, in vivo. J Athl Train 2005;40(2):S43.
13. Draper DO, Castel JC, Castel D. Rate of temperature increase in human muscle during 1 MHz and 3 MHz continuous ultrasound. J Orthop Sports Phys Ther 1995;22:142–150.
14. Anderson M, Eggett D, Draper D. Combining topical analgesics and ultrasound, Part 2. Athl Ther Today 2005;10:45–47.

15. Rose S, Draper DO, Schulthies SS, Durrant E. The stretching window, Part two: Rate of thermal decay in deep muscle following 1-MHz ultrasound. J Athl Train 1996;31:139–143.

16. Ashton DF, Draper DO, Myrer JW. Temperature rise in human muscle during ultrasound treatments using flex-all as a coupling agent. J Athl Train 1998;33:136–140.

17. Draper DO, Schulthies S, Sorvisto P, Hautala A-M. Temperature changes in deep muscles of humans during ice and ultrasound therapies: An in vivo study. J Orthop Sports Phys Ther 1995;21:153–157.

18. Draper D, Sunderland S. Examination of the law of Grotthus-Draper: Does ultrasound penetrate subcutaneous fat in humans? J Athl Train 1993;28:246–250.

19. Chudleigh D, Schulthies S, Draper D, Myrer J. Muscle temperature rise during 1 MHz ultrasound treatments of two and six times the effective radiating areas of the transducer. J Athl Train 1998;33:S11.

20. Rimington SJ, Draper DO, Durrant E, Fellingham G. Temperature changes during therapeutic ultrasound in the precooled human gastrocnemius muscle. J Athl Train 1994;29:325–327.

21. Draper DO. A breakthrough on comfortable ultrasound treatments: Beam non-uniformity ratio is only half of the equation [S-25]. Paper presented at the annual symposium of the National Athletic Trainer's Association, Kansas City, MO, 1999.

22. Draper D, Abergel P, Castel J. Rate of temperature change in human fat during external ultrasound: Implications for liposuction. Am J Cosmet Surg 1998;15:361–367.

23. Chan AK, Myrer JW, Measom GJ, Draper DO. Temperature changes in human patellar tendon in response to therapeutic ultrasound. J Athl Train 1998;33:130–135.

24. Bishop S, Draper DO, Knight KL, et al. Human-tissue temperature rise during ultrasound treatments with the Aquaflex gel pad. J Athl Train 2004;39:25–30.

25. Wells A, Draper D, Vincent W. The regression equation of the Omnisound 3000P is valid: Ultrasound treatments should be temperature dependent not time dependent. J Athl Train 2004;39:S24.

26. Draper DO, Ricard MD. Rate of temperature decay in human muscle following 3 MHz ultrasound: The stretching window revealed. J Athl Train 1995;30:304–307.

27. Fang H-Y., ed. Environmental Geotechnology Dictionary Available at: www.iseg.giees.uncc.edu/dictionary.cfm. Accessed Apr 2007.

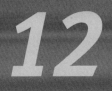
Application Procedures: Superficial Thermotherapy

OPENING SCENE

There are several ways to apply therapeutic heat. Your grandfather tells you he applies a heating ointment to his arthritic knees each morning. He says that although the ointment seems to help, he is curious whether there are other ways to heat his painful knees. You tell him that there are several heating modalities, but you wonder why so many exist. There must be advantages and disadvantages for using each heating agent. Which heat modality would be the best to use under certain circumstances? Is the ointment your grandfather applies to his knees actually producing heat?

Superficial Thermotherapy

Superficial thermotherapy includes modalities that effectively heat only the surface tissues, to ~1 cm deep. The most commonly used modalities are the whirlpool, hot pack, paraffin bath, and electrical heating pads. Infrared lamps are sometimes used as heat modalities, although we do not recommend them because they burn too easily. Although most of the research on these modalities was conducted before 1970, some work has been done since then, and it is included, as appropriate, throughout this chapter.

In general, these modalities heat the surface 6–8°F (3–5°C) and muscles 3–5°F (2–3°C) at depths <2 cm (see Table 11.1). Blood flow doubles, and metabolism increases. Superficial thermotherapy decreases pain but not enough to facilitate active exercise. Soreness, however, is decreased during resting and activity.

Application of Whirlpool

STEP 1: FOUNDATION

A. Definition. A **whirlpool** is a large body of either hot or cold water that is forcibly circulated or "whirled" about in its container (Fig. 12.1).

B. Effects
1. *Hydrotherapy:* The buoyancy of water supports the body or body part, providing a sort of suspended animation, thereby allowing easy exercise.
2. Physical massage, provided by the whirling water and air
3. Convective heating or cooling provided by whirling water
4. Temperature effects
   a. Hot water will cause
      i. Conductive heating, a superficial increase in temperature
      ii. A superficial increase in blood flow
      iii. Decreased muscle spasm through analgesia
      iv. Whole-body relaxation through analgesia (if the whole body is treated)
      v. Increased metabolism
   b. Cold water will cause
      i. Conductive cooling, a decreased temperature that will penetrate farther than heat
      ii. Decreased blood flow
      iii. Contraction or tightness of connective tissue around muscles and joints
5. A decrease in pain
6. Decreased metabolism

C. Advantages
1. Can treat the whole body
2. Provides irregular surfaces with total contact

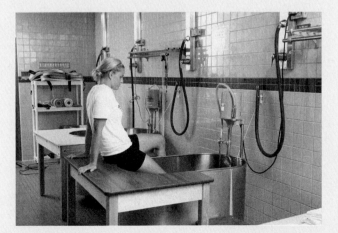

FIGURE 12.1. A typical whirlpool.

3. Temperature stability of water. It loses (or gains) heat very slowly.
4. Can provide multiple treatments simultaneously, if treatments involve the limbs (e.g., two to four patients can dangle their legs in the whirlpool at the same time)
5. The force of the water massage can be regulated from quite vigorous to very gentle.
6. Allows range of motion exercises during treatment

D. Disadvantages
1. Causes a person to feel weak or lethargic (if the majority of the body is treated with heat)
2. Increased edema (if hot water is used) when a limb is in a dependent position (lower than the rest of the body)
3. Possibility of infection
4. Messy and noisy
5. Not portable

E. Indications
1. General whole-limb or whole-body stiffness or soreness (e.g., early in a sports season, when practice sessions occur two or three times daily or when you perform an unaccustomed activity for 3–4 days)
2. Whenever superficial heat is desired
3. As a supplement to other treatments

F. Contraindications
1. General heat contraindications. Avoid using
   a. Within 24–48 hr after an acute injury
   b. If circulation is compromised
   c. If sensation to the area is compromised
2. Avoid treating a person with a high fever (>101°F; 38.3°C).

G. Precautions
1. Do not leave a patient in the whirlpool unattended; she might become lethargic enough to faint and drown.
2. Do not allow a patient to turn the whirlpool on or off while in the whirlpool.
3. Clean the tank before and after treating someone with an infectious wound.
4. Keep clothing and bandages out of the whirlpool.
5. Do not let a whirlpool treatment substitute for a more beneficial treatment (e.g., therapeutic exercise).

STEP 2: PREAPPLICATION TASKS

A. Make sure whirlpool is the proper modality for this situation.

1. Reevaluate the injury or problem. Make sure you understand the patient's condition.
2. If whirlpool was previously used, review the patient's response to that treatment.
3. Confirm that the objectives of therapy are compatible with whirlpool.
4. Make sure whirlpool is not contraindicated in this situation.

B. Preparing the equipment. *Prepare the equipment before preparing the patient.*
   1. Close the drain.
   2. Select the temperature
      a. For cryotherapy: 50–60°F (10–15.5°C).
      b. For thermotherapy: whole body, 100–108°F (37.7–42.2°C); extremity, 105–112°F (40.5–44.4°C).
   3. Fill the whirlpool approximately two thirds full of water; the level depends on the body part being treated.
      a. Cover the agitator intakes by at least 2 in. (5 cm) of water.
      b. Plan ahead; if someone is going to sit down in the whirlpool, this will raise the level of the water. Don't fill so high that it will overflow.
      c. Agitator pressure will raise the level of the water.
      d. Check the temperature while filling, and adjust the hot or cold water as necessary.
   4. If the whirlpool is already filled, check the temperature and adjust as necessary.
   5. Check the whirlpool electrical system (Box 12.1).
      a. It must be grounded via a ground-fault interrupter (GFI) (Box 12.2).
      b. The electrical cord must be intact; no cracked or frayed sections.
      c. The electrical cord must be off the floor.
      d. Make sure the on–off switch is insulated and out of reach of a patient in the whirlpool.
   6. Add disinfectant if necessary.
      a. Especially if treating a person with open wounds.
      b. It can be a psychological aid to patients who are anxious about catching something from patients who previously used the whirlpool. *Note:* Disinfectants react with extremely hard water to form clusters of scummy bubbles. The scum is not unsanitary, but it gives the appearance of being so. This can be eliminated by adding an antacid to the water.
   7. Check the equipment operation before allowing the patient to get into the tank (unless you have just used the equipment to treat another patient).

      a. Turn on the turbine.
         i. Make sure the water intakes are well covered.
         ii. Adjust the water pressure and air bubbles to soft flow.
         iii. Make sure the air intakes on the motor are not covered.
      b. Turn off the turbine.

C. Preparing the patient psychologically
   1. Explain the procedure to the patient, including the following:
      a. The combining effects of water and massage action
      b. The physiological effects of heat or cold
      c. The water will be warm (or cold).
      d. The water should be comfortable (unless very cold).

BOX 12.1 *THE WHIRLPOOL ELECTRICAL SYSTEM*

A whirlpool must be hard-wired into an electrical supply. Observe the following guidelines:

- The on–off switch should be on a wall remote from the whirlpool, far enough away that a patient cannot reach the switch from within the whirlpool.
- The electrical cord connecting a whirlpool to an electrical source should be hard-wired into the source rather than plugged into an outlet.
- The cord between the whirlpool and electrical source should be enclosed in electrical conduit.

These measures will minimize damage to the electrical system, which could result in an electrical fault and possibly cause a patient's death. Although these measures and a GFI may be redundant, with electricity and water, it is best to be safe.

BOX 12.2 *GFIS FOR PREVENTING ELECTROCUTION*

All therapeutic modalities involving electricity and water must be plugged into a GFI-protected outlet (see Figs. 9.3 and 9.4). As explained in Chapter 9, GFIs detect ground faults and interrupt the flow of current. Patients have been electrocuted during whirlpool treatments (usually when the whirlpool was turned on while the patient was in the water). Never give a whirlpool treatment unless the whirlpool is plugged into a GFI. (See Chapter 9 to review how GFIs work.)

e.   The massage should be comfortable.

f.   The action of the turbine is to add air to the water and to force water to move (whirl) in the tank.

2.   Check for, and warn the patient about, precautions.

D.   Preparing the patient physically

1.   Have the patient remove clothing as necessary.

   a.   A rolled-up shirt sleeve or pants leg will often get wet.

   b.   Gym shorts and T-shirt or swimming suit are best.

2.   Remove all bandages, tape, braces, etc.

3.   Position the patient in the whirlpool tank.

   a.   Make sure the seat is secure, if a seat is being used.

   b.   If the patient is sitting outside the tank, make sure the edge of the tank is padded to prevent cutting off the circulation to an arm or a leg.

   c.   The patient should be comfortable.

3 STEP 3: APPLICATION PARAMETERS

A.   Procedures

1.   Turn on the turbine before the patient gets into the water.

2.   Help the patient into the whirlpool tank, if necessary.

3.   Adjust the turbine height and re-adjust the patient (Fig. 12.2).

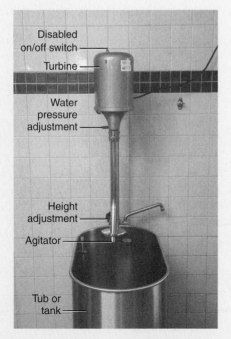

Disabled on/off switch

Turbine

Water pressure adjustment

Height adjustment

Agitator

Tub or tank

FIGURE 12.2. Components of a whirlpool agitator unit.

4.   Adjust the flow of the water (Fig. 12.2).

   a.   For maximum force, position the body part directly in line with and about 1 ft. (30 cm) from the turbine.

   b.   For minimum force, direct the turbine to the side of the tank opposite the body part to be treated.

   c.   Adjust the water pressure.

   d.   Adjust the air flow.

5.   Do not leave the patient unattended. If two or more patients are using the whirlpool simultaneously, they can watch each other for signs of lethargy.

6.   Turn off the turbine before the patient gets out of the water. The water level may fall below the intake hole when the patient gets out.

B.   Dosage. See temperature selection in step 2.

C.   Length of application

1.   Treatments usually last 10–20 min.

2.   If the patient becomes dizzy, tired, nauseated, or overheated, terminate the treatment.

D.   Frequency of application. One or two times daily.

E.   Duration of therapy. Varies, depending on phase of injury and desired effects.

4 STEP 4: POSTAPPLICATION TASKS

A.   Instructions to the patient

1.   Schedule the next treatment.

2.   Instruct the patient about the level of activity and/or self-treatment before the next formal treatment.

3.   If the patient has just finished a warm full-body whirlpool, he should rehydrate.

B.   Record of treatment, including unique patient responses

C.   Whirlpool and area cleanup

1.   Wipe water off benches and clean up the floor.

2.   Drain the tank at the end of the day, after cleaning the inside of the turbine shaft. Clean the inside of the turbine shaft by adding disinfectant to the water, lowering the shaft to its lowest position, and turning on the motor for 5 min, causing the disinfected water to flow through the inside of the shaft.

3.   Clean and disinfect the whirlpool daily or after five to eight treatments, if used infrequently.

5 STEP 5: MAINTENANCE

A.   Keep the equipment clean and polished. Do not use an abrasive cleaner on the whirlpool tank; it will scratch the stainless steel, causing tiny grooves in which staphylococci (bacteria) can grow.

B.   Check the electrical cord for fraying.

Application of Hot Packs

5 STEPS

STEP 1: FOUNDATION

A. Definition. A **hot pack** is a form of moist superficial heat applied with one of the following (Fig. 12.3):
   1. *Hot water bottle:* Used for centuries, but it does not stay warm long (<5 min).
   2. *Kenny pack:* A wool pack that is steam heated and spun dry. It has intense initial heat but cools quickly (5 min).
   3. *Hot towel:* A towel dipped in hot water and wrung out. Stays warm 5–10 min. Effectiveness time has been increased by adding a heat source such as an electric pad (plastic coated) or heat lamp. *Caution:* This is not recommended; it burns too easily.
   4. **Hydrocolator pack:** A canvas pack that encases silica gel.
      a. The gel absorbs great amounts of water and thus retains heat for long periods of time (Fig. 12.4).
      b. Can hold heat up to 30 min if heated to 140–160°F (60–70°C).
      c. Towel wrapping provides a temperature of about 115°F (45°C) to the skin.
      d. As the pack cools, layers of towel are removed. Thus the temperature presented to the skin remains at about 115°F (45°C).

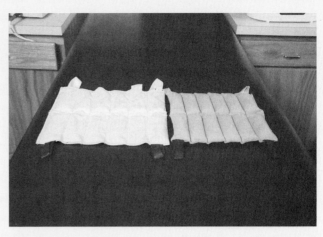

FIGURE 12.4. Hot packs before hydration *(left)* and after hydration *(right)*. Notice the difference in volume, indicating the amount of water absorbed by the silica.

B. Effects. Those of conductive heating:
   1. Superficial increase (100%) in circulation
   2. Increased metabolism
   3. Muscle relaxation through analgesia.
C. Advantages
   1. Ease of application.
   2. Local heat without heating the whole body.
   3. Can provide multiple treatments.
   4. Relatively inexpensive.
   5. Can treat over an open wound without fear of spreading germs to others.
   6. Durability.
   7. Portable; the patient can move around.
   8. Heats surface and intramuscular tissues more than paraffin[1]
D. Disadvantages
   1. Weight of the pack may be uncomfortable in some situations
   2. Time-consuming; packs must be reheated between uses.
   3. Packs are difficult to contour to some body parts.
   4. Effects are only superficial: a temperature increase of 6.5°F (3.6°C) at 1 cm deep; a tissue temperature increase of 1.4°F (.8°C) at 3 cm deep[2]
   5. Difficult to perform range-of-motion exercises with the pack on the body
   6. The effects of heat are short lived; the tissue cools quickly.[1,3–5]
E. Indications
   1. Any place local heat is desired
   2. As a supplement to other treatment
F. Contraindications. General heat contraindications

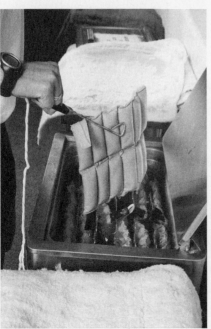

FIGURE 12.3. A hot pack being removed from its heating unit.

G. Precautions
    1. Never place a bare (unwrapped) pack on a patient.
    2. Do not prepare a hot pack on a patient; the initial single layer of towel is not enough insulation, and you might burn the patient.
    3. Do not let a patient sit or lie on a hot pack; the heat will not be able to dissipate into the atmosphere, and the pack will become too hot. The patient might get burned.
    4. Keep checking on the patient to make sure the pack does not get too hot (packs are initially cool until the heat penetrates through).
    5. Keep removing layers of toweling as the hot pack cools.
    6. Hot packs should be comfortably warm but not hot; may burn if blood does not carry heat away
    7. It usually takes several minutes for a person to feel the warmth.
    8. Report immediately if the hot packs become too hot.

STEP 2: PREAPPLICATION TASKS

A. Make sure hot packs are the proper modality for this situation.
    1. Reevaluate the injury or problem. Make sure you understand the patient's condition.
    2. If a hot pack was applied previously, review the patient's response to that treatment.
    3. Confirm that the objectives of therapy are compatible with hot packs.
    4. Make sure hot packs are not contraindicated in this situation.
B. Preparing the patient psychologically
    1. Explain the procedure to the patient, including the following:
        a. Heat will increase blood flow and relax the muscles.
        b. It should be comfortable.
        c. Relax and enjoy it.
    2. Check for, and warn the patient about, precautions.
C. Preparing the patient physically
    1. Clothing need not be removed but it will get damp if the hot pack is placed over it. Let the patient decide.
    2. Position the patient in a comfortable position, one that she can remain in for 15–20 min. Lying down is usually best.
D. Preparing the equipment
    1. Make sure the heating unit is set at the proper temperature, 140–160°F (60–70°C). The warmer it is, the more it can heat the skin but the more toweling you must have initially so the *interface temperature* (temperature presented to the skin) is ~115°F (45°C).
    2. Have adequate toweling available (terry cloth towels and/or terry cloth hydrocolator pack covers) (Fig. 12.5).
        a. Hot pack covers are more convenient than towels because you do not have to spend time preparing them. But layers cannot be removed as the hot pack cools, so the treatment cannot last as long.
        b. Individual towels give greater control because you can remove layers of toweling as the hot pack cools, thus maintaining the interface temperature at 115°F (45°C) longer.
    3. Several hours before treatment:
        a. Presoak new packs for 12–24 hr to absorb a sufficient amount of water.
        b. Water should cover the packs at all times. (Add water only when there is time for it to heat up; end of day or first thing in the morning is a convenient time.)
        c. Preheat the packs for 2–3 hr if the water is cold, 30 min if the water is hot.[5]
    4. Immediately before treatment:
        a. Decide whether to use a towel or hot pack cover.
        b. Place a towel or hot pack cover on the table, not on the patient.

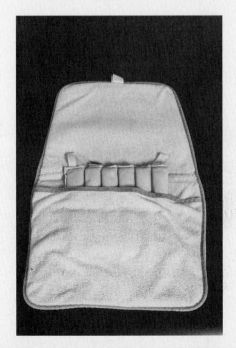

FIGURE 12.5. Hot pack covers contain four layers of terry cloth. They are folded over a hot pack and secured with Velcro straps.

c. Remove the pack from the heating unit.
   i. Do not reach into the water; use tongs or a hook to lift the pack out of the water.
   ii. Allow the excess water to drip into the tank.
   iii. Close the lid of the heating unit so that other packs will stay hot.
d. Prepare the pack on the table, not on the patient.
   i. Place the hot pack in the middle of the cover, fold the other side over and attach the Velcro fasteners.
   ii. Alternatively, place the hot pack in the middle and at the end of the towel (Fig. 12.6a).
   iii. Fold the sides of towel lengthwise over the pack (Fig. 12.6b).
   iv. Fold the towel end over end over the hot pack to form a bundle (Fig. 12.6c).

STEP 3: APPLICATION PARAMETERS

A. Procedures
   1. Place the folded pack on the patient. *Caution:* Never let a patient lie or sit on a hot pack; the heat cannot dissipate and can cause burning.

2. Place another towel over the pack to keep the heat from dissipating into the air.
3. Check the patient every 4–5 min.
   a. Add an extra towel between the pack and the patient if the pack is too hot.
   b. Remove a layer of toweling if the pack is too cool or change the hot pack if using a hot pack cover.
B. Dosage. Within the comfort limits of the patient.
C. Length of application. 20–25 min.
D. Frequency of application. Application can be repeated two or three times per day if separated by 3–4 hr.
E. Duration of therapy. Varies, depending on phase of injury and desired effects.

STEP 4: POSTAPPLICATION TASKS

A. Instructions to the patient
   1. Schedule the next treatment.
   2. Instruct the patient about the level of activity and/or self-treatment before the next formal treatment.
B. Record of treatment, including unique patient responses
C. Equipment replacement and cleanup

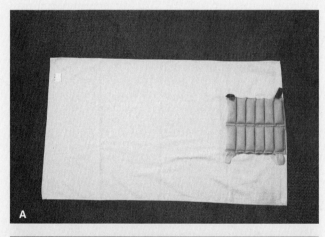
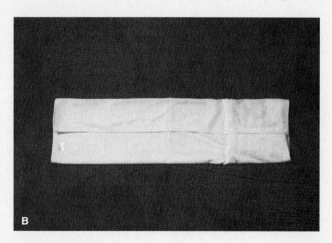
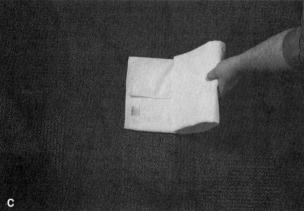

FIGURE 12.6. Preparing a hot pack for application. **(a)** Place the pack at the end of the towel. **(b)** Fold the sides of the towel lengthwise over the pack or **(c)** fold the towel end over end around the hot pack to make a bundle.

BOX 12.3 *A HOT PACK ROTATION SYSTEM*

A system for rotating the use of hot packs is essential for ensuring that each treatment involves the pack that has warmed or rewarmed the longest. This is especially important in busy clinics. Without such a system, a single hot pack might be used over and over again without adequately rewarming between treatments, while packs that are at maximum temperature remain unused.

An effective system is the use of colored tabs on one side of the hot packs (use a laundry pen to color the tabs). The following instructions apply to a four-pack heating unit, but the same system can be used for eight-pack units:

- Remember two principles:
  - Orientation is front to back of the heating unit.
  - Look for the first color change.
- Start the day with all four hot packs placed in the heating unit so the same color tabs are sticking up.
- For a treatment, select the first hot pack after a color change. For example, for the first treatment of the day, all tabs will be the same color and so you take the first one. But later in the day, if the first two packs are black and the third and fourth are white, you would select the third one. If you have two black-tabbed packs, a blank slot (one is in use), and a white-tabbed pack in slot four, you would choose the white-tabbed pack (Fig. 12.7).
- After a treatment, return the pack to the first open slot so that the tabs on top are the same color as the packs before it (toward the front) and opposite of the packs after it (toward the back) (Fig. 12.8).

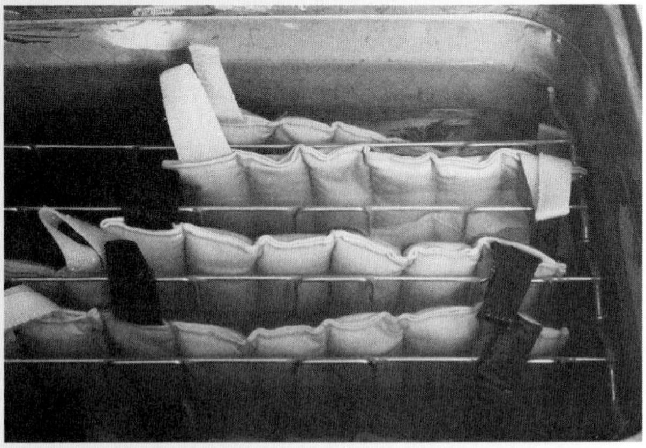

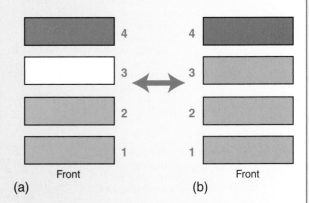

FIGURE 12.7. Hot packs in a heating unit. Note the difference in colors of the first two and last two tabs.

FIGURE 12.8. A used hot pack is returned to the heating unit with the same tab orientation as the packs in front of it. *Note:* A four-pack heating unit is shown here, but the same principles apply for an eight-pack unit.

---

1. Return the hot pack to the heating unit immediately after the treatment. Delaying its return will prolong reheating. Return packs to the heating unit according to a specific rotation system (Box 12.3).
2. Return the towels (or covers) to the drying rack. Exceptions:
   a. If treating a patient with an infectious disease, launder the towel before using it on another person.
   b. If it is the end of the day, all towels must be laundered.

STEP 5: MAINTENANCE

A. Regular equipment cleaning. Clean the heating unit at least once a month.

1. Remove the packs and rack.
2. Drain the water.
3. Clean the tank with a mild disinfectant and soap; do not use abrasives.
4. Replace the rack, packs, and water.

B. Routine maintenance
1. Keep the water level in the heating unit above the top of the packs. Always add water at the end of the day so it has time to heat. Adding water during the day may reduce the temperature of the bath and hot packs.
2. Do not allow the packs to dry out. Always return them to the heating unit.
3. Check the thermostat yearly for proper operation by inserting an external thermometer in the heated water.

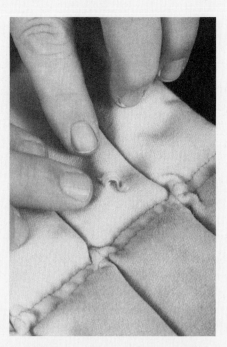

FIGURE 12.9. Hot packs can lose gel, from tears in the canvas pack.

C. Simple repairs. Watch the packs for loss of gel, usually as a result of wear to, or ripping of, the canvas pack cover (Fig. 12.9).
  1. When this occurs, slit the individual damaged cell, remove the gel by squeezing, wash the inside of the cell with water, and rewarm the pack for continued use.
  2. Hot packs can be used with up to three or four missing cells.

Application of Paraffin Bath

5 STEPS

STEP 1: FOUNDATION

A. Definition. A **paraffin bath** is a form of moist superficial heat applied by forming a paraffin glove around the affected body part (Fig. 12.10).
B. Effects. Those of conductive heating:
  1. Superficial increase in circulation.
  2. Increased metabolism
  3. Muscle relaxation through analgesia.
C. Advantages
  1. Ease of application.
  2. Local heat without heating the whole body.
  3. Softens the skin; water tends to dry it.

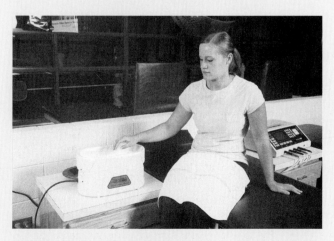

FIGURE 12.10. A paraffin bath treatment.

  4. Uniform heating; all surfaces of the treated part are heated at one time.
  5. Relatively inexpensive.
D. Disadvantages
  1. Hand heating is less than with a hot pack, even in the web spaces between fingers[1]
  2. Can treat only hands and feet
  3. Messy and has a somewhat unpleasant odor
  4. Tends to accumulate dirt and debris from the skin
  5. Cannot observe the treated area during treatment
  6. Effects are not long lasting
  7. Cannot perform range-of-motion exercises during treatment
E. Indications
  1. Local heat to the feet and hands
  2. As a supplement to other treatment
F. Contraindications
  1. General heat contraindications
  2. Cannot apply over infections, rashes, open lesions, burns, or new scars
G. Precautions
  1. Check the temperature of the paraffin before applying.
  2. The skin must be dry; water droplets may result in burns.

3. Small scratches must be covered.
4. Avoid the seepage of hot paraffin beneath the initial application. This can occur in the following situations:
   a. If you go above the first immersion line on subsequent immersions.
   b. If cracks develop in the glove, usually caused by moving the body part.

2 STEP 2: **PREAPPLICATION TASKS**

A. Make sure a paraffin bath is the proper modality for this situation.
   1. Reevaluate the injury or problem. Make sure you understand the patient's condition.
   2. If a paraffin bath was used previously, review the patient response to that treatment.
   3. Confirm that the objectives of therapy are compatible with paraffin.
   4. Make sure a paraffin bath is not contraindicated in this situation.
B. Preparing the patient psychologically
   1. Explain the procedure to the patient, including the following:
      a. The paraffin will feel hot, but it will not burn.
      b. It should be comfortable
   2. Check for, and warn the patient about, precautions.
C. Preparing the patient physically
   1. Remove all clothing, jewelry, bandages, etc. from the area to be treated. (If a ring cannot be removed, cover it with several layers of gauze and then tape it.)
   2. Make sure the skin is clean and dry.
   3. Cover any small scratches.
   4. Place a towel over any clothing that may get soiled from treatment.
D. Preparing the equipment
   1. Several hours before treatment
      a. Prepare the paraffin by either of these two methods:
         i. Mix seven parts wax with one part mineral oil. The mineral oil lowers the melting point of the wax to about 126°F (52°C). Paraffin above 130°F (55.4°C) will burn.
         ii. Purchase premixed paraffin. It comes in blocks (about the size of a gallon of milk) or chips (about the size of potato chips). Place in the heated container and the solid wax will slowly melt.
      b. Use a candy thermometer to check the temperature after all the wax is melted (Fig. 12.11).

   c. Adjust the temperature if it is too hot (add mineral oil) or too cool (add wax). A light scum will form if the temperature is right.
   2. Immediately before treatment, check the temperature.

3 STEP 3: **APPLICATION PARAMETERS**

A. Procedures
   1. Dip the body part into the paraffin bath and quickly pull it out.
   2. Allow the paraffin to cool until it solidifies (it will turn milky white in color within 10 sec) (Fig. 12.12).
   3. Repeat steps 1 and 2 until there are 7–12 layers of paraffin.
   4. Cover the area with cellophane wrap or a plastic bag and then with a towel.
B. Dosage. Between 7 and 12 layers of paraffin.
C. Length of application. From 20 to 25 min.
D. Frequency of application. Application can be repeated two or three times per day if separated by 3–4 hr.
E. Duration of therapy. Varies, depending on phase of injury and desired effects.

4 STEP 4: **POSTAPPLICATION TASKS**

A. Instructions to the patient
   1. Schedule the next treatment.
   2. Instruct the patient about the level of activity and/or self-treatment before the next formal treatment.

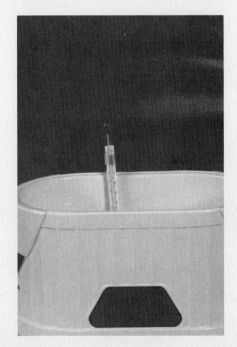

FIGURE 12.11. Use a candy thermometer to check the temperature of a paraffin bath. Note the light scum on top of the paraffin.

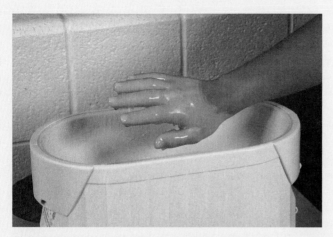

FIGURE 12.12. Paraffin cooling on the hand of a patient.

B. Record of treatment, including unique patient responses
C. Equipment removal; patient cleanup. Peel the paraffin from the body part, and discard it or put it into the bath. Some consider the used paraffin soiled and unsuitable for further use.

STEP 5: MAINTENANCE

A. Check the paraffin bath periodically for scum or foreign material. Remove any foreign material.
B. Replace the paraffin as it is used.

Application of Infrared Lamp

STEP 1: FOUNDATION

A. Definition. Heat from an **infrared (IR) lamp** is a form of superficial heat that radiates from a heat lamp or an IR lamp. Two types, called *near IR* and *far IR,* have been used therapeutically.
B. Effects. Those of conductive heating:
   1. Superficial increase in circulation
   2. Increased metabolism
   3. Muscle relaxation through analgesia
C. Advantages
   1. Ease of application
   2. Local heat without heating the whole body
   3. Very inexpensive. An IR bulb can be purchased in any department store

D. Disadvantages
   1. Burning. It is very easy to burn someone with an IR lamp.
   2. Not as effective as hot packs and paraffin baths
   3. Not portable
E. Indications. None; it is too easy to burn.
F. Contraindications. The danger of easily burning patients and the availability of better forms of superficial heat contraindicate the use of this modality.
G. Precautions
   1. We recommend against using an infrared lamp.
   2. If you choose to use an IR lamp, make sure you have a full understanding of the inverse square law and the cosine law (see Chapter 11).

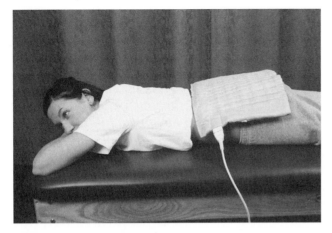

FIGURE 12.13. An electrical heating pad.

CRITICAL THINKING 12.1 *A gymnast is experiencing some general soreness in her shoulder and desires some heat application before practice. Which would be the most appropriate modality and why?*

CRITICAL THINKING 12.2 *A concert pianist is experiencing some general soreness in his right hand and desires a heat application before tonight's concert. Which would be the most appropriate modality and why?*

Other Superficial Heating Devices

There are many other types of devices for applying superficial heat. The most prominent of these for orthopedic and sports medicine use are electrical heating pads, portable heat pads, and analgesic balms.

ELECTRICAL HEATING PADS

Electrical heating pads are an economical (~$30), alternative to a moist hot pack (Fig. 12.13). Once heated, it heats tissue about the same as a moist hot pack,[6] but does not need a hot water bath to prepare it for application, and you don't have to worry about rewarming between applications. It also is an excellent device to send home with a patient who needs additional treatments.

It is commonly believed that moist heating devices heat better than dry heating devices. This was not the case in our single research study.[6] Further investigation will clarify this point.

Caution is advised when using electrical heating pads. Many cases of death and burning have been reported to the U.S. Product Safety Commission and the U.S. Food and Drug Administration.[7] Most problems appear to occur as a result of one of the following:

- Cracked or frayed electrical cords
- Cracked or worn pads
- Use in infants or the elderly
- Left on while the patient is sleeping

PORTABLE HEATING PRODUCTS

Portable heating devices (e.g., ThermaCare) use chemical reactions to produce long-lasting, low-level heating.[8] ThermaCare heat wraps are disks composed of iron, charcoal, and salt in a paper wrap (Fig. 12.14). When the wrap is exposed to oxygen in the air, an *exothermic reaction* occurs, which produces a low level of heat (104°F, or 40°C) on the skin that lasts for 8 hr (Fig. 12.15).[9]

FIGURE 12.14. The results of a 2-hr treatment with a topical analgesic patch that claims to heat muscle and a portable heat wrap. (Adapted with permission from Trowbridge et al.[9])

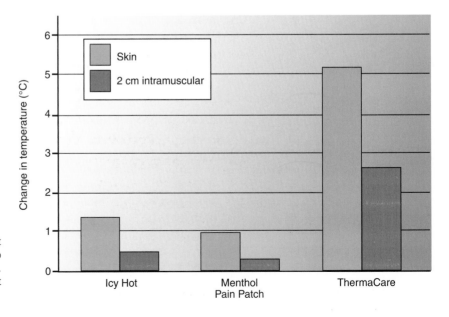

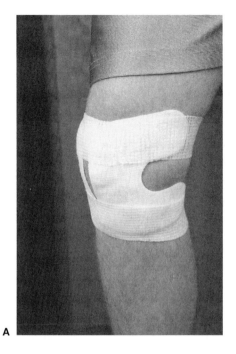

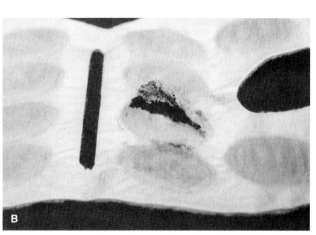

FIGURE 12.15. **(a)** A ThermaCare portable heat wrap applied to the knee. **(b)** It is composed of disks of iron, charcoal, and salt woven into a paper wrap.

TOPICAL ANALGESICS

Several over-the-counter topical analgesics (e.g., Ben-Gay, Icy Hot) claim to provide heat to muscles. These products contain menthol or hot pepper plant extracts (capsaicin), substances that cause a sensation of warmth on the skin and a slight increased blood flow to the skin. These products, however, do not substantially increase skin or muscle temperature (see Fig. 12.14). Intramuscular temperature at 2 cm deep and skin temperature and were $<1°F$ ($<0.5°C$) and $<2.7°F$ ($<1.5°C$), respectively.[9]

CLOSING SCENE

In response to your grandfather's questions in the chapter opening scene, you explain that the ingredients in the topical ointment he uses do not actually heat or cool muscles, they just provide a hot or cool sensation. This irritation, in a sense, stimulates nerves that help override the pain signals. You tell him about thermal agents that actually produce heat, such as whirlpool, hot packs, and portable heat wraps. By analyzing the advantages and disadvantages of each modality, you can provide some sources of heat that are appropriate for his arthritic knees.

CHAPTER REFLECTIONS

1. Read and ponder each of the following points. Do you feel you have a clear understanding of each concept? If not, reread the appropriate section of the chapter.
   - Discuss whirlpool application, including foundational information, preapplication tasks, application procedures, postapplication tasks, and maintenance.
   - Discuss hot pack application, including foundational information, preapplication tasks, application procedures, postapplication tasks, and maintenance.
   - Discuss paraffin bath application, including foundational information, preapplication tasks, application procedures, postapplication tasks, and maintenance.
   - Why are infrared lamps contraindicated as a heating modality?
   - Discuss portable heating devices and how they compare with other superficial heating devices.

- Discuss why it is incorrect to classify topical analgesics as heating devices.

2. Write three to five questions for discussion with your class instructor, clinical instructor, classmates, and clinical colleagues.

3. Get together with classmates and quiz each other on the concepts of this chapter. Use the points in exercise 1 and questions you wrote for exercise 2 as a beginning. Explaining concepts out loud to others requires a deeper grasp of the material than feeling you understand it as you read.

4. Once you feel you understand the principles of application of whirlpools, hot packs, and paraffin baths, practice applying them using the five-step approach with a classmate or clinical colleague. Alternate applying the modalities to each other. When it is being applied to you, listen and observe carefully to determine whether your classmate is using proper application. Consult your notes when the modality is applied to you and for the first few times you apply the modality to another person. Continue practicing the application until you can do so without using your notes.

CRITICAL THINKING RESPONSES

Critical Thinking 12.1

Probably the best form of heat for the shoulder is a hot pack. Paraffin would be very messy to apply to this area, and the patient would need to immerse her whole body in a whirlpool to target the shoulder.

Critical Thinking 12.2

Many would answer a paraffin glove because it can treat the peaks (knuckles) and valleys (palm and between knuckles) of the hand. Others would answer a small whirlpool because it can treat the peaks and valleys of the hand. However, a hot pack is the best answer. It warms the hand, including the peaks and valleys, more than a paraffin glove and is easier to use.

REFERENCES

1. Wilson J, Knight KL. Hot packs heat hands more effectively than paraffin baths. Undergraduate research paper, Brigham Young University, 2006.
2. Draper DO, Harris ST, Schulthies SS, et al. Hotpack and 1 MHz ultrasound treatments have an additive effect on muscle temperature increase. J Athl Train 1998;33:21–24.
3. Morris AK. Moist heat pack re-warming following 10, 20, 30 min application Masters thesis, Brigham Young University, 2003.
4. Smith K. The effect of silicate gel hot packs on human muscle temperature. Masters thesis, Brigham Young University, 1994 .
5. Kaiser DA, Knight KL, Huff JM, et al. Hot-pack warming in 4- and 8-pack hydrocollator units. J Sports Rehabil 2004;13:103–113.
6. Wood C. Dry and moist heat application and the subsequent rise in tissue temperatures. Undergraduate research paper, Brigham Young University, 2004.
7. U.S. Consumer Product Safety Commission. Safety advisory—Hazards association with the use of electric heating pads [SA:020]. Rockville, MD: Federal Drug Administration, June 15, 1996.
8. Draper DO, Trowbridge CA. Continuous low-level heat therapy: What works, what doesn't. Athl Ther Today 2003;8:46–48.
9. Trowbridge C, Draper DO, Feland JB, Eggett D. Paraspinal musculature and skin temperature changes: Comparing the ThermaCare Heat Wrap, the Johnson & Johnson Back Plaster, and the ABC Warme-Pflaster. J Orthop Sports Phys Ther 2004;34: 549–558.

CHAPTER OUTLINE

OPENING SCENE

You have traveled with your supervising athletic trainer (AT) to a basketball game. During the game, your shooting guard sprains his ankle. After a through evaluation, the AT diagnoses it as a moderate ankle sprain. You then apply an ice pack and elastic wrap to the area. The AT tells you to stay with the athlete while he goes back to check on the game. After 15 min, an AT student from the host team comes into the room and asks if you need any help. He then asks how long you are going to ice the ankle. You say 30–45 min. The student's eyes get wide and he says, "You're kidding. Don't you know about the hunting response?" When you shake your head no, he continues, "After about 15 minutes of ice application, the blood vessels will dilate, so you don't want to ice the area for any longer than 15 minutes to avoid vasodilation." You ask yourself as you scratch your head, "Is he right?"

Cryotherapy: Not Just Immediate Care

The common misconception that you treat injuries with cold for the first 24–72 hr and then treat them with heat is not true. For many injuries, cryotherapy extends beyond immediate care. Rehabilitation progresses more quickly because therapeutic exercises can be used earlier and are more effective when they are alternated with cold application. In addition, spasticity is reduced, surgical complications are minimized, and organs are preserved for transplantation. However, cold is used differently during rehabilitative cryotherapy than during immediate care RICES (rest, ice, compression, elevation, stabilization) treatments.

MODALITY MYTH

CRYOTHERAPY

There are numerous myths about the use of cryotherapy, some of which were presented in Chapter 5. Additional myths are exposed in this chapter, including the following:

- The major reason for cryotherapy is to decrease blood flow.
- Acute injuries are treated with cold for the first 24–72 hr and then with heat.
- Cold should always be applied for _____. [fill in the blank]
- The application of cryotherapy is essentially the same regardless of why it is being applied.
- Cold increases circulation, if applied for longer than 15–20 min, through the process of cold-induced vasodilation, or the hunting reaction.

- Research proves that cold-induced vasodilation occurs during athletic injury rehabilitation.
- Contrast bath therapy reduces swelling through a milking action caused by alternating vasodilation (from the heat) and vasoconstriction (from the cold).
- Heat applications decrease pain and allow active exercise during the early acute stages of orthopedic injury.

CRYOTHERAPY CONFUSION

The versatility of cryotherapy has caused great confusion among those who use it with an inadequate understanding of its scientific and theoretical basis. Confusion has resulted in various definitions and in numerous opinions about why certain cryotherapeutic techniques should be used, their proper application, and the response of body tissues when they are used. See Box 13.1 for one example.

The debate over how long ice should be applied illustrates how confusion has led to the improper use of cryotherapy. Some clinicians claim cryotherapy should be applied for only 20 min, while others claim treatments of <30 min are ineffective. Both are correct, depending on when and why the cold is applied. Cold is used during immediate care to limit secondary injury (see Chapter 5); therefore, applications of 30 min or longer are needed to lower metabolism in the underlying tissues. However, the goal in intermediate care is to decrease pain to facilitate active exercise, and localized numbing can be achieved in 12–20 min.

 CRITICAL THINKING 13.1 *How is using cold to reduce swelling an example of cryotherapy confusion?*

BOX 13.1 *HEAT OR COLD? PATIENT EXPECTATIONS*

"Quack, quack, quack," is a phrase I (KK) have heard at two stages in my career. In both cases, it was uttered by patients under my care as a commentary on my incompetence in treating their athletic injuries. The comment was first expressed in the early 1970s when I began using cryokinetics to rehabilitate joint sprains. Many Weber State athletes were convinced I was incompetent. "Everyone knows you use heat after the first 24–72 hours to treat injuries," they would say. I hasten to add, however, that none of my cryokinetics patients was among the detractors.

In the early 1980s, after the cryotherapy revolution, I was again accused of being incompetent when I applied a hot pack to an Indiana State patient with an extremely sore ankle. "Don't you know you treat injuries with cold?" I was asked. It had come full circle.

My philosophy had not changed in the intervening years, but my philosophy has been more comprehensive than that of the athletes I treat. Thus my actions sometimes don't meet my patients' expectations. The use of therapeutic heat or cold depends on the situation.

As in all modalities, it is essential that any cryotherapy begin with a clear understanding of the goal of the therapy and of the differing physiological responses of the body to cold applications. To obtain the maximum benefit from any therapeutic modality, you must understand the specific needs of the patient and the physiological response to specific modalities. You must also understand that cryotherapy involves more than cold applications and that both the cold and the noncold portions of the therapy differ, depending on the therapeutic goals. There are numerous local physiological responses to cold applications, including decreased temperature, metabolism, inflammation, circulation, pain, and spasm and increased tissue stiffness. Some of these responses are beneficial, others are detrimental, depending on the phase of injury management.

Cryotherapeutic modalities are used for a wide range of objectives, and referring to an individual specific technique as cryotherapy leads to confusion and ambiguity. To avoid the confusion, refer to individual techniques by their names. Think of the term *cryotherapy* only in a broad sense, as an umbrella covering a group of specific techniques.

EXAMPLES OF CRYOTHERAPY

Cryotherapy literally means "cold therapy," and therefore any use of ice or cold application for therapeutic purposes can be considered cryotherapy. Stated another way, cryotherapy is the therapeutic application of any device or substance to the body that results in the withdrawal of heat, thereby lowering tissue temperature. Thus each of the following techniques is a type of cryotherapy:

- Ice or cold pack application for the immediate care of acute injuries
- Running cold water over a burn
- Cryokinetics (alternating cold applications with active exercise)
- Cryostretch (alternating cold applications with muscle stretching)
- Cold water baths (cold whirlpool or immersion in a slush bucket)
- Ice massage
- Treating trigger points with ice massage
- Ice or cold pack application after orthopedic surgery
- Lowering whole-body temperature to induce hypothermia before organ transplant surgery
- Cryosurgery (applying $-76°F$ [$-60°C$] probes or spraying liquid nitrogen on tissue to freeze and destroy it)

CRYOTHERAPEUTIC TECHNIQUES

Cryotherapeutic techniques can be grouped into five major categories, based on the objectives for using them:

- *Immediate care:* cooling acutely injured musculoskeletal tissue immediately after the injury as part of first aid (see Chapters 4 and 5)
- *Post–immediate care:* cooling tissue during rehabilitation of various musculoskeletal pathologies as an adjunct to other therapy, usually exercise
- *Surgical adjunct:* cooling tissue before, during, or after surgical procedures
- *Cryosurgery:* freezing tissue for surgical purposes
- *Miscellaneous:* techniques that don't fit into one of the other four categories

Immediate Care Cryotherapy

The objective during immediate care procedures is twofold: removing the cause of the injury and minimizing the adverse sequelae. A **sequela** is an effect that follows, or results from, an injury, disease, or treatment. Except in the case of a burn, cold applications have no effect in removing the cause of the injury, but they have a great effect on minimizing secondary injury and thereby deceasing total injury (see Chapter 5).[1]

Post-Immediate Care Cryotherapy

The main benefit of cold application during post–immediate care is that it decreases pain and/or muscle spasm and thereby allows earlier mobilization. The sooner therapeutic exercise begins, the better the patient is for three reasons:

- The proper use of exercise speeds the healing process.[2–4]
- The lack of exercise during the early stages of rehabilitation may result in permanent disability.[5,6]
- Function is restored sooner, which is beneficial physically and psychologically.

Caution must be observed though; too vigorous exercise can also result in permanent disability. The optimum conditions for healing depend on the very fine balance between returning to full normal function at the earliest possible time and protecting the injury from overstress and reinjury[6] (see Fig. 1.5).

The major cryotherapeutic techniques used during post–immediate care are

- Cryokinetics
- Cryostretch
- Connective tissue stretch
- Cold compression devices
- Contrast baths

These will be explained in greater detail later in this chapter. Detailed application procedures are in Chapter 14.

Surgical Adjunct Cryotherapy

Cryotherapy is often used before, during, and after surgical procedures. The objective is the same as during immediate care of acute injuries: lowering metabolism to minimize secondary injury.

Cryosurgery

Cryosurgery is a surgical technique that uses ultra-low-temperature probes (−4 to −94°F [−20 to −70°C]) to freeze tissue and thereby destroy it.[7,8] Its use is beyond the scope of this book.

Miscellaneous Techniques

Techniques for decreasing menstrual cramps and pain, reducing cold sores, and easing painful injections are examples of miscellaneous cryotherapeutic techniques. Descriptions are outside the scope of this book; they can be found elsewhere.[1]

The Physiological Effects of Cold Application

The physiological responses to cold can be summarized or grouped into nine categories:[1]

- Decreased temperature
- Tissue destruction
- Increased or decreased inflammation
- Decreased metabolism
- Decreased or increased pain
- Decreased muscle spasm
- Increased tissue stiffness
- Decreased arthrogenic muscle inhibition
- Decreased circulation

DECREASED TEMPERATURE

Immediately upon the application of cold, heat begins moving from the tissue into the cold modality, resulting in decreased tissue temperature. In severe cooling (−4 to −94°F [−20°C to −70°C]), tissue is destroyed, as in cryosurgery. For treating orthopedic injuries, the tissue is usually cooled to a surface temperature of 33–50°F (1–10°C). This degree of cooling causes the tissue responses listed earlier, except for tissue destruction.

Temperature changes are neither immediate nor uniform throughout the tissue. Heat moves by conduction (see Chapter 11), which means that heat moves from the surface into the cold modality first. As the surface temperature decreases, heat is withdrawn from subcutaneous tissues, which then withdraw heat from intermediate tissues, and so on until heat is being withdrawn from the very deep tissues (if the cold modality remains on long enough and doesn't warm up too quickly).

After a few minutes, a thermal gradient develops in the tissue (see Fig. 11.1) . This gradient remains after the cold modality is removed. In fact, because of the gradient and heat conduction, deeper tissue temperature continues to decrease after the modality is removed or the body is removed from the modality, as is the case with ice water immersion.

Thermal gradients can also develop in the modality. The clinician should shake a cold pack and swirl the water in an ice immersion bucket every 5 min or so to break up the gradient. Patients will notice the difference.

 CRITICAL THINKING 13.2 *Why might a patient complain of increased pain when he moves his foot during an ice water bath treatment?*

TISSUE DESTRUCTION

Tissue destruction occurs at extreme temperatures (−4 to −94°F [−20 to −70°C]), such as with liquid nitrogen. This cold application is used to remove unwanted tissue, such as warts.

INCREASED OR DECREASED INFLAMMATION

It is commonly thought that one of the benefits of cryotherapy in treating acute injury is to decrease inflammation. This is probably not true for two reasons: (1) inflammation is necessary for resolution of the injury (see Chapter 5) and (2) there has been very little research on the acute inflammatory response.

Cryotherapy research involving inflammation has concentrated on arthritis, the healing of surgical wounds, and inflammation induced by injecting various substances under the skin. In these situations, inflammation has been decreased[9–11] or delayed—that is, it is reduced during cryotherapy but then runs its full course after rewarming.[12–15] But these situations are quite different from the inflammatory response during acute trauma.

DECREASED METABOLISM

There is a direct relationship between tissue temperature and metabolism (see Fig. 5.3). The more the cooling, the greater the decrease in metabolism.[1]

DECREASED OR INCREASED PAIN

Cold is the most effective and underused modality for pain.[16] Although there is clear experimental evidence that cold decreases pain,[17] many clinicians do not appreciate its value, especially during acute injury care. By numbing a muscle or joint, active exercise can be used earlier in the rehabilitation process.[18–21]

Understanding the relationship between cryotherapy and pain begins with the recognition that pain from three origins is involved:

- *Cold pain:* Caused by the cold application, usually ice water immersion. Patients quickly habituate to it, so it is a problem only during the first few treatment sessions. Cold pain is a nuisance; it serves no useful purpose.
- *Residual pain:* Caused by the injury (damaged tissue and pressure on nerve endings by swelling and by inflammatory chemicals, such as bradykinins and prostaglandins). Residual pain precludes exercising and can be neutralized by cold-induced numbness.
- *Reinjury pain:* Caused by stressing the tissues to the point of reinjuring them. Reinjury pain will not be affected by numbness. This is your safety valve. Respect it and respond to it. Reduce the intensity of the patient's activity when she feels reinjury pain.

Cold pain rarely occurs during immersion in water lower than 59°F (15°C) and rarely during other cold applications, such as ice massage and ice packs. Immersion in water near 32°F (0°C) is very painful during its first use.[1] Patients quickly habituate to cold pain, however, so it is a manageable problem. Efforts to minimize cold pain during ice immersion have led to the following application adjustments:

- The development of a neoprene toe cap.[22] The toe cap eliminates pain in the toes and forefoot, which accounts for >50% of the pain during ice immersion.[23] We recommend them.
- Refraining from using cryokinetics. This is unfortunate because cryokinetics is a powerful tool, and cold pain is temporary. Its intensity decreases dramatically after the first immersion and continues to decrease after subsequent immersions.
- The use of warmer water. Although warmer water is less painful, it is not as effective in numbing the injured limb,[24] and so the effectiveness of the treatment is decreased.

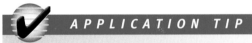

APPLICATION TIP

ICE WATER IMMERSION SHOULD BE IN 32–33°F (0–1°C) WATER. Pain is most effectively reduced with immersion in 32–33°F (0–1°C) ice water. Always have your patient wear a toe cap to moderate the cold-induced pain.

DECREASED MUSCLE SPASM

Muscle spasm is not muscle cramping. A **muscle cramp**, commonly called a *charley horse,* is a sudden, intense, painful, tetanic muscle contraction. It is short-lived, usually lasting less than 20 sec. In contrast, a **muscle spasm** is a tightness; it is of gradual onset and usually not particularly painful. Muscle spasm results from an increase in the baseline tone (neurological activity) of the muscle.

Muscle spasm is decreased by cold applications, although the specific mechanism is unknown.[1] Three mechanisms have been suggested, each of which probably plays a role:

- Decreased nerve conduction[1,25–27]
- Breaking the pain–spasm–pain cycle.[28–31] This mechanism is undoubtedly effective and part of the explana-

tion: Remove the cause of the spasm, and the spasm disappears.
- A reflex mechanism. This hypothesis is based on the following:
  - Cooling a skin flap (cut in a U and lifted from the body) without cooling the underlying muscle causes a decrease in tonic stretch reflexes in the muscle.[32]
  - Reflex responses decrease quickly after cold application.[33,34]
  - Sympathetic nervous system stimulation causes a significant decrease in *muscle spindle* afferent discharge during stretching.[35]

Whatever the mechanism, cold is effective in diminishing the muscle spasm that accompanies most acute strains and sprains. Its effectiveness is increased when combined with stretching, as is the case with the cryostretch technique.

INCREASED TISSUE STIFFNESS

Cooling tissues causes them to become more stiff (less elastic) and more resistant to movement, owing to a combination[36] of increased viscosity of joint synovial fluid,[37–40] decreased muscle power,[40,41] and decreased connective tissue elasticity.[41–43] Some feel this contraindicates exercise after cryotherapy, fearing tissues will tear. We disagree. Fine motor skills are hindered, but gross motor movement is not.[1,44]

DECREASED ARTHROGENIC MUSCLE INHIBITION

Arthrogenic muscle inhibition (AMI) is an ongoing reflex inhibition of muscles surrounding a joint, caused by distension or damage to that joint.[45] AMI from injecting saline in the knee occurs in the absence of pain[45] and is reversed or disinhibited by transcutaneous electrical nerve stimulation (TENS) and cryotherapy.[46] In this model, cryotherapy also facilitates the motor neuron pool, but TENS does not.[46] Perhaps one of the most exciting results of this research is that cryotherapy facilitated the resting motor neuron pool (motor neurons available to be stimulated) above baseline measures during cooling and during the 30 min[47,48] and 60 min after cryotherapy.[48]

It appears that cryotherapy not only may reverse inhibition following injury but also may facilitate muscular activity above normal levels. This research is still in its infancy, and much remains to be discovered concerning the effects of cryotherapy on muscle inhibition. The possibilities are exciting to contemplate.[49]

DECREASED CIRCULATION

There is great confusion concerning the circulatory effects of cold applications. Some reports indicate that cold applications result in both increased and decreased blood flow, although those who have proposed increased blood flow have had either nonexistent or arbitrary explanations for when blood flow increases and decreases.

Most of the confusion about the circulatory response of cold has resulted from an inappropriate application of the concept of **cold-induced vasodilation (CIVD)**. Even though there is ample evidence that cryotherapy used in treating orthopedic injuries deceases rather than increases blood flow, the concept of CIVD persists. Because of the resilience of the CIVD concept, a detailed discussion follows.

Cold-Induced Vasodilation: Facts and Fallacies

Cold-induced vasodilation is the dilation of blood vessels (increase in circumference) as a result of cold applications. Popular thought, however, is that CIVD causes an increase in blood flow as a result of cold applications.[1] Although some have claimed that CIVD increases blood flow more than do heat applications, this is not the case.[50]

The term CIVD was coined by Lewis[51] in 1930 to explain temperature fluctuations in the finger during and after ice water immersion. The success of cryokinetics, the alternating of cold applications and active exercise, in the mid-1960s led to claims that CIVD caused increased blood flow in one of two possible times (Fig. 13.1):

- During application, sometimes called the **hunting response.**
- After application, sometimes called the *rebound effect.*

Many accepted the CIVD concept without question and despite the confusion about when CIVD occurs.

There is also confusion about when during injury management CIVD occurs. Most clinicians accept that cold applications during immediate care cause vasoconstriction and decreased blood flow. Yet others believe that postacute cold applications cause vasodilation and increased blood flow. How does the body know what your therapeutic goal is?

THE HISTORY AND DEVELOPMENT OF THE CIVD CONCEPT

A brief timeline of the CIVD concept is shown in Box 13.2. Grant[18], an army physiatrist and Hayden,[19] a physical therapist, introduced cryokinetics in 1965 for rehabilitating acute musculoskeletal injuries occurring during army basic training. Their articles included dramatic statistics of the "striking" success of CIVD. Grant proposed that early movement and restoring normal function are the keys to reducing symptoms and that using ice is simply an added measure for relieving pain and allowing such early movement.[18]

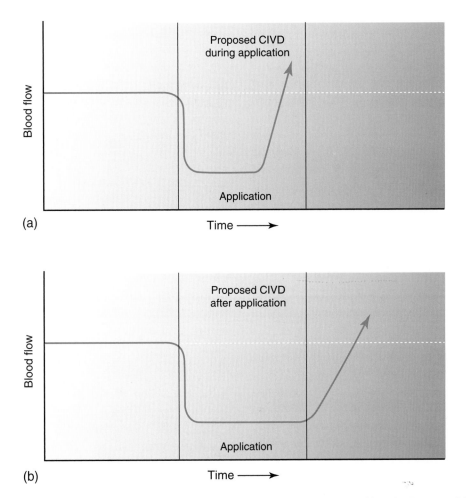

FIGURE 13.1. Proponents of CIVD as an explanation for enhanced rehabilitation have suggested that cold applications cause blood flow to increase, either **(a)** during application or **(b)** after application. We disagree with both hypotheses, as explained in the text. (Adapted with permission from Knight.[1] © 1995 by Kenneth L. Knight. Reprinted with permission from Human Kinetics [Champaign, IL].)

Athletic trainers began using the technique, and they experienced much quicker rehabilitation than with traditional heat applications.[52–54] One AT reported on a football player who returned to full contact with no limitation of motion in <72 hr after a sprained ankle, which normally would have kept the player sidelined for 2–3 weeks.[53] In one of the first attempts to explain mecha-

nisms to account for this quicker rehabilitation, Moore et al.[52] stated that cold prepares the area for exercise and that exercise was important to the success of cryokinetics. They also introduced the idea that CIVD might be involved, even though they were not able to provide adequate evidence to substantiate CIVD as the physiological rationale for cryokinetics.[52]

BOX 13.2 A TIMELINE OF THE CIVD CONCEPT TO EXPLAIN THE SUCCESS OF CRYOTHERAPY

1930	Lewis[51] coined term to explain finger temperature fluctuations during and after cold water immersions
1965	Grant[18] and Hayden[19] developed cryokinetics but did not explain why it worked
1967	Moore et al.[52] suggested CIVD as a possibility but offered no evidence to support the suggestion
Late 1960s	Considered an extreme idea
Middle 1970s	Probable; too much success with cryokinetics to ignore the possibility
Early 1980s	Absolute; cryotherapy had swept the athletic training world and was popular in physical therapy
Middle 1980s	Doubtful; research did not support the concept but did support the theory that exercise was the key
Early 1990s	Improbable; evidence against CIVD continued to build
Today	Many still believe; apparently they have not read, or they ignore, the evidence

During the next 7 years, the technique became a standard in orthopedic and sports medicine. By the mid-1970s, the concept of CIVD became the standard explanation for the success of cryokinetics, apparently because CIVD more closely resembled the previous theory that heat applications promote healing by increasing blood flow to carry away debris and bring nutrients to the healing wound (see Chapter 11). Numerous clinicians wrote as if CIVD were a proven fact.[29,55–59] However, they did not present original data; they quoted the research and opinions of others. The major points of evidence quoted include the following:

- Research of Lewis[51]
- Research of Clarke et al.[60]
- A feeling of warmth occurs during ice water immersion.
- Cold applications cause the tissue to turn red.
- Rehabilitation is quicker with cryokinetics than with thermotherapy.

Because thermotherapy promotes healing by increasing blood flow, cryokinetics must also, many thought.

One of the first attempts to substantiate the occurrence of CIVD during cryokinetics involved measuring blood flow to the ankle during six combinations of heat, cold, and exercise[50] with strain-gauge plethysmography (Box 13.3). There was no CIVD, in fact just the opposite—blood flow decreased during a 25-min cold pack application and remained depressed for 20 min after application (blood flow was measured for only 20 min after application) (Fig. 13.2). Blood flow during combined

---

BOX 13.3 *STRAIN-GAUGE PLETHYSMOGRAPHY FOR MEASURING BLOOD FLOW*

Strain-gauge plethysmography is a standard technique for measuring total blood flow to a limb. Plethysmography involves occluding a limb's venous return (without hindering arterial inflow), causing it to expand.[61] The rate of expansion is a function of the rate of arterial flow. Various methods have been used to measure the rate of expansion, including strain gauges.

Strain-gauge plethysmography uses a very thin rubber tube filled with mercury and attached to electrical wires. The strain gauge is 5–10% less than the circumference of the limb to be measured, so it is on stretch when placed around the limb. A small electrical current is passed through the strain gauge. When it is lengthened (as when the limb expands), its resistance changes. Through calibration and mathematical equations, blood flow can be calculated as a percent change in limb volume.

---

cold and exercise (cryokinetics) had greater increases than with cold alone, with control (meaning no treatment), and with heat pack application, therefore supporting Grant's hypothesis that exercise is the key to cryokinetics success and that cold acts only to facilitate exercise. This study[50] stimulated a reexamination of the studies of Lewis[51] and Clarke et al.[60] to determine why the results differed.

LEWIS CIVD REEXAMINED

As noted, Lewis[51] introduced the concept of CIVD. In his 1930 paper, he reported a series of experiments in which he measured finger temperature—not blood flow—in a single individual. A typical experiment involved one finger, with adjacent fingers as controls (Fig. 13.3). The fingers rested on a cork platform above a beaker of ice water, and then the experimental finger was immersed into the beaker through a hole in the cork. Resulting data were neither combined nor statistically analyzed. Here are the key points of this paper:

- At 6 min after 15 min of immersion in 44.6°F (7°C) water, the right second finger (R2) temperature was 50°F (10°C) warmer than the control (R3) finger. The temperature remained at this level for 10 min and then gradually returned toward control, but it was still 35.6°F (2°C) above control 1 hr after immersion.
- These data appear to provide unquestionable support for CIVD. A closer evaluation of the data, however, after work by Knight et al.,[62] revealed that the control finger was maintained at 66.2°F (19°C), probably because the room temperature (RT) was quite cold (see Fig. 13.3, bottom right. The experimental finger rose to 84.2°F (29°C). Normal finger temperature is 86–93.2°F (30–34°C). Therefore, the experimental finger warmed toward normal but began cooling without ever reaching what would be considered normal temperature.

Lewis recognized that the aftereffect occurred only when the fingers and room were at what he called a "suitable" initial temperature, which was much colder than what would be considered normal.

After three studies using Lewis's methods, except at room temperature and involving the finger and other body parts, we concluded that:

- The finger returns to normal within 10–20 min, but ankle temperature remains depressed (average of 50°F, or 10°C) for an extended period of time.[62]
- After 30 min[63] and 40 min[64] of immersion, the forearm and ankle require in excess of 2.5 hr to return to within 1.8°F (1°C) of the contralateral control limb (Fig. 13.4).

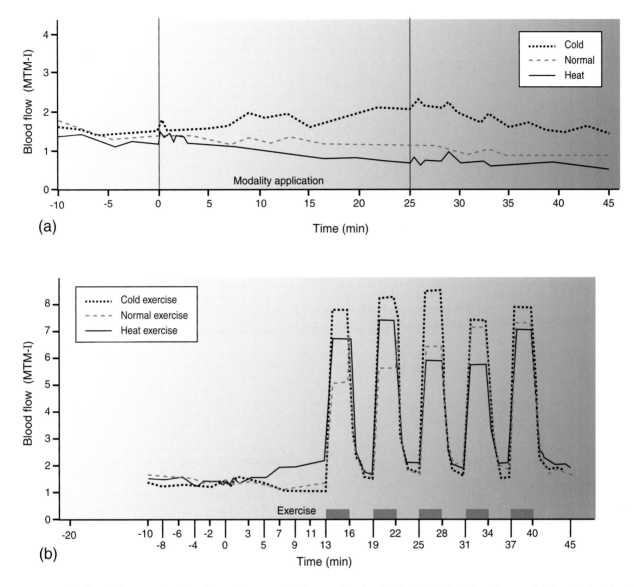

FIGURE 13.2. The first challenge to the idea that CIVD occurred during cryokinetics. **(a)** Note that blood flow decreased during the 25-min cold pack application and remained depressed for 20 min after application. **(b)** Blood flow during the exercise conditions was much greater than during hot pack application. *MTM-I,* blood flow (in millimeters) per 100 mm of tissue, or percent blood flow, at the specific time of measurement. (Adapted with permission from Knight and Londeree.[50])

Lewis also reported that during prolonged cold water immersion (for 2 hr), finger temperature oscillated, a phenomenon he called the hunting reaction, also known as the hunting response. At one time, he reported, there was a sixfold increase. [This caused some[57] to conclude that cold caused greater blood flow than did heat applications.] A close examination of the data indicates this interpretation was in error (Fig. 13.5). The sixfold oscillation was from 35.6°F to 53.6°F (2°C to 12°C) and occurred only after an initial decrease from ~88°F (31°C). Moreover, most oscillations were between 35.6°F and 42.8°F (2°C and 6°C).

The hunting response may be only a measurement artifact. In the course of one experiment, Knight et al.[62] noticed that finger temperature rose, as Lewis had described, but quickly fell when the finger was moved. We incorporated this into another experiment in which we asked subjects to hold their ankles very still for 20 min of immersion.[23] Then when they moved their ankles (while still in the water), the temperature decreased (Fig. 13.6, toe cap group). The hunting response is the result of a water temperature gradient, not a physiological response, and it does not result in increased blood flow to the immersed body part.

CRITICAL THINKING 13.3 *Aside from the hunting response trends, why is there more oscillation in the data of Lewis (Figs. 13.3 and 13.5) than in the data of Nimchick and Knight (Fig. 13.6)? Both involve digit temperature during immersion in a cold water bath. In the former, the temperature is bouncing up and down, while in the later it is a smooth line. Why?*

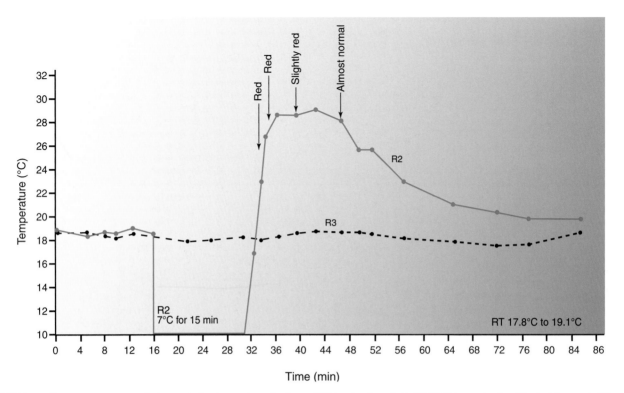

FIGURE 13.3. Finger temperatures during and after immersion of a finger (*R2*) in a beaker of 44.6°F (7°C) ice water for 15 min. The control finger (*R3*) remained on a cork platform above the beaker. *RT,* room temperature (Adapted with permission from Lewis.[51] Reproduced with permission from the BMJ Publishing Group.)

Misinterpreting the Lewis Data

Were Lewis's data faulty? No. Did he try to deceive the scientific community? No. His methods and conclusions were solid. The problem was that his data were misinterpreted by those who claimed his results support the concept that CIVD substantially increases blood flow during orthopedic injury rehabilitation. Consider the following.

- Lewis's CIVD does not occur in warm fingers—that is, fingers whose temperature is what would be considered normal (>90°F [>32.2°C]).
- There is no direct correlation between blood flow and finger temperature.[65]
- Apparently the enthusiasm to explain the rapid rehabilitation, coupled with the pervading theory that rehabilitation was the result of blood flow, overshadowed careful examination of his work.
- The hunting response is a measurement artifact, occurring when a thermal gradient builds and then is interrupted.

CRITICAL THINKING 13.4 *How can you prevent making errors in judgment when interpreting research related to clinical techniques?*

DILATION: A PROCESS, NOT A PRODUCT

Dilation is the process of an organ, orifice, or vessel expanding; it is the opposite of constriction. The final result

of the process is a matter of perspective. For example, consider a structure whose circumference is 10 (units are arbitrary). If the circumference goes from 10 to 2, it has constricted. Then if it goes from 2 to 5, it has dilated 250%. Or you could argue that the second stage was a partial reversal of the original constriction, because even after the "250% dilation," it is still 50% smaller than it was at the start (Fig. 13.7). To conclude, therefore, that blood flow is greater or less than normal after dilation or constriction at a particular point during the application is unfounded.

CLARKE ET AL. REVISITED

Clarke et al.[60] measured blood flow to the forearm with strain-gauge plethysmography during 45 min of immersion in ice water of 33.8°F (1°C), 42.8°F (6°C), and 50°F (10°C) (Fig. 13.8). They reported that blood flow during immersion in 10°C water was little changed from pre-immersion levels. During the 42.8°F (6°C) immersion, however, blood flow gradually increased above pre-immersion levels, and during the 33.8°F (1°C) immersion it increased substantially above pre-immersion levels.

The results of Clarke et al. are in sharp contrast to those of others who have reported blood flow to be less than normal during the following:

- Forearm immersion in 39.2°F (4°C) water for 192 min[66]
- Cold packs applied to the ankle for 25 min[50] (see Fig. 13.2)

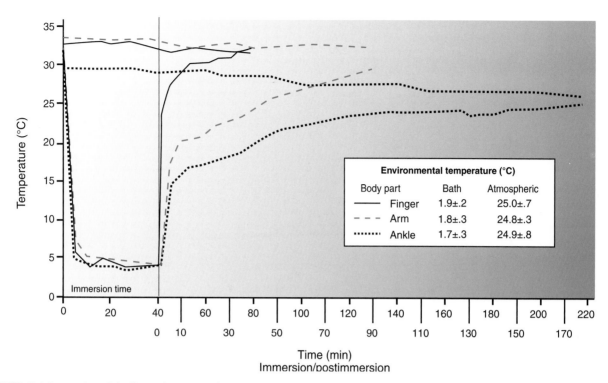

FIGURE 13.4. Rewarming of the finger, forearm, and ankle after 40 min of immersion in 35.6°F (2°C) water. At no time did the temperature exceed either the control (contralateral limb) or pre-immersion temperatures. Note that the finger rewarmed much more quickly (~20 min) than either the forearm or the ankle, which required more than 2.5 hr to return to within 33.8°F (1°C) of the contralateral control. (Adapted with permission from Knight and Elam.[64])

- Forearm immersion in 33.8°F (1°C), 42.8°F (6°C), 50°F (10°C), and 59°F (15°C) water baths for 45 min[67] (Fig. 13.9)
- Gel pack application to the ankle for 20 min[68]

A major problem with the data of Clarke et al. is that there was no initial vasoconstriction, as has been reported by others.[61,66,69–73] One explanation for discrepancies is that the researchers shifted their data to compensate for the effects of the cold on the strain gauge. (Fig. 13.10).

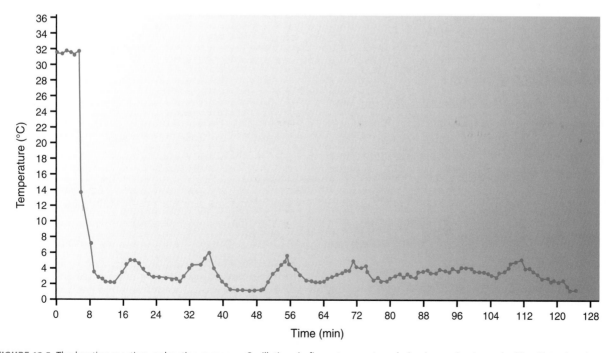

FIGURE 13.5. The hunting reaction, or hunting response. Oscillations in finger temperature during immersion in crushed ice. Note that the oscillations occur only after a profound decrease in temperature, and their magnitude is small compared to the pre-immersion temperature. (Adapted with permission from Lewis.[51] Reproduced with permission from the BMJ Publishing Group.)

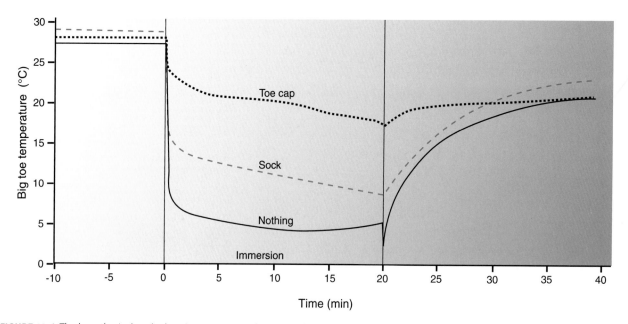

FIGURE 13.6. The hypothesis that the hunting response is the result of developing and then disrupting the thermal gradient is illustrated in the toe cap group. See the text for details. (Adapted with permission from Nimchick and Knight.[23])

This is not an accusation of scientific misconduct, rather speculation about a possible methodological decision on the part of the researchers. Scientists using strain-gauge plethysmography now adjust for the cold with an electronic compensation. Clarke et al. may have adjusted for the cold by adjusting the baseline. The possibility that they shifted the data is based on two facts: First, they did not report blood flow during the first 3 min of immersion. Second, data from an experiment by Knight et al.[67] using similar conditions (Fig. 13.9) look much like the data from Clarke et al. would have if latter had "returned" their data to a preshifted position (compare Figs. 13.9 and 13.10). This explanation also accounts for the lack of initial vasoconstriction.

FEELING OF WARMTH

Most people experience four sensations during cold application: pain, warming or burning, aching or tingling, and numbness.[1] The warming sensation has been attributed to CIVD.[57] But neither a surface nor a subcutaneous temperature increase accompanies changes in sensation during ankle immersion in ice water (Fig. 13.11).[74] Both temperatures decreased throughout the time that subjects reported feeling a warming sensation. Apparently, the feeling of warmth is a psychological sensation rather than a physiological sensation.

SKIN REDNESS

The skin turns bright red during cold application, which some attribute to CIVD.[57] This phenomenon has not been investigated, so any explanation is speculative. One proposed explanation is that owing to lowered tissue metab-

olism during cold applications, oxygen exchange between the tissues and capillaries is decreased. The result is more highly oxygenated blood (which appears redder) in the skin's venous system.[38]

INCREASED RATE OF HEALING

The success of cryokinetics is owing to exercise. Exercise increases blood flow to a greater degree than either heat or

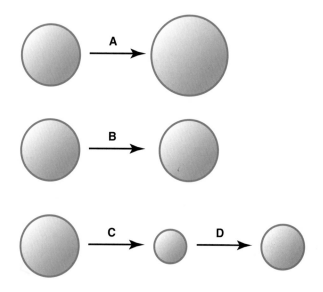

FIGURE 13.7. Constriction and dilation are processes without specific end results. Here, changing from A to B is constriction and moving from B to C is dilation, if considered as isolated events. But if the move from B to C is considered in relation to A, the later process is a partial reversal of the original constriction. Confusion about these processes contributed to the confusion that led to the erroneous idea that CIVD leads to increased blood flow. (Adapted with permission from Knight.[1] © 1995 by Kenneth L. Knight. Reprinted with permission from Human Kinetics [Champaign, IL].)

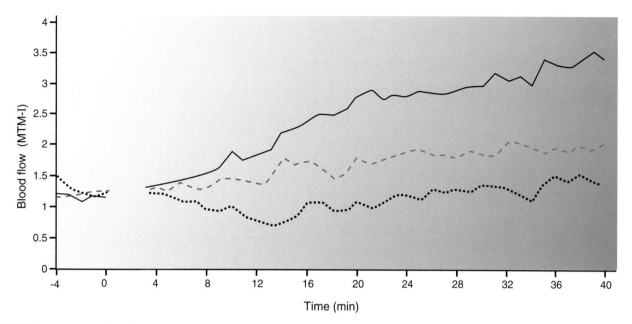

FIGURE 13.8. Forearm blood flow during 40 min of immersion in ice water baths. Note the lack of a control condition and the 3-min gap at the beginning of immersion. This is a composite graph drawn from data obtained by averaging four individual graphs (each representing a single subject).[60] *MTM-I,* blood flow (in millimeters) per 100 mm of tissue, or percent blood flow, at the specific time of measurement. (Adapted with permission from Knight.[1] © 1995 by Kenneth L. Knight. Reprinted with permission from Human Kinetics [Champaign, IL] and Blackwell Publishing.)

cold applications (Fig. 13.12).[50] But in addition to increased blood flow, exercise stimulates healing in other ways as well (see Chapter 6).

CONCLUSIONS ABOUT CIVD AND CRYOKINETICS

Based on a critical reexamination of the literature concerning CIVD after a series of studies by Knight and associates, we conclude the following:

- CIVD does not lead to increased blood flow during or after therapeutic applications of cold. Those who claimed it did were too hasty in developing a theory to explain the success of cryokinetics.
- The purpose of cold applications post–immediate care is to facilitate pain-free exercise. Injury pain and muscle spasm are decreased, thereby allowing exercise to begin earlier and progress faster.

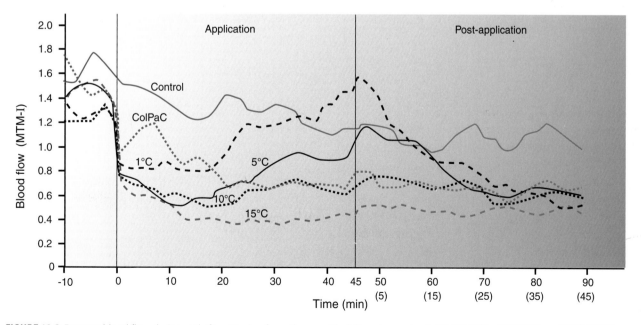

FIGURE 13.9. Forearm blood flow during and after 45 min of cryotherapy. *Black lines,* immersion in 33.8°F (1°C), 41°F (5°C), and 50°F (10°C) water baths; *blue lines,* immersion in 59°F (15°C) water, gel pack, and control; *MTM-I,* blood flow (in millimeters) per 100 mm of tissue, or percent blood flow, at the specific time of measurement. (Adapted with permission from Knight et al.[67])

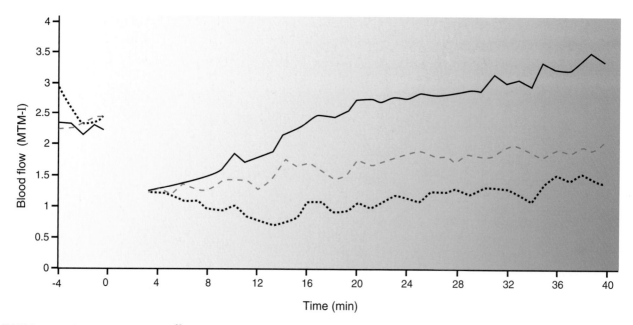

FIGURE 13.10. The data of Clarke et al.[60] as they may have appeared before being adjusted. See the text for details. Note the similarity between these data and the black lines in Figure 13.9. *MTM-I,* blood flow (in millimeters) per 100 mm of tissue, or percent blood flow, at the specific time of measurement. (Adapted with permission from Knight.[1] © 1995 by Kenneth L. Knight. Reprinted with permission from Human Kinetics [Champaign, IL].)

- Exercise is the key to rehabilitation. Without properly executed therapeutic exercise, cold applications will hinder rather than promote rehabilitation.
- Moore et al.[52] stated that one of the purposes of their paper was to encourage other researchers to continue studying the physiological mechanisms involved in cryokinetics. It has.
- Nathan,[75] commenting on the gate control theory of pain, stated that ideas need to be fruitful, but they don't necessarily have to be right. The same can be said about CIVD during therapeutic applications of cold. Although the idea that CIVD results in increased blood

flow has proven to be false, it has been very fruitful. It has led to a greater understanding of the physiological basis of cold and rehabilitation and has, therefore, served us well.

Heat vs. Cold: When and Why

Each of the physiological responses discussed so far occurs when cold is applied to the body. As mentioned earlier, not all of them are beneficial, however, and a response that helps reach one therapeutic goal may not be

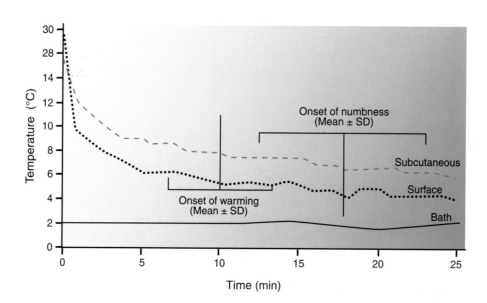

FIGURE 13.11. Although patients may report a warming sensation during ice immersion, these data clearly indicate no increase in tissue temperature during the warming sensation. *SD,* standard deviation. (Reprinted with permission from Johannes.[74])

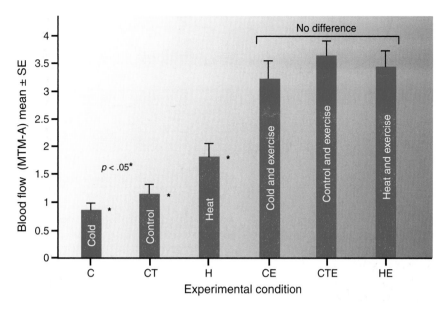

FIGURE 13.12. Average blood flow during six treatments clearly demonstrates that exercise is more effective than either heat or cold in increasing blood flow. Data are averages of 45-min treatments that included 25 min of modality application each. *MTM-A,* average blood flow (in millimeters) per 100 mm of tissue, or percent blood flow; *SE,* standard error of the mean. Data are the same as in Figure 13.2. (Adapted with permission from Knight and Londeree.[50])

desirable or useful for reaching another goal. The specific modality you use and how you apply it will make a difference in the physiological response and thus the therapeutic effect. Therefore, it is important to understand both the response and its efficacy (desirability) during various phases of orthopedic injury care. Table 13.1 presents the physiological responses of local tissue to therapeutic applications of heat and cold, along with their efficacy during various phases of orthopedic injury management.

IMMEDIATE CARE OF ACUTE INJURIES

Decreased metabolism is the most important physiological response to cold during immediate care procedures because it limits secondary injury.[1,76,77] Decreasing circulation is actually detrimental at this time, because it reduces oxygen delivery and, therefore, contributes to secondary metabolic injury. The benefits from decreased metabolism, however, are so much greater than the detrimental effects of decreased circulation that the net result of cold applications is positive. In addition, cold is beneficial during these procedures because it decreases muscle spasm and pain.

Heat applications are contraindicated during immediate care because increased metabolism will promote secondary metabolic injury, thereby increasing the total injury.

SUBACUTE CARE OF ACUTE INJURIES

Decreased circulation, metabolism, and inflammation and increased tissue stiffness are detrimental to acute injury rehabilitation.[15,78] During this period, the tissue needs in-

creased circulation and metabolism. Decreased pain and spasm are, of course, desirable. From a mathematical standpoint (summing the positive and negative effects), there is no benefit to using cryotherapy during rehabilitation. This is true for some cryotherapeutic techniques; however, the exercise component of cryokinetics provides benefits that more than compensate for the decrease in circulation and metabolism caused by the cold.[6,28,50,79]

Exercise does the following:

- Increases blood flow to a much greater extent than that which results from heat applications[50]
- Retards the development of adhesions
- Reverses neural inhibitions[80] and thus facilitates increased activity
- Activates the lymphatic system,[81–83] the primary system for removing tissue debris from injured tissue.[84] Because lymphatic flow requires muscular action to pump the fluid, active exercise is essential for proper functioning.

INCREASED TISSUE STIFFNESS

Pain usually prevents active exercise for many days after even minor joint sprains.[28,80,85] Therefore, cold-induced pain relief enables the performance of active exercise much earlier than would otherwise be possible.[28,86,87] Because increased tissue stiffness hinders active exercise, it is considered a negative effect during rehabilitation.

Heat applications are not as effective as cold applications in facilitating exercise after an acute orthopedic injury.[88] Exercise after heat applications usually causes a return of the pain and muscle spasm that were present

TABLE 13.1   *The Efficacy of Heat and Cold Applications during Orthopedic Injury Care*

PHYSIOLOGICAL RESPONSE	EFFICACY DURING IMMEDIATE CARE OF ACUTE INJURIES*	EFFICACY DURING REHABILITATION	
		Acute Injuries	Chronic Injuries
OF COLD			
Decreased circulation	Nil	Negative	Negative
Decreased metabolism	Very positive[†]	Negative	Negative
Decreased inflammation	Negative	Negative	Positive
Decreased pain (anesthesia)	Positive	Positive[‡]	Positive
Decreased muscle spasm	Positive	Positive	Nil
Increased tissue stiffness	Nil	Negative	Negative
Overall	Positive[†]	Positive[‡]	?
OF HEAT			
Increased circulation	Nil	Positive	Positive
Increased metabolism	Very negative[§]	Nil	Nil
Increased inflammation	Positive	Positive	Negative
Decreased pain (anesthesia)	Positive	Nil[¶]	Positive
Decreased muscle spasm	Positive	Positive	Nil
Decreased tissue stiffness	Nil	Nil	Positive
Overall	Negative	Nil	?

*There is no immediate care of chronic injuries.
[†]Inhibits secondary metabolic injury.
[‡]Allows/requires active exercise.
[§]Promotes secondary metabolic injury.
[¶]Often does not facilitate active exercise.

beforehand. This does not seem to be true with chronic injuries. In addition, heat is effective in relieving general muscle soreness.

Cryokinetics can begin much earlier than thermal therapy.[86,89,90] Thermotherapy requires waiting until the circulation is restored, to avoid causing additional secondary metabolic injury. This usually takes 48–72 hr after an injury, whereas cryokinetics can begin 1–24 hr postinjury.[89]

LATE SUBACUTE CARE

Within 10–15 days after an acute injury, pain becomes more of a dull soreness than a sharp stabbing pain. Soreness responds better to heat than cold. Decreased range of motion can result from either muscle spasm or contracted connective tissue. Therefore, treat muscle spasm with cold; and treat connective tissue with a combination of heat, stretching, and cold.

CHRONIC OR OVERUSE INJURIES

There is no immediate care for overuse injuries. Because the onset of these injuries is gradual, there is little vascular collapse and, therefore, little fear of secondary metabolic

injury. Issues surrounding the rehabilitation of chronic injuries are a source of confusion.[91–93] Generally, there is minimal or no muscle spasm, and pain occurs only during extended activity. An overactive inflammatory response indicates cold applications to decrease the inflammation. However, there is no evidence that cold is beneficial.

A popular therapy for tendinitis is the application of hot packs before, and cold packs after, practice or exercise. But evidence neither supports nor refutes this regimen. Although ultrasound applications applied twice daily for 10 days might be effective, there is no documented evidence to support the claim; it is strictly our clinical impression, based on experience with baseball players and gymnasts.

Cryotherapeutic Techniques for Transition and Subacute Care

The five most popular cryotherapy techniques used for transition and subacute care of acute orthopedic injury are discussed in this section. Each has specific indications; the techniques are not interchangeable. Specific application procedures for four of the techniques are in Chapter 14.

CRYOKINETICS FOR ACUTE JOINT SPRAIN REHABILITATION

Cryokinetics is a systematic combination of cold applications to numb the injured body part and graded, progressive, active exercise.[20,52] Cryokinetics is the most effective form of cryotherapy for rehabilitating ligament sprains. Especially effective for ankle sprains, the technique can be used for any acute musculoskeletal joint injury. Cryokinetics allows rehabilitation to begin much sooner than traditional thermotherapy, and it can shorten rehabilitation time by days or even weeks.[18,19,94,95]

Pain-Free Exercise

Pain-free exercise is the key to cryokinetics.[1,20,52] The purpose of cold applications is pain reduction to make active exercise possible.

Safety Valve

Unlike local anesthetic injections of pain-numbing drugs, such as procaine, cold does not totally inhibit the body's pain-sensing mechanism. Cold relieves residual pain (pain from damaged tissue, pressure from swelling on nerves, etc.), thereby facilitating active exercise. But if the exercise becomes so vigorous that further damage might result, the body responds with a pain sensation. Thus cryokinetics has a built-in safety valve: Pain during numbness indicates the exercise is too vigorous and the activity level must be decreased (as long as the limb is properly numbed with ice application).

Psychological Preparation

The initial numbing during the first treatment session is usually difficult for the patient, and he will experience intense pain before the body part numbs. But the body quickly adapts to the pain, so subsequent ice applications are much less intense.[96,97] You must prepare the patient for the initial intense pain. Make sure he understands these important points:

- The pain is only temporary; it will not occur during subsequent cold applications.
- The benefits of the treatment, primarily decreased disability time, greatly outweigh the temporary discomfort.
- Shorter disability time is the main benefit of the cold.

Patients who are not prepared for the intense cold and pain at the first immersion sometimes refuse to continue the treatment. (See Chapter 14 for cryokinetics application procedures.)

CRYOSTRETCH FOR ACUTE MUSCLE INJURIES

Although cryokinetics is especially effective for treating acute joint sprains, it is not the best treatment for acute muscle strains. Muscle strains should be passively stretched. The cryostretch technique combines cold and passive stretching. It should be used during the early phases of muscle strain rehabilitation and followed by cryokinetics, as explained later in this chapter.

The cryostretch technique is dynamite for reducing low-grade muscle spasm, and most muscle injuries (strains and contusions) result in some degree of muscle spasm or tightness. In fact, many mild muscle "pulls" are actually muscles in spasm rather than torn muscle fibers.[98] In either case, the first step in rehabilitation is reducing the spasm and reestablishing pain-free range of motion.

Cryostretch combines three techniques for reducing muscle spasm: cold application, static stretching, and isometric contraction—the hold–relax technique of *proprioceptive neuromuscular facilitation* (PNF).[99,100] Although cryostretch is similar to cryokinetics in that exercise is performed while the body part is numbed, it differs in the number of exercise sets (three in cryostretch vs. five in cryokinetics) and in the exercise itself. During cryostretch exercises, the injured muscle is alternately statically stretched and isometrically contracted.

Cryostretch begins with cold application, typically ice massage, ice packs, or large cold packs. After numbness, interspersed with renumbing, are three exercise bouts of about 2.5 min. Each *exercise bout* consists of two 65-sec sets of exercise with a 20-sec relaxation period between sets. An *exercise set* consists of alternating static stretch with three repetitions of isometric contractions (hold–relax). See Chapter 14 for application procedures.

CONNECTIVE TISSUE STRETCH

The **connective tissue stretch** is a combination of heat application, long-term passive stretch, and cold applications. It is used to increase joint flexibility after prolonged immobilization during which connective tissue contractures have developed. Heat causes collagen fibers to relax, stretch lengthens the collagen fibers, and cold enables the collagen fibers to reattach in a lengthened position. See Chapter 14 for application procedures.

LYMPHEDEMA PUMPS

Lymphedema pumps, known formerly as *intermittent compression pumps, cold compression devices, pneumatic compression pumps,* and *intermittent compression devices* are devices for providing intermittent compression to a body segment. The device consists of a boot or sleeve that fits over an extremity, a pump, hoses connecting the pump to the sleeve, and often a small ice water bath. The pump forces air or chilled water into the sleeve, applying pressure to the joint. The pump is controlled by a timing mechanism that turns it on and off, causing the sleeve or boot to intermittently inflate and deflate. The changes in sleeve pressure force lymphatic and venous drainage and thus reduce edema.

Cryokinetics is preferred for edema reduction because the rate of inflation–deflation of lymphedema pumps is much slower than the muscle pump provided by cryokinetics. Also, with cryokinetics you get the additional benefits of active exercise. See Chapter 14 for application procedures.

CONTRAST BATH THERAPY

Contrast bath therapy involves alternating immersion of the injured body part in hot and cold water baths. The traditional theory is that the alternating hot and cold baths cause alternating vasodilation and vasoconstriction, which pumps edema from the tissue. The time of application of the two baths varies greatly. Numerous ratios of hot to cold have been suggested, including 4:1, 3:1, 3:2, 5:2, and 5:5 min.[1,101]

The theory that contrast therapy helps pump out edema has so many holes in it that we do not recommend the technique. For example:

- Edema is reduced by removing free protein from the tissue. This is done via the lymphatic system, not the vascular system (see Chapter 5).
- Even if edema were reduced via the vascular system, the tissue temperature changes would not be great enough to cause significant vascular reactions.[101–103]

- Even if the temperature changes were great enough to effect vascular changes, neither the venules, the capillaries, nor the lymph vessels contain muscles to be effected by the temperature changes. They, therefore, could not constrict and dilate with contrasting temperatures.
- Even if the technique caused vascular or lymphatic pumping, cryokinetics would cause many more pumps. Consider: A ratio of 3:1 would induce a pump each 4 min, or 15 pumps per hour. During 1 hr of cryokinetics, a patient would actively exercise for 15 min. During each exercise repetition, muscle contraction will pump the venous and lymphatic systems. The patient would perform 20–30 pumps per minute, or 20–30 times more than each minute in a contrast bath.

Another theory is that alternating sensations during the alternating applications of heat and cold cause a decrease in pain that allows more activity after the contrast bath therapy. This theory is flawed, however.[1] There is no change in numbness in uninjured subjects when contrast therapy is used.[99]

Comparing Heat and Cold for Rehabilitation

Some clinicians feel that cryotherapy is better than thermotherapy during rehabilitation because the temperature change during application is many times greater with cold than with heat. This is not true. This false idea developed because core temperature was used to compute the changes. But therapeutic modalities are applied most often to the extremities, so the differential should be com-

TABLE 13.2 *Temperature Differentials During Cryotherapy and Thermotherapy*

BODY PART/MODALITY	NORMAL TEMPERATURE	CHANGE IN TEMPERATURE FROM	
		Core	Extremities
Core	98.6°F (37°C)		
Human extremities	86 to 93°F (30 to 34°C)		
SUPERFICIAL HEAT			
Hot packs	115°F (45°C)	+16.4°F (+8°C)	+22 to 29°F (+11 to 15°C)
Whirlpool	105°F (40°C)	+6.4°F (+3°C)	+12 to 19°F (+6 to 10°C)
SUPERFICIAL COLD			
Immersion	34°F (1°C)	−64.6°F (−36°C)	−52 to 59°F (−29 to 33°C)
Cold pack	41°F (5°C)	−57.6°F (−32°C)	−45 to 52°F (−25 to 29°C)
Whirlpool	65°F (18°C)	−33.6°F (−19°C)	−21 to 28°F (−12 to 16°C)

puted from extremity temperature, which is lower than core temperature (Table 13.2). For instance, the absolute change in temperature between a cold whirlpool and the core is 6.3 times as great as the change from a warm whirlpool and core: 66.2°F vs. 37.4°F (19°C vs. 3°C). When computing the difference between extremity temperature and hot and cold whirlpool temperatures, the change with cold is only twice as great: 42.8°F vs. 53.6°F (6°C vs. 12°C).

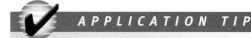

APPLICATION TIP

CRYOTHERAPY: POWERFUL THERAPY BEYOND IMMEDIATE CARE. Cryotherapy is extremely powerful during immediate care and beyond. But we don't want to give the impression that it is the answer to rehabilitation of all orthopedic injuries. For acute sprains and strains, cryotherapy, in the form of cryokinetics or cryostretch, should follow RICES treatments and continue well into the postacute phase of rehabilitation. Heat helps reduce general soreness and must be used to prepare collagen tissue for stretching and joint mobilization. Both thermotherapy and extended cryotherapy have their place.

WHEN TO USE COLD AND WHEN TO USE HEAT

Based on our personal research, reading, and clinical experience, we offer the following opinions:

- Cold applications must always be used for the immediate care of acute injuries.

- Cold applications are more effective in facilitating exercise during the rehabilitation of acute orthopedic injuries.
- Muscle spasm is relieved more quickly with cold and stretching than with heat and stretching.
- Chronic inflammatory conditions should respond well to ultrasound (twice a day) and with either superficial heat or cold. Some individuals respond better to superficial cold, whereas others respond better to superficial heat. Treat the symptoms with whatever modality is most comfortable for the patient.
- Connective tissue contractures resulting from immobilization (2 weeks or longer) must be treated with heat followed by stretching or mobilization.
- General soreness is best treated with a warm whirlpool.
- Subacute joint sprains (4–14 days postinjury) that remain sore but that allow the patient to exercise should be treated with heat before exercise or practice and cold afterward.

APPLICATION TIP

THERAPEUTIC GOALS DETERMINE SELECTION OF THERAPEUTIC MODALITIES. The recommendations for when to use cold and when to use heat illustrate the principle that the choice of what therapeutic modality to use should be a matter of matching therapeutic goals with the body's response to the modality. Remember the SAID (specific adaptation to imposed demands) principle from Chapter 1?

CLOSING SCENE

The AT student in the opening scene tells you to apply ice to an injured player's ankle for no longer than 15 min. His rationale was that after 15 min, cold-induced vasodilation will occur and this might add to the swelling. You correct him and explain why CIVD is a flawed theory but that this does not negate the use of cryotherapy beyond immediate care. Further, you explain why facilitating therapeutic exercise is much more powerful than inducing increased blood flow.

CHAPTER REFLECTIONS

1. Read and ponder each of the following points. Do you feel you have a clear understanding of each concept? If not, reread the appropriate section of the chapter.
   - Define cryotherapy.
   - Why is there confusion concerning cryotherapy?
   - Explain the profile of temperature changes during cold applications, including differences between surface and deep temperatures, and thermal gradients in the tissue and modality.
   - Describe the relationship between immediate care and post–immediate care cryotherapy during orthopedic injury management. Include the theory, goals, and application of cryotherapy during each phase.
   - Why is there confusion about cryotherapy during immediate care and post-immediate care of orthopedic injuries?
   - Consider the relationship between pain and cryotherapy: How can cryotherapy both cause and relieve pain?
   - Name the nine major physiological responses to cryotherapy and briefly explain the mechanism of each.
   - Discuss strategies to minimize pain during cryotherapy.
   - What is the difference between coping with and habituation to cold-induced pain? Discuss strategies for both during cryotherapy.

   - Describe CIVD—what it is, when it occurs, and why clinicians are confused about its role in orthopedic injury management.
   - Discuss the efficacy of heat and cold (including the influence of each physiological response) when used during immediate care and acute care of orthopedic injuries.
   - What are the criteria for selecting which therapeutic modality to use?
   - Define and briefly discuss when and how you would use cryokinetics, cryostretch, connective tissue stretch, contrast bath therapy, and lymphedema pumps.

2. Write three to five questions for discussion with your class instructor, clinical instructor, classmates, and clinical colleagues.

3. Get together with classmates and quiz each other on the concepts of this chapter. Use the points in exercise 1 and questions you wrote for exercise 2 as a beginning. Explaining concepts out loud to others requires a deeper grasp of the material than feeling you understand it as you read.

CRITICAL THINKING RESPONSES

Critical Thinking 13.1

Cold (RICES) is essential immediately after an injury and extending for 10–24 hr to decrease secondary injury. Many continue to use it for days after the injury in an effort to reduce the swelling. The later efforts are futile, however. First of all, swelling is a process, not an entity. Swelling is the result of a shift in capillary filtration pressure owing to extracellular free protein. To reduce the swelling, you must remove the excess extracellular free protein. This requires stimulating the lymphatic system via some type of intermittent compression, such as active exercise, massage, a lymphedema pump, or electrical muscle stimulation.

Critical Thinking 13.2

If the foot is held still in an ice water bath, a temperature gradient develops in the water, making the water near the body warmer than the rest of ice water bath. If the patient then moves his foot (or if you swirl the water), the gradient is broken up and the water near the foot becomes colder. The decrease in temperature of the local environment elicits a pain response.

Critical Thinking 13.3

Figures 13.3 and 13.4 represent data from a single subject; Figure 13.6 presents averaged data from 12 subjects. Temperatures of individual subjects in the later study oscillated just as much as in the former, but because the fluctuation occurred at slightly different times, averaging them together smoothed the line. For example, consider three consecutive measurements in each of three subjects: subject A = 2, 4, 2; subject B = 3, 3, 4; and subject C = 4, 2, 3. The measure for each of the three subjects is oscillating; in fact, the second reading of subject A is twice as much as the first and third readings. When the data are averaged, however, they are 3, 3, 3, which would graph as a straight line. Remember when reading experimental results that the data presented represent an average of many individuals. A second important consideration is that patients are not average, meaning that individual patients are not going to respond exactly like the average.

Critical Thinking 13.4

You can prevent interpretation errors by actively thinking. Don't be naive or cynical. As the sixteenth-century philosopher Francis Bacon taught, "Read not to contradict and refute, nor to believe and take for granted, . . . but to weigh and consider."

We all want to be able to justify or explain why we do something, not only for our own curiosity but to explain what we are doing to our patients. Unfortunately, many clinicians accept dubious claims of theory and pass them on. This is especially true of claims by salespeople. Most are honorable, but there are snake-oil peddlers among

them. And even the honorable inadvertently share misinformation.

Be sure to check references when you read journal articles. References are sometimes misinterpreted and then passed on. For example, McMaster[104] is often quoted as a source for applying cold for 20 min during immediate care, but his source is an article by Knight and Londeree[50] about cryokinetics. So research concerning cryotherapy for pain control was improperly used to reference cryotherapy for immediate care, for which the goal is decreased metabolism, and then passed on by many others who did not check the original reference.

Another point about references is their content. A reference to specific research on a topic is stronger than to an opinion, even if the opinion is by a prominent scientist or clinician.

REFERENCES

1. Knight KL. Cryotherapy in Sport Injury Management. Champaign, IL: Human Kinetics; 1995.
2. Jarvinen M. Immobilization effect on the tensile properties of striated muscle: An experimental study in the rat. Arch Phys Med Rehabil. 1977;58:123–127.
3. Jarvinen M. Healing of a crush injury in rat striated muscle. 2. A histological study of the effect of early mobilization and immobilization on the repair processes. Acta Pathol Microbiol Scand [A] 1975;83: 269–282.
4. Hurme T, Kalimo H, Lehto M, Jarvinen M. Healing of skeletal muscle injury: An ultrastructural and immunohistochemical study. Med Sci Sports Exerc 1991;23:801–810.
5. Kvist H, Jarvinen M, Sorvari T. Effect of mobilization and immobilization on the healing of contusion injury in muscle. A preliminary report of a histological study in rats. Scand J Rehabil Med 1974;6: 134–140.
6. Dehne E. The rationale of early functional loading in the healing of fractures: A comprehensive gate control concept of repair. Clin Orthop 1980;146:18–27.
7. Buch B, Papert AI, Shear M. Microscopic changes in rat tongue following experimental cryosurgery. J Oral Pathol 1979;8:94–102.
8. Marcove RC, Weis LD, Vaghaiwalla MR, Pearson R. Cryosurgery in the treatment of giant cell tumors of bone: A report of 52 consecutive cases. Clin Orthop 1978;134:275–289.
9. Boykin JV Jr, Crute SL. Mechanisms of burn shock protection after severe scald injury by cold-water treatment. J Trauma 1982;22: 859–866.
10. Rippe B, Grega GJ. Effects of isoprenaline and cooling on histamine induced changes of capillary permeability in the rat hindquarter vascular bed. Acta Physiol Scand 1978;103:252–262.
11. Harris ED Jr, McCroskery PA. The influence of temperature and fibril stability on degradation of cartilage collagen by rheumatoid synovial collagenase. N Engl J Med 1974;290:1–6.
12. Svanes K. Studies in hypothermia I. The influence of deep hypothermia on the formation of cellular exudate in acute inflammation in mice. Acta Anaesth Scand 1964;8:143–156.
13. Svanes K. Studies in hypothermia II. The influence of deep hypothermia on the formation of fluid exudate in acute inflammation in mice. Acta Anaesth Scand 1964;8:157–166.
14. Dorwart BB, Hansell JR, Schumacher HR. Effects of heat, cold and mechanical agitation on crystal-induced synovitis in the dog. Arthritis Rheum 1974;17(5):563–571.
15. Abakumova E. Effect of hypothermia on wound healing. Stomatologiia 1978;57:19–21.
16. McCaffery M. Nursing Management of the Patient with Pain. Philadelphia: Lippincott, 1979.
17. Chapman CE. Can the use of physical modalities for pain control be rationalized by the research evidence? Can J Physiol Pharmacol 1991;69:704–712.
18. Grant AE. Massage with ice (cryokinetics) in the treatment of painful conditions of the musculoskeletal system. Arch Phys Med Rehabil 1964;44:233–238.
19. Hayden CA. Cryokinetics in an early treatment program. J Am Phys Ther Assoc 1964;44:990–993.
20. Knight KL. Ankle rehabilitation with cryokinetics. Physician Sportsmed 1979;7:113.
21. Knight KL. Cryokinetics in rehabilitation of joint sprains. J Can Athl Ther Assoc 1981;8:17–18.
22. Tovel J. Ice immersion toe cap. Athl Train 1980;15:33.
23. Nimchick PSR, Knight KL. Effects of wearing a toe cap or a sock on temperature and perceived pain during ice water immersion. Athl Train 1983;18:144–147.
24. Jutte LS, Konz S. A 15 min immersion in 1°C water produces greater numbness than immersion in 4°C or 10°C water. J Athl Train: In review.
25. Everall M. Cold therapy. Nursing Times 1976;70:144–145.
26. Haines J. A study into a report on cold therapy. Physiotherapy. 1970;56:501–502.
27. Raptou AD. Cryotherapy: A brief review. South Med J 1968;61: 625–627.
28. Kraus H. Prevention and treatment of skiing injuries. J Trauma 1961; 1:457–463.
29. Chu DA, Lutt CJ. The rationale of ice therapy. J Natl Athl Train Assoc 1969;4:8–9.
30. Travell J, Rinzler SH. The myofascial genesis of pain. Postgrad Med 1952;11:425–434.
31. Ashby EC. Abdominal pain of spinal origin. Ann R Coll Surg Engl 1977;59:242–246.
32. Wolf SL, Knutsson E. Effects of skin cooling on stretch reflex activity in triceps surae of the decerebate cat. Exp Neurol 1975;49: 22–35.
33. Lane L. Localized hypothermia for relief of pain in musculoskeletal injuries. Phys Ther 1971;51:182–183.
34. Wolf SL, Letbetter WD. Effect of skin cooling on spontaneous EMG activity in triceps surae of the decerebrate cat. Brain Res 1975;91: 151–155.

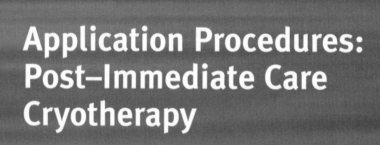

Application Procedures: Post–Immediate Care Cryotherapy

After reading about cryokinetics in the previous chapter, you decide to give it a try on Andrew, one of your patients, who suffered a second-degree ankle sprain yesterday. You prepare the container of ice water and slowly have him immerse his foot in the slush. You are not prepared for what happens next! He lifts his leg out of the water and yells, "This is too cold!" You have read about how effective cryokinetics is and you want to continue the treatment. What can you do to help Andrew get through the session effectively?

Transition and Subacute Care Cryotherapy Techniques

In Chapters 5 and 13, we discussed the differences between cryotherapy for immediate care and for transition and post-immediate care. In Chapter 5, we discussed rest, ice, compression, elevation, stabilization (RICES) application techniques for immediate care. In this chapter, we present application techniques for transition and post–immediate care.

Acute transition care begins once secondary injury stops. The goal is to facilitate therapeutic exercise by numbing the body so that active exercise can proceed pain free. The two most common methods for local numbing are ice water immersion and ice massage. Occasionally an ice bag is used; its construction and application are covered in Chapter 5.

ICE WATER IMMERSION

Ice water immersion also called *ice bath immersion* and sometimes inappropriately called *ice water submersion,* is not simply immersing an extremity in a pail of ice water. Although proper use of the technique is not complicated, there are a few tricks that improve its usefulness:

- Use a container that is large enough for the extremity to fit but that is not big and bulky. Also, a plastic or rubber container works better than a metal container. Because the metal container gets very cold, it is painful if the extremity comes in contact with the edge of the metal container.
- Fill the container with ice first and then add water. This will result in a bath temperature between 32°F and 34°F (0° and 1°C). Warmer water may be less painful during the initial treatment, but does not numb the tissue as well.[1]
- Help the patient adapt to the initial cold pain. She may become discouraged with the treatment if you leave her alone to think about the pain. Here are strategies that will diminish the pain sensation.

- Give the patient a choice before beginning the treatment. For example, "We can use cryokinetics, which will be quite painful during the initial immersion but will get you back in 2–4 days. Or we can use the traditional heat treatments, which will not be painful and get you back in 2–3 weeks. Which would you prefer?"
- Assure the patient that subsequent bouts of this session and subsequent sessions will be much less painful.[2] Point out that after a few days, she will feel little or no pain from the cold.
- Use a toe cap when treating foot, ankle, or lower leg sprains (Fig. 14.1). It will minimize the pain if worn during immersion.[3,4] Most of the pain during ankle immersion is in the toes. The toe cap keeps the toes warm—and, therefore, relatively pain free—but has no effect on the uncovered portions of the foot and ankle.[4] Thus it does not interfere

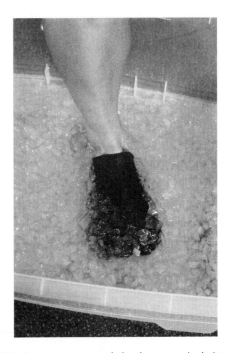

FIGURE 14.1. A neoprene toe cap helps decrease pain during ice water immersion.

with the benefits of the treatment. Patients are much more comfortable with a toe cap than without it.

- Talk to the patient continuously during the initial immersion.[5] Any topic that will take her mind off the cold is appropriate. It doesn't matter if you exaggerate or downplay the potential pain; just talk about something.[5]
- Make sure the patient goes through multiple immersion bouts during the first session. Subsequent bouts are much less painful than the first immersion.[2] After realizing this, patients are more likely to continue the treatments.

ICE MASSAGE

Ice massage is massage with ice, consisting of stroking a body part (usually a muscle) with a large ice cube or "ice pop" (6–8 oz). Here are tips for using ice massage:

- Prepare ice cubes or ice pops by freezing water in paper drinking cups. The only difference between the two is that one has a tongue depressor inserted before freezing (Fig. 14.2).
  - To keep the patient from eating the ice, put a few drops of liquid soap into the cup before freezing.

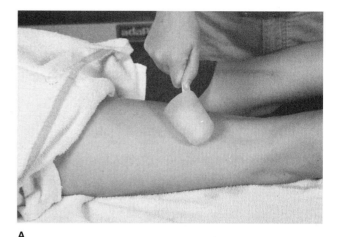

A

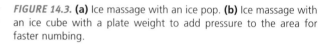

B

FIGURE 14.3. (a) Ice massage with an ice pop. **(b)** Ice massage with an ice cube with a plate weight to add pressure to the area for faster numbing.

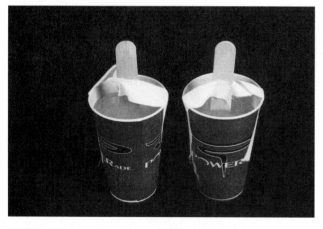

FIGURE 14.2. Preparing an ice massage ice pop by inserting a tongue depressor into the water before freezing. Note the tape used to hold the handle in the center during freezing.

- Massage the muscle by grasping the ice cube with a towel or the tongue depressor handle and slowly stroking the muscle (Fig. 14.3a). Discontinue when the muscle is numb (10–20 min).
- Numbness can be increased by adding resistance to the massage.[6] Do this by placing a 5–10 lb Olympic plate weight over the ice cube. Use the weight as a handle to maneuver the ice over the muscle (Fig. 14.3b).

Application of Cryokinetics for Joint Sprains

STEP 1: FOUNDATION

A. Definition. **Cryokinetics** is a combination of cold applications and active exercise. (Fig. 14.4).[7]
B. Effects
   1. Cold decreases pain and arthrogenic muscle inhibition, thus allowing exercise.
   2. Ice moderates arthrogenic muscle inhibition.
   3. Exercise stimulates increased blood flow.
   4. Exercise reestablishes neuromuscular functioning.
   5. Stresses induced by exercise influence collagen deposition and fiber orientation during repair.
C. Advantages
   1. It allows exercise much sooner than normally would be the case.
   2. Exercise
      a. Retards muscular atrophy
      b. Retards neural inhibitions
      c. Reduces swelling dramatically through muscular milking action
   3. Ice is inexpensive; exercise is free.
D. Disadvantages
   1. The extreme cold is very painful during the initial ice immersion of the first session. (The patient usually adapts, and subsequent immersions of the specific body part are not as painful.)

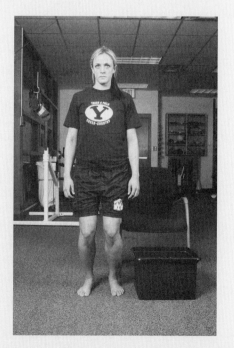

FIGURE 14.4. In a cryokinetics treatment, a patient actively exercises after undergoing cold-induced numbing.

   2. Melting ice can be messy.
E. Indications
   1. Ankle sprains
      a. Cryokinetics is more effective on ankle sprains than any other injury.
      b. Cryokinetics is more effective on ankle sprains than any other technique for treating the ankle.
   2. Finger sprains
   3. Shoulder sprains
   4. Other joint sprains
F. Contraindications
   1. Any exercise or activity that causes pain.
   2. Use of ice on a person who is hypersensitive to cold.
G. Precautions
   1. Pain must be used as a guideline. The patient should not consciously or willfully overcome or gut out pain.
   2. When treating lower extremity injuries, the patient might limp if he is not regularly reminded to refrain from limping. Limping could lead to overuse injuries to surrounding and contralateral structures.
   3. There may be an increase in pain 4–8 hr after treatment.

STEP 2: PREAPPLICATION TASKS

A. Make sure cryokinetics is the proper modality for this situation.
   1. Reevaluate the injury or problem. Make sure you understand the patient's condition.
   2. If cryokinetics was applied previously, review the patient's response to that treatment.
   3. Confirm that the objectives of therapy are compatible with cryokinetics.
   4. Make sure cryokinetics is not contraindicated in this situation.
B. Preparing the patient psychologically
   1. Explain the four sensations that the person will go through during ice immersion:
      a. Pain will be very intense during the first application but will lessen considerably during subsequent treatments.
      b. Warming (in some patients)
      c. Ache or tingling
      d. Numbness or relative anesthesia
   2. Explain that the advantages of the treatment compensate for the discomfort (exercise will be

possible, so rehabilitation will proceed much more quickly.)

C. Preparing the patient physically
1. Remove necessary clothing (if ice massage is used, the ice will melt and create a puddle of water).
2. Position the patient so he is comfortable.

D. Equipment preparation
1. Have a container and ice or an ice pop available.
2. A toe cap is helpful, but not necessary.
3. Have a towel if ice massage is used, to sop up the melting ice.

3 STEP 3: APPLICATION PARAMETERS

A. Procedures
1. Numb the body part by applying ice to the injured area.
   a. Immersion in ice water is preferred, but if that method is not possible, use
      i. Massage with ice cubes (made in 6–8 oz paper cups)
      ii. Ice bag (ice in a plastic bag)
      iii. Ice packs (ice folded in a towel)
   b. The ice application lasts through four sensations (listed in step 2) and takes 10–20 min.
      i. The patient's sensation is more important than the length of application. When the patient reports numbness, begin exercising; continued cold application wastes time.
      ii. Some people (10–20%) cannot judge when they are numb. If the patient does not report numbness after 20 min (5 min when renumbing), assume that pain is sufficiently decreased and proceed with the exercise phase of the treatment.
   c. Help the patient endure the initial cold pain. He might become discouraged if left alone to think about the pain. Avoid this by talking continuously during the initial immersion to distract attention from the discomfort.[5]
   d. Use a toe cap when treating lower limb injuries. It will substantially reduce pain.
   e. Alternative: If cold applications fail to provide enough pain relief for exercise, try transcutaneous electrical nerve stimulation (TENS) or neuromuscular electrical stimulation (NEMS).
2. Exercise the area, as explained later in this step, for as long as it remains numb (about 3 min).
3. Reapply the ice until numbness is again reached (3–5 min).
4. Exercise the injured area, alternating with ice immersion and numbness at least five times during each treatment.
5. Exercising, not the ice, causes rehabilitation. Remember, numbing serves no purpose other than to allow the body part to exercise actively.
6. Principles of cryokinetic exercises
   a. All exercise should be
      i. Active—performed by the patient
      ii. Progressive—increasing in both intensity and complexity
      iii. Pain free—Never use an exercise or motion that causes pain. If a particular exercise does cause pain, return to the former activity level.
   b. Exercise as long as the body part is numb, usually 2–3 min. As the numbness begins to wear off, reapply the cold. (Renumbing will take only 3–5 min.)
   c. Begin with simple range-of-motion (ROM) activities and progress through full activity or sport-specific drills.
   d. Exercise must be performed without pain and in a normal, rhythmic, coordinated fashion.
   e. Constantly encourage the patient to progress to the next level of activity (as long as all exercises are performed properly). With some injuries, progression through full activity will take place in a single treatment session; but for others, it may take a week or more.
   f. The time spent performing an activity or the number of repetitions is not important. The key to cryokinetics is the ability to perform exercise of increasing difficulty properly and without pain.
7. An exercise progression for an ankle sprain can be used as a model for similar progressions for other joints. The exercise progression begins with a basic ROM movement and successively becomes more difficult until full activity is achieved. For an athlete, this means full sport activity, without restrictions.
   a. Non-weight-bearing ROM (Fig. 14.5a)
      i. Perform plantar flexion, dorsiflexion, inversion, eversion, and circumduction (pointing toes to ground, toward nose, to right, to left, and moving in a circle) with the ankle to the limits of motion and/or pain. Exercises such as writing the alphabet with the big toe or picking up a marble with the toes are other ways

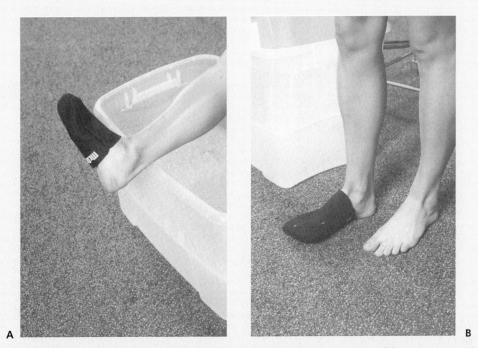

A   B

FIGURE 14.5. **(a)** Begin cryokinetic exercising with non-weight-bearing active range-of-motion exercises. **(b)** Progress to weight-bearing ROM exercises with crouching and toe raises, and then shift weight back and forth between injured and uninjured foot.

of requiring the patient to go through an active ROM.[8]

ii. Move on to the next step when full pain-free ROM is achieved.

b. Bearing weight

i. The patient stands with most of his weight on the uninjured leg. He then slowly shifts his weight back and forth between the uninjured and the injured leg, while progressively bearing more weight on the injured leg.

ii. When he can bear his full body weight on the injured leg, progress to the next step.

c. Weight-bearing ROM

i. With his weight on both legs (Fig. 14.5b), perform plantar flexion and dorsiflexion on the ankle by alternatively crouching and raising up on the toes.

ii. If dorsiflexion is difficult or extremely limited, have him perform Achilles tendon (heel cord) stretches (Fig. 14.6) as part of each subsequent treatment session.[8]

d. Walking

i. Begin with short steps (heel to toe) and walk straight ahead, gradually lengthening the steps (Fig. 14.7). Once normal stride length is achieved, walk in gentle

arcs or large circles. Progress to making sharper cuts on turns.

ii. Do not allow the patient to limp.

(a) Limping is subconscious, and simply telling him not to limp will not help. You must constantly supervise the walking (and subsequent running), looking for limping or any

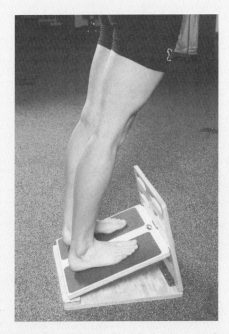

FIGURE 14.6. Achilles tendon (heel cord) stretching is indicated if the patient lacks dorsiflexion.

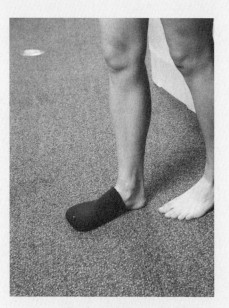

FIGURE 14.7. Walking begins with baby steps (heel to toe as shown) and progresses to medium-length steps and then to large steps.

other unnatural gait pattern. If limping persists, work with him to eliminate it.

(b) If the limb is sufficiently numbed and he still experiences pain during walking or running, he is not ready for this level of activity and should return to a former activity level (short-step walking or weight-bearing ROM).

(c) Limping can also occur if the patient has one shoe on and one off; be sure both shoes are off before the patient begins to walk.

e. Strengthening the ankle muscles

i. Perform inversion, eversion, and dorsiflexion on an ankle machine (Fig. 14.8) or with a weighted boot, using the daily

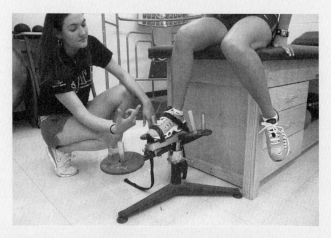

FIGURE 14.8. Resistive ankle strengthening begins as soon as the patient can walk. Ankle strengthening is done without numbness, after a cryokinetic session. (Courtesy of Jody Brucker.)

adjustable progressive resistive exercise (DAPRE) technique.[9,10] Plantar flexion exercises on a weight machine are not necessary. Walking and normal toe raises are adequate to develop plantar flexion strength.

ii. Perform the muscle-strengthening exercises once a day, after one of the cryokinetic sessions. Using cold applications before or during weight training is unnecessary.

f. Jogging

i. Once the patient can walk briskly, with turns and without pain or limping, gradually increase speed until he is jogging. Initial jogging should be slow and straight ahead. As tolerance increases, progress to jogging in a lazy S or figure-eight pattern, then a sharp Z pattern.

ii. A hallway is a convenient location for jogging. The patient can begin the S pattern jogging with large sweeps from side to side in the hallway (Fig. 14.9). The S is gradually tightened until the pattern is a sharp Z. Progress to sprinting, hopping, and jogging.

g. Hopping and jumping (performed simultaneously with sprinting)

i. Any type of hopping and jumping is acceptable, as long as it is pain free. We like the *four-square program*[11] because it provides excellent guidelines for progressing through hopping and jumping with increasing complexity (Fig. 14.10). Make a large plus sign (+) on the floor with adhesive tape. Instruct (and demonstrate if necessary) the patient to jump from square to square (delineated by the plus sign) in the following progression, as tolerated: both feet forward and back, side to side, then diagonally; one foot (injured) forward and back, side to side, then diagonally. Progress from short, shallow hops to long, high hops.

ii. After the patient has mastered the four-square program, have him hop on the injured foot back and forth across a crack, a taped line, or an imaginary line in the floor while progressing forward across the room (Fig. 14.11).

h. Sprinting (performed simultaneously with hopping and jumping)

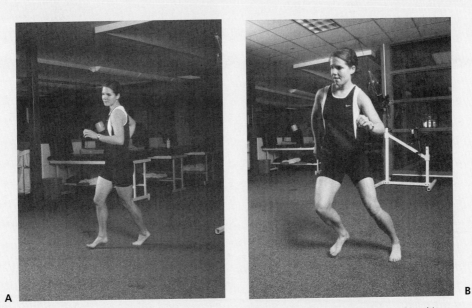

A   B

FIGURE 14.9. Jogging begins slowly and straight ahead. It progresses to **(a)** lazy S and **(b)** sharp Z patterns. Speed increases until the patient is jogging.

i. Begin with short (5–10 yd.) straight-ahead, slow sprints. Start and stop slowly at first, then progress gradually to distinct starts and stops (e.g., an explosive push-off and stopping on a dime).

ii. Progress to sprinting in a lazy S or figure-eight pattern, then in a sharp Z pattern.

i. Hopping and sprinting without ice numbing.

Gradually increase the duration of hopping, jumping, and sprinting beyond the period of numbing until the patient can perform these activities without the aid of numbing.

j. Ankle taping

i. The ankle should be taped during the following phases of team drills and practices (Fig. 14.12). During earlier phases of cryokinetic exercising, the ankle need

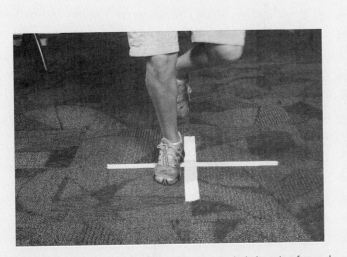

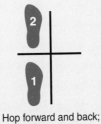

Hop forward and back;
1 - 2 - 1 - 2, etc.

Hop side to side;
1 - 2 - 1 - 2, etc.

Hop four square;
1 - 2 - 3 - 4 -1, etc.
1 - 4 - 3 - 2 -1, etc.

Hop forward and back;
1 - 2 - 3 - 1, etc.
1 - 3 - 2 - 1, etc.

Hop side to side;
1 - 2 - 3 - 1, etc.
1 - 3 - 2 - 1, etc.

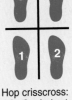

Hop crisscross:
1 - 2 - 3 - 4 -1, etc.
1 - 4 - 3 - 2 -1, etc.

FIGURE 14.10. Four-square hopping exercises include hopping forward and back, side to side, in a square, and diagonally—first using both feet and then using only the injured foot. Patients should perform the exercises in the order given here, mastering each exercise before performing the next exercise.

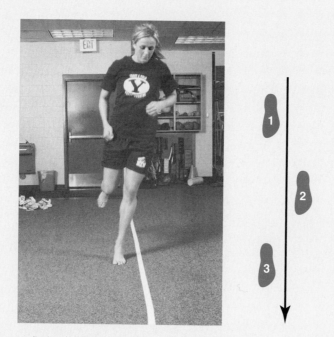

FIGURE 14.11. A line-hopping exercise involves hopping back and forth across a center line, on the injured foot, while progressing forward.

not—in fact, *should not*—be taped. The earlier exercises are performed indoors, on a smooth surface (such as a hall floor) where there is little chance of reinjury.

ii. Taping is unnecessary; in fact, it will interfere with treatment. If you tape the ankle before numbing, the tape will insulate the ankle and thereby reduce the effects of the ice. If you tape the ankle after numbing it, you will waste valuable exercising time. You only have 2–3 min of numbness to work with.

k. Team drills

i. Team drills are a natural progression from hopping, jumping, and sprinting.

Begin them at half speed, then progress to three-quarter speed, and finally to full speed (Fig. 14.13).

ii. As with all aspects of cryokinetics, pay particular attention during team drills and practice to how the patient performs. All activities must be performed with proper mechanics. Any pain, hesitancy, or irregular movement indicates he is not ready for the complexity of the

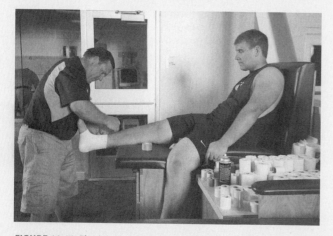

FIGURE 14.12. The injury should be taped once the patient progresses beyond sprinting drills in a hallway or gym.

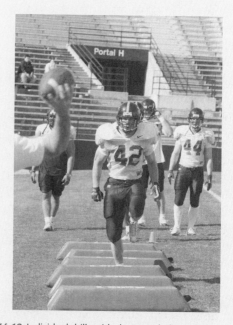

FIGURE 14.13. Individual drills with the team help patients progress beyond running and improve their mental state.

activity. In that case, have him perform at a lower level for a while.

   iii. Patients who are not fully rehabilitated must be protected while performing reduced-intensity team drills. One way of doing so is to have them wear an off-color jersey so they are easily distinguished by coaches and teammates. (Red or green jerseys are good colors to use, as long as they are not the school colors.) This reminds coaches and teammates that the injured athlete should be treated carefully. Excessive aggression by either a teammate or the recovering athlete himself in response to an overly demanding coach might cause reinjury.

   l. Team practice. Begin at reduced speed and intensity the first day and progress to full speed, complexity, and intensity as quickly as possible.

  8. A complete cryokinetic session consists of:
   a. 10–20 min ice application for initial numbness
   b. Five exercise bouts with numbness in between
   c. Each exercise bout consists of active exercises during the numbness (~3 min)

B. Dosage
  1. Exercise as vigorously as possible but within the limits of pain.
  2. Most new clinicians will not encourage their patients to progress as rapidly as possible.

C. Length of application. Five exercise bouts per treatment session

D. Frequency of application. Two or three times per day.

E. Duration of therapy. Until patient returns to full, unhindered activity.

STEP 4: POSTAPPLICATION TASKS

A. Instructions to the patient
  1. Instruct the patient to use whatever supportive devices (elastic wrap, crutches, sling, etc.) that were used before the treatment. Many patients will have a false sense of security because of the numbing; they may feel no pain during activities of daily living while undergoing treatment, but once the joint fully rewarms, such activities may be painful. Our rule of thumb is that patients should leave with the same joint support they came with. If after a few hours the support is not needed, the patient can discontinue using it.
  2. Instruct the patient about the level of activity and/or self-treatment before the next formal treatment.
  3. Explain that the patient might feel pain in 4–8 hr. If so, apply an ice pack for 30 min.
  4. Schedule the next treatment.

B. Record of treatment, including unique patient responses

C. Area cleanup
  1. Put away the ice container, towel, etc.
  2. Wipe up any water from the floor

STEP 5: MAINTENANCE

A. Replace the slush container when it cracks.
B. Sew the sides of the toe caps if they rip.

Application of Cryostretch for Muscle Injuries

STEP 1: FOUNDATION

A. Definition. **Cryostretch** includes three techniques: cold application, static stretching, and the hold–relax technique of proprioceptive neuromuscular facilitation (PNF).[12] It is used after muscle strains to increase flexibility by decreasing muscle spasm (Fig. 14.14).

B. Effects
  1. Ice decreases pain and muscle spasm.
  2. Static stretching overcomes the stretch reflex, thereby reducing muscle spasm.
  3. A muscle or muscle group will often relax after a near-maximal contraction to a state of relaxation greater than was achieved before the contraction.

C. Advantages

  1. Combining the three techniques (icing, static stretching, and contraction–relaxing) in one procedure is more effective than applying any of the techniques independently.
  2. Ice is inexpensive, and exercise is free.

D. Disadvantages
  1. Ice is sometimes painful to some people, but the techniques used with cryostretch (ice massage and ice bag) are not as painful as ice immersion, which is preferred with cryokinetics.
  2. Melting ice can be messy.

E. Indications
  1. Any muscle with residual, low-grade muscle spasm.

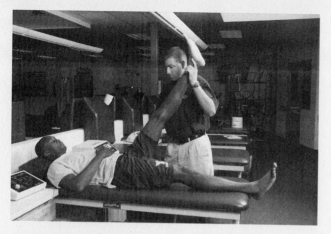

FIGURE 14.14. A hamstring is statically stretched as part of a cryostretch treatment.

2. Any first-degree muscle strain.
3. A muscle that is stiff from prolonged disuse (immobilization). Do not confuse this with decreased ROM owing to connective tissue contractures. Cryostretch is contraindicated for the latter.

F. Contraindications
1. Any exercise or activity that causes pain.
2. Use of ice on a person who is hypersensitive to cold (see Chapter 5).
3. Decreased ROM owing to connective tissue contractures.

G. Precautions
1. Pain must be used as a guideline. The patient should not consciously or willfully overcome or gut out the pain.
2. There may be an increase in pain 4–8 hr after treatment.
3. Tearing or pulling a muscle is a possibility if the static exercise begins too quickly or suddenly. It must be a gradual buildup to a maximal contraction.

STEP 2: PREAPPLICATION TASKS

See step 2 for "Application of Cryokinetics for Joint Sprain" (earlier in this chapter).

STEP 3: APPLICATION PARAMETERS

A. Procedures
1. Apply ice to the injured muscle(s) by:
   a. Ice massage (with 6–8 oz ice cubes or ice pop) (see Figs. 14.2 and 14.3)
   b. Ice bag (crushed ice in a plastic bag)
   c. Ice pack (commercial gel pack)
2. Continue the ice application until the body part is numb (10–20 min).
   a. The goal is numbness, not 10–20 min of application.

b. Some people, however, cannot judge when they are numb. Therefore, stop the application after 20 min, whether or not the patient reports numbness.
3. Stretch the muscle(s), as explained later in this step, for as long as numbness remains (~3 min).
4. Reapply the ice until numbness is again reached (3–5 min).
5. A complete treatment consists of three bouts of stretching alternating with ice and numbness. Each stretching bout consists of two 60-sec sets of stretching (Box 14.1).
6. Both stretching and the ice result in muscle relaxation, but the stretching is more important than the ice.
7. Each set of stretching consists of passive stretching and static contraction of the muscle(s) needing to be relaxed, as follows:
   a. (Part of the first bout only.) Help the patient get the feel of using the affected muscle by actively contacting it and moving the appropriate joint through as great a range of motion as possible (Fig. 14.15). Offer no resistance—this is demonstration only. Repeat the motion two or three times, making sure the affected muscle performs the majority of the work.
   b. Passively stretch the muscle by moving the affected limb until the patient begins to feel tightness and/or pain. If pain is felt, back off just slightly.
   c. Hold the position for 20 sec.
   d. Explain to the patient that in a few moments you will tell her to contract the muscle. At this time:
      i. She attempts to perform the same motion that she practiced earlier.
      ii. Explain that no motion will be possible, however, because you will be holding the limb/body part to resist the motion.

BOX 14.1 *A SUMMARIZED CRYOSTRETCH EXERCISE SET*

- Static stretch: 20 sec
- Isometric contraction: 5 sec
- Static stretch: 10 sec
- Isometric contraction: 5 sec
- Static stretch: 10 sec
- Isometric contraction: 5 sec
- Static stretch: 10 sec

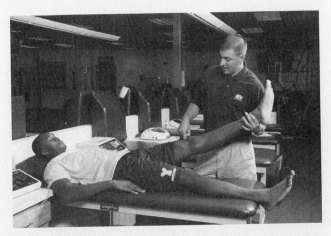

FIGURE 14.15. Before the first exercise bout, the patient must learn to contract the proper muscle.

   iii. State: "Do not contract the muscle quickly or suddenly." Emphasize that the contraction must start slowly and build up to a maximal contraction.
   e. The patient contracts the affected muscle for 5 sec, beginning slowly and building up to a maximal contraction while you resist the movement (it should be an isometric contraction).
   f. The patient relaxes the contraction. You then move the limb until she feels tightness and/or pain. (The ROM should be greater than in step b.) Hold this passive stretch for 10 sec.
   g. Repeat steps d–f twice more.
   h. Return the limb to the anatomical position and rest for 20 sec.
   i. Perform the second bout of stretching by repeating steps b–g.
8. A complete cryostretch session consists of:
   a. 10–20 min ice application for initial numbness
   b. Three exercise bouts with numbness in between (see Box 14.1).

   c. Each exercise bout consists of two 65 sec sets of passive stretch and isometric contractions, with a 20 sec rest between sets.
B. Dosage. Stretch as much as possible but within the limits of pain.
C. Length of application. Three exercise bouts per treatment session
D. Frequency of application. Two or three times per day
E. Duration of therapy. Until the muscle spasm or tightness diminishes. At that point, transition into a combination of cryostretch and cryokinetics.

4 STEP 4: **POSTAPPLICATION TASKS**

A. Instructions to the patient
   1. Instruct the patient to use whatever supportive devices (elastic wrap, crutches, sling, etc.) as were used before the treatment. Many patients will have a false sense of security because of the numbing; they may feel no pain during activities of daily living while undergoing treatment, but once the joint fully rewarms, such activities may be painful. Our rule of thumb is that patients should leave with the same joint support they came with. If after a few hours the support is not needed, the patient can discontinue using it.
   2. Instruct the patient about the level of activity and/or self-treatment before the next formal treatment.
   3. Explain that the patient might feel pain in 4–8 hr. If so, apply an ice pack for 30 min.
   4. Schedule the next treatment
B. Record of treatment, including unique patient responses
C. Area cleanup
   1. Put away the ice container, towel, etc.
   2. Wipe up any water from the floor.

5 STEP 5: **MAINTENANCE**

None

Application of Combined Cryostretch and Cryokinetics

5 STEPS

A. This combination of modalities is used to treat muscle strains once spasm is relieved and joint ROM is within 90% of normal.
B. Administer the same as for cryostretch, *except:*
   1. During the second set of the first stretching bout, after the initial 20 sec stretch, the patient performs 6–10 repetitions of full ROM contraction against manual resistance.
   2. The patient performs only one set during each of the second and third exercise bouts. This set is the same as the second set of the first bout—that is, a 20 sec passive stretch followed by 6–10 full ROM repetitions against manual resistance.
C. Encourage the patient to work hard during the muscle contraction, especially at the end of the ROM.
D. Once the strength begins to return (2–4 days), switch the patient to some type of isotonic weight lifting, preferably using the DAPRE technique.[9,10]

Application of Connective Tissue Stretch

STEP 1: FOUNDATION

A. Definition. The **connective tissue stretch** is a combination of heat application, long-term passive stretch, and cold applications (Fig. 14.16). It is used to increase joint flexibility after prolonged immobilization during which connective tissue contractures have developed.

B. Effects
1. Heat causes collagen fibers to relax.
2. Stretch lengthens the collagen fibers.
3. Cold causes the collagen fibers to reattach in a lengthened position if the stretch is held.[12]

C. Advantages
1. Heat applications minimize collagen tearing by inducing fiber relaxation.
2. Cold applications cause the fiber to reform in a lengthened position, thus preserving the gains made during stretching.
3. Minimal equipment needed.

D. Disadvantages. The 30 min of stretching is boring

E. Indications. Reduced joint flexibility owing to immobilization

F. Contraindications
1. Any exercise or activity that causes pain
2. Use of ice on a person who is hypersensitive to cold

G. Precautions. Avoid pain during stretching; it usually occurs because resistance is too great.

H. Alternatives. Thermal ultrasound or diathermy and mobilization (see Chapters 15 and 16)

STEP 2: PREAPPLICATION TASKS

See step 2 for "Application of Cryokinetics for Joint Sprain" (earlier in this chapter).

STEP 3: APPLICATION PARAMETERS

A. Procedures
1. Heat the injured joint for 10–30 min, depending on the modality used:
   a. Shortwave pulsed diathermy is preferred for heating large areas.
   b. Use moist hot packs if diathermy is unavailable.
      i. Apply the hot packs to both sides if it is a large joint.
      ii. Change the hot packs after 15 min to compensate for their cooling.
2. Stretch the joint with a low-level continuous passive force for 15 min.
   a. Begin stretching after 15 min of heating (Fig. 14.17)
   b. Use an external force such as 3–15 lb of weight. Manual resistance is unacceptable because it ties up a clinician for 15 min, it is quite tiring for the clinician, and a clinician will not be able to provide consistent constant pressure.
   c. There is no specific way to apply the resistance. Use your ingenuity. Attach one end of a rope or cord to the limb and the other end to the weight. Then place the rope over a fulcrum so the weight hangs down (Fig. 14.17).
3. Discontinue heating and begin cooling the joint while maintaining the stretch. The collagen fibers that detached during the heating will reattach during cooling. If the joint is held in the stretched position during reattachment, the fibers will reattach in a lengthened position.

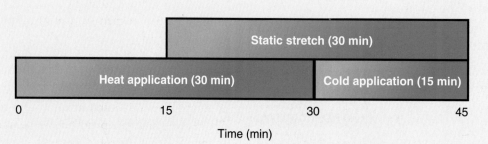

FIGURE 14.16. An outline of the connective tissue stretch. Note the timing, length of, and interaction among the three elements: heating, static stretch, and cooling.

B. Dosage. Use as much resistance as is comfortable.

C. Length of application. For 45 min

D. Frequency of application. Daily

E. Duration of therapy. For 1–2 weeks

STEP 4: POSTAPPLICATION TASKS

A. Instructions to the patient
   1. Schedule the next treatment
   2. Instruct the patient about the level of activity and/or self-treatment before the next formal treatment.

B. Record of treatment, including unique patient responses

C. Equipment removal

STEP 5: MAINTENANCE

None

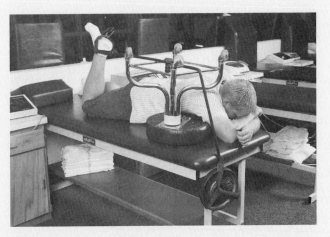

FIGURE 14.17. The quadriceps is statically stretched during a connective tissue stretch treatment.

Application of Lymphedema Pumps

STEP 1: FOUNDATION

A. Definition. **Lymphedema pumps** (known formerly as *intermittent compression pumps, cold compression devices, pneumatic compression pumps,* and *intermittent compression devices*) are pumps attached to a boot or sleeve that forces air or water (usually chilled water) into the sleeve. The boot or sleeve is fitted around a joint so that when it inflates, it applies pressure to the joint (Fig. 14.18). A timing mechanism turns the pump on and off so the sleeve alternates inflating and deflating, thus providing intermittent compression. Classified as:
   1. Pneumatic (air)
   2. Cryocompression (chilled water)

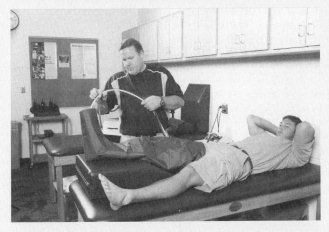

FIGURE 14.18. A lymphedema pump helps reduce swelling by forcing tissue debris from the injured tissue via the lymphatic system.

   3. Circumferential (all at once)
   4. Sequential (distal to proximal)

B. Effects
   1. The changes in sleeve pressure force lymphatic and venous drainage and thus reduces edema. Permanent reduction of edema occurs only after free protein from cellular debris is removed from the tissue and capillary filtration pressure is normalized (see Chapter 4).
   2. Both the lymphatic system and the venous system contain one-way valves that allow contents to move proximally but block distal movement.

C. Advantages. Requires minimal clinician time

D. Disadvantages
   1. The slow rate of boot or sleeve inflation
   2. The rate of compression is much faster with either active exercise or massage.

E. Indications
   1. Posttraumatic edema
   2. Postoperative edema
   3. Chronic edema; primary and secondary lymphedema
   4. Venous stasis ulcers
   5. Persistent swelling caused by venous insufficiency

F. Contraindications. Intermittent compression should not be applied to a patient suffering from the following conditions (it could aggravate the condition):
   1. Compartment syndrome
   2. Peripheral vascular disease

3. Arteriosclerosis
4. Deep vein thrombosis
5. Local superficial infection
6. Edema secondary to congestive heart failure
7. Ischemic vascular disease
8. Gangrene
9. Dermatitis
10. Acute pulmonary edema
11. Displaced fractures

G. Precautions. Pain must be used as a guideline.
H. Alternatives
1. Active muscle activity
2. Massage

2 STEP 2: PREAPPLICATION TASKS

See step 2 for "Application of Cryokinetics for Joint Sprain" (earlier in this chapter).

3 STEP 3: APPLICATION PARAMETERS

A. Procedures
1. Apply the sleeve or boot to the extremity and tighten it so it is snug but doesn't apply pressure to the limb.
2. Attach the sleeve tube to the pump.
3. If using a water device, fill the water container with ice and water.
4. Select on and off times.
5. Turn on the device.

B. Dosage
1. Inflation pressure
    a. Between 40 and 60 mm Hg for upper extremity
    b. Between 60 and 100 mm Hg for lower extremity, but no greater than the patient's diastolic pressure
2. On–off time sequence (45–15 sec; 3:1 duty cycle)
C. Length of application. For 20 min
D. Frequency of application. Two or three times per day
E. Duration of therapy. Until the condition is resolved

4 STEP 4: POSTAPPLICATION TASKS

A. Instructions to the patient
1. Schedule the next treatment
2. Instruct the patient about the level of activity and/or self-treatment before the next formal treatment.
B. Record of treatment, including unique patient responses
C. Area cleanup
    a. Equipment removal
    b. Clean the inside of the cuff or boot with a disinfectant

5 STEP 5: MAINTENANCE:

Periodically check hoses, valves, boots, and sleeves for leaks.

CLOSING SCENE

You're attempting to use cryokinetics on Andrew 48 hr after an ankle sprain. Because this is his first time receiving ice immersion, you gently immerse his ankle in the water. As described in the opening scene, within about 5 sec he pulls his leg from the water and yells, "This is too cold!" You now know some strategies to use to help him complete the treatment:

- *Use a toe cap.*
- *Explain that using cryokinetics will get him back in 2–4 days (several times faster than using traditional heat treatments).*
- *Assure him that subsequent treatments will be much less painful.*
- *Explain that he will soon adapt to the cold.*
- *Talk to him about anything to take his mind off of the pain, such as asking him about his family or his studies.*

Andrew places his ankle back in the slush; and after about 18 min, he informs you that his ankle feels numb. He then goes through several sessions of weight bearing, gentle walking, and renumbing. He returns twice a day for cryokinetics and a week later plays in a basketball game, in which he scores the winning basket. He thanks you for your wisdom and gives you the game ball.

CHAPTER REFLECTIONS

1. Read and ponder each of the following points. Do you feel you have a clear understanding of each concept? If not, reread the appropriate section of the chapter.

   • Discuss the use of ice water immersion in transitional acute care. Explain how it is different from crushed ice packs and why this is important to this stage of rehabilitation.

   • Explain when and how ice massage is used in transitional acute care.

   • Discuss the use of cryokinetics for joint sprain rehabilitation, including what it is, why it is used and a brief overview of how to apply the therapy.

   • Discuss the use of cryostretch for muscle injury rehabilitation, including what it is, why it is used and a brief overview of how to apply the therapy.

   • Explain why and when you should use combined cryostretch and cryokinetics.

   • Discuss the use of connective tissue stretch in rehabilitation, including what kinds of injuries would you use this technique with and how you would apply it.

   • Discuss why, when, and how you would use intermittent compression during rehabilitation.

2. Write three to five questions for discussion with your class instructor, clinical instructor, classmates, and clinical colleagues.

3. Get together with classmates and quiz each other on the concepts of this chapter. Use the points in exercise 1 and questions you wrote for exercise 2 as a beginning. Explaining concepts out loud to others requires a deeper grasp of the material than feeling you understand it as you read.

4. Once you feel you understand the principles of application of cryokinetics, cryostretch, connective tissue stretch, and intermittent compression treatments, practice applying them using the five-step approach with a classmate or clinical colleague. Alternate applying the modalities to each other. When it is being applied to you, listen and observe carefully to determine whether your classmate is using proper application. Consult your notes when the modality is applied to you and for the first few times you apply the modality to another person. Continue practicing the application until you can do so without using your notes.

REFERENCES

1. Jutte LS, Konz S. A 15 min immersion in 1°C water produces greater numbness than immersion in 4°C or 10°C water. J Athl Train: In review.
2. Carman KW, Knight KL. Habituation to cold-pain during repeated cryokinetic sessions. J Athl Train 1992;27:223–230.
3. Tovell J. Ice immersion toe cap. Athl Train 1980;15:33.
4. Nimchick PSR, Knight KL. Effects of wearing a toe cap or a sock on temperature and perceived pain during ice water immersion. Athl Train 1983;18:144–147.
5. Streator SS, Ingersoll CD, Knight KL. The effects of sensory information on the perception of cold-induced pain. J Athl Train 1995; 30:293–296.
6. Rogers J. Increased pressure of application during ice massage results in an increase in calf skin numbing. Master's thesis, Brigham Young University, 2000.
7. Knight KL. Ankle rehabilitation with cryotherapy. Physician Sportsmed 1979;7:133.
8. McCluskey GM, Blackburn TA Jr, Lewis T. A treatment for ankle sprains. Am J Sports Med 1976;4:158–161.
9. Knight KL. Knee rehabilitation by the daily adjustable progressive resistive exercise technique. Am J Sports Med 1979;7:336–337.
10. Knight KL. Quadriceps strengthening with the DAPRE technique: Case studies with neurological implications. Med Sci Sports Exerc 1985;17:646–650.
11. Toomey SJ. Four-square ankle rehabilitation exercises. Physician Sportsmed 1986;14(3):81.
12. Knight KL. Cryostretch for muscle injuries. Physician Sportsmed 1980;8:126.

Therapeutic Ultrasound

OPENING SCENE

During a clinical rotation, Nancy, an athletic training student, overhears some patients talking about previous ultrasound treatments they experienced. One says, "I don't think ultrasound works—I mean, I never feel anything." Another responds, "You're not supposed to feel anything during an ultrasound treatment, at least that's what I've heard." The third replies, "I feel some heat when my knee tendon is treated, but not when my low back is treated." They see Nancy and direct their questions to her. What should she tell them?

Introducing Therapeutic Ultrasound

Ultrasound is one of the most commonly used modalities by athletic trainers, physical therapists, occupational therapists and chiropractors, typically employed to bring about deep heating (Fig. 15.1). It is one of the most misunderstood and, therefore, one of the most misused modalities. When placed in the hands of a competent clinician, it can provide positive outcomes; however, when used improperly, there are few benefits from this modality.

ORIGINS AND USE IN MEDICAL PRACTICE

Before World War II, German scientists were experimenting with sonar in submarines. Sound was emitted from the vessel to detect objects in the surrounding water. The scientists noticed that fish were destroyed in the process. Thus the idea of ultrasound producing biological effects was born.

In the health professions, ultrasound is used for a number of different purposes: for the destruction of tissue, for diagnosing fetal development, and as a therapeutic agent.

Ultrasound has been used to destroy tumors in the breast, liver, kidney, pancreas, abdomen, pelvis, uterus, and lungs (some treatments use a combination of chemotherapy and ultrasound).[1] Ultrasound has been used during surgery as recently as 2002 to seal air leaks in the lungs, destroy blood clots, obliterate kidney stones, and seal blood vessels. Experiments are under way in using ultrasound for male sterilization[2] and for treating some brain disorders.[3] In pregnant women, diagnostic ultrasound can be used to monitor the development of the fetus and determine its gender. Ultrasound is also used in plastic surgery, to heat and soften fat pockets under the eyes and chin before liposuction.[4] These various applications use ultrasound with very different characteristics; in this chapter we are concerned only with ultrasound for treating musculoskeletal injuries.

Clinical Therapeutic Ultrasound

Therapeutic **ultrasound** is inaudible, acoustic vibrations of high frequency that produce thermal and/or nonthermal physiologic effects. It is not a form of electromagnetic energy. It is a valuable tool for the rehabilitation of many different injuries, primarily for the purpose of stimulating the repair of soft tissue injuries and relieving pain.[5] Although ultrasound has effects on both normal and damaged tissues, damaged tissue may be more responsive to ultrasound than is normal tissue.[6]

The primary advantage of ultrasound over other nonacoustic heating modalities is that tissues high in collagen—such as tendons, muscles, ligaments, joint capsules, joint menisci, intermuscular interfaces, nerve roots, periosteum, and cortical bone—and other deep tissues may be selectively heated to a therapeutic range without causing a significant tissue temperature increase in skin or fat.[7,8]

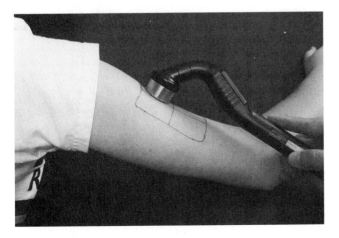

FIGURE 15.1. Ultrasound treatment of the biceps muscle.

MODALITY MYTH

WHIRLPOOL, PARAFFIN BATHS, AND HOT PACKS ARE JUST AS EFFECTIVE FOR HEAT TREATMENTS AS ULTRASOUND

Warm whirlpools, paraffin baths, and silica gel hot packs all produce therapeutic heat, but their depth of penetration is superficial—at best only 1–2 cm.[9] At 1 cm below the fat surface, a 4 min warm whirlpool (105°F [40.6°C]) raises the temperature 2.0°F (1.1°C).[10] At this same depth, 3 MHz ultrasound increases the temperature >10.8°F (6°C).[11,12] For deep heating, use an ultrasound device.

Components of an Ultrasound Device

An ultrasound device is made up of four main parts: generator, crystal, soundhead, and applicator.

THE GENERATOR

The largest part of an ultrasound device is the generator. It is typically a rectangular box consisting of a high-frequency electrical generator linked through an oscillator circuit and a transformer. The oscillator circuit produces a specific frequency electrical current at the frequency requirements of the crystal. A coaxial cable connects the generator to the crystal, which is housed in an insulated applicator handle.

The generator also houses a control panel with buttons or switches that regulate the following parameters: on–off, power, time, intensity, duty cycle, continuous or pulsed mode, 1 or 3 MHz frequency, and automatic shutoff if the crystal overheats.

THE CRYSTAL

The crystal is a thin (2–3 mm thick) synthetic ceramic, usually made of lead zirconate or titanate. Decades ago, most ultrasound crystals were made of quart;, but quartz is expensive, and does not produce a uniform beam. Thus the crystals used today are ceramic.

The **crystal** is a transducer that converts electrical energy to acoustic energy through mechanical deformation of the crystal. When an alternating electrical current is passed through the crystal, it expands and contracts, creating what is referred to as the **piezoelectric effect**. There are two forms:

- *Direct piezoelectric effect:* The creation of an electrical voltage across a substance (the crystal) as it is compressed or expanded

- *Reverse piezoelectric effect:* An effect created from an alternating current running through a crystal, resulting in compression or expansion of the crystal (Fig. 15.2)

 The expansion and contraction of the crystal creates a vibration at the frequency of the electrical oscillation received from the generator. The vibration of the crystal causes the soundhead to vibrate and results in the mechanical production of high-frequency sound waves.

THE SOUNDHEAD

The **soundhead** transfers the acoustic energy (sound waves) from the crystal to the tissues, where it causes the tissue to vibrate (Fig. 15.3). It is a ceramic, aluminum, or stainless-steel plate attached to the crystal. Stainless-steel soundheads last longer than do those made of aluminum or ceramic and are, therefore, one of the features of higher-quality ultrasound devices. Imagine the beating that the soundhead takes as a crystal expands and contracts at a speed of 1–3 million times per second.

Soundheads and crystals are manufactured to be matched to a particular generator, so they are generally not interchangeable among generators. Recently, however, dual-frequency crystals and soundheads have become standard equipment on ultrasound devices, so clinicians have a greater choice of treatment parameters.

MODALITY MYTH

THE SOUNDHEAD IS A TRANSDUCER

Many clinicians, scientists, and marketing people refer to the soundhead as a transducer. This is incorrect because a **transducer** is a device that converts variations in a physical quantity (such as pressure or brightness) into an electrical signal, or vice versa. So the crystal is a transducer that converts electricity to acoustic energy and the soundhead is a transmitter that transfers the acoustic energy to the body.

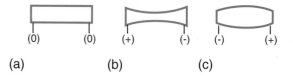

FIGURE 15.2. The contraction or expansion of a crystal is caused by passing an alternating current through it. **(a)** With no current flow, the crystal is normally shaped. **(b)** Current flow in one direction causes the crystal to become concave. **(c)** Current flow in the opposite direction causes the crystal to become convex.

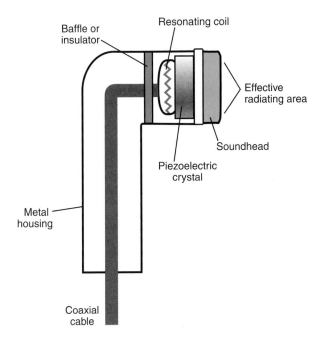

FIGURE 15.3. A typical ultrasound applicator. (Adapted with permission from Prentice WE. Therapeutic Modalities for Sports Medicine and Athletic Training. 5th ed. New York. McGraw Hill, 2003.)

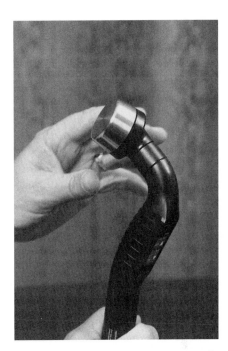

FIGURE 15.4. An applicator with a 360° rotating soundhead enables the clinician to hold the wrist in a neutral position. Notice the convenient location of the control buttons on the handle.

THE APPLICATOR

The applicator, which is the housing for the crystal and soundhead, is a device that facilitates application of the ultrasound to patients (see Fig. 15.3). The soundhead must be in constant motion during treatment, so the design of the applicator is important. It should allow the clinician to keep the wrist and hand in a neutral position, to avoid a repetitive stress injury, especially because clinicians often give several ultrasound treatments a day (Box 15.1.).

BOX 15.1 *A USER-FRIENDLY APPLICATOR*

Because some ultrasound treatments may take >10 min, it is important that the applicator fits comfortably in your hand. Ergonomics is very important, and some manufacturers of ultrasound devices have hired design engineers to create a user-friendly applicator for clinicians. The result is a transducer with a 360° rotating soundhead so that the wrist can always be held in a neutral position. Fig. 15.4 shows an ultrasound applicator with a rotating soundhead and control buttons on the handle. This makes it possible for the clinician to increase or decrease the intensity without having to look over to the generator switches and lose eye contact with the treatment area.

The applicator is usually made of a hard, insulated plastic. Some newer applicators also have controls on them so the clinician can vary the treatment characteristics during the treatment.

The Physics of Ultrasound

Now that you have been introduced to the components of an ultrasound device, let's explore the physics behind how ultrasound works.

WHAT IS SOUND?

Solids and liquids are made of molecules held together by forces that act like rubber bands, connecting each molecule to its next-door neighbor. When a force acts on one molecule, it causes it to vibrate back and forth a small distance from its original position. This movement causes the molecule next door to vibrate, and eventually the whole neighborhood is set in motion. This vibrational energy travels over millions of molecules in the tissue. This transfer or spreading of vibrational motion is basically what sound is. Unlike electromagnetic energy, which travels most effectively through a vacuum, acoustic energy is transmitted by molecules bumping against each other. As stated earlier, ultrasound is a mechanical wave in which energy is passed by the vibrations of the molecules of a biological medium through which the wave is traveling.

The human ear can hear sound waves that vibrate 16,000–20,000 times per second. Sound waves that vibrate faster than the human ear can hear are termed *ultrasound*. Therapeutic ultrasound ranges from 750,000 to 3 million vibrations per second (0.75–3.0 MHz). If the wavelength of the sound is larger than the source that produced it, then the sound will spread in all directions.[13] Such is the case with audible sound, thus explaining why it is possible for a person behind you to hear your voice almost as well as a person in front of you. In the case of therapeutic ultrasound, the sound is less divergent, and energy is concentrated in a limited area.

TYPES OF WAVES

Imagine you are at the beach and decide to go for a swim in the ocean. As you swim out from the shore, waves crash against you and push you back. Ultrasound has a similar effect on tissues as the sound waves travel through them.

Waves travel through solids in two ways: as longitudinal and as transverse waves. In a **longitudinal wave**, molecular displacement or vibration is along the direction in which the wave travels (somewhat like a stretched Bungee cord). In a **transverse wave**, the molecules are transferred, or vibrate, in a direction perpendicular to that in which the wave is traveling.

Within a longitudinal wave pathway, there are regions of:

- **Compressions**: areas of high molecular density and high pressure as the molecules are squeezed together.
- **Rarefactions**: areas of lower molecular density as the molecules are pulled apart (Fig. 15.5).

Although longitudinal waves travel in solids and liquids, transverse waves travel only in solids. Ultrasound travels as a longitudinal wave through soft tissue. It becomes a transverse wave as it bounces back or rebounds when it hits bone. The compressions and rarefactions are similar to the squeezing together and pulling apart of a Slinky toy.

WAVE TRANSMISSION FREQUENCY

The higher the frequency of the sound waves emitted from a sound source, the less the sound will diverge (spread out), and thus a more focused beam of sound is produced. Therapeutic ultrasound produces a very focused or **collimated beam**, but not as focused as a laser beam, which has little divergence (see Chapter 19).

Whether an ultrasound wave is absorbed locally or transmitted to deeper tissues is also a function of sound frequency. In tissues of the body, ultrasound energy absorption increases as the frequency increases, thus less energy is transmitted to the deeper tissues. For example, most 3 MHz ultrasound waves are absorbed superficially and transmitted 2–3 cm deep. This amount of absorption occurs in one third the time of 1 MHz. On the other hand, 1 MHz ultrasound is absorbed deeper than 3 MHz and is transmitted up to 6 cm deep.

The majority of therapeutic ultrasound devices have a frequency between 0.75 and 3.0 MHz. Recently, low-frequency or long-wave ultrasound (45 kHz and 90 kHz) has been introduced. It is used for deep muscle heating and for phonophoresis (a technique that is discussed later in this chapter). It is thought that this frequency will provide the greatest depth of penetration in biological tissues, possibly up to 10 cm.

ATTENUATION

Ultrasound transducers produce a sound wave at a preset frequency. As this sound wave passes through various tis-

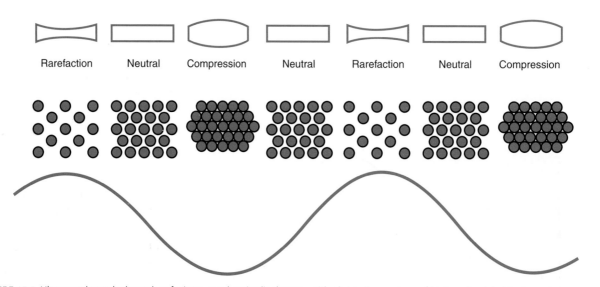

FIGURE 15.5. Ultrasound travels through soft tissue as a longitudinal wave, with alternating regions of high molecular density and pressure called *compressions* and regions of low molecular density called *rarefactions*. Thus the molecules are squeezed together and pulled apart.

sues, **attenuation,** or a decrease in energy, occurs as a result of absorption, reflection, and refraction of the wave (Fig. 15.6). Some of the energy is absorbed in the tissues. The remaining energy passes through tissues to deeper layers, where it is later absorbed, or else it bounces off tissues. This bouncing off the tissues is known as *dispersion* and *scattering* of the sound wave. When a sound wave encounters a boundary or an interface between different tissues (e.g., fascia), some of the energy will also scatter.

The ability of acoustic energy to penetrate or be transmitted to deeper tissues depends, in part, on the type of tissue being treated. In the case of therapeutic ultrasound, the following tissue types have these responses:

- *Tissue that is high in water content:* Energy penetrates easily.
- *Fat:* Energy is absorbed very little and is transmitted to deeper tissues.
- *Dense tissue that is high in protein:* Energy is absorbed well.
- *Muscle:* Energy is absorbed in high amounts.
- *Peripheral nerves:* Energy is absorbed at twice the rate as muscle.
- *Superficial bone:* Energy is absorbed more efficiently than any other type of tissue.

CRYSTAL CHARACTERISTICS

Another factor that determines how well ultrasound will penetrate tissues is the crystal quality. Some manufacturers of ultrasound devices purchase hundreds of crystals, scan each one, and throw away three out of every four that do not meet certain specifications. Crystal quality is partially determined by the effective radiating area and the beam nonuniformity ratio.

The Effective Radiating Area

The **effective radiating area (ERA)** of a soundhead is the surface area that transmits a sound wave from the crystal to the tissues. It is determined by scanning the crystal at a distance of 5 mm from the radiating surface and recording all areas producing >5% of the maximum power output found on the surface of the soundhead (Fig. 15.7).[5]

The ERA is always smaller than the crystal and soundhead; sometimes significantly smaller than the soundhead. If the manufacturer produces a device that houses a 5 cm² crystal and states that the ERA is also 5 cm², you can be sure that the individual crystal has not been scanned for quality.[14] No crystal is 100% active. This is not as big a concern as the relative sizes of the crystal and soundhead.

As we stated earlier, the size of the soundhead does not indicate the actual radiating surface. A common mistake is to assume the entire surface radiates ultrasound output. This is generally not true, particularly with the larger (10 cm²) soundheads (slightly smaller than the size of a doorknob).

There is no point in having a large soundhead with a small radiating surface because it mechanically limits the treatment in smaller areas. The ERA should match the total size of the crystal and soundhead surface as closely as possible for ease of application to various body surfaces and to maintain the most effective contact (Fig. 15.8).

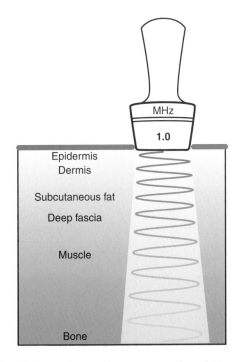

FIGURE 15.6. As an ultrasound wave passes through tissues, a decrease in energy, known as attenuation, results from the absorption, reflection, and refraction of energy. (Adapted with permission from Castel D, International Academy of Physio Therapeutics, clip art.)

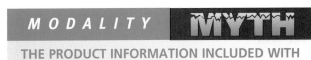

THE PRODUCT INFORMATION INCLUDED WITH ULTRASOUND DEVICES ACCURATELY LISTS THE SIZE OF THE SURFACE AREA OF THE SOUNDHEAD

Unfortunately, there is a gray area in ultrasound advertising. The majority of ultrasound devices are reported as having a 5 cm² soundhead; however, this is the size of the crystal inside the soundhead. Soundheads listed as 5 cm² have been found to have surface areas between 7 and 11 cm².[15] Thus if a soundhead surface is larger than the size of the crystal, the clinician might think a larger area is being treated than actually is. We suggest that, in the future, ultrasound manufacturers list the size of the surface area of the soundhead and the size of the crystal (Fig. 15.9).

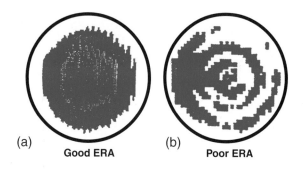

(a) **Good ERA** (b) **Poor ERA**

FIGURE 15.7. The effective radiating area (*ERA*) is the surface area of a soundhead that transmits a sound wave. **(a)** The ERA is always smaller than the soundhead because the crystal is smaller than the soundhead. **(b)** A bad crystal has dead spots, where no sound is transmitted, so its ERA is much smaller than the ERA of an equal-size good crystal. (Adapted with permission from Castel D, International Academy of Physio Therapeutics, clip art.)

The Beam Nonuniformity Ratio

Ultrasound beams are not completely uniform; they have small peaks and valleys in them. Some points are of higher intensity (peaks) than others away from the soundhead surface. The **beam nonuniformity ratio (BNR)** is an indicator of the variability of intensity within an ultrasound beam. The BNR is the ratio of the **spacial peak intensity**, highest intensity in the beam, to the **spacial average intensity (SAI)**, the average intensity across the beam, both of which are measured with an underwater microphone. For example, a BNR of 5:1 means when the average output intensity is 1 W/cm^2, the highest intensity of the beam is 5 W. Figure 15.10 shows the peaks and valleys of a beam scan of a high and low BNR.

An optimal BNR is 1:1 (a smooth line with no peaks and valleys); however, this is not possible. The BNR should fall between 2 and 5. The lower the BNR, the more

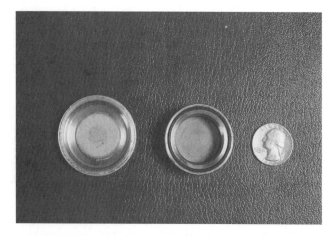

FIGURE 15.8. Note how the size of the soundhead faceplate does not determine treatment size. At the left, a quarter-size crystal is mounted to the inside of a large soundhead. In the middle, a quarter-size crystal is placed inside a medium soundhead. Ideally, the crystal and the soundhead should be close to the same size, as shown in the middle. The quarter provides a relative scale.

uniform the output and, therefore, the lower the chance of developing hot spots. A **hot spot** is an area at tissue interfaces that may become overheated from too much energy being concentrated in one area. Hot spots often result in pain, and they can damage tissues. A low BNR allows the clinician to deliver ultrasound at a higher energy level without causing discomfort to the patient.

The U.S. Food and Drug Administration (FDA) Center for Devices and Radiological Health requires that the BNR be indicated on all ultrasound devices. Manufacturers do not have to report the BNR of individual crystals, so the BNR of the soundhead being used may be different from that indicated on the label. The FDA allows companies to randomly sample their crystals and report the maximum BNR.[16] Thus a company might label their crystals as "6:1 BNR max." If a 6:1 BNR is used at an intensity of 1.5 W/cm^2, then at least one peak would be 9 W and tissue damage could occur because peak intensities of only 8 W have been shown to damage tissue.

The high peak intensities associated with high BNRs cause much of the discomfort often associated with ultrasound treatment.[17] From personal experience, this feels like a dull ache on the outer layer of the bone (*periosteal pain*). Therefore, the higher the BNR the more important it is to use lower intensities or to move the soundhead faster during treatment to avoid hot spots and areas of tissue damage.

The PAMBNR

Some ultrasound manufacturers include another aspect to the definition of BNR: the **peak area of the maximum**

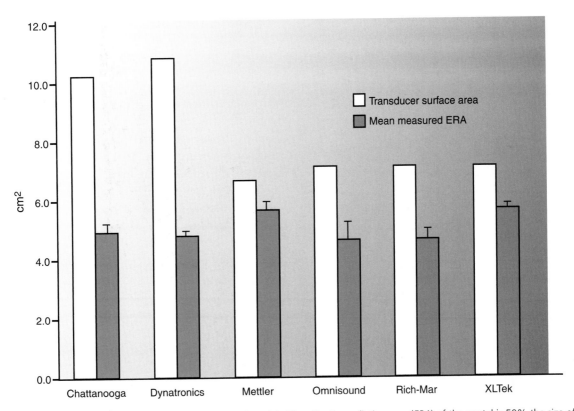

FIGURE 15.9. Note the variability that exists among ultrasound models. The effective radiating area (*ERA*) of the crystal is 50% the size of the surface of the soundhead in the first two devices. The ERA size should be closer to the transducer surface size, such as the four devices on the right. (Adapted with permission from Johns et al.[15])

BNR (PAMBNR). This concept was developed during research in which subjects reported that one of two ultrasound devices with identical BNRs (7:1) was more comfortable than the other. Why? The scientists concluded that peak intensity is only half the equation. The other half is the area of the crystal that produces the peak intensity, or the beam profile. Thus one crystal with a BNR of 7:1 over only 1 mm of the crystal will cause less discomfort than a crystal with a BNR of 7:1 over 5 mm of the crystal. This conclusion led to the concept of PAMBNR (Fig. 15.11).[18]

Other scientists have examined lateral beam profiles. So far, they believe, as we do, that nonuniform heating rates may exist even with low BNRs.[19]

As you can see, crystal quality is an important factor for ultrasound, but it is not the only factor. Box 15.2 lists the components of an optimal ultrasound device; note that crystal quality is only one criterion. Of course, having a good ultrasound device is of no value unless you use it properly, so you need to understand the correct treatment parameters.

Treatment Parameters

Can you imagine how ineffective an ice pack treatment would be if applied for only 1–2 min immediately after an acute injury? No therapeutic modality is therapeutic unless correct treatment parameters are used. Essential treat-

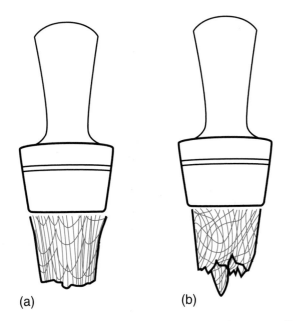

(a)   (b)

FIGURE 15.10. The BNR represented on a beam scan. The amount of intensity variability within the ultrasound beam is indicated by the BNR. **(a)** A low BNR of 2:1. **(b)** A high BNR of 6:1. (Adapted with permission from Castel D, International Academy of Physio Therapeutics, clip art.)

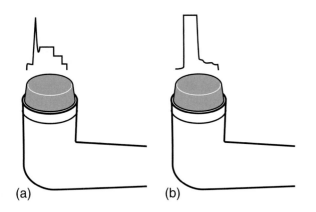

(a) (b)

FIGURE 15.11. The PAMBNR represents the size of the peak intensity. **(a)** A small PAMBNR means there is a small, if any, hot spot. **(b)** A large BNR means there is a large hot spot.

ment parameters for therapeutic ultrasound include the following:

- Mode
- Frequency
- Intensity
- Treatment length
- Treatment area size

BOX 15.2 TEN COMPONENTS OF A STATE-OF-THE-ART ULTRASOUND DEVICE

1. High-quality synthetic crystal:
   a. Low BNR ≤4:1; small PAMBNR
   b. High ERA (nearly matches the size of the soundhead)
   c. BNR and ERA scans provided by the manufacturer or distributor, not estimates
2. Multiple frequencies (1 and 3 MHz; possibly 90 kHz or lower for phonophoresis)
3. Multiple sizes of soundheads
4. Sensing device that shuts off the unit when overheating occurs
5. Insulation for underwater use
6. Input jack for combination therapy
7. Several pulsed duty cycles
8. Applicator handle that maintains the operator's wrist in a natural, relaxed position
9. Durable soundhead that will protect the crystal if dropped
10. Computer-controlled timer that makes adjustments in treatment duration as the intensity is adjusted (similar to iontophoresis, in which the treatment time adjusts according to the dose applied)

MODE

Practically all therapeutic ultrasound devices can produce either continuous or pulsed ultrasound. With **continuous ultrasound**, the sound energy remains constant throughout the treatment—that is, the ultrasound energy is produced 100% of the time (Fig. 15.12a). With **pulsed ultrasound**, the energy is periodically interrupted, and no ultrasound energy is produced during the off period (Fig. 15.12b). Pulsed ultrasound reduces the average intensity of the output over time. The term **temporal average intensity (TAI)** is used to describe the power of ultrasonic energy over a given period of time. The percentage of time that ultrasound is generated (pulse duration) over one pulse period is referred to as the **duty cycle**:

$$\text{Duty cycle} = \frac{\text{Pulse duration (on time)} \times 100}{\text{Pulse period (on time + off time)}}$$

For example, if the pulse duration is 10 msec and the total pulse period is 40 msec, the duty cycle would be 25%. Therefore, the total amount of energy delivered to the tissues would be only 25% of the energy delivered if a continuous wave were used.

> **CRITICAL THINKING 15.1** *What would be the duty cycle if the pulse duration is 20 msec and the total pulse period is 40 msec?*

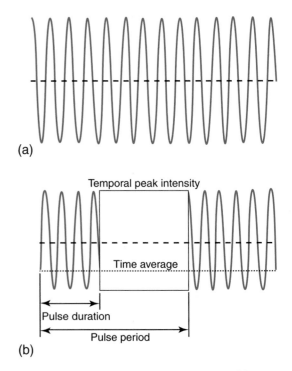

FIGURE 15.12. Ultrasound can be delivered in either **(a)** continuous mode or **(b)** pulsed mode. The temporal peak intensity is the same in both modes, but the average intensity is less in the pulsed mode. (Adapted with permission from Castel D, International Academy of Physio Therapeutics, clip art.)

Many ultrasound devices have preset duty cycles at either 20% or 50%. Some provide several optional duty cycles. Continuous ultrasound is most commonly used when thermal effects are desired, whereas pulsed ultrasound is typically used when nonthermal effects are desired. Thus pulsed ultrasound typically results in a reduced average heating of the tissues.

MODALITY MYTH

PULSED ULTRASOUND DOES NOT HEAT TISSUES

Some clinicians think that pulsed ultrasound does not produce heat. This is too simplistic, however, because heating is a function of the total energy delivered to the tissue, which in turn is a function of intensity, mode, and ERA. For example, applying the same intensity continuously over an area four times the soundhead surface area and a pulsed application at a 50% duty cycle to an area two times the soundhead area will impart the same energy. Also keeping the treatment area constant, application of ultrasound at 0.5 W/cm² continuously and application of ultrasound at 1 W/cm² pulsed 50% both impart the same energy. In a recent study we applied 3 MHz at two times the soundhead surface continuously at 0.5 W/cm², and 50% pulsed 50% at 1 W/cm². Both protocols produced peak temperature increases of nearly 5.4°F (3°C), with no statistical difference between protocols.[20] Thus pulsed ultrasound can produce heat when the average intensity is 0.5 W/cm².

FREQUENCY

Therapeutic ultrasound has a frequency range of 0.75–3.0 MHz. Most therapeutic ultrasound devices produced before 1990 were set at a frequency of 1 MHz. After 1990, several manufacturers added a 3 MHz frequency. A generator that can be set between 1 and 3 MHz provides the greatest treatment flexibility, because ultrasound frequency determines the depth of tissue penetration and the rate of tissue heating.

MODALITY MYTH

INCREASING THE ULTRASOUND POWER INCREASES THE DEPTH OF TISSUE PENETRATION

The frequency of the ultrasound determines the depth of penetration into the body's tissues. Turning up the power (intensity) simply sends more energy to the same depth.[14]

Depth of Tissue Penetration

The depth of ultrasound penetration is described in terms of the *half-value layer,* the depth by which 50% of the ultrasound beam is absorbed in tissue. Temperature effects are expected to be highest at the half-value layer and less at greater depths.[21] Thus when it is stated that 1 MHz ultrasound will go as deep as 6 cm into the tissue, according to the half-value layer principle, theoretically it will have a higher temperature at half that depth (3 cm).

When a high ultrasound frequency (such as 3 MHz) enters the tissues, some of it is absorbed superficially. The energy that has not been absorbed and used by the superficial tissues will penetrate to deeper tissues. Scientists have measured significant heat increases at 2.5 cm in human muscle.[22] Thus 3 MHz is ideal for treating superficial conditions such as plantar fasciitis, Achilles tendinitis, and epicondylitis (tennis elbow).[23]

Ultrasound energy generated at 1 MHz is transmitted through the more superficial tissues and absorbed primarily in the deeper tissues at depths of 2–6 cm (Fig. 15.13).[8,11] A 1 MHz frequency is most useful in patients with a high percentage of cutaneous body fat and whenever desired effects are in the deeper structures, such as the soleus, piriformis, and hip adductor muscles.[24] Recently low-frequency ultrasound (45 kHz and 90 kHz) has been introduced as a possible modality in orthopedic medicine. The very low frequencies will provide the greatest depth of penetration in body tissues, possibly generating ultrasound energy to deep bone.

CRITICAL THINKING 15.2 A patient is complaining of pain at the tendon just distal to the kneecap and has been diagnosed with chronic patellar tendinitis. Which frequency of ultrasound should you use to treat this condition: 1 MHz or 3 MHz?

Rate of Heating

The rate of absorption, and therefore attenuation, increases as the frequency of the ultrasound increases.[25] The 3 MHz frequency is not only absorbed more superficially but is also absorbed three times faster than 1 MHz ultrasound.[11] This faster rate of absorption results in faster peak heating in tissues. Both 45 kHz and 90 kHz ultrasound are absorbed so slowly that little or no heating occurs; therefore, these lower frequencies are used primarily for nonthermal effects. The size of the area treated also affects the amount of heating, as will be discussed later in this chapter.

INTENSITY

Power is a function of both pulse width and pulse frequency, measured in watts. **Intensity** is the rate at which energy is being delivered per unit area. Ultrasound power

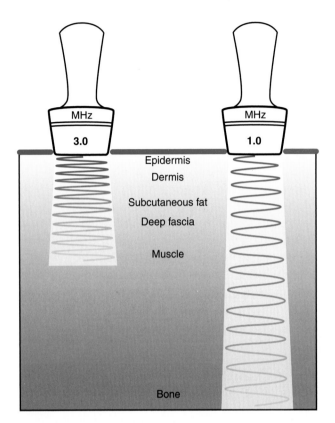

FIGURE 15.13. The depth of tissue penetration is determined by ultrasound frequency. The effects of 3 MHz occur more superficially (2.5 cm deep) than those of 1 MHz (6 cm deep). (Adapted with permission from Castel D, International Academy of Physio Therapeutics, clip art.)

and intensity are usually expressed in watts per square centimeter. Intensity is also referred to as spatial average intensity (SAI), the intensity of the ultrasound beam averaged over the area of the soundhead. It usually occurs in the central third of the ERA. SAI is calculated by dividing the power output in watts by the total effective radiating area of the sound head in square centimeters:

$$SAI = \frac{Total\ watts\ (W)}{Effective\ radiating\ area\ (cm^2)}$$

If ultrasound is produced at a power of 8 W and the ERA of the soundhead is 4 cm^2, the SAI would be 2.0 W/cm^2. On many ultrasound devices, both the power (W) and the SAI (W/cm^2) are displayed. If the power output is constant, increasing the size of the soundhead surface will decrease the SAI.

According to the World Health Organization's guidelines, an SAI of 3.0 W/cm^2 is the safe limit for therapeutic treatment. Intensities >10 W/cm^2 are used to destroy tissue surgically, whereas intensities <0.1 W/cm^2 are used for diagnostic purposes. There are no definitive guidelines for selecting specific ultrasound intensities during treatment; however, if the intensity is too high, tissue damage can occur.[13] We suggest that you use the lowest intensity possible to achieve a desired therapeutic effect.

PATIENTS DO NOT FEEL ANYTHING DURING ULTRASOUND TREATMENTS

Only when nonthermal ultrasound is being delivered with a low duty cycle and/or low intensity (low SAI) will patients not feel a thing. Thermal ultrasound treatments should feel slightly warm. Remember that each person's tolerance to heat is different, so ultrasound intensity should always be adjusted to patient tolerance.[17] At the beginning of the treatment, turn the intensity to the point at which the patient feels deep warmth, and then lower the intensity slightly until gentle heating is felt.[14] During the treatment, ask the patient for feedback and make the necessary intensity adjustments. If the patient complains that the soundhead feels hot at the skin surface, the crystal has been damaged, the soundhead is overheating, or there isn't enough ultrasound gel between the skin and the soundhead to conduct the energy into the tissues.

The goal of continuous ultrasound treatments should be a specified temperature increase. Thermal ultrasound is used to bring about certain therapeutic effects, and tissues respond according to the amount of heat they receive.[26] Therefore, any significant adjustment in the intensity should be countered with an adjustment in the treatment time. It is possible that ultrasound treatments in the future will be like iontophoresis, in which the treatment time depends on the dosage delivered (or the amount of heat absorbed by the tissues). For this reason, one manufacturer of ultrasound devices places a microchip in the generator that makes adjustments in treatment time corresponding to the operator's thermal goals of a 1.8°, 3.6°, or 7.2°F (1°, 2°, or 4°C) increase (based on research means). If the intensity is increased, treatment time is reduced; if intensity is reduced, treatment time is increased.[27] Table 15.1 shows treatment goals based on temperature increases.

TREATMENT LENGTH

In the 1980s, most textbooks stated that an ultrasound treatment should last 5–10 min. In 2006 many insurance companies would deny payment for ultrasound treatments lasting <8 min. It is a mistake to use a predetermined length for all ultrasound treatments. Setting a specific treatment length for all thermal ultrasound treatments would be as ridiculous as saying it takes exactly 3 hr to fly from Salt Lake City to Chicago. Just as travel time from city to city depends on several factors (speed, tailwind, route, size of plane), ultrasound treatment length also depends on several factors.

TABLE 15.1 *Temperature Increases Theorized to Bring About Desired Effects in Tissues*

TEMPERATURE INCREASE	EFFECT
1.8°F (1°C); mild heat	Increases metabolism, reduces mild inflammation
3.6–5.4°F (2–3°C); moderate heat	Reduces pain and muscle spasm, increases blood flow
7.2°F (4°C); vigorous heat	Increases ROM and tissue extensibility*

*This works best when heat and stretch or heat and mobilization are used in combination.
ROM, range of motion.

The length of the treatment is made according to the size of the area to be treated, the ultrasound frequency, the intensity (W/cm²), and the desired temperature increase.[14] We suggest that ultrasound be administered in an area two to three times the ERA (roughly twice the size of the soundhead surface). If you desire deep thermal effects in an area larger than this, obviously the treatment time needs to be increased or you should consider short-wave diathermy (see Chapter 16).

As stated earlier, higher ultrasound frequencies require a shorter treatment length than lower frequencies. Ultrasound at 3 MHz consistently heats tissues three times faster than 1 MHz, thus reducing the required treatment length by one third.[11,28] The lower the intensity, the longer the treatment time, and vice versa. It does not make sense to treat one patient at 1 W/cm² and another at 2 W/cm² for *identical treatment lengths* when both patients require vigorous heating. In this scenario, the second patient will experience tissue temperature increases of twice that of the first one.

Temperature Increase

The desired temperature increase is also a factor in determining the length of an ultrasound treatment. Table 15.2 shows research results on the rate of muscle temperature increases at various intensities and frequencies.[11] These are average temperature increases recorded for about 50 subjects using what many consider to be the best ultrasound device available. Such data are difficult to obtain with many ultrasound devices; therefore, the table should be used only as a rough estimate.[30,31]

APPLICATION TIP

USE ONE OF THESE TWO METHODS TO DETERMINE ULTRASOUND TREATMENT LENGTH

METHOD A
Based on the information in Table 15.2, you can guesstimate the appropriate duration of an ultrasound treatment. For example, if a patient has tennis elbow and chronic pain in the wrist extensor group,

you may want to heat the area before some massage or stretching. An appropriate goal would be to vigorously heat the muscle–tendon junction (an increase of 7.2°F [4°C]). If 3 MHz ultrasound were used at an intensity of 1 W/cm², the 7.2°F (4°C) increase would take ~7 min (1 W = 0.6°C/min × 7 min = 7.6°F or 4.2°C). If at 5 min into the treatment, however, the patient complains that the treatment is too hot, decrease the intensity until it is comfortable. Because you have decreased the total dosage, it would be wise to counter this by adding a minute or so to the treatment time, if possible. Now you are ready to massage the muscle or perform the passive stretch. Although this tip might not apply to your device, it can be used as an estimate for setting treatment goals with a desired temperature increase, instead of giving a 5 min treatment all the time.

METHOD B
Use the heating sensation reported by patients as a guide for peak heating. Experimental subjects reported discomfort from ultrasound as the intramuscular temperature reached 40°C. Therefore, this should signal the end of the treatment. Note that a device with a poor PAMBNR will cause discomfort long before peak heating is reached.

APPLICATION TIP

IF ULTRASOUND DOESN'T SEEM TO BE WORKING, TRY SOMETHING ELSE. Some clinicians will give an unlimited number of ultrasound treatments to a patient. The usual recommendation is to limit ultrasound to 14 treatments, because more than 14 can reduce both red and white blood cell counts. After 14 treatments, it is advisable to avoid ultrasound use for 2 weeks.[24] If no improvement is noted after 4 or 5 treatments, discontinue the ultrasound or use different treatment parameters.

TABLE 15.2	Rates of Muscle Heating Using Ultrasound (per min)*	
INTENSITY (W/CM²)	**FREQUENCY**	
	1 MHZ	**3 MHZ**
0.5	0.07°F (0.04°C)	0.54°F (0.3°C)
1.0	0.36°F (0.2°C)	1.08°F (0.6°C)
1.5	0.54°F (0.3°C)	1.62°F (0.9°C)
2.0	0.72°F (0.4°C)	2.52°F (1.4°C)

*Data obtained with Omnisound ultrasound devices (Accelerated Care Plus, Reno, NV). Data from Draper et al.,[11] Wells and Draper,[27] and Anderson et al.[29]

TREATMENT AREA SIZE

It is not uncommon to see ultrasound used on large areas, such as the hamstrings and low-back muscles. The non-thermal effects may benefit the patient, but research has shown that no heating will occur in this large an area.[32] Scientists have tested the heating capacity of ultrasound over areas of six and four times the size of the sound-head.[33,34] Although the temperature increased 2.3°F (1.3°C) and 3.6°F (2°C), respectively, this is only mild to moderate heating. The appropriate size of the area to be treated using ultrasound is two or three times the size of the ERA of the crystal[35,36] or twice the size of the sound-head surface (Fig. 15.14a). Thus ultrasound is most effec-

tively used for treating small areas.[28] Hot packs, whirlpools, and shortwave diathermy have an advantage over ultrasound in that they can be used to heat much larger areas.[32,37]

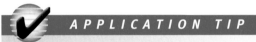

APPLICATION TIP

FOR OPTIMAL HEATING, DIVIDE AND CONQUER.
If you have an area four times the size of the soundhead, treat half of the area first, and then treat the second half (Fig. 15.15). If you need to heat much larger areas, consider using whirlpools or hot packs if your target is superficial or pulsed shortwave diathermy if the target tissue is deeper than 1–2 cm.

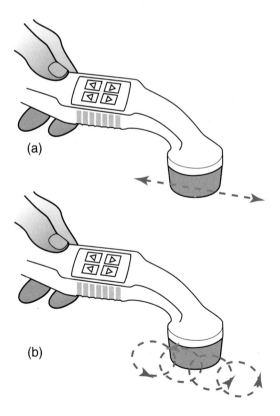

FIGURE 15.14. Ultrasound can be applied in either **(a)** a longitudinal or **(b)** a circular motion. In either case, if heating is desired, the total area covered should not be more than twice the size of the soundhead.

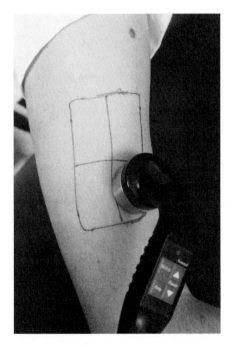

FIGURE 15.15. If you have an area four times the size of the sound-head, treat half of it first, and then treat the second half.

CRITICAL THINKING 15.3 *You are visiting another clinic and notice that the clinician is treating a patient who has a chronic hamstring strain. He is applying ultrasound to the patient's entire leg. Is this the best treatment choice for heating?*

Application Techniques

While administering an ultrasound treatment, it is important to keep the soundhead's surface flat with the surface you are treating at all times. The greatest amount of reflection of ultrasonic energy occurs at the air–tissue interface. If you lift the soundhead from the skin at an angle of >15°, a large percentage of the energy will be reflected, and the treatment effects will be minimal.

COUPLING MEDIA

Ultrasound beams are not transmitted through the air, but require a medium to send the energy from the soundhead to the patient.[13] A substance that facilitates the transmission of ultrasound energy by decreasing impedance at the air–skin interface is referred to as a **coupling medium**, or *couplant*. There are three main types of ultrasound coupling media:

- Gels, for direct application
- Water, for the immersion technique
- Gel pads, for use over bony prominences

The most commonly used coupling medium is ultrasound gel. It is composed mainly of distilled water and an inert, nonreflective material that increases the viscosity of the mixture. A thin layer of coupling medium or gel between the skin and the soundhead has two purposes:

- It allows ultrasonic energy to enter the target tissue at the desired intensity by minimizing the air between the soundhead surface and the tissue.
- It serves as a lubricant.

A common practice is to mix ultrasound gel with an analgesic cream for use as an ultrasound couplant. Although petroleum-based creams will actually impede the transmission of the sound energy, water-based creams can be beneficial. In 1995, a 50/50 mixture of Flexall was compared with 100% ultrasound gel as a coupling medium; the study concluded that ultrasound gel was the best couplant.[38] In 2004 the study was repeated, and this time 100% ultrasound gel was compared to a 25% Flexall/75% ultrasound gel mixture.[29,39] The muscle temperatures reached during treatment were nearly identical. Thus this commonly used sports cream was found to be an excellent couplant when mixed with ultrasound gel at a 1:3 ratio.

DIRECT CONTACT APPLICATION

The majority of ultrasound treatments are direct applications, in which the soundhead comes in contact with the skin (with a thin film of couplant in between). A layer of gel is applied to the treatment area in sufficient amounts to maintain good contact and lubrication between the soundhead and the skin, but not so much that air pockets form from movement of the soundhead. A direct technique of exposure may be used as long as the surface being treated is larger than the diameter of the soundhead. If a smaller surface area is being treated, use a soundhead with a smaller surface so that direct application can still be performed. In the absence of a smaller soundhead, use the immersion technique.

THE IMMERSION TECHNIQUE

Water is a great coupling medium, but it is not suited for surface application because it will not stay in one place, like gel. There are, however, some instances in which you might want to use the underwater technique. The immersion technique is recommended if the area to be treated is smaller than the diameter of the available soundhead, or if the treatment area is irregular with bony prominences (Fig. 15.16).

Use a plastic, ceramic, or rubber basin, because a metal basin or whirlpool will reflect some of the ultrasound, thereby increasing the intensity near the basin walls. Tap water seems to be just as effective as degassed water as a coupling medium for the immersion technique[40] and less likely to produce surface heating than mineral oil or glycerin.[38] The soundhead should be moved parallel to the

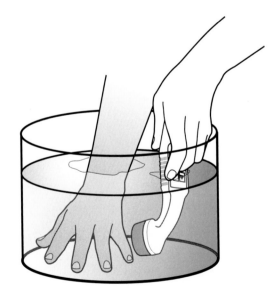

FIGURE 15.16. The immersion technique is recommended if the area to be treated is smaller than the diameter of the soundhead or if the treatment area is irregular with bony prominences.

surface being treated at a distance of 0.5–1 cm.[23] If air bubbles accumulate on the soundhead or over the treatment area, wipe them away quickly during the treatment. To ensure adequate heating, increase the intensity, possibly as much as 50%.[41,42]

✔ **A P P L I C A T I O N   T I P**

CONSIDER THESE POINTS WHEN ADMINISTERING UNDERWATER ULTRASOUND

- *If thermal effects are desired, don't use room temperature water; use a water bath at least as warm as body core temperature 98.6°F (37°C).*
- *Ask yourself if the condition would be better served by using an ultrasound gel pad.*

THE GEL PAD TECHNIQUE

If the treatment area is irregular but cannot be immersed in water, you can use a gel pad as a medium. Companies have recently been manufacturing ultrasound gel packs, which consist of gel housed in a thin plastic envelope, or gel pads, which resemble gel-filled clear hockey pucks.

A few studies have been performed on the efficacy of gel pads. One study suggests that ultrasound gel pads are as effective as ultrasound gel.[43] When the gel pad is used over bony prominences, such as the lateral malleolus of the ankle or the knuckles of the hand, you need to apply a thin layer of ultrasound gel on both sides of the gel pad.[44] The bottom layer ensures that no air is trapped between the bony prominences and the gel pad, and the top layer helps the soundhead glide smoothly on the gel pad (Fig. 15.17).

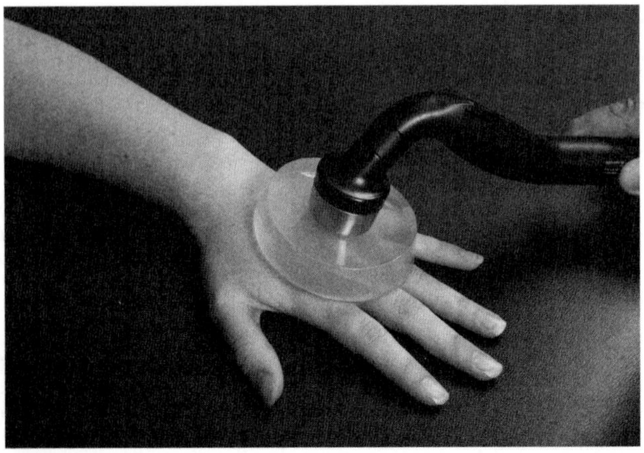

FIGURE 15.17. The use of a gel pad over bony prominences requires a layer of gel on both sides of the pad to avoid trapping air and to lubricate the soundhead.

CRITICAL THINKING 15.4 A patient reports to you for ultrasound treatment 5 days after getting a cast taken off her hand. You can see that it will be difficult to apply ultrasound over her knuckles and maintain good direct contact over the treatment area. What alternative coupling techniques could you use?

SOUNDHEAD MOVEMENT

The ultrasound soundhead is usually moved on the skin in small, overlapping circular motions, or back and forth strokes (see Fig. 15.14). The movement is slow, 3–4 cm per second.[9] If the patient starts to experience pain during the treatment, move the soundhead faster to avoid periosteal irritation or overheating of the tissue.[17,35] Turn the intensity down, and then resume the speed of 3–4 cm/sec.

M O D A L I T Y   MYTH

TISSUES HEAT THE SAME REGARDLESS OF THE SPEED OF SOUNDHEAD MOVEMENT

Soundhead movement doesn't affect the heating of tissues if you can limit the treatment size to a small area.[45] For example, you can use a template to keep the treatment size at 2–3 ERA. Moving the soundhead slowly enables you to control the treatment area. If you move it too rapidly (>4 cm/sec), you run the risk of slipping into treating too large an area (especially if you are carrying on a conversation during treatment) and the desired temperatures might not be attained.

Recording Treatment Parameters

Record the specific treatment parameters whenever you use ultrasound or any other therapeutic modality. There have been several malpractice cases involving the alleged misuse of ultrasound (personal experience as expert witnesses). During the discovery deposition in one such case, the clinician was asked to provide the treatment records of the claimant. Under ultrasound treatment, all that was listed was, "10 minutes of ultrasound application." This is irresponsible record keeping. We recommend that you report or record the specific parameters used in an ultrasound treatment to ensure that:

- The treatment can be reproduced.
- The treatment can be adapted to the patient's needs.
- The records can stand alone when challenged.

The parameters that should be recorded include frequency, intensity, mode, duty cycle (if pulsed), type of coupling medium, area treated, and treatment length. For example, a typical treatment might be recorded as "3 MHz, at 1.2 W/cm², continuous, 2–3 ERA (lateral elbow), ultrasound gel, 6 min."

Thermal Effects

In orthopedic medicine, ultrasound is primarily used to produce a tissue temperature increase. The clinical effects of thermal ultrasound include, but are not limited to:[26]

- Increased extensibility of collagen fibers in tendons and joint capsules
- Reduced viscosity of fluid elements in the tissues
- Decreased joint stiffness
- Reduced muscle spasm
- Diminished pain perception
- Increased metabolism
- Increased blood flow

As previously mentioned, the primary advantage of ultrasound over nonacoustic heating modalities is that collagen-rich tissues such as tendons, muscles, ligaments, joint capsules, joint menisci, intermuscular interfaces, nerve roots, periosteum, and cortical bone as well as other deep tissues can be selectively heated to the therapeutic range without causing a significant tissue temperature increase in skin or fat.[7] Ultrasound will penetrate skin and fat with little attenuation.[41]

OPTIMAL HEATING

One source indicates that tissue temperature must be raised to a level of 104–113°F (40–45°C) for a minimum of 5 min for most thermal effects to occur.[45] Temperatures >113°F (45°C) can cause tissue damage, and 113°F (45°C) is a very high temperature. In our 17 years of laboratory experience with ultrasound, we have never raised human muscle temperature higher than 109.4°F (43°C). Our research subjects usually start to experience mild pain at temperatures above 104–105.8°F (40–41°C) even when a unit with a low BNR is used.[11,27] This agrees with the published recommendation of Merrick et al.[30]

Others are of the opinion that absolute temperatures are not the key but rather how much the temperature rises above baseline.[26,35] They suggest that tissue temperature increases of 1.8°F (1°C) over baseline increase metabolism and healing, increases of 3.6–5.4°F (2–3°C) decrease pain and muscle spasm, and increases of 7.2°F (4°C) or greater increase the extensibility of collagen and decrease joint stiffness (see Table 15.1).[26,35]

In human muscle, which is quite vascular, 1 MHz and 3 MHz ultrasound at 1 W/cm² increased the temperature, on average, 0.36°F (0.2°C) and 1.08°F (0.6°C) per minute, respectively.[11,27] If the intensity is <0.2 W/cm², the intensity is too low to produce a tissue temperature increase, and only nonthermal effects will occur.[46]

In tissues with a poor vascular supply, ultrasound at 1 MHz with an intensity of 1 W/cm² has been reported to raise soft tissue temperature by as much as 1.5°F (0.86°C) per minute.[13] Caution must be used in evaluating the results of one tendon study (ultrasound at 3 MHz and 1 W/cm² intensity) that raised patellar tendon temperatures 3.6°F (2°C) per minute.[47] This increase could have been owing to some of the sound energy rebounding off the tibia. Tendon heats faster than muscle; but more research, perhaps in deeper tendons, needs to be performed to better explain the rate of ultrasound heating in tendon.

Nonthermal Effects

Regardless of whether thermal effects are produced with ultrasound, nonthermal changes do occur.[48] The nonthermal effects of therapeutic ultrasound in the treatment of injured tissues may be as important if not more important than, the thermal effects. They include[49,50]

- Increased histamine release
- Calcium ion influx
- Increased phagocytic activity of macrophages
- Increased protein synthesis
- Increased capillary density of ischemic tissue
- Tissue regeneration
- Wound healing
- Cell membrane alteration
- Attraction of immune cells to the injured area
- Increased fibroblasts
- Vascular regeneration

These nonthermal or mechanical effects of therapeutic ultrasound are thought to originate at the cell membrane. As the ultrasound wave exerts pressure against the cell wall, the membrane deforms slightly. This cell deformation, often referred to as *micromassage*, occurs from processes known as cavitation and microstreaming. **Cavitation** is the formation of gas-filled bubbles that expand and contract as a result of ultrasonically induced pressures in tissue fluids.[46] As the sound waves propagate through the medium, the characteristic compressions and rarefactions cause microscopic gas bubbles in the tissue fluid to contract and expand.

Cavitation can produce both positive and negative effects. Positive effects occur from *stable cavitation*, by which the bubbles expand and contract in response to regularly repeated pressure changes over many acoustic cycles. Negative effects are produced when unstable cavitation occurs. With *unstable or transient cavitation,* tissue can be damaged from increased bubble volume, implosion, and collapse. Apparently, the rapid changes in pressure in and around the cell can result in cell damage caused by the leading and lagging edges of the sound wave. Considerable injury to the cell can occur when gas bubbles expand then collapse rapidly, resulting in a microexplosion. The pulsation of gas bubbles can disrupt cell activity, thereby altering the function of the cell; however, true microexplosions apparently do not occur at therapeutic levels.[49]

Acoustic microstreaming is the unidirectional movement of fluids along the boundaries of cell membranes. It results from the pressures of sound waves that displace ions and small molecules.[46,59] While many cellular organelles and molecules of different molecular weights are stationary, many are also free floating and can be driven to move around the stationary structures. The mechanical pressure from ultrasound waves produces unidirectional movement of fluid along and/or around the cell membrane. Microstreaming produces stresses that can alter the cell membrane's structure and function, thereby affecting the healing process. As long as the cell membrane is not damaged, acoustic microstreaming can be of therapeutic value in accelerating healing.[46,49]

Clinical Applications of Therapeutic Ultrasound

As with many medical devices, research on ultrasound began and continues to be performed on animal models. Results from animal studies have driven much of our human applications for ultrasound. There are a few studies and case reports on humans that continue to point to the efficacy of this modality. We cannot predict what evidence-based research will demonstrate about the future use of therapeutic ultrasound. Yet we can tell you what we know now and in what direction the research is pointing.

Therapeutic ultrasound research has been an ongoing process since the 1960s. Although there was little research during the 1970s and 1980s, it picked up somewhat in the 1990s. This is important because the ultrasound devices manufactured in the 1990s are of much higher quality than previous ones. We now have a vast amount of information regarding heating rates and treatment parameters for using continuous ultrasound. What is lacking, however, is recent research on the healing effects of ultrasound. Thus many of the decisions about how ultrasound should be used are based on personal experience and opinion. In this section we summarize the various clinical

applications of therapeutic ultrasound based on research findings of others and ourselves.

AIDING THE INFLAMMATORY RESPONSE TO INJURY

There is nothing mysterious about ultrasound—it isn't a magic wand. It is theorized that it stimulates bodily functions to perform better. When an injury occurs, some biological mechanisms shut down, and apparently ultrasound can stimulate normal functioning.[51,52]

Scientists have shown that ultrasound stimulated collagen synthesis and cellular proliferation.[52] Macrophages, the main cell type present in wounds 4–5 days after injury, secrete substances that stimulate fibroblast proliferation. Using a culture model, Young and Dyson[53] showed that when macrophages were treated with ultrasound, they had a positive effect on fibroblast proliferation.

Ultrasound has been shown to stimulate the release of histamine from mast cells.[54] Histamine is one of the primary initiators of the acute phase inflammatory response. Histamine attracts leukocytes, which clean up debris from the injured area. Histamine also draws monocytes into the area to release agents that stimulate fibroblasts and endothelial cells to form a collagen-rich, well-vascularized tissue for the development of new connective tissue. Thus ultrasound can be effective in facilitating inflammation and healing.[46,52,55] scientists suggest that the best parameters to use include pulsed ultrasound at a 20% duty cycle, at 0.5 W/cm^2, for 5 min, or continuous ultrasound at 0.1 W/cm^2 for 5 min.[48]

APPLICATION TIP

BEGIN NONTHERMAL ULTRASOUND SOON AFTER AN INJURY. To maximize the effects on the healing process, ultrasound treatments, in a nonthermal mode, can begin as soon as possible after an injury, ideally within a few hours but definitely within 72 hr.[40] Acute conditions may be treated using nonthermal ultrasound once or even twice daily until acute symptoms, such as pain and swelling, subside.

Johns[49] reports that 1 MHz, 3 MHz, and 45 kHz ultrasound stimulate cellular and molecular effects that are centrally involved in the inflammatory and healing processes. However, he concludes that no clear protocols exist for optimum times and parameters for administration during healing.

SUPERFICIAL WOUND HEALING

During the healing process, a connective tissue matrix forms into which new blood vessels will grow. Fibroblasts are the main formative component of connective tissue.

Fibroblasts exposed to therapeutic ultrasound are stimulated to produce more collagen, which gives connective tissue most of its strength.[56] Rat incisions treated with ultrasound displayed more new blood vessel development than areas not treated with ultrasound.[57]

Research has shown increased strength of incisional wounds and collagen deposition when ultrasound is applied.[58] Ultrasound increases smooth muscle cell activity, which is thought to enhance wound contraction.[59] Contraction is an advantage in tissue repair because it means less scar tissue is required to fill the wound gap. The centralizing tug on healthy collagen fibers at the edge of the lesion pulls the wound together. This process is attributed to myofibroblast activity.

CONNECTIVE TISSUE HEALING

Like many studies, the majority of research of ultrasound on connective tissue healing has been performed on animals. Low-intensity ultrasound has been used to stimulate articular cartilage for healing-induced arthritis in animals.[60,61] Muscles of injured rats have shown more healing and force production after ultrasound treatments compared to no treatment.[62,63]

When rabbits and rats with surgically induced Achilles tendon tears were treated with ultrasound, they displayed more parallel collagen orientation, and greater strength, than controls.[64,65] Ultrasound was used on dogs with ruptured Achilles tendons. They showed more advanced healing and a faster return to normal gait than did dogs not treated with ultrasound.[66] Turner and Powell[67] studied the effects of ultrasound treatment on torn, then repaired, tendons of chickens. There was no difference in tendon strength between the group treated with ultrasound and the control group.

Scientists have used rats to study ultrasound effects on healing of either cut or crushed sciatic nerves.[68,69] In both cases, rats treated with ultrasound showed improvements over the control group. In one study, quantity and diameter of regenerating nerve fibers increased; and in the other study, function of the foot increased, owing to the healing of the sciatic nerve.

Torn medial collateral ligaments of rats showed superior healing when ultrasound was used.[70] Unfortunately, there was no improvement noted when ultrasound applications were given to humans with ankle sprains.[71] We point out, however, that no human studies are reported in the literature when low-intensity ultrasound has been used on acute tendon and ligament injury. Thus more evidence-based research on humans is needed in this area.

BONE HEALING

Bone goes through basically the same stages of healing as other soft tissues. Over the past decade, low-intensity pulsed ultrasound to assist fracture healing has increased in orthopedic medicine. Using a 1 MHz therapeutic ultrasound device commonly used by therapists and clinicians, Da Cunha et al.[72] treated damaged rat Achilles tendons and reporting superior healing when the pulsed mode was used (20% duty cycle, 0.5 W/cm^2, 5 min, 12 days). Pulsed low-intensity ultrasound using similar parameters has been shown to assist bone healing in patients with nonunion fractures who failed previous treatments.[73,74] Compared to controls, rat femur fractures treated with diagnostic ultrasound (7.5 MHz, 11.8 mW/cm^2, 10 min) responded well (between 3 and 8 treatments).[60]

BONE GROWTH STIMULATORS

Bear in mind that most of the bone healing performed is with bone growth stimulators, not the typical ultrasound device (Fig. 15.18). The Sonic Accelerated Fracture Healing System (SAFHS) of the Exogen uses the following parameters for bone growth stimulation:

- Duty cycle: 20%
- Frequency: 1.5 MHz
- Intensity: 30 mW/cm^2
- Time: 20 min

Animal Studies

There have been several animal studies with positive outcomes when the SAFHS was used at these parameters. Scientists reported a faster healing rate and stronger bones compared to the opposite limb when the SAFHS was used on surgically induced femur fractures in rats.[75,76] Rabbit fibula fractures treated with the SAFHS healed faster when compared to sham treatments on the opposite limb.[77]

Human Studies

The SAFHS has also had success in stimulating bone growth in human patients. Tibial shaft fractures have shown a 38% reduction in healing time.[78] Distal radius fractures treated with the SAFHS have also healed 38% faster than normal.[79] Compared to a control group, scaphoid fractures treated

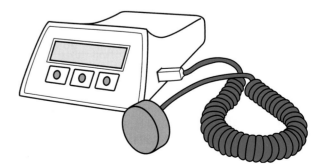

FIGURE 15.18. A low-intensity pulsed ultrasound stimulator for the acceleration of fracture healing.

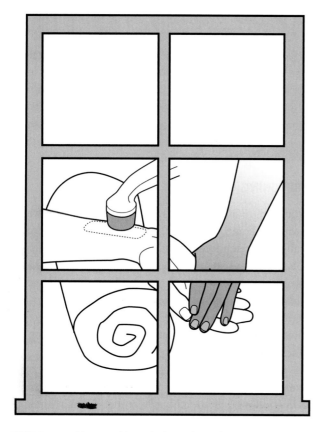

FIGURE 15.19. The stretching window. This is the period of vigorous heating, when tissues undergo the greatest degree of extensibility and elongation.

CRITICAL THINKING 15.5 *A patient is recovering successfully from knee surgery, except that his patella isn't moving well. The physician prescribes patellar mobilizations. How could you use ultrasound to assist you in obtaining normal ROM of the patella?*

TREATING CHRONIC INFLAMMATION

One of the biggest challenges for any clinician is treating chronic injuries that just don't want to go away. Two key ingredients in treating chronic conditions are increased blood flow and decreased pain, both of which result from continuous ultrasound.[23] It might prove beneficial to heat the area with ultrasound and then perform cross-friction massage to break up the adhesions and allow the tendon to glide more smoothly on the surrounding structures. There are few clinical or experimental studies that discuss the effects of therapeutic ultrasound on chronic inflammation (i.e., tendinitis, bursitis, epicondylitis), and the results are mixed. Ultrasound treatments have proven to be beneficial for treating tibial periostitis[88] and epicondilytis.[89]

Phonophoresis

Phonophoresis is the use of ultrasound to help move a topical medication into the tissues. The theory is that ul-

trasound enhances transdermal drug delivery by dilating hair follicles and sweat glands, increasing circulation and kinetic energy of the local cells.[90] Many think that ultrasound drives the medicine into the tissues, but this is not correct. In ultrasound, **sonoporation** occurs, in which the sound waves increase cell membrane permeability, thereby facilitating the delivery of molecules to precise locations in the body.[90,91] The success of the delivery of the medication is limited by the inability of the molecules to cross biological barriers, such as the cell membrane. An advantage of phonophoresis is that medication can be delivered via a safe, painless, noninvasive technique.

DRUG AND MODE DECISIONS

Which medications work well during phonophoresis still remains somewhat of a mystery. Scientists have found that hydrocortisone gels and many salicylate preparations actually block ultrasound wave transmission, whereas other gels and creams serve as good ultrasound transmitters.[92,93] For treating orthopedic injuries, the most commonly used medications in phonophoresis are either anti-

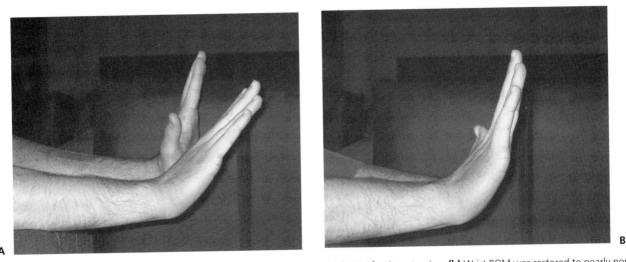

FIGURE 15.20 **(a)** Owing to prolonged immobilization, the patient's wrist lacked 30° of wrist extension. **(b)** Wrist ROM was restored to nearly normal after ultrasound and joint mobilizations.

inflammatories—such as cortisol, salicylates, and dexamethasone—and analgesics—such as lidocaine. With phonophoresis, it is important to select the appropriate drug for the condition. Because phonophoresis can increase drug penetration, it could also increase the clinical benefits as well as the risks of topical drug application.[93]

Both pulsed and continuous ultrasound have been used in phonophoresis. Strapp et al.[94] report greater levels of dexamethasone sodium phosphate in the bloodstream after continuous ultrasound application of that medication. However, continuous ultrasound at an intensity great enough to produce thermal effects may induce a proinflammatory response.[48] If the goal is to decrease inflammation, phonophoresis using pulsed ultrasound at a low intensity might be the best choice.[24]

TOPICAL PREPARATIONS

Earlier, we discussed the ability of various coupling media to actually penetrate the skin barrier. Adding an active ingredient into the coupling medium is common practice; however, topical pharmacologic products are usually not formulated to optimize their efficiency as ultrasound coupling media.[95] For example, 1% or 10% hydrocortisone usually comes in a thick white cream base, which is a poor ultrasound couplant. Clinicians have tried mixing this preparation with ultrasound gel without improvement in transmission capabilities.

The use of topical preparations with poor transmission capabilities may decrease the effectiveness of ultrasound therapy. Unfortunately only a few suitable products are available, and there is clearly a need for appropriate active ingredients in gel form. Because research has shown some of these medications to impede the sound,[96] we recommend applying the medication and gel separately. This is done by rubbing the medication into the skin, then applying an ultrasound gel couplant, followed by an ultrasound treatment.

EFFECTIVENESS OF PHONOPHORESIS

The effectiveness of phonophoresis is inconclusive, especially at the frequencies commonly used in orthopedic medicine (1 MHz and 3 MHz). Evidence indicates that little medication actually reaches the target tissue. The answer might not come from clinicians who work in physical medicine and rehabilitation but from chemical engineering, where phonophoresis is being used on animals and humans with some positive results.[97–99]

In chemical engineering, the positive results for phonophoresis are being obtained at low frequencies, such as 45 kHz and 20 kHz. Scientists measured the ability of both 1 MHz and 20 kHz ultrasound to facilitate the delivery of butanol, corticosterone, salicylic acid, and sucrose across human cadaver skin.[100] The result: 20 kHz increased skin permeability a thousand-fold over that of 1 MHz. Scientists have also been successful at transdermal transport of corticosterone, insulin, interferon, and erythropoietin across human skin using 20 kHz ultrasound.[101] These results indicate that lower frequencies might be useful in treating orthopedic injuries.[102]

Using Ultrasound and Other Modalities Collectively

In an orthopedic setting, it is not uncommon to combine modalities to accomplish a specific treatment goal. Although you want to avoid the shotgun approach, ultrasound is frequently used with other modalities, including hot packs and electrical stimulating currents. Unfortunately there is very little documented evidence to substantiate the effectiveness of ultrasound and electrical currents; however, studies of heating or cooling the area before ultrasound application have produced interesting results.[103–105]

HOT PACKS

Hot packs, like continuous or high-intensity ultrasound, are used primarily for their thermal effects. Heat is effective in reducing muscle spasm and muscle guarding and useful in relieving pain. For these reasons, heat and ultrasound in combination can be effective for accomplishing these treatment goals. In one study, a 15-min hot pack application before ultrasound had an additive heating effect.[105] Based on this finding, we recommend that the ultrasound treatment duration can be decreased by 3–5 min when tissues are preheated with hot packs.

MODALITY MYTH

APPLYING COLD BEFORE ULTRASOUND ENHANCES HEATING

Although the theory sounds good, this approach doesn't work. According to this premise, applying a cold pack to the tissues increases the density of the tissue to be heated. Because ultrasound transmission is directly related to tissue density, this facilitates transmission to deeper tissues, thereby enhancing the thermal effects of ultrasound. But studies refute such claims. Applying an ice pack for 5 min before ultrasound caused the temperature to drop so much that the ultrasound failed to raise the muscle temperature to even 50% of that of subjects who did not receive an ice application before ultrasound.[103] Applying an ice pack for 15 min before ultrasound caused the temperature to drop so much that the ultrasound failed to raise the muscle temperature back to the previous baseline temperature.[104] It just doesn't make sense to cool something that you immediately want to heat.[14]

ULTRASOUND AND ELECTROTHERAPY

Ultrasound and electrotherapy techniques, also known as combination therapy, are frequently used (Fig. 15.21). Understand that when combination therapy is used, the ultrasound soundhead acts as an electrode. The muscles will be stimulated to contract and you will have the effects of the ultrasound. The electrical stimulating currents will cause analgesia and muscle contraction. Combination therapy has been recommended in the treatment of myofascial trigger points.[106] We have had success in treating ilio-tibial band tightness with combination therapy. Both modalities provide analgesic effects, and both have been shown to be effective in reducing the pain–spasm–pain cycle, although the underlying mechanisms are not clearly understood.

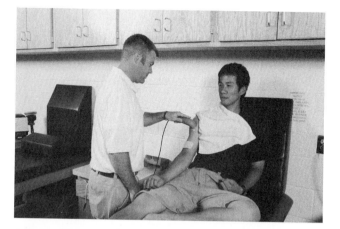

FIGURE 15.21. Ultrasound is frequently used in combination with electrotherapy. The ultrasound head serves as one electrode. Note the second electrode attached to the bicep.

Treatment Precautions and Concerns

As with all therapeutic modalities, specific safety precautions must be observed when using ultrasound:

- Avoid using thermal ultrasound whenever a tissue temperature rise is contraindicated.
- Avoid using high-intensity continuous ultrasound in acute and postacute conditions because of the associated thermal effects.
- Use caution when treating areas of decreased sensation, particularly when the patient has difficulty perceiving pain and temperature.
- Exercise caution in areas of decreased circulation, because excessive heat buildup can potentially damage tissues.
- Individuals with vascular problems involving thrombophlebitis should not receive ultrasound because of the possibility of dislodging a clot and creating an embolus.
- Ultrasound should not be applied around the eyes where heat is not dissipated well; the lens and retina can be damaged.
- Do not apply ultrasound over reproductive organs, especially the testes; temporary sterility can result. Although the ovaries are fairly deep and well protected, use caution (lower intensities and 3 MHz) when treating the female abdominal region during the reproductive years or immediately after menstruation.
- The use of ultrasound to the abdominal region or lower back is contraindicated during pregnancy because of potential damage to the fetus. Diagnostic ultrasound for tracking maturation of the fetus is delivered in doses >0.1 W/cm^2 at 2.5 MHz and thus is safe.
- Use precaution when treating areas around the heart, because of potential changes in electrocardiographic (EKG) activity.

- Avoid using ultrasound below the ribs, directed toward the heart.
- Ultrasound can interfere with the normal functioning of a pacemaker and should not be applied directly over the device.
- Do not use ultrasound over malignant tissue; it could cause cell detachment and metastasis.
- Do not apply ultrasound over an active infection, as it may cause it to spread.
- Use caution when applying ultrasound over epiphyseal areas in young children. It appears that low-intensity treatment (<1 W/cm^2) can be used but only for a few treatment sessions.[59]
- Ultrasound can be used relatively safely over metal implants. According to theory, there is little increase in the temperature of tissue adjacent to the implant because metal has high thermal conductivity, so heat is removed from the area faster than it can be absorbed. However, metal reflects about 90% of ultrasound energy, and adjacent tissues can absorb some of the reflected waves. Regardless, when performing ultrasound on an area with metal implants (or any area for that matter), if the patient complains of pain, reduce the intensity. Be aware that in cases of total joint replacement, the cement used (methyl methacrylate) absorbs heat rapidly, and overheating can damage surrounding soft tissues.

Challenges to the Efficacy of Therapeutic Ultrasound

Some clinicians believe that ultrasound has no therapeutic value. In two recent publications, the authors took a comprehensive look at ultrasound based on previously published studies and determined that the modality did not work.[107,108] We studied the two articles in depth. After systematically analyzing the data and research methods, we came to the conclusion that these studies were not based on reliable, quantifiable proof.

In another article, Robertson and Baker[108] reviewed 35 ultrasound studies performed between 1975 and 1999. Using a model to determine whether the original scientists were rigorous enough in the original research design, the authors eliminated studies because of one or more of the following factors: small sample size; nonclinical condition; inadequate controls; no comparison to placebo; and nonblinding of observers, subjects, or scientists. In all, 25 studies did not match up to this model, leaving just 10 studies to examine. In 8 of these, active ultrasound performed no better than placebo ultrasound. From this, the authors concluded that active ultrasound is no more effective than placebo or sham ultrasound.

We analyzed the same 8 articles in depth and found several research errors from which the authors drew their conclusion. In fact, many of the original scientists made the same mistakes therapists and athletic trainers make in everyday use of this often-misunderstood modality.[109,110] These errors include

- Treating too large an area for thermal goals (4 studies)[111–114]
- Using the wrong frequency for superficial tissues (1 study)[111]
- Inadequate treatment duration (5 studies)[113,114]

It appears that the papers from which Robertson and Baker[108] drew their conclusions were flawed; they mistakenly compared placebo ultrasound with placebo ultrasound. In other words, a study is flawed to begin with if the research doesn't use correct treatment parameters. The authors' impressions that ultrasound is not effective is based on less than adequate research.[109,110] Until more controlled studies using correct parameters are performed, we cannot rule out ultrasound as a therapeutic modality. Although it can't do everything, when used correctly, it can be a valuable tool for you and your patients.

5 STEPS   *Application of Therapeutic Ultrasound*

1 STEP 1: FOUNDATION

A. Definition. Therapeutic ultrasound is inaudible, acoustic vibrations of high frequency that produce either thermal or nonthermal physiologic effects in tissues.

B. Effects
   1. Thermal effects include:
      a. Diminished pain perception
      b. Increased metabolism
      c. Increased blood flow
   2. Nonthermal effects include:
      a. Tissue regeneration
      b. Wound healing
      c. Cell membrane alteration

C. Advantages
   1. Can heat deep tissues without overheating the surface
   2. Heats the deepest of all modalities (except diathermy)

D. Disadvantages
   1. Can only heat small areas; approximately twice the size of the soundhead surface
   2. Variability in the quality of ultrasound devices

E. Indications
   1. Acute and postacute conditions (ultrasound with nonthermal effects)
   2. Soft tissue healing and repair
   3. Scar tissue
   4. Joint contracture
   5. Chronic inflammation
   6. Increase extensibility of collagen
   7. Reduction of muscle spasm
   8. Pain modulation
   9. Increase blood flow
   10. Soft tissue repair
   11. Increase protein synthesis
   12. Tissue regeneration
   13. Bone healing
   14. Repair of non-union fractures
   15. Inflammation associated with myositis ossificans
   16. Plantar warts
   17. Myofascial trigger points

F. Contraindications
   1. Acute and postacute conditions (ultrasound with thermal effects)
   2. Vascular insufficiency
   3. Thrombophlebitis
   4. Eyes
   5. Reproductive organs
   6. Pelvis immediately after menstruation
   7. Pregnancy
   8. Pacemaker
   9. Malignancy
   10. Infection

G. Precautions
   1. Epiphyseal areas in young children
   2. Metal implants
   3. Areas of decreased temperature sensation
   4. Areas of decreased circulation
   5. Total joint replacements

2 STEP 2: PREAPPLICATION TASKS

A. Make sure ultrasound is the proper modality for this situation.
   1. Reevaluate the injury or problem. Make sure you understand the patient's condition.
   2. If ultrasound was applied previously, review the patient's response to that treatment.
   3. Confirm that the objectives of therapy are compatible with ultrasound.
   4. Make sure ultrasound is not contraindicated in this situation.

B. Preparing the equipment. Prepare the equipment before preparing the patient.
   1. Make sure the soundhead is clean.
   2. Make sure you have enough coupling medium available for treatment.

C. Preparing the patient psychologically
   1. Explain the procedure.
      a. Sound waves generated into the body cause an increased movement of molecules, which results in heat, or a type of micromassage of the tissues.
      b. Gentle warmth should be felt during the treatment (unless it is a nonthermal treatment).
      c. Demonstrate the procedure on yourself if the patient is apprehensive.
   2. Check for, and warn the patient about, precautions. Ask the patient to let you know if the treatment starts to feel too warm.

D. Preparing the patient physically
   1. Remove any metal or jewelry from the part to be treated.
   2. Inspect the area to be treated for rashes or open wounds.
   3. Position the patient in a manner that will be comfortable, yet allow accessibility to the ultrasound device.

STEP 3: APPLICATION PARAMETERS

A. Procedures
 1. Obtain the appropriate soundhead size
 2. Apply the coupling medium to the area
B. Dosage
 1. Determine the appropriate frequency
   a. 1 MHz for deep to moderate
   b. 3 MHz for moderate to superficial
 2. Set the duty cycle (choose either continuous or pulsed setting)
 3. Set the treatment duration (vigorous heat: 10–15 min at 1 MHz; 3–7 min at 3 Mhz)
   a. Maintain contact between the skin and the applicator
   b. Move at a rate of 4 cm/sec for 2–3 ERA
 4. Adjust the intensity to the patient's perception of heat. If it gets too hot, move the applicator slightly faster as you turn down the intensity.
 5. If the treatment goal is increased joint ROM, put the body part on stretch for the last 2–3 min of the ultrasound application and maintain stretch or friction massage for 5 min after the ultrasound application.
C. Length of application. Varies according to treatment goals
D. Frequency of application. One or two times daily
E. Duration of therapy. 14 treatments

STEP 4: POSTAPPLICATION TASKS

A. Equipment removal; patient cleanup
 1. When the timer shuts off or the patient can no longer tolerate the treatment even at low intensity, remove the soundhead and clean it off.
 2. Wipe any ultrasound gel off the patient.
B. Instructions to the patient
 1. Schedule the next treatment.
 2. Instruct the patient about the level of activity and/or self-treatment before the next formal treatment.
 3. Instruct the patient about what he should feel after treatment.
C. Record of treatment, including unique patient responses
D. Equipment replacement
 1. Towels
 2. Coupling medium

STEP 5: MAINTENANCE

A. Clean the equipment regularly.
B. An ultrasound device that is used daily should be calibrated every 6 months.

CLOSING SCENE

Recall from the chapter opening scene that several patients asked Nancy some difficult questions about ultrasound. She told them that there are two types of ultrasound: thermal and nonthermal. A patient should feel gentle warmth during a thermal treatment but nothing during a nonthermal treatment. As for the patient who could feel an ultrasound treatment on his patellar tendon but not on his back, Nancy informed him that ultrasound is correctly used to heat small areas. That's why he felt the gentle heat on his knee but couldn't feel it on his low back—an area too large to benefit from ultrasound. Hot packs, whirlpools, or—even better—pulsed shortwave diathermy should be used to heat his back. Nancy seems to know her stuff about ultrasound.

CHAPTER REFLECTIONS

1. Read and ponder each of the following points. Do you feel you have a clear understanding of each concept? If not, reread the appropriate section of the chapter.
   - Name the key components of an ultrasound device.
   - What happens when ultrasound enters the body's tissues?
   - Explain the thermal effects of therapeutic ultrasound.
   - Discuss the nonthermal effects of therapeutic ultrasound.
   - Describe the different techniques of ultrasound application.
   - List several parameters associated with ultrasound use.
   - Itemize the contraindications and precautions of using therapeutic ultrasound.
   - Compare and contrast ultrasound with other heating agents.
   - What is the stretching window? Explain how it would be most effectively used with ultrasound.

2. Write three to five questions for discussion with your class instructor, clinical instructor, classmates, and clinical colleagues.

3. Get together with classmates and quiz each other on the concepts of this chapter. Use the points in exercise 1 and questions you wrote for exercise 2 as a beginning. Explaining concepts out loud to others requires a deeper grasp of the material than feeling you understand it as you read.

4. Once you feel you understand the principles of application of ultrasound, practice applying them using the five-step approach with a classmate or clinical colleague. Alternate applying the modalities to each other. When it is being applied to you, listen and observe carefully to determine whether your classmate is using proper application. Consult your notes when the modality is applied to you and for the first few times you apply the modality to another person. Continue practicing the application until you can do so without using your notes.

CRITICAL THINKING RESPONSES

Critical Thinking 15.1

The duty cycle would be 50%.

Critical Thinking 15.2

The higher the frequency, the more the energy is absorbed in the superficial tissues. The majority of the sound waves generated from the 3 MHz treatment would be absorbed in the tendon, whereas 1 MHz goes much deeper and might rebound off the bone, causing some discomfort.

Critical Thinking 15.3

In this case the best treatment choice is not to use ultrasound at all. A better decision would be to use either hydrocollator packs or shortwave diathermy, both of which are more useful in treating larger areas. If depth of penetration is a concern, then shortwave diathermy would be the treatment modality of choice.

Critical Thinking 15.4

When using a large soundhead over bony prominences, the immersion technique done in a plastic or rubber tub can be effective. Also, the gel pad technique could be used to ensure that there is consistent contact between the soundhead and the coupling medium. Remember to have a small amount of gel on both sides of the pad.

Critical Thinking 15.5

Application of 3 MHz ultrasound to patient tolerance for 4–5 min on the lateral side and 4–5 min on the medial side. Immediately apply patellar glides in all directions.

REFERENCES

1. Andrew MA, Crum LA, Vaezy S. 2nd International Symposium on Therapeutic Ultrasound. Vol 2. Seattle: Center for Industrial and Medical Ultrasound Applied Physics Laboratory, University of Washington, 2002.
2. Fried NM, Roberts WW, Wright EJ, Solomon SB. Noninvasive male sterilization: Thermal occlusion of the vas deferens and epididymis in a canine model using a therapeutic focused ultrasound clip. Paper presented at the second International Symposium on Therapeutic Ultrasound, Seattle, 2002.
3. Mourad PD, Nemecek A, Mesiwala A, et al. Ultrasound treatment of brain disorders. Paper presented at the second International Symposium on Therapeutic Ultrasound, Seattle, 2002.
4. Draper D, Abergel P, Castel J. Rate of temperature change in human fat during external ultrasound: Implications for liposuction. Am J Cosmet Surg 1998;15:361–367.

5. Dyson M. The use of ultrasound in sports physiotherapy. In: Grisogono V, ed. Sports Injuries (International Perspectives in Physiotherapy). Edinburgh, UK: Churchill Livingstone; 1989.

6. Dyson M, Luke DA. Induction of mast cell degranulation in skin by ultrasound. IEEE Trans UFFC 1986;33:194.

7. ter Haar G. Basic physics of therapeutic ultrasound. Physiotherapy 1987;64:100–103.

8. Draper D, Sunderland S. Examination of the law of Grotthus-Draper: Does ultrasound penetrate subcutaneous fat in humans? J Athl Train. 1993;28:246–250.

9. Michlovitz S. Thermal Agents in Rehabilitation. Philadelphia: Davis. 1996.

10. Myrer JW, Draper DO, Durrant E. Contrast therapy and intramuscular temperature in the human leg. J Athl Train 1994;29:318–322.

11. Draper DO, Castel JC, Castel D. Rate of temperature increase in human muscle during 1 MHz and 3 MHz continuous ultrasound. J Orthop Sports Phys Ther 1995;22:142–150.

12. Draper DO, Ricard MD. Rate of temperature decay in human muscle following 3 MHz ultrasound: The stretching window revealed. J Athl Train 1995;30:304–307.

13. Williams R. Production and transmission of ultrasound. Physiotherapy 1987;73:113–116.

14. Draper D. Ten mistakes commonly made with ultrasound use: Current research sheds light on myths. Athl Train Sports Health Care Perspect 1996;2:95–107.

15. Johns LD, Straub SJ, Howard SM. Variability in effective radiating area and power output of new ultrasound transducers at 3 MHz. J Athl Train 2007;42(3):22–28.

16. Ferguson BA. A practitioners' guide to ultrasonic therapy equipment standard. Washington DC: U.S. Department of Health and Human Service, U.S. Public Health Service, U.S. Food and Drug Administration, 1985.

17. Hecox B, Mehreteax TA, Weisberg J. Physical Agents. Norwalk, CT: Appleton & Lange, 1994.

18. Draper D. A breakthrough on comfortable ultrasound treatments: Beam non-uniformity ratio is only half of the equation. Paper presented at the annual symposium of the National Athletic Trainers' Association, Kansas City, MO, June 1999.

19. Johns LD, Straub SJ, LeDet EG. Ultrasound beam profiling: Comparative analysis of 4 new ultrasound heads a both 1 and 3.3 MHz variability within a manufacturer. J Athl Train 2004;39:S26.

20. Gallo JA, Draper DO, Thein-Body L, Fellingham GW. Continuous and pulsed ultrasound produce similar increases in human muscle temperature when equivalent temporal average intensities are used. J Orthop Sports Phys Ther 2004;34:339–401.

21. Stewart H. Ultrasound therapy. In: Repacholi M, Benwell D, eds. Essentials of Medical Ultrasound. Clifton, NJ: Humana Press, 1982.

22. Hayes BT, Merrick MA, Sandrey MA, Cordova ML. 3MHz ultrasound heats deeper into the tissues than originally theorized. J Athl Train 2004;39:230–234.

23. Ziskin M, McDiarmid T, Michlovitz S. Therapeutic ultrasound. In: Michlovitz S, ed. Thermal agents in rehabilitation. Philadelphia: Davis, 1996.

24. Gann N. Ultrasound: Current concepts. Clin Manage 1991;11: 64–69.

25. Kitchen S, Partridge C. A review of therapeutic ultrasound: Part 2, The efficacy of ultrasound. Physiotherapy 1990;79:595–599.

26. Lehmann JF. Therapeutic Heat and Cold. 4th ed. Baltimore: Williams & Wilkins, 1990.

27. Wells A, Draper D, Vincent W. The regression equation of the Omnisound 3000P is valid: Ultrasound treatments should be temperature dependent not time dependent. J Athl Train 2004;39: S24.

28. Draper DO. Current research on therapeutic ultrasound and pulsed short-wave diathermy. Paper presented at the Physio Therapy Research Seminars, Sendai, Japan, Nov 1996.

29. Anderson M, Eggett D, Draper D. Combining topical analgesics and ultrasound, Part 2. Athl Ther Today 2005;10:45–47.

30. Merrick MA, Bernard KD, Devor ST, Williams MJ. Identical 3-MHz ultrasound treatments with different devices produce different intramuscular temperatures. J Orthop Sports Phys Ther 2003; 33:379–385.

31. Holcomb WR, Joyce CJ. A Comparison of temperature increases produced by 2 commonly used ultrasound units. J Athl Train 2003;38:24–27.

32. Garrett CL, Draper DO, Knight KL. Heat distribution in the lower leg from pulsed short-wave diathermy and ultrasound treatments. J Athl Train 2000;35:13–22.

33. Chudleigh D, Schulthies S, Draper D, Myrer J. Muscle temperature rise during 1 MHz ultrasound treatments of two and six times the effective radiating areas of the transducer. J Athl Train 2006 1998; 33:S11.

34. Demchak T, Meyer L, Stemmans C, Brucker J. Therapeutic benefits of ultrasound can be achieved and maintained with a 20-minutes 1 MHz, 4-ERA ultrasound treatment. J Athl Train 2006;41:S42.

35. Castel D. Electrotherapy and Ultrasound Update. 2nd ed. Reno, NV: International Academy of Physio Therapeutics, 1996.

36. Reid DC, Cummings GE. Factors in selection the dosage of ultrasound with particular reference to the use of various coupling agents. Physiother Can 1973;63:255.

37. Draper DO, Harris ST, Schulthies SS, et al. Hotpack and 1 MHz ultrasound treatments have an additive effect on muscle temperature increase. J Athl Train 1998;33:21–24.

38. Ashton DF, Draper DO, Myrer JW. Temperature rise in human muscle during ultrasound treatments using flex-all as a coupling agent. J Athl Train 1998;33:136–140.

39. Draper D, Anderson M. Combining topical analgesics and ultrasound, Part 1. Athl Ther Today. 2005;10:26–27.

40. Fyfe MC, Chahl LA. The effect of single or repeated applications of "therapeutic" ultrasound on plasma extravasation during silver nitrate induced inflammation of the rat hindpaw ankle joint in vivo. Ultrasound Med Biol 1985;11:273–283.

41. Draper DO, Sunderland S, Kirkendall DT, Ricard MD. A comparison of temperature rise in the human calf muscles following applications of underwater and topical gel ultrasound. J Orthop Sports Phys Ther 1993;17:247–251.

42. Klucinec B, Scheidler M, Denegar C, et al. Transmissivity of common coupling agents used to deliver ultrasound through indirect methods. J Orthop Sports Phys Ther 2000;30:263–269.

43. Merrick MA, Mihalyov MR, Roethemeier JL, et al. A comparison of intramuscular temperatures during ultrasound treatments with coupling gel or gel pads. J Orthop Sports Phys Ther 2002;32:216–220.

44. Bishop S, Draper DO, Knight KL, et al. Human-tissue temperature rise during ultrasound treatments with the Aquaflex gel pad. J Athl Train 2004;39:25–30.

45. Weaver SL, Demchak TJ, Stone MB, et al. Effect of transducer velocity on intramuscular temperature during a 1-MHz ultrasound treatment. J Orthop Sports Phys Ther 2006;36:320–325.

46. Dyson M. Mechanisms involved in therapeutic ultrasound. Physiotherapy 1987;73:116–120.

47. Chan AK, Myrer JW, Measom GJ, Draper DO. Temperature changes in human patellar tendon in response to therapeutic ultrasound. J Athl Train 1998;33:130–134.

48. Dyson M. Therapeutic application of ultrasound. In: Nyborg WL, Ziskin MC, eds. Biological Effects of Ultrasound. Edinburgh, UK: Churchill Livingstone, 1985.

49. Johns LD. Nonthermal effects of therapeutic ultrasound: The frequency resonance hypothesis. J Athl Train 2002;37:293–299.

50. Kimmel E, Dines M, Elad D, et al. Shear-like response of endothelial cells to therapeutic ultrasound. Paper presented at the second International Symposium on Therapeutic Ultrasound, Seattle, 2002.

51. Watson T. Therapeutic Ultrasound. Available at: www.electrotherapy.org. Accessed Apr 2007.

52. Ramirez A, Schwane JA, McFarland C, Starcher B. The effect of ultrasound on collagen synthesis and fibroblast proliferation in vitro. Med Sci Sports Exerc 1997;29:326–332.

53. Young S, Dyson M. Macrophage responsiveness to therapeutic ultrasound. Ultrasound Med Biol 1990;16:326–332.

54. Hashish I, Harvey W, Harris M. Anti-inflammatory effects of ultrasound therapy: Evidence for a major placebo effect. Br J Rheumatol 1986;25:77–81.

55. Draper DO, Karns PB, Sokolowski MS. Chronic ankle and foot injuries in professional ice hockey players: Jumpstarting inflammation to re-direct healing. J Athl Train 2001;2:S90.

56. Harvey W, Dyson M, Pond JB, Grahame R. The stimulation of protein synthesis in human fibroblasts by therapeutic ultrasound. Rheumatol Rehabil 1975;14:237.

57. Young S, Dyson M. The effect of therapeutic ultrasound on angiogenesis. Ultrasound Med Biol 1990;16:261–269.

58. Byl NN, McKenzie A, Wong T, et al. Incisional wound healing: A controlled study of low and high dose ultrasound. J Orthop Sports Phys Ther 1993;18:619–628.

59. Behrens BJ, Michlovitz SL. Physical Agents: Theory and Practice for the Physical Therapist Assistant. Philadelphia: Davis, 1996.

60. Heybeli N, Yesildag A, Oyar O, et al. Diagnostic ultrasound treatment increases the bone fracture-healing rate in an internally fixed rat femoral osteotomy model. J Ultrasound Med 2002;21:1357–1363.

61. Huang MH, Ding HJ, Chai CY, et al. Effects of sonication on articular cartilage in experimental osteoarthritis. J Rheumatol 1997;24:1978–1984.

62. Rantanen J, Thorsson O, Wollmer P, et al. Effects of therapeutic ultrasound on the regeneration of skeletal myofibers after experimental injury. Am J Sports Med 1999;27:54–59.

63. Karnes J, Burton H. Continuous therapeutic ultrasound accelerates repair of contraction-induced skeletal muscle damage in rats. Arch Phys Med Rehabil 2002;83:1–4.

64. Jackson BA, Schwane JA, Starcher BC. Effect of ultrasound therapy on the repair of Achilles tendon injuries in rats. Med Sci Sports Exerc 1991;23:171–176.

65. Enwemeka CS, Rodriguez O, Mendosa S. The biomechanical effects of low-intensity ultrasound on healing tendons. Ultrasound Med Biol 1990;16:801–807.

66. Saini NS, Roy KS, Bansal PS, et al. A preliminary study on the effect of ultrasound therapy on the healing of surgically severed Achilles tendons in five dogs. J Vet Med A Physiol Pathol Clin Med 2002;49:321–328.

67. Turner SM, Powell ES, Ng CS. The effect of ultrasound on the healing of repaired cockerel tendon: Is collagen cross-linking a factor? J Hand Surg [Br] 1989;14:428–433.

68. Crisci A, Ferreira A. Low-intensity pulsed ultrasound accelerates the regeneration of the sciatic nerve after neurotomy in rats. Ultrasound Med Biol 2002;28:1335–1341.

69. Mourad P, Lazar D, Curra F, et al. Ultrasound accelerates functional recovery after peripheral nerve damage. Neurosurgery 2001;48:1136–1140.

70. Takakura Y, Matsui N, Yoshiya S, et al. Low-intensity pulsed ultrasound enhances early healing of medial collateral ligament injuries in rats. J Ultrasound Med 2002;21:283–288.

71. Van Der Windt DA, Van Der Heijden GJ, Van Den Berg SG, et al. Ultrasound therapy for acute ankle sprains. Cochrane Database Syst Rev 2002:CD001250.

72. da Cunha A, Parizotto NA, Vidal Bde C. The effect of therapeutic ultrasound on repair of the Achilles tendon (tendo calcaneus) of the rat. Ultrasound Med Biol 2001;27:1691–1696.

73. Nolte PA, van der Krans A, Patka P, et al. Low-intensity pulsed ultrasound in the treatment of nonunions. J Trauma 2001;51:693–702; discussion 702–693.

74. Mayr E, Frankel V, Ruter A. Ultrasound—An alternative healing method for nonunions? Arch Orthop Trauma Surg 2000;120:1–8.

75. Azuma Y, Ito M, Harada Y, et al. Low-intensity pulsed ultrasound accelerates rat femoral fracture healing by acting on the various cellular reactions in the fracture callus. J Bone Miner Res 2001;16:671–680.

76. Wang SJ, Lewallen DG, Bolander ME, et al. Low intensity ultrasound treatment increases strength in a rat femoral fracture model. J Orthop Res 1994;12:40–47.

77. Pilla AA, Mont MA, Nasser PR, et al. Non-invasive low-intensity pulsed ultrasound accelerates bone healing in the rabbit. J Orthop Trauma 1990;4:246–253.

78. Heckman JD, Ryaby JP, McCabe J, et al. Acceleration of tibial fracture-healing by non-invasive, low-intensity pulsed ultrasound. J Bone Joint Surg Am 1994;76:26–34.

79. Kristiansen TK, Ryaby JP, McCabe J, et al. Accelerated healing of distal radial fractures with the use of specific, low-intensity ultrasound. A multicenter, prospective, randomized, double-blind, placebo-controlled study. J Bone Joint Surg Am 1997;79:961–973.

80. Mayr E, Rudzki MM, Rudzki M, et al. Does low intensity, pulsed ultrasound speed healing of scaphoid fractures? Handchir Mikrochir Plast Chir 2000;32:115–122.

81. Michlovitz SL, Nolan T. Modalities for Therapeutic Intervention. Philadelphia: Davis, 2005.

82. Lowden A. Application of ultrasound to assess stress fractures. Physiotherapy 1986;72:160–161.

83. Kitchen S, Partridge C. A review of therapeutic ultrasound: Part 1, Background and physiological effects. Physiotherapy 1990;79:593–594.

84. Lehmann JF, Masock AJ, Warren CG, Koblanski JN. Effect of therapeutic temperatures on tendon extensibility. Arch Phys Med Rehabil 1970;51:481–487.

85. Rose S, Draper DO, Schulthies SS, Durrant E. The stretching window. Part two: Rate of thermal decay in deep muscle following 1-MHz ultrasound. J Athl Train 1996;31:139–143.

86. Oates D, Draper D. Restoring wrist range of motion using ultrasound and mobilization: A case study. Athl Ther Today 2006;11:57–59.

87. Patrick MK. Applications of therapeutic pulsed ultrasound. Physiotherapy 1978;64:103–104.

88. Smith W, Winn F, Parette R. Comparative study using four modalities in shinsplint treatments. J Orthop Sports Phys Ther 1986;8:77–80.

89. Davidson JH, Vandervoort AA, Lessard LA, Miller L. The effect of acupuncture versus ultrasound on pain level, grip strength and disability in individuals with lateral epicondylitis: A pilot study. Physiother Can 2001;53:195–202.

90. Byl NN. The use of ultrasound as an enhancer for transcutaneous drug delivery: Phonophoresis. Phys Ther 1995;75:539–553.

91. van Wamel A, Bouakaz A, ten Cate F, et al. Effects of diagnostic ultrasound parameters on molecular uptake and cell viability. Paper presented at the second International Symposium on Therapeutic Ultrasound, Seattle, 2002.

92. Darrow H, Schulthies S, Draper D, et al. Serum dexamethasone levels after Decadron phonophoresis. J Athl Train 1999;34:338–341.

93. Cameron MH, Monroe LG. Relative transmission of ultrasound by media customarily used for phonophoresis. Phys Ther 1992;72:142–148.

94. Strapp EJ, Guskiewicz KM, Hirth C, et al. The cumulative effect of multiple phonophoresis treatments on dexamethasone and cortisol concentrations in the blood. J Athl Train 2002;35:S47.

95. Benson HAE, McElnay IC. Transmission of ultrasound energy through topical pharmaceutical products. Physiotherapy 1988;74:587.

96. Draper DO, Ashton DF, Cosgrove C, et al. Comparison of Flex-all 4554 and Biofreeze as ultrasound couplants. Paper presented at the annual symposium of the National Athletic Trainers' Association, Orlando, FL, June 1996.

97. Le L, Kost J, Mitragotri S. Combined effect of low-frequency ultrasound and iontophoresis: Applications for transdermal heparin delivery. Pharm Res 2000;17:1151–1154.

98. Tang H, Mitragotri S, Blankschtein D, Langer R. Theoretical description of transdermal transport of hydrophilic permeants: Application to low-frequency sonophoresis. J Pharm Sci 2001;90:545–568.

99. Tang H, Wang CC, Blankschtein D, Langer R. An investigation of the role of cavitation in low-frequency ultrasound-mediated transdermal drug transport. Pharm Res 2002;19:1160–1169.

100. Mitragotri S, Blankschtein D, Langer R. Transdermal drug delivery using low-frequency sonophoresis. Pharm Res 1996;13:411–420.

101. Mitragotri S, Blankschtein D, Langer R. Ultrasound-mediated transdermal protein delivery. Science 1995;269:850–853.

102. Mitragotri S, Kost J. Low-frequency sonophoresis: A review. Adv Drug Deliv Rev 2004;56:589–601.

103. Draper DO, Schulthies S, Sorvisto P, Hautala A-M. Temperature changes in deep muscles of humans during ice and ultrasound therapies: an in vivo study. J Orthop Sports Phys Ther 1995;21:153–157.

104. Rimington SJ, Draper DO, Durrant E, Fellingham G. Temperature changes during therapeutic ultrasound in the precooled human gastrocnemius muscle. J Athl Train 1994;29:325–327.

105. Smith K. The effect of silicate gel hot packs on human muscle temperature. Master's thesis, Brigham Young University, 1994.

106. Girardi CQ, Seaborne D, Savard-Goulet F. The analgesic effect of high voltage galvanic stimulation combined with ultrasound in the treatment of low back pain: a one group pretest/posttest study. Physiother Can 1984;36:327–333.

107. Baker KG, Robertson VJ, Duck FA. A review of therapeutic ultrasound: Biophysical effects. Phys Ther 2001;81:1351–1358.

108. Robertson VJ, Baker KG. A review of therapeutic ultrasound: Effectiveness studies. Phys Ther 2001;81:1339–1350.

109. Draper D. Facts first: Contrary to recent reports, ultrasound is an effective modality: Part I. Advr Directors Rehabil 2002(Feb): 75–87.

110. Draper D. Ultrasound is more than a placebo: Part II. Adv Directors Rehabil 2002(Mar):67–70.

111. Lundeberg T, Abrahamsson P, Haker E. A comparative study of continuous ultrasound, placebo ultrasound and rest in epicondylalgia. Scand J Rehabil Med 1988;20:99–101.

112. McLachlan Z. Ultrasound treatment for breast engorgement: A randomized double blind trial. Austral J Physiother 1991;37:23–28.

113. Falconer J, Hayes KW, Chang RW. Effect of ultrasound on mobility in osteoarthritis of the knee. A randomized clinical trial. Arthritis Care Res 1992;5:29–35.

114. ter Riet G, Kessels AG, Knipschild P. A randomized clinical trial of ultrasound in the treatment of pressure ulcers. Phys Ther 1996;76: 1301–1311.

CHAPTER OUTLINE

Joel, a cross-country skier reports to you with pain in the buttocks. When you question him about his recent skiing regimen, he states that he has been doing a lot of uphill work. Because you know that this type of activity stresses the external rotators of the hip, and through other evaluative measures, you determine that he has piriformis syndrome. Your treatment regimen involves a heat-and-stretch-routine of the piriformis. Which modality would be most appropriate to heat this area before or during stretching of the piriformis muscle? Why?

Introducing Diathermy

The word *diathermy* means "through heat" (*dia* + *therm*). **Diathermy** is therapeutically defined as a modality that uses high-frequency electromagnetic waves to heat deep tissues. Heat is produced by the resistance of tissue to the passage of the energy.[1,2]

DIATHERMY AS A THERAPEUTIC MODALITY

Diathermy is used quite frequently in the United Kingdom, but it has fallen out of favor among many health care professionals in other parts of the world. Physical therapists in Australia[3] and more recently in Canada[4] were surveyed about their ultrasound and diathermy use. Ultrasound was used daily by 93% and 94%, respectively, yet only 8% and 0.6% of them administered daily diathermy treatments. As I (DD) travel to speak at different regional and national conventions of athletic trainers and physical therapists, I often ask attendees how many use diathermy. Usually 1% or 2% raise their hands, yet >90% typically raise their hands when the follow-up question involves the regular use of ultrasound.

Diathermy is not used often in therapeutic settings in the United States for several reasons:

- Expense
- Infamous folklore and misinformation
- Lack of research

Shortwave diathermy units are expensive, ranging from $3,000 to $25,000. Their high cost is prohibitive for many situations, especially a high school, college, or university on a limited budget. For those in private practice, there is a risk that the device will not pay for itself. Many insurance claim forms do not include billing codes for diathermy treatment.

Another reason for limited diathermy use can be attributed to rumor and folklore, which have led many clinicians to put their diathermy machines in a locked closet. Many of the contraindications regarding diathermy use are untested and have been based on speculation and shallow research. For example, authors of a 1993 paper concluded that a possible reason physical therapists were having miscarriages was proximity to their patients being treated with diathermy.[5] Rumors spread that if a pregnant woman was even in the same room as an operating diathermy unit, she risked losing her baby. The facts are that all of those surveyed who had experienced a miscarriage worked in an office in which *microwave* diathermy was in use, not the safer *shortwave* diathermy. Also, the paper concluded that the miscarriage rate of respondents to this survey was no greater than the national average.

There has also been speculation concerning the leak of electromagnetic waves during diathermy use. Whether this is true, manufacturers responded by improving the design and safety of the equipment since the 1990s. These improvements include shielding from electromagnetic waves, which not only protects the patient but also safeguards the clinician.[6,7]

Lack of research on diathermy has also contributed to ignorance about this modality. Many of the diathermy studies were performed before 1970 on equipment that is not the caliber of that currently produced. The latest research was performed on updated and improved equipment.[8–16]

Types of Diathermy

There are two main classifications of diathermy: medical for therapeutic purposes and surgical for cauterizing or burning tissue. The three types of medical or therapeutic diathermy, including their most common frequencies, are:

- *Longwave* (1 MHz; 300 m): This is the oldest method of diathermy but is not used any longer.
- *Shortwave* (27.12 MHz; 11 m): The wave is identical to shortwave radio; therefore, it is regulated by the government to specific frequencies. Shortwave diathermy forms mainly magnetic fields in the tissues.[2]
- *Microwave* (2450 MHz; 0.12 m): This is similar to radar, and it mainly produces electrical fields in the tissues.[2] It is seldom used today in the United States, partly because of its long list of contraindications[5] (Fig. 16.1).

MICROWAVE DIATHERMY

Microwave diathermy (MWD) is a modality that uses high-frequency (300 MHz–300 GHz) electromagnetic waves to heat tissues. A 1984 survey by the U.S. Food and Drug Administration (FDA) indicated that clinics were using **shortwave diathermy (SWD)** <6 hr per week and microwave even less. Here are a few reasons why MWD is so rarely used:

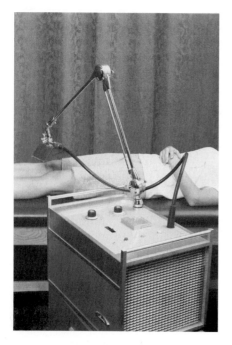

FIGURE 16.1. A microwave diathermy device, rarely used today in the United States.

- *Metals in the vicinity:* Just as with microwave ovens, most metals in contact with MWD will reflect the rays. When this occurs outside the body, these rays may reflect back to the *director* (the part of the device that emits the waves), the patient, or the clinician, thereby resulting in burns. When metal implants are within the body, the reflected rays may overheat adjacent tissues. No metal should be closer than 4 ft. during MWD use.
- *Skin burning:* The higher frequency that MWD uses results in more absorption of the electromagnetic energy in the shallow, fatty tissues. This may result in overheating and superficial burning of the skin and underlying tissues.
- *Overheating of superficial tissues:* The most common frequency used with MWD is 2450 MHz. This higher frequency heats fat and skin but heats muscle at only about one third the temperature of SWD. Another frequency for MWD is being studied. This 915 MHz MWD is capable of deeper heating, yet because it is similar to the frequency of cellular phones (840–880 MHz) the risk of tumors has not been ruled out.
- *Increased reflection at tissue interfaces:* As MWD energy enters the tissues, much of the energy is reflected at tissue interfaces, creating a standing wave (concentrated area of energy) that might lead to hot spots and burning.
- *Lost effects:* At 2450 MHz, the wave director is placed a certain distance from the body part it is treating, so some of the energy is emitted into the surrounding environment. Thus some of the therapeutic effects could be lost. The power must be high enough to heat the tissues but low enough so that skin and fat are not overheated. These calculations can be complicated.
- *Hot spots:* Little MWD energy is reflected at the bone's surface, which can lead to hot spots.

Ongoing work is being done to produce a lower frequency (750 MHz) microwave diathermy that might heat deep tissues as well as does SWD. However, because the majority of treatments in the United States and Europe include SWD and because most of the recent research has been performed on SWD, we will focus on shortwave diathermy in this chapter. Table 16.1 compares microwave and shortwave diathermy as used clinically.

SHORTWAVE DIATHERMY

SWD is a modality that uses high-frequency (10–100 MHz) electromagnetic waves, similar to radio waves, to heat deep tissues. An SWD device is basically a radio transmitter. Three frequencies have been assigned to SWD devices by the U.S. Federal Communications Commission (FCC): 13.56, 40.68, and 27.12 MHz; the latter is the most common and has a wavelength of 11 m.

TABLE 16.1 *Shortwave and Microwave Diathermy Compared*	
SHORTWAVE (SWD)	**MICROWAVE (MWD)**
10–50 MHz frequency	2456–915 MHz frequency
Heating mainly due to magnetic fields	Heating mainly owing to electrical fields
Penetrates fat layer easily	Difficult penetration of fat (if fat layer is >0.5 cm, penetration is only one third of SWD)
Unlikely to create hot spots	Can create hot spots
Can apply directly to skin	Spacing required between skin and applicator
Does not heat metal as much as MWD	No metal can be within 4 ft. of applicators
Most commonly used in orthopedics	Becoming obsolete

COMPONENTS OF A SHORTWAVE DIATHERMY DEVICE

An SWD device has two main parts (Fig. 16.2):

- *Generator:* This box-shaped unit (about the size of a miniature refrigerator) contains all of the electrical components of the machine. Usually on the top of the generator is a control panel that houses buttons, knobs, and switches for operating the machine.
- *Drum:* The drum, (or applicator) is made up of one or more flat spiral copper coils that are rigidly fixed inside a hard plastic housing (Fig. 16.3). The surface area of the drum is about 200 cm², but the size varies by manufacturer. If this size area is to be treated, particularly a small flat area, then a one-drum setup is appropriate. Some manufacturers of SWD produce a device with two drums attached on a hinged arm for treating large or contoured areas (Fig. 16.4).

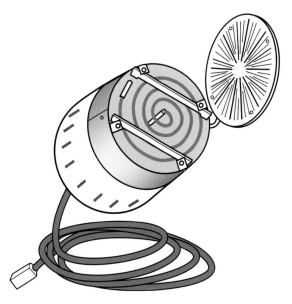

FIGURE 16.3. A shortwave diathermy drum includes a specifically designed coil of wire through which an electrical current flows, creating a magnetic field that causes an induction field in the tissues to which the drum is applied. (Adapted with permission from Castel D. International Academy of Physio Therapeutics, clip art.)

A diathermy drum is like a giant ultrasound transducer soundhead. The soundhead helps deliver sound energy to the tissues, whereas a diathermy drum helps transmit electromagnetic energy to the tissues.

In the past, shortwave diathermy devices housed several types of applicators, including air space plates, pad electrodes, and cable electrodes, many of which are outdated. By far the most common type of SWD applicator in use today is the induction drum; it is the only one discussed in this chapter.

How Shortwave Diathermy Works

An SWD device runs on 110 V electricity from a wall outlet. The generator takes the alternating current (AC) electricity and converts it to radio frequency, usually 27.12

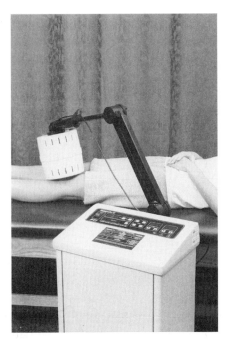

FIGURE 16.2. A shortwave diathermy generator and drum.

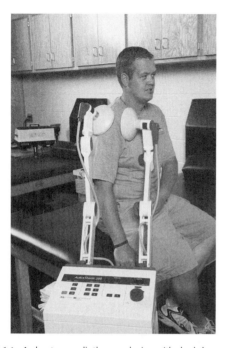

FIGURE 16.4. A shortwave diathermy device with dual drums can treat a larger area than conventional one-drum units. It can also be used to treat two patients at the same time.

MHz. The radio frequency then passes into a flat, spiral copper coil housed in an inductive applicator, or drum. When the radio frequency is applied to the coil, a fluctuating magnetic field is generated around the coil. As the radio frequency exits the drum, an oscillating magnetic field is produced in the body. As the magnetic field passes through the tissues, two things occur. There is an increase in the random motion and kinetic energy among atoms, ions, and molecules and *eddy currents* are created in the tissues. This increased kinetic and eddy current energy results in the thermal and mechanical effects of SWD (Fig. 16.5).

Current Flow

The greatest current flow is through the tissues with the smallest resistance. When SWD produces a magnetic field, adipose tissue (fat) does not provide much resistance to the flow of energy, but it will heat up to some extent.[9] Thus tissues that are high in electrolytes (i.e., muscle and blood) respond best to a magnetic field and produce heat.[17] The greatest amount of heating occurs in tissues with low impedance, especially muscle[17] (Fig. 16.6).

Continuous and Pulsed Shortwave Diathermy

Shortwave diathermy can be applied in either continuous or pulsed mode. *Continuous shortwave diathermy* (CSWD), by which a continuous current is generated, has been used in the treatment of a variety of conditions for some time. In the 1930s, it was used in the United States for treating infections, but its use declined in the 1950s with the introduction of antibiotics to fight infection and with concerns about safety of the device. CSWD is rarely used today because it causes too rapid and too much heating in the patient and can be quite uncomfortable. It has been replaced by pulsed shortwave diathermy.

Pulsed shortwave diathermy (PSWD) uses high-frequency (10–100 MHz) electromagnetic waves in a pulsed mode to produce nonthermal and thermal effects in deep tissues. The modality was first developed in 1940.[7] Although its use has declined, PSWD has recently been the subject of renewed interest, and research documenting its clinical efficacy continues to grow.[6,8,9,14,16]

The electromagnetic waves create a sine wave current that is interrupted (pulsed) at regular intervals. Each series of *pulses*, or *pulse trains*, similar to those used in electricity (see Chapter 9) can be adjusted to the point at which nonthermal or thermal effects are received by the tissues. In much the same way that a pulsed electrical current is created by periodically interrupting continuous current flow, PSWD is created by interrupting the 27.12

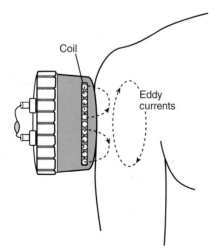

FIGURE 16.5. The magnetic field induced by short wave diathermy creates small eddy currents in the body tissues, resulting in heat.

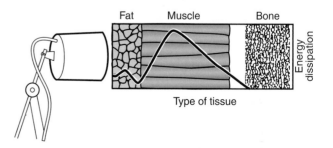

FIGURE 16.6. The greatest amount of shortwave diathermy heating is in tissues with low impedance, especially muscle.

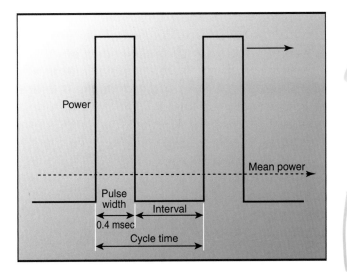

FIGURE 16.7. PSWD results from interrupting continuous shortwave output.

MHz output of CSWD at consistent intervals and having distinct on and off times (Fig. 16.7).

Three factors determine how much heat a PSWD device produces: pulse width, pulse rate, and power.

- **Pulse width,** also known as *pulse duration,* is the time required for each pulse to complete its cycle. The interval between pulses is the off time. A wide pulse generates more energy to tissues than a narrow pulse. Pulse widths are very short. They are measured in microseconds (millionths of a second), with ranges from 20 to 400 μsec. Each manufacturer provides several preset options. For example, the Megapulse II has pulse widths of 20, 40, 65, 100, 200, and 400 μsec, and the Curapulse 403 offers pulse widths of 65, 82, 110, 150, 200, 300, and 400 μsec.
- **Pulse rate,** or pulse repetition rate, is the number of pulses delivered per second (pps, in Hz). The greater the number of pulses per second, the greater the energy produced. Pulse rate ranges from 1 to 7000 Hz. Each manufacturer provides several preset options. For example, the

Megapulse II has pulse rates of 100, 200, 400, 600, and 800 pps, and the Curapulse 403 offers pulse rates of 26, 35, 46, 62, 82, 110, 150, 200, 300, and 400 pps.

- **Power,** also referred to as *intensity,* is measured in watts. It is the power delivered from the machine and is a function of both pulse width and pulse frequency. Shortwave diathermy with a long pulse width and a high pulse frequency generates more power than that with a short pulse width and low pulse frequency.

When PSWD is used, energy is transmitted to the tissues in a series of high-frequency pulse trains. Pulse width is generally short, ranging from 20 to 400 μsec with an intensity of up to 1000 W per pulse. For example, if PSWD is used at 400 Hz with a pulse duration of 400 μsec, the machine is on ~0.16 sec per second or 16% of the time.

The pulse repetition rate is chosen using the pulse–frequency button on the generator control panel.[7,18] Typically the on time is shorter than the off time. This has led many to believe that even if heat is produced during the on time, the long off-time interval allows blood flow to disperse the heat and thereby reduce the likelihood of any significant tissue temperature increase. This assumption is not correct, because researchers have found significant temperature increases of >104°F (40°C) in human muscle when PSWD was applied at 400 and 800 Hz (or just 48 W average power).[8,10,14]

When PSWD is used at intensities that create an increase in tissue temperature, its effects are no different from those of CSWD. Successful treatments have largely resulted from the application of higher intensities and longer treatment times. To increase temperature in tissues, the average intensity needs to be >12 W. In general, PSWD produces lower intensities than CSWD (80–120 W).

Table 16.2 lists the common pulse width and pulse rate settings available on many PSWD devices. Note that we often refer to 48 W average power in this chapter. It is simply because the 7.2°F (4°C) increase in muscle temper-

TABLE 16.2	*PSWD Parameters Based on Treatment Goals*				
DOSE	**TEMPERATURE SENSATION**	**INDICATIONS**	**PULSE WIDTH**	**PULSE RATE**	**AVERAGE WATTS**
N/A	Nonthermal	Acute trauma, nonoticeable inflammation	65 μsec	100–200 pps	N/A
		Edema reduction Cell repolarization and repair			
1°C	Mild warmth	Subacute inflammation	100 μsec 200 μsec	800 pps or 400 pps	12
2°C	Moderate warmth	Pain reduction, muscle spasm Chronic inflammation	200 μsec 400 μsec	800 pps or 400 pps	24
4°C	Vigorous heating	Stretching collagen-rich tissues	400 μsec	800 pps	48

N/A, not applicable.

ature that we have repeatedly obtained in 15–20 min using the parameters of 400 μsec and 800 pps.

Physiological Effects of Diathermy

The physiological effects of shortwave diathermy are categorized as thermal and nonthermal. Whenever diathermy is applied, nonthermal effects occur. When enough energy is absorbed by the tissue, both nonthermal and thermal effects occur.

According to Bricknell and Watson,[19] mild heating can occur with an average power of just 10.88 W. In our experience, 12 W PSWD will produce a mild temperature increase of 1.8°F (1°C). For nonthermal effects (i.e., when the effects of heat are not desired [as with acute swelling] but when mechanical effects are desired for the treatment of soft tissue injuries), we suggest using an average power of 10 W or less.[7,20]

NONTHERMAL EFFECTS

To put it simply, when a patient has an injury, cells are affected. We refer to the cells that are unable to perform their normal function as "sick cells." Basically electromagnetic energy from PSWD helps sick cells get better and return to their normal function. The nonthermal effects of PSWD appear to be at the cell membrane level. They are caused by changes in the way ions bind to the cell membrane as well as changes in cell function caused by the electromagnetic waves.[21] The nonthermal effects include:

- Repolarization of damaged cells, enabling them to return to normal function.[22] Although the mechanism behind this is not well understood, some speculate that it has to do with cell membrane potential.[23] Injured cells experience depolarization, which may cause the cell to lose its ability to divide, multiply, and regenerate. It is thought that both PSWD and ultrasound can stimulate increased macrophage activity.
- Acceleration of cell growth and division when it is too slow, and inhibition of cell growth when it is too fast[24]
- Reestablishment of the sodium pump. During injury, energy deficiencies occur in the cell, and the sodium pump slows down (see Chapter 4). Thus an excess of sodium is deposited in the cell, producing a negatively charged environment. When a magnetic field is induced, the sodium pump speeds up, thereby allowing the cell to regain normal ionic levels.
- Increased microvascular perfusion.[26,27] This increase in local circulation can increase oxygen uptake in local tissues, increase nutrient availability, and promote phagocytosis.

- Improved cell function. A cell involved in the inflammatory process demonstrates a reduced cell membrane potential, thus cell function is disturbed. The altered potential affects ion transport across the membrane; and the resulting ionic balance alters cellular osmotic pressures, often resulting in pain and edema. Apparently, application of PSWD to these cells restores cell membrane potential to their normal values and also restores normal membrane transport and ionic balance.
- Increased number of white cells in a wound[19]

THERMAL EFFECTS

PSWD can cause significant temperature increases up to 4–5 cm deep in the muscle when the drum is placed directly on the skin.[8,10,14] The physiological effects of PSWD at ≥12 W average power are primarily thermal and include

- Tissue temperature rise[8,6,14,28–31]
- Increased blood flow[28–31]
- Vasodilation[32]
- Relaxation[32]
- Decreased joint stiffness[33]
- Increased membrane filtration and diffusion
- Increased tissue metabolic rate
- Changes in some enzyme reactions[34]
- Alterations in the physical properties of fibrous tissues[35,36] (tendons, joints, and scars)
- Muscle relaxation[35]
- Pain reduction[28,29,31,33,35,37]
- Reduction of knee synovitis in arthritic patients[28]
- Reduction of the inflammatory process[19]
- Encouragement of collagen layering at an early stage[19]
- Hematoma absorption[19]

Optimal Tissue Temperatures

Views regarding the temperature required to bring about the various physiological effects are diverse. Some are of the opinion that a 7.2°F (4°C) increase above baseline produces optimal thermal effects[18] (see Table 15.1). Others believe that the temperature must reach at least 100.4–104°F (38–40°C).[35] Most researchers believe the temperature of deep tissues with a baseline temperature of 98.6°F (37°C) should be raised as close as possible to 104°F (40°C) for diathermy to reach its optimal therapeutic effectiveness.[8,38,39] Too rapid or too great a temperature increase can be detrimental. As temperature rises past 113°F (45°C), it alters the structural characteristics of protein, as occurs when such tissue is burned.[1]

As with all modalities, you should experience for yourself the effects of thermal and nonthermal PSWD. Compare them to the sensation of other heating devices, such as hot packs, whirlpools, ultrasound, and even paraffin baths.

Treatment Time

Vigorous heating (104°F [40°C] from a baseline temperature of 98.6°F [37°C]) 3–5 cm deep in the lower leg can be reached in as little as 15–20 min when treated with PSWD at 48 W average power.[8,10] A 20 min treatment for one body area is probably all that is necessary to reach maximum physiological effects. In fact, in two studies, the temperature actually started to drop slightly (0.54°F [0.3°C]) during the last 5 min of a 20 min treatment.[8,14] Apparently, as the tissue temperature reaches 104–105.8°F (40–41°C), the thermoregulatory aspect of the cerebral cortex responds to this high localized temperature, and blood flow increases to the area in an attempt to cool the tissues. Increased blood flow is one of the benefits of using any thermal modality.[40,41]

Trying to determine the correct parameters such as time, pulse frequency, and duration to reach specific treatment goals can be overwhelming. Box 16.1 describes a user-friendly PSWD machine.

Clinical Applications of Shortwave Diathermy

There are several situations in which PSWD is considered appropriate or, in some cases, optimal:

- Heating is required before passive stretch or joint mobilizations of any joint larger than the wrist.

- Nonthermal effects are desired in deep tissue over a large area.
- The skin or some underlying soft tissue is very sensitive and will not bear the pressure of a moist heat pack or the jet from a whirlpool.
- A tissue temperature rise is desired in tissues deeper than 1–2 cm beneath the skin.
- Nonthermal effects are desired in tissues deeper than 1–2 cm beneath the skin.
- The treatment goal is to increase deep tissue temperatures over a large area (approximately the size of the drum), such as the shoulder girdle, low back, or the hamstring or triceps surae muscle belly.
- Heating is required in areas of moderate subcutaneous fat and deep muscle.
- Treatment is desired over irregular or uneven surfaces, such as the hand or foot.

CRITICAL THINKING 16.1 *A lean patient comes to you with some muscular back pain over a large area. He can pinpoint two or three silver dollar–size tender areas, but the rest of his back is generally sore. Unfortunately, you don't have a PSWD device. What can you do to heat the area?*

HEATING JOINT CAPSULES BEFORE STRETCHING OR MOBILIZATIONS

Some of the most promising uses of PSWD have been with stretching or joint mobilizations to increase range of motion (ROM).[11,15,16,33,42] A heat-and-stretch regimen using PSWD has been successful in increasing the flexibility of

---

BOX 16.1 *A USER-FRIENDLY PSWD DEVICE*

In Chapter 15 we described an ultrasound device that enabled the clinician to use temperature increases for treatment goals, instead of a clock to measure treatment time. A PSWD device has been developed in much the same way. The research involved measuring the temperature in the leg muscles of >50 subjects to determine the pulse rate and pulse width required to raise muscle temperature 1.8°F (1°C) for mild heat, 3.6°F (2°C) for moderate heat, and 7.2°F (4°C) for vigorous heat. Based on this research, a diathermy device was equipped with a keypad that included these three levels of heat (Fig. 16.8). After setting up the device over the area to be treated, the clinician selects the heating level that best achieves the treatment goal. The device auto-

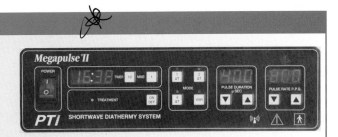

FIGURE 16.8. The control panel on a typical PSWD device.

matically tunes into the preprogrammed settings (pulse width, pulse rate) to reach that goal. The device shuts off when the desired temperature is theoretically reached (*theoretical* because the device does not measure the patient's temperature but is based on the means of study subjects).

subjects with tight hamstrings[11] and increasing ankle dorsiflexion ROM.[15] This effect probably results from:

- Local relaxation by decreasing muscle guarding and pain[39]
- Decreased stiffness of tissues[23]
- Increased extensibility of the collagen fibers and the resilience of contracted soft tissues[23,33,39]

 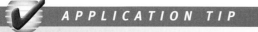

USE PSWD BEFORE STRETCHING. *If you have a patient who has a joint capsule with adhesions that won't seem to allow normal ROM, consider using PSWD before stretching. Box 16.2 provides an example of how this can be accomplished.*

According to Kaltenborn,[43] joint mobilizations should always be preceded by some form of heat. Joint mobilizations, preceded by PSWD are not only beneficial at restoring ROM but are much more comfortable for the patient. Boxes 16.2–16.5 present some of our many successful cases using PSWD with joint mobilizations to restore ROM in a patient with a frozen joint.

APPLICATION TIP

USE PSWD BEFORE JOINT MOBILIZATIONS. *We agree with joint mobilization specialist Kaltenborn:*[43] *Joint mobilizations should be preceded by some form of heat. Then why not use deep heat aimed right at the source? PSWD for 15–20 min before joint mobilizations will not only help heat the tissues to be stressed but will reduce the discomfort patients often experience during mobilizations.*

Diathermy Treatment Contraindications and Precautions

There are more precautions and contraindications for the use of microwave diathermy than for shortwave diathermy. In addition, there are apparently more treatment precautions and contraindications for the use of PSWD than any of the other physical modalities used in a clinical setting. However, don't let this discourage you from using it. Many prescription medications have a long

BOX 16.2 *REGIMEN OF PSWD AND STRETCHING RESTORES ROM TO ANKLE*

In 1995, 34-year-old Brian rolled his Jeep and was stabbed in the calf by the knobless gear-shift shaft, which caused significant muscle damage and a fractured tibia. After surgery and some physical therapy, he had 0° dorsiflexion ROM. About 4 years later (1999), he was treated with a regimen of 20 min PSWD at 800 Hz, at a pulse width of 400 μsec (48 W average power). Then 10 min into the heat treatment, stretch was applied for 10 min. By the seventh treatment Brian reached 16° of dorsiflexion (20° is normal). Even 7 years after his treatments (2006), he still has all the ROM he gained from the diathermy and stretching regimen (Fig. 16.9).

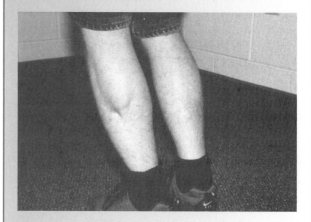

FIGURE 16.9. Dorsiflexion was restored in the left ankle with PSWD and stretching 4 years after an accident that caused significant muscle damage and a fractured tibia. (Note the divot in the calf, a residual of the accident.)

list of contraindications; but when used appropriately, the benefits far outweigh the risks. This same approach should be taken with shortwave diathermy. It is a powerful tool when used correctly.

Remember that the power meter on a diathermy device does not indicate the actual amount of energy that is being absorbed in the tissues. Thus you must rely on the sensation of pain for a warning that the patient's tolerance level has been exceeded.

CONTRAINDICATIONS

The contraindications of PSWD include the following:

- *Implanted pacemaker, neurostimulator, or defibrillator:*[44] The lead wires can act as antennas and provide intensely focused fields at the tissue–lead junction, causing significant tissue damage that could lead to serious

When Erin was 12 years old, she fell from a height of 8 ft. and fractured her elbow. She had surgery and was immobilized in a cast for >3 months. At age 20, while she was a college student, her professor (DD) noticed that she couldn't extend her elbow very far (she lacked 23° of full extension). He put her on a regimen of PSWD (48 W) and joint mobilizations every other day (Fig. 16.10). She gained 8° of extension from the first treatment and all but 2° of full extension after five treatments, which is very acceptable in an elbow.

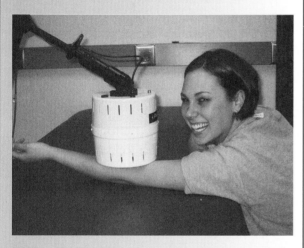

FIGURE 16.10. PSWD before joint mobilizations to treat adhesive capsulitis of the elbow.

injury or death. People with a pacemaker should not even be in the direct vicinity of PSWD.

- *Some surgically implanted metals:* Don't use PSWD over metal implants that form closed loops, such as might occur with wires used for fixating rods and plates in surgical fracture repairs. The current can flow in the wire loops, resulting in heating.[2]
- *Pregnancy:* Avoid treating the abdomen, pelvis, or back in view of the probable effect that PSWD might have on embryonic tissue and the placenta.[39]
- *Over tumors:* Some physicians use very high power PSWD to destroy cancerous cells; however, owing to the possibility that PSWD increases the activity of tumor cells, this is beyond the scope of the athletic trainer or therapist.[39,45]
- *Fever:* PSWD can cause the temperature to increase even more.[45]
- *Infection:* PSWD can increase metabolism, thereby causing the infection to spread.

- *Growth plates:* Although this has not been tested in humans, we surmise that a rapid increase in temperature may damage epiphyseal plates.
- *Testes:* A rapid increase in temperature might lead to sterility.
- *Eyes:* Do not use on or near the eyes or contact lenses for prolonged time.
- *Joint effusion*
- *Protruded nucleus pulposus*[45]

MODALITY MYTH

PSWD CANNOT BE USED NEAR METAL

Metal is highly conductive when an electrical current is applied, and it is thought to become very hot when diathermy is applied. This is true with MWD and CSWD but not true for PSWD. We list it as a precaution with PSWD. In the past, it was considered unsafe to treat a patient with PSWD on a wooden table or a plastic chair if it had been constructed with metal screws.[2] But it is safe. The energy will not heat up the screws, nor will it be transmitted to the patient.

PRECAUTIONS

Care should be taken when using PSWD:

- For conditions in which increased temperature is not desired
- Over traumatic musculoskeletal injuries with acute bleeding
- For acute inflammatory conditions[39]
- On areas with reduced blood supply
- Over areas with reduced sensitivity to temperature or pain[23]
- Over fluid-filled areas or organs
- During menstruation. PSWD applied to the abdomen, pelvis, or low back could increase bleeding[39]
- Over wound dressings. If the wound is dry and not infected, PSWD is safe.
- Over some implanted metals.[46] PSWD can be used to treat soft tissue adjacent to most metal implants that don't form a loop, without much increase in the temperature of the metal. Before treating any patient with metal implants, be aware of what type of implant is involved. If you do proceed with a treatment, and the patient complains of too much heat, turn the machine off.
- Near other equipment. Some of the newer PSWD devices are shielded from emitting stray electromagnetic

waves and are probably safe to use around other equipment. If your unit was manufactured before 1993, it may be wise to use it at a safe distance from other types of medical electrical devices or equipment that is transistorized. Transcutaneous electrical nerve stimulation (TENS) units and other low-frequency current units often have transistor-type circuits, and these can be damaged by the reflected or stray radiation that might be produced by PSWD devices.

MODALITY **MYTH**

PSWD CANNOT BE USED OVER ANY METAL

Many are of the opinion that PSWD can't be used on a patient with braces in her mouth. This is safe, unless the face is being treated. For treating the temporomandibular joint (TMJ), we suggest ultrasound. Several journal articles and texts state that it is absolutely contraindicated to use PSWD on a patient with surgically implanted pins, rods, or screws in a joint. Some machines at 48 W have proven to be safe and effective, as long as the metal implant is not a circular wire or loop.[2,16,47] As of the writing of this text, we have tested only the Megapulse II (Accelerated Care Plus, Reno, NV).

PSWD USE ON PATIENTS WITH SURGICALLY IMPLANTED METAL

Perhaps the greatest controversy regarding the use of shortwave diathermy is surgically implanted metal plates, screws, and pins in the area being treated. In a recent survey of physiotherapists in Ireland, 49% considered PSWD to always be contraindicated for use on patients with metal implants.[48] It is thought that the shunting of the radio frequency field through a metal implant may increase the current density around the implant and cause a more local temperature increase.[6,12,14,16] This is, however, a definite contraindication for microwave diathermy.

Metals, however, do concentrate electromagnetic energy and can be heated with continuous shortwave diathermy. Therefore, all metals (pins, screws, etc.) are also contraindicated for use with CSWD. But can a patient with pins, rods, or screws in a joint be treated with low-watt PSWD? We have had great success in treating such patients with 48 W PSWD for the purpose of restoring ROM with joint mobilizations.[12,16] Boxes 16.4 and 16.5 describe two of the many patients treated in our laboratory.

MODALITY **MYTH**

A FOLDED TOWEL MUST BE PLACED BETWEEN THE DIATHERMY DRUM AND THE PATIENT

In the past, the clinician would place a single layer of toweling between the drum and the skin to absorb perspiration. With the newer developments in PSWD, this practice is necessary only in humid climates or when the tissue temperature becomes a little uncomfortable for the patient. Also, toweling might be used in areas of the body where moisture accumulates (such as the axillas or gluteal cleft). The results are best when the drum is placed directly on the skin, but the area treated must remain dry. Clinicians used to think it was important to remove clothing from the treatment area. Although this is true with synthetic fabrics that do not allow moisture to evaporate, shortwave diathermy can safely be applied over cotton clothing. This is a great advantage for modest patients.

The Advantages of PSWD Over Ultrasound

There are several advantages to using PSWD instead of ultrasound (Fig. 16.15):

- *A larger area is heated:* The surface of a diathermy drum is about the size of a small salad plate, whereas

---

BOX 16.4 *LAUREL'S LONG ROAD TO RECOVERY*

In 2002, Laurel fractured her elbow in several places during an automobile accident.[12] During two surgeries, physicians installed plates, pins, and screws to repair her arm (Fig. 16.11). After 10 weeks of immobilization, she started physical therapy. Within several months, some of the ROM was restored. However, during the next 2 months, little progress was made and she lacked the last 12° of flexion and 28° of extension. She reported to our laboratory, where PSWD (48 W) and joint mobilizations were applied to her elbow. She gained 5° flexion and 7° extension on the first visit. By her fourth visit, all of her flexion had returned; and by her sixth visit, she had regained all but 3° of extension (Fig. 16.12). Upon evaluation a few months later, she had full active elbow extension. And 3 years later (2006), she still had full ROM.

BOX 16.4 *(continued)*

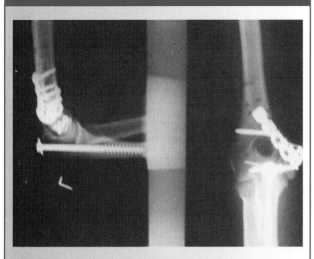

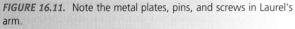

FIGURE 16.11. Note the metal plates, pins, and screws in Laurel's arm.

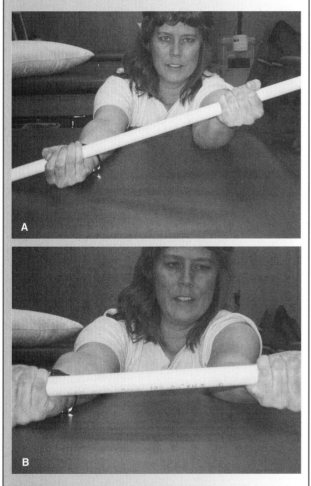

FIGURE 16.12. **(a)** Laurel lacked 28° of elbow extension before PSWD and joint mobilizations. **(b)** She gained 25° of elbow extension when treated every other day for six visits.

BOX 16.5 *PSWD AND JOINT MOBILIZATIONS TO RESTORE ANKLE ROM*

Figure 16.13 is an x-ray of the leg of a 48-year-old woman who suffered a severe automobile accident. The injury was so bad that the physician suggested amputation. Instead, surgery was performed using extensive metal plates, pins, and screws to repair the leg. About 1 year later she reported to our laboratory with very little ROM in the ankle. After several treatments of PSWD and joint mobilizations, she returned to pain-free gait and improved her dorsiflexion 15° (Fig. 16.14).

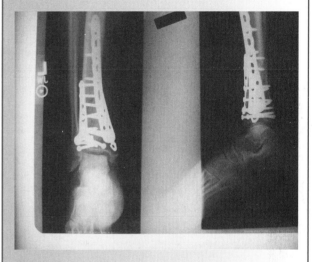

FIGURE 16.13. Note the surgical repair of a severely injured leg, which required metal plates, pins, and screws.

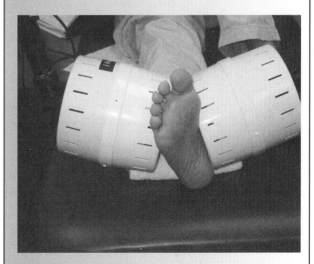

FIGURE 16.14. Two PSWD drums being applied to the patient before joint mobilizations.

the ultrasound treatment size is about the size of a tablespoon. Thus the diathermy drum is often 25–30 times larger than the treatment area for ultrasound (50–60 times larger if a two-drum applicator is used).

- *A diathermy drum remains stationary during the treatment:* Thus there are no hot spots in the tissue. The ultrasound applicator is constantly moving, thus creating the possibility for uneven heating and hot spots.
- *The heat provided by diathermy lasts two or three times longer than that provided by ultrasound:* This enables the clinician to perform low-load, long-duration stretching for 10–15 min while the tissue is still warm.
- *No messy gels or couplants are required*

- *The treatment can be applied over some clothing.*
- *Ultrasound application requires a clinician or aide to be present during the entire treatment:* PSWD application requires only periodic monitoring by the clinician or aid, so the clinician is free to work with multiple patients at a time.

CRITICAL THINKING 16.2 *Now you have read both the ultrasound and the diathermy chapters and have just finished reading about some of the advantages of PSWD use over ultrasound. Can you think of some advantages of ultrasound use over PSWD?*

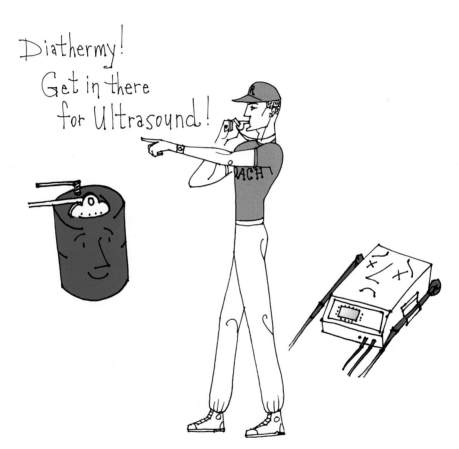

FIGURE 16.15. Shortwave diathermy has many advantages over ultrasound, especially when the area to be heated is more than two times the size of the ultrasound soundhead.

Application of Diathermy

STEP 1: FOUNDATION

A. Definition. Pulsed shortwave diathermy (PSWD) uses high-frequency (10–100 MHz) electromagnetic waves in a pulsed mode to produce nonthermal and thermal effects in deep tissues.

B. Effects
   1. Thermal effects include
      a. Increased metabolism
      b. Increased blood flow
      c. Tissue temperature rise
      d. Diminished pain perception
      e. General muscle relaxation
   2. Nonthermal effects include soft tissue healing

C. Advantages
   1. Heats deeper than all other modalities (except 1 MHz ultrasound)
   2. Heats an area 25–30 times larger than ultrasound

D. Disadvantages
   1. Expensive ($3,000–$25,000 for a machine)
   2. Big, bulky, and heavy; not portable

E. Indications
   1. Muscle strain
   2. Sprain
   3. Contusion
   4. Tendinitis
   5. Tenosynovitis
   6. Bursitis
   7. Myofascial trigger points
   8. Pain
   9. Removal of the byproducts of the inflammatory process
   10. Joint contracture

F. Contraindications
   1. Cardiac pacemaker
   2. Pregnancy
   3. Malignant tumor
   4. Fever
   5. Ischemic areas
   6. Peripheral vascular disease
   7. Tuberculosis
   8. Sites of infection
   9. Eyes
   11. Genitals
   12. Epiphyseal plates in children
   13. Protruded nucleus pulposus

G. Precautions
   1. Surgically implanted metals (especially circular, or loops)
   2. Pelvic or lumbar exposure during menstruation
   3. Arterial and venous circulatory disorders (thrombosis, atherosclerosis, etc.)
   4. Osteoporosis
   5. Wound dressings
   6. Over tissues or organs with high fluid volume
   7. Acute inflammation
   8. Active hemorrhage
   9. Sensory impairment

STEP 2: PREAPPLICATION TASKS

A. Make sure PSWD is the proper modality for this situation.
   1. Re-evaluate the injury or problem. Make sure you understand the patient's condition.
   2. If PSWD was applied previously, review the patient's response to that treatment.
   3. Confirm that the objectives of therapy are compatible with PSWD.

B. Preparing the equipment. Prepare the equipment before preparing the patient. Make sure the drum is clean and dry.

C. Preparing the patient psychologically
   1. Explain the procedure.
      a. Safe electromagnetic energy enters the body tissues and causes the molecules to rotate and move about faster, resulting in heat.
      b. Gentle warmth should be felt during the treatment (unless it is a nonthermal treatment).
      c. Demonstrate the procedure on yourself if the patient is apprehensive.
   2. Check for, and warn the patient about, precautions. If the treatment starts to feel too warm, ask the patient to let you know.

D. Preparing the patient physically
   1. Remove any metal or jewelry from the part to be treated.
   2. Remove any synthetic fabrics that might trap heat in the area to be treated.
   3. Position the patient in a comfortable yet modest position, while allowing accessibility to the diathermy device.
   4. Inspect the area to be treated. If there are rashes or moist open wounds, do not proceed.

STEP 3: APPLICATION PARAMETERS

A. Procedures
   1. Place the drum on the area (place a towel between the drum and the skin if desired).

2. Turn the device on.
B. Dosage
   1. Set the pulse duration (low for acute, nonthermal; high for thermal).
   2. Set the pulse frequency (low for acute, nonthermal; high for thermal).
   3. Set the treatment time (15–30 min).
   4. Depress the start button.
   5. Adjust the intensity according to the patient's comfort. Recheck in 4–5 min as the tissues heat up.
C. Length of application. For 15–30 min
D. Frequency of application. Use 1–2 times daily.
E. Duration of therapy. Until treatment goals are reached

4️⃣ STEP 4: POSTAPPLICATION TASKS

A. Equipment removal and replacement. When the timer shuts off, signaling the end of the treatment, make sure all knobs and buttons are returned to zero.

B. Instructions to the patient
   1. Schedule the next treatment.
   2. Instruct the patient about level of activity and/or self-treatment before the next formal treatment.
   3. Instruct the patient about the what she should feel after treatment.
C. Record of treatment, including unique patient responses
D. Equipment cleaning and replacement
   1. Clean off the table, removing any sweat or moisture.
   2. If you used a towel, replace it with a clean one.

5️⃣ STEP 5: MAINTENANCE

A. Clean the equipment regularly.
B. Make sure all cables and connections are in good repair.

CLOSING SCENE

Recall from the chapter opening scene that Joel, a cross-country skier who has piriformis syndrome, came to see you. In applying a heat-and-stretch routine of the piriformis, you were asked which modality would be most appropriate to heat this area and why. After reading this chapter and previous chapters, you know that hot packs and whirlpools, though convenient, can penetrate only the superficial structures from 1 to 2 cm deep. To penetrate the gluteal muscles and get at the source of the problem (piriformis), you must use a deep-heating modality. Although ultrasound is a deep-heating modality, it is not appropriate in this situation because it heats only a small area.[14] Diathermy heats deep tissues and heats an area as large as the applicator drum, so PSWD is the modality of choice in this situation.[10,14]

CHAPTER REFLECTIONS

1. Read and ponder each of the following points. Do you feel you have a clear understanding of each concept? If not, reread the appropriate section of the chapter.
   - What is diathermy?
   - Name two types of diathermy.
   - Identify the most popular type of diathermy in the United States and explain the reasons for its popularity.
   - List the effects of diathermy.
   - Describe the indications of diathermy.
   - List several contraindications of diathermy.
   - Compare and contrast diathermy with ultrasound.
   - Discuss some diathermy myths.
2. Write three to five questions for discussion with your class instructor, clinical instructor, classmates, and clinical colleagues.
3. Get together with classmates and quiz each other on the concepts of this chapter. Use the points in exercise 1 and questions you wrote for exercise 2 as a beginning. Explaining concepts out loud to others requires a deeper grasp of the material than feeling you understand it as you read.

4. Once you feel you understand the principles of application of PSWD, practice applying them using the five-step approach with a classmate or clinical colleague. Alternate applying the modalities to each other. When it is being applied to you, listen and observe carefully to determine whether your classmate is using proper application. Consult your notes when the modality is applied to you and for the first few times you apply the modality to another person. Continue practicing the application until you can do so without using your notes.

CRITICAL THINKING RESPONSES

Critical Thinking 16.1

The key here is that the patient is lean, so you can apply hot packs to the general sore areas. On the silver dollar–size tender areas, consider using ultrasound. The treatment size is perfect, and the 1 MHz setting will penetrate deep enough to get at the problem.

Critical Thinking 16.2

Therapeutic ultrasound has the following advantages over shortwave diathermy:

- It is less expensive.
- There are fewer contraindications.
- The devise is smaller and portable.
- It has variable frequencies for treating various tissue depths.
- It can be used under water.
- It can provide phonophoresis.
- Servicing is easier (there are more distributors).

REFERENCES

1. Michlovitz S. Thermal Agents in Rehabilitation. Philadelphia: Davis, 1996.
2. Cameron M. Physical Agents in Rehabilitation: From Research to Practice. St. Louis: Saunders, 2003.
3. Lindsay DM, Dearness J, Richardson C, et al. A survey of electromodality usage in private physiotherapy practices. Aust J Physiother 1990;36:249–256.
4. Lindsay DM, Dearness J, McGinley CC. Electrotherapy usage trends in private physiotherapy practice in Alberta. Physiother Can 1995;47:30–34.
5. Hellstrom RO, Stewart WF. Miscarriages among female physical therapists who report using radio- and microwave-frequency electromagnetic fields. Am J Epidemiol 1993;138:775–785.
6. Draper DO. Interest in diathermy heats up again. Biomechanics 2001;8:77–83.
7. Kitchen S, Partridge C. Review of shortwave diathermy continuous and pulsed patterns. Physiotherapy 1992;78:243–252.
8. Draper DO, Knight KL, Fujiwara T, Castel JC. Temperature change in human muscle during and after pulsed short-wave diathermy. J Orthop Sports Phys Ther 1999;29:13–18; discussion 19–22.
9. Draper DO, Abergel PA, Castel JC, Schlaak C. Pulsed shortwave diathermy restricts swelling and bruising of liposuction patients. Am J Cosmet Surg 2000;17:17–22.
10. Draper DO, Garrett C. Pulsed shortwave diathermy heats a considerably larger area than 1 MHz ultrasound treatments. J Athl Train 1999;34:S23.
11. Draper DO, Castro J, Feland JB, et al. Shortwave diathermy and prolonged stretching increase flexibility more than prolonged stretching alone. J Ortho Sports Phys Ther 2003;34:13–20.
12. Draper DO, Castel JC, Castel D. Low-watt pulsed shortwave diathermy and metal-plate fixation of the elbow. Athl Ther Today 2004;9:27–31.
13. Draper DO. Shortwave diathermy in the athletic training room. Paper presented at the annual symposium of the National Athletic Trainers' Association, Los Angeles, June 2001.
14. Garrett CL, Draper DO, Knight KL. Heat distribution in the lower leg from pulsed short-wave diathermy and ultrasound treatments. J Athl Train 2000;35:13–22.
15. Peres SE, Draper DO, Knight KL, Ricard MD. Pulsed shortwave diathermy and prolonged long-duration stretching increase dorsiflexion range of motion more than identical stretching without diathermy. J Athl Train 2002;37:43–50.
16. Seiger C, Draper DO. Pulsed shortwave diathermy and joint mobilizations increase range of motion to normal in fractured ankles with surgical implanted metal: A case series. J Orthop Sports Phys Ther 2006;36:669–677.
17. Van der Esch M, Hoogland R. Pulsed Shortwave Diathermy with the Curapuls 419. Delft, The Netherlands: Delft Instruments Physical Medicine, 1990.
18. Castel D. Electrotherapy and Ultrasound Update. 2nd ed. Reno, NV: International Academy of Physio Therapeutics, 1996.
19. Bricknell R, Watson T. The thermal effects of pulsed shortwave therapy. Br J Ther Rehabil 1995;2:430–434.
20. Brown M, Baker RD. Effect of pulsed short wave diathermy on skeletal muscle injury in rabbits. Phys Ther 1987;67:208–214.
21. Pilla AA, Markov MS. Bioeffects of weak electromagnetic fields. Rev Environ Health 1994;10:155–169.
22. Low JL. Dosage of some pulsed shortwave clinical trial. Physiotherapy 1995;81:611–616.
23. Kloth L, Ziskin M. Diathermy and pulsed electromagnetic fields. In: Michlovitz SL, ed. Thermal Agents in Rehabilitation. 2nd ed. Philadelphia: Davis, 1990.
24. Canaday D, Lee R. Scientific basis for clinical application of electric fields in soft tissue repair. In: Brighton C, Pollack S, eds. Electromagnetics in Biology Medicine. San Francisco: San Francisco Press, 1991.
25. Sanseverino EG. Membrane phenomena and cellular processes under the action of pulsating magnetic fields. Presented at the 2nd International Congress of Magneto Medicine. Rome, Italy, 1980.
26. Mayrovitz H, Larsen P. A preliminary study to evaluate the effect of pulsed radio frequency field treatment on lower extremity peri-ulcer skin microcirculation of diabetic patients. Wounds 1995;7:90–93.

Chapter 12

1. Which of the following is the most common type of superficial heat used in an athletic training clinic?
    a. whirlpool
    b. hot pack
    c. paraffin bath
    d. infrared lamp
    e. ultraviolet light

2. Which of the following is a disadvantage of a paraffin bath?
    a. It doesn't allow for range of motion during treatment.
    b. It feels too hot.
    c. The mineral oil can irritate the skin.
    d. It is messy.
    e. both a and d

3. Which of the following is a disadvantage of whirlpool?
    a. can treat the whole body
    b. provides irregular surfaces with total contact
    c. loses (or gains) heat very slowly
    d. can provide multiple treatments simultaneously
    e. difficult to keep the treatment area clean and sanitary

4. Which of the following is essential to have when using a whirlpool?
    a. IFC
    b. GFI
    c. RICES
    d. DC
    e. rubber duck

5. Which of the following is not an advantage of hot packs?
    a. easy to apply
    b. relatively expensive
    c. can treat over an open wound without fear of spreading germs to others
    d. durable
    e. portable

6. Which of the following is an advantage of topical heat wraps, such as the ThermaCare wrap?
    a. easy to apply
    b. difficult to keep the treatment area clean and sanitary
    c. heat lasts for only 15 min
    d. portable
    e. both a and d

7. The appropriate water temperature for treating a limb in a warm whirlpool is _____.
    a. 100–108°F (37.7–42.2°C)
    b. 105–112°F (40.5–44.4°C)
    c. 95–100°F (35–38°C)
    d. 112–117°F (44.4–47.2°C)
    e. none of the above

8. The appropriate water temperature for treating a full body in a warm whirlpool is _____.
    a. 100–108°F (37.7–42.2°C)
    b. 105–112°F (40.5–44.4°C)
    c. 95–100°F (35–38°C)
    d. 112–117°F (44.4–47.2°C)
    e. none of the above

Chapter 13

1. Which of the following is not a physiological effect of cold application?
    a. decreased temperature
    b. increased metabolism
    c. decreased or increased pain
    d. decreased muscle spasm
    e. increased tissue stiffness

2. Which of the following are not suggested hot-to-cold ratios (in minutes) for contrast therapy?
    a. 4:1
    b. 3:1
    c. 3:2
    d. 5:5
    e. all of the above have been suggested

3. A sudden, intense, painful, tetanic muscle contraction that is short lived, usually lasting <20 sec, is called a _____.
    a. muscle spasm
    b. muscle cramp
    c. charley horse
    d. muscle strain
    e. two of the above

4. A gradual onset of tightness in a muscle, usually not particularly painful, is known as a _____.
    a. muscle spasm
    b. muscle cramp
    c. charley horse
    d. muscle strain
    e. two of the above

5. The increase in vascular circumference of blood vessels as a result of cold applications is known as _____.
   a. cryostretch
   b. cryotherapy
   c. cold-induced vasodilation
   d. cold-induced vasoconstriction
   e. the Lewis effect

6. Cryokinetics is _____.
   a. alternating of cold applications to numb an area, followed by active graded exercise
   b. three techniques for reducing muscle spasm: cold application, static stretching, and isometric contraction (the hold–relax technique of PNF)
   c. a combination of heat application, long-term passive stretch, and then cold applications, used to increase joint flexibility after prolonged immobilization
   d. a therapeutic agent that uses a pump attached to a boot or sleeve that intermittently forces air or chilled water into the sleeve for the purpose of decreasing lymphedema
   e. alternating immersion of the injured body part in hot and cold water baths

7. Which of the following is the best to use to increase joint flexibility after prolonged immobilization during which connective tissue contractures have developed?
   a. cryostretch
   b. connective tissue stretch
   c. lymphedema pump
   d. contrast bath stretch
   e. cryokinetics

8. Which of the following is the best to use to increase joint flexibility following an acute muscle strain?
   a. cryostretch
   b. connective tissue stretch
   c. lymphedema pump
   d. contrast bath stretch
   e. cryokinetics

Chapter 14

1. During ice massage, numbness can be increased by _____.
   a. applying more pressure with the ice
   b. moving the ice faster
   c. using an ice bag
   d. heating the area with ultrasound before icing
   e. applying a compression wrap

2. A toe cap is used during the application of which modality?
   a. RICES
   b. ice bag
   c. ice massage
   d. ice water immersion
   e. hot whirlpool

3. Which of the following is *not* a beneficial effect of cryokinetics?
   a. decreased pain, thus allowing exercise
   b. exercise increases blood flow
   c. exercise reestablishes neuromuscular functioning
   d. decreased metabolism
   e. none of the above, all are beneficial

4. Which of the following is *not* a contraindication for intermittent compression pumps?
   a. compartment syndrome
   b. peripheral vascular disease
   c. arteriosclerosis
   d. lymphedema
   e. local superficial infection

5. Which of the following is the reason an ice pack is used after connective tissue stretch?
   a. Ice causes collagen fibers to relax.
   b. Ice lengthens the collagen fibers.
   c. Ice causes the collagen fibers to reattach in a lengthened position.
   d. Ice helps cause plastic elongation.
   e. two of the above

6. Which of the following includes five sets of exercise?
   a. cryostretch
   b. cryokinetics
   c. lymphedema pump
   d. ice massage
   e. two of the above

Chapter 15

1. Within ultrasound waves are regions of high molecular density called _____ and regions of low molecular density called _____.
   a. compressions; reflections
   b. compressions; refractions
   c. refractions; compressions
   d. absorptions; transmissions
   e. none of the above

2. Which of the following would be the best crystal BNR?
   a. 3:1
   b. 1:3
   c. 4:1
   d. 1:4
   e. 6:1

3. Spatial average intensity is the amount of energy passing through a specified area, such as an ultrasound transducer soundhead. If 8 W are being delivered through a 5 cm soundhead, the SAI is _____.
   a. 2 W/cm^2
   b. 1.8 W/cm^2
   c. 1.6 W/cm^2
   d. 1.4 W/cm^2
   e. 0.62 W/cm^2

4. Which of the following is *true* with respect to temporal average intensity?
   a. It is the amount of energy passing through a specified area.
   b. It is the power of ultrasonic energy over a given period of time.
   c. It refers to continuous ultrasound.
   d. two of the above
   e. none of the above

5. A low PAMBNR provides for _____.
   a. a more comfortable treatment
   b. more even heating of tissue layers
   c. greater depth of penetration
   d. all of the above
   e. two of the above

6. During the ultrasound application, unstable cavitation can occur from _____.
   a. moving the soundhead too slow
   b. moving the soundhead too fast
   c. using a high intensity
   d. using a poor conducting medium
   e. both a and c
   f. both b and d

7. When reading your ultrasound manual, it says that during the pulsed mode, your unit has a 1:5 duty cycle. This means that the current is _____.
   a. off 80% of the time
   b. off 75% of the time
   c. on 30% of the time
   d. on 25% of the time
   e. none of the above

8. Which of the following is the least effective ultrasound couplant?
   a. water
   b. ultrasound gel pad
   c. ultrasound gel
   d. massage lotion
   e. petroleum jelly

9. The abbreviation W refers to the _____.
   a. power or intensity of the treatment
   b. pulse duration (width)
   c. number of pulses per second
   d. type of current (alternating or direct)
   e. stretching window

10. The decrease of energy contained within a sound wave as it travels through tissue is known as _____.
    a. the Ardnt-Schultz principle
    b. the law of Grotthus-Draper
    c. attenuation
    d. the piezoelectric effect
    e. rarefaction

11. According to the text, a state-of-the-art ultrasound device would contain which of the following?
    a. a high-quality natural crystal
    b. a pause button
    c. a high BNR
    d. a high ERA
    e. a gel warmer

12. Which of the following is a contraindication for ultrasound?
    a. pain
    b. skin anesthesia
    c. muscle spasm
    d. heat before stretching
    e. orthopedic implanted metal

Chapter 16

1. Which of the following is true with respect to microwave diathermy?
   a. If fat is <1 cm, it can penetrate up to 5 cm.
   b. Spacing is required between the applicator and the skin.
   c. It heats by the production of magnetic fields.
   d. all of the above
   e. both a and b

2. Which of the following is true with respect to short-wave diathermy?
   a. It heats fat more than muscle.
   b. Spacing is required between the applicator and the skin.
   c. It heats by the production of magnetic fields.
   d. all of the above
   e. both a and b

3. Which of the following is not part of a SWD machine?
   a. generator
   b. copper coil
   c. drum
   d. power switch
   e. transducer

4. The term *diathermy* means _____.
   a. excessive fluid in cells
   b. changing from one energy form into another
   c. loss of sensation
   d. heat loss or gain through direct contact
   e. to heat through

5. Which is the most common type of diathermy applicator?
   a. induction coil
   b. drum
   c. pad
   d. pancake cable
   e. air space plates

6. Which of the following is a contraindication for PSWD?
   a. myofascial trigger points
   b. pain
   c. removal of the byproducts of the inflammatory process
   d. joint contracture
   e. cardiac pacemaker

7. Which of the following pulsed SWD treatments would provide the most heat?
   a. pps = 400; μsec = 200
   b. pps = 200; μsec = 400
   c. pps = 600; μsec = 200
   d. pps = 800; μsec = 100
   e. All of the above produce the same amount of heat.

8. Which of the following has the greatest effect on increasing ROM in a contracted joint?
   a. diathermy
   b. ultrasound
   c. diathermy and passive stretch
   d. ultrasound and passive stretch
   e. diathermy and joint mobilizations

9. What is the most commonly used frequency for microwave diathermy?
   a. 2450 MHz
   b. 27.12 MHz
   c. 915 MHz
   d. 40.68 MHz
   e. 11 m

10. What is the most commonly used frequency for shortwave diathermy?
   a. 2450 MHz
   b. 27.12 MHz
   c. 915 MHz
   d. 40.68 MHz
   e. 11 m

Therapeutic Massage

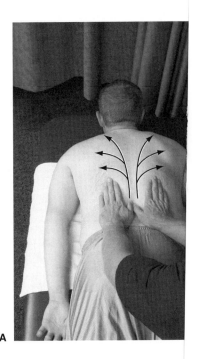

- Applying more or less pressure
- Using different parts of the hand
- Changing the direction of the strol
- Changing the rhythm and speed o

EFFLEURAGE

Effleurage is a gliding manipulation p
sure (directed toward the heart) th
neous tissue down to the deep fascia.
as *stroking* (Fig. 17.1). A massage sl
with light effleurage. It relaxes the |
ning; and at the end, it calms any n
tated during the massage.

Following are the keys for applyir

- Rhythmically stroke the skin.
- Use either light or deep pressure.
  motes relaxation and sensory refl
  promotes mechanical effects, suck
  ficial blood and lymphatic flow.
- When deep stroking, follow the
  lymph vessels to direct fluids tow
- When superficial stroking, follov
  body or the underlying tissue.
- Use the palms of both hands in a
  fashion.
- Maintain contact with the skin at
  in one direction with both hands :
  the beginning with light fingertip
  D (right hand) and reverse D (le
  Alternatively, stagger the hands,

A

You are an athletic training student who has been assigned to track and field for the semester. You approach your clinical instructor and ask her what is involved in working with track and field. She chuckles a little and then says, "We do a lot of massage because the coaches and athletes insist on it. But I try to educate them on the appropriateness of massage—when they need it and when they don't." You think to yourself, "I have had some classroom theory on massage, but I've never given a real sports massage, and I don't even know where to start. It must involve more than giving the athlete's legs a good rubdown." This chapter will help you understand how and when to deliver a therapeutic sports massage.

Massage as a Therapeutic Modality

Many people think a therapeutic modality is a black box that you plug into the wall. It has blinking lights and all the bells and whistles to help patients think they are being treated with a modern medical device. This might be why some textbooks on therapeutic modalities don't include massage. We are of the opinion that massage is an important modality if used appropriately. But therein lies the rub! (Pun intended.) How often is massage used appropriately in a sports medicine environment? We have worked as athletic trainers in many settings—some in which massage is rarely used, some in which it is used appropriately, and some in which it is overused. Let's face it, massage feels good and can be psychologically relaxing. If you could lay down on a comfortable table for a half hour or so every day and have someone use trained hands to gently (or not so gently) rub your sore, aching muscles and relieve your stress, would you do it? Most people would. In fact, many people pay $40 to $50 for a 30-min massage.

Therapeutic massage is the systematic manual manipulation of the body's tissues to restore normal function. Currently in North America, massage is considered to be a complementary therapy to conventional medical practice. Elsewhere in the world, and throughout much of medical history, massage has been regarded as an important component of mainstream health care. In fact, many of the greatest proponents of the clinical use of massage include such respected physicians as Cyriax, Mennell, Travell, and Hippocrates,[1] although it could be argued that all Hippocrates had to work with was his hands. Massage is one of the oldest and most widespread healing techniques. It is practiced in most cultures, and there are many variations. It is a skill-based technique and is licensed in many states.

Facts and Misconceptions About Massage

For decades, there has been some debate about the physiological effects of massage. Some question any use of a passive modality in treating injuries. Remember, one of the purposes of a therapeutic modality is to assist the body in recovery. Therefore, therapeutic massage has a definite role as a modality; when applied correctly, positive effects can occur.[1]

THE THERAPEUTIC EFFECTS OF MASSAGE

Depending on the type, speed, and pressure of the strokes, the benefits of massage can be described as follows:

- Invigorates the body before athletic competition[1]
- Promotes relaxation before and after competition[1]
- Promotes blood flow in the skin.[2]
- Decreases pain by interrupting muscle spasm and reducing edema, increasing blood and lymph flow to rid tissue of cellular wastes, and activating cutaneous receptors to close the gate to pain[1] (see Chapter 7)
- Mild promotion of lymph flow, but no greater than active or passive movement of the limbs (in dogs)[3]
- Increases muscle flexibility after a routine of deep effleurage, circular friction, and transverse friction. Massage might aid in short-term flexibility, especially if applied to an area where an accumulation of scar tissue has resulted in lost range of motion (ROM).
- Decreases scar tissue in tendintitis.[4,5] Friction massage is often the manual intervention of choice for repetitive strain injuries, such as tendinitis, in which there is ongoing microtrauma, low-grade inflammation, and pain.

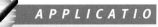

APPLICATIO

USE FRICTION MASSAGE TO BO(
of friction massage as rebooting
computer. In much the same way
computer enables the machine t(
ately, friction massage might he|
flammatory process so that the a
progress normally through the p.

MISCONCEPTIONS ABOUT MA(

For a long time, many clinicians us
would remove lactic acid from
Today, however, we now know th
Massage has also been used to in(
this belief is only partially correct.
blood flow to the skin, but not t(
muscle recovering from a bout of e
thus be problematic. If massage in(
but not arterial blood flow, the blo(
the skin from the skeletal muscles.
recovery process.

Massage also carries with it a la
is difficult to differentiate between
chological effects. Here is a list of
sage does *not* have on the body,
search:

- Stride frequency or length in sp
- Muscular fatigue is unaffected
  bouts (sprinter's legs and pitch(
- Recovery after exercise is unaff(
- Cardiac output, blood pressure,
  lation is not changed during
  running after precompetition m
- Blood lactate is not removed.[2,6]
- Endorphin release is not prom(
- Arterial blood flow is not incre(
- Muscle temperature is not incr(

Indications and Contrair

Indications for therapeutic massag
quiring local blood flow and in(
pain relief, muscle spasm reducti(
systemic relaxation is desired. T
contraindicated in some situations
formed over acute sprains and stra
disease conditions, and sites where
heal. Massage should also not be u

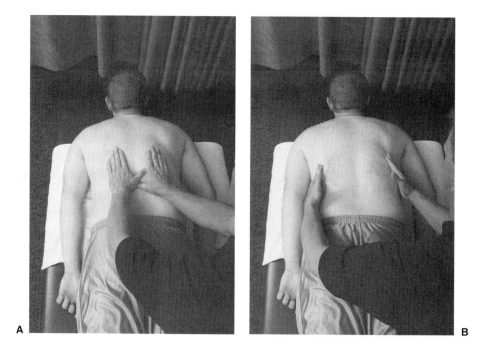

FIGURE 17.2. During effleurage, always maintain contact with the skin, by using **(a)** a D pattern with both hands or **(b)** alternating hands.

go through the normal stages of inflammation and healing. The purpose of friction massage is to increase inflammation (jump-start it) to a point at which the inflammatory process will run its normal course and the injury can progress to the later stages of healing. This is why cross-friction massage is often used for repetitive strain injuries such as tendinitis, where there is ongoing microtrauma, inflammation, and tissue remodeling.[1,4,12]

Do not use friction massage on acute injury, because the pressure could cause more damage. This technique is usually painful, especially when treating trigger points.

Following are the keys for applying friction massage:

- Use friction in a circular or transverse fashion. If circular, work the thumbs in a circular motion. If transverse, the thumbs stroke the tissue from opposite directions.
- Apply the strokes across fibers when treating a ligament or tendon (Fig. 17.5).
- When treating scar tissue in which the collagen has irregular organization, alternate the directions or apply the strokes in a circular motion.
- Use your elbow on large muscles.
- Place the muscle in a relaxed position.
- Apply sufficient pressure so that it will reach deep into the tissue.
- Follow it with stretching to increase ROM.

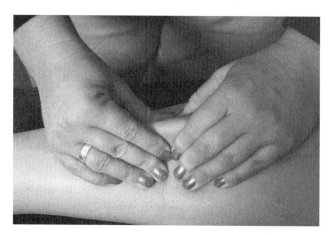

FIGURE 17.3. Kneading. This type of pétrissage involves grasping the muscle between the thumb and the fingers or between the fingers and the palm and lifting and rolling the muscle.

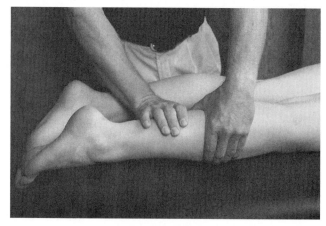

FIGURE 17.4. Wringing. This type of pétrissage involves resting your hands on opposite sides of the circumference of the body segment (your hands are facing each other). You then compress the muscle between your hands and wring out the muscle with a shearing force as your hands move toward each other.

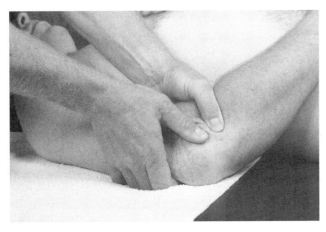

FIGURE 17.5. Friction massage being applied to the wrist extensor tendons to treat lateral epicondylitis (tennis elbow).

PERCUSSION

Percussion, also referred to as *tapotement*, is repeated, rhythmical, light striking of the skin. Techniques include gentle tapping, pounding, cupping, hacking, and slapping the skin. The two main uses of percussion massage are for respiratory ailments to promote phlegm mobilization and to stimulate an athlete during precompetition preparation.

Following are the keys for applying percussion:

• Hack with the ulnar (pinky) side of the hand with wrist and fingers limp (karate chop) (Fig. 17.6a).

• With cupping, allow only the rim of the hand to come in contact with the body (Fig. 17.6b).

• Use raindrops, a variation to promote relaxation and desensitization of irritated nerve endings, by lightly touching the skin with the fingers in an alternating manner, like typing (Fig. 17.6c).

VIBRATION

Vibration, also referred to as *shaking*, is repetitively moving soft tissue (usually muscle) back and forth over the underlying bone with minimal joint motion (Fig. 17.7). The main uses of vibration massage are to relax skeletal muscle and as a stimulus for precompetition and intercompetition, owing to its effects of systemic arousal and enhanced awareness.

Following are the keys for applying vibration:

• Apply moderate to rapid shaking strokes to the skin. Use rapid strokes for precompetition and moderate strokes after competition.

• Apply with the hands or with a machine (Fig. 17.8).

CRITICAL THINKING 17.1 *A soccer player comes into the athletic therapy clinic and tells you about a knot she has in her hamstring that won't go away. It has been bothering her for the past 2 weeks and seems to be related to an old strain. What type of massage stroke will be the most effective at relaxing the knot?*

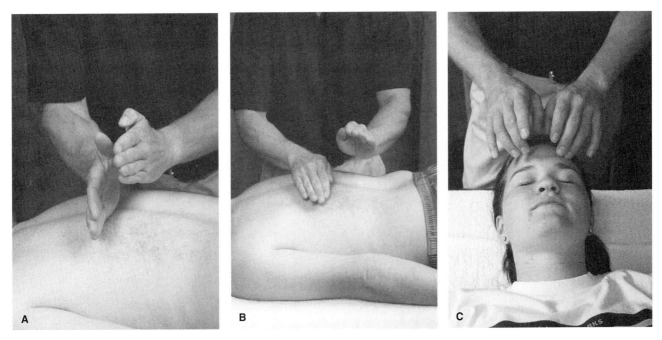

FIGURE 17.6. Percussion techniques. **(a)** Hacking is performed with the ulnar side of hand with the wrist and fingers limp (karate chop). **(b)** Cupping uses only the rim of the hand in contact with the patient's body. **(c)** The raindrops technique is applied by lightly touching the skin with the fingers in an alternating manner.

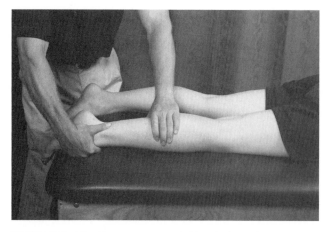

FIGURE 17.7. Vibration massage, or shaking the lower leg.

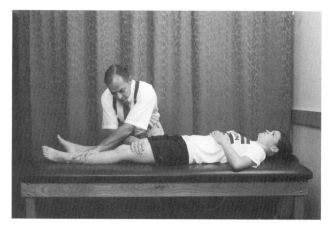

FIGURE 17.9. A myofascial release technique. This advanced method combines traction with varying amounts of stretch to produce a moderate sustained force on the muscle and associated fascia.

Myofascial Release

Myofascial release combines traction with varying amounts of stretch to produce a moderate sustained force on the muscle and its associated fascia. The goal is to produce viscoelastic lengthening and plastic deformation of the fascia[1,13] (Fig. 17.9). In other words, this technique is used to help lengthen the muscle and fascial layers and enable them to remain in the lengthened state.

Myofascial release is indicated to lengthen fascial layers, to restore mobility between fascial layers, and to decrease the effects of adhesions on the muscular system. This technique is indicated for a wide variety of conditions in which chronic fascial shortening results in limited joint ROM and ease of movement.[1]

Clinical training and supervised practice are critical for proper application of this technique.[1] These subjects are beyond the scope of this text. We suggest that anyone interested in learning myofascial release enroll in a workshop or course in which proper instruction and clinical skills in this technique are taught. You can also read articles and texts on the subject.[1,14–17]

Massage Lubricants

The purpose of a **massage lubricant** is to decrease friction and control the amount of glide and drag that occurs between the clinician's moving hands and the client's skin. Lubricants aid some techniques (e.g., where gliding is required) but are actually a hindrance for other techniques (e.g., friction massage). Lubricants should be hypoallergenic and dispensed from a squeeze bottle, pump, or shaker that prevents contamination. There are four main types of massage lubricants: lotions, oils, creams, and powders.

LOTIONS

Massage lotions are probably the most commonly used in orthopedic injury rehabilitation. They are opaque, liquid suspensions of particles in either oil or water. They rapidly lose their ability to lubricate because they absorb into the skin quickly and thus have to be reapplied often during a treatment. Rapid absorption, however, can be advantageous when you are preparing for more deeper or vigorous strokes when little or no lotion is desired. Lotions clean up easily with soap and water.[1]

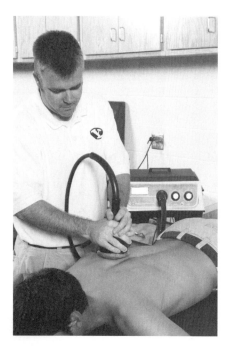

FIGURE 17.8. Vibration massage can also be performed with a machine.

OILS

Massage oils are not used as much in injury rehabilitation as lotions; however, they are the lubricant of choice among massage therapists.[1] Mineral oil is popular, but any high-quality vegetable oil can be used, such as sunflower, olive, almond, safflower, coconut, or jojoba. One advantage of oil is that it does not absorb into the skin very quickly, so the clinician does not have to keep adding more.

There are a few disadvantages to using oils. First, they are messy and leave a stain. It is a good idea to cover any clothing (yours and the patient's) that is in the direct vicinity of the treatment. Also, the patient will need to shower after the treatment, and the area will need to be wiped off with (disposable) towels because the residue may stain the patient's clothing.[1]

CREAMS

Massage creams are thicker suspensions that fall midway between oils and lotions in their absorption rate. Some creams contain more oil to promote gliding techniques. Other creams contain sticky substances such as lanolin or beeswax to reduce glide for treating tissue release techniques.[1] Creams often include menthol, capsaicin, or aloe vera as one of their active ingredients.

POWDERS

Powders can be used when patients prefer not to use lotions, creams, or oils. Unscented baby powder or cornstarch are commonly used. The weaknesses of using powders are that they are not very lubricating and require a lot of cleanup.[1]

CRITICAL THINKING 17.2 *What massage stroke does not require the use of a lubricant? Why?*

Application of Therapeutic Massage

STEP 1: FOUNDATION

A. Definition. Therapeutic massage is a systematic manual manipulation of the body's tissues.
B. Effects
   1. Depends on type, pressure, and speed of stroke
   2. Invigorates the body before athletic competition, promotes relaxation and blood flow in the skin; decreases pain
C. Advantages
   1. Patients feel that you are actively involved in their healing.
   2. Tactile contact by a clinician's hands can be enjoyable, relaxing, and soothing.
   3. The laying on of hands demonstrates concern, compassion, and care.
   4. Requires no special equipment
   5. Easily learned; extensive background is not required. The clinician can instruct individuals, family, or friends to do their own massage. However, it does require much practice to become skilled in this area.
D. Disadvantages
   1. Time-consuming
   2. Lotions, oils, and powders can get messy.
E. Indications
   1. Increase venous return
   2. Break the pain–spasm–pain cycle
   3. Evoke systemic relaxation
   4. Improve or stimulate local blood flow
F. Contraindications
   1. Acute sprains and strains; massage can:
      i. Increase the inflammatory response
      ii. Cause myositis ossificans
   2. Over skin with lesions or disease conditions; may spread disease over the patient or to the clinician
   3. Sites where fractures have failed to heal
   4. People who are hypersensitive to touch
G. Precautions
   1. Pitting edema
   2. Hypertension

STEP 2: PREAPPLICATION TASKS

A. Selecting the proper modality. Make sure massage is the proper modality for this situation.
B. Preparing the patient psychologically
   1. Explain the benefits of massage.
   2. State that at no time will any private body parts be touched or undraped.

C. Preparing the patient physically. Ensure a suitable environment that includes:
   1. A comfortable room temperature 68–75°F (20–24°C)
   2. Upholstered table to protect pressure points and bony prominences (pelvic bones, ankles, head, etc.)
   3. A relaxed atmosphere; perhaps relaxing music
   4. Positioning the patient
      a. So that both patient and clinician are comfortable
      b. With a rolled-up towel under the body parts (e.g., the ankle) to increase comfort
      c. Making sure the patient is properly draped with towels to observe modesty (if the massage involves body parts where nudity may be a concern)
D. Equipment preparation
   1. Determine the type of massage you want to give, including what strokes you will use and in what order.
   2. Determine whether you will use lubricants.

STEP 3: APPLICATION PARAMETERS

A. Instead of standard procedures, a massage application is designed to meet the individual patient's needs. A typical sports massage application is as follows:
   1. Light effleurage (superficial stroking)
   2. Deep effleurage (deep stroking)
   3. Pétrissage (kneading, wringing, and lifting)
   4. Optional friction or percussion
   5. Deep effleurage (deep stroking)
   6. Light effleurage (superficial stroking)
B. Dosage (varies according to patient tolerance). During the treatment, seek feedback about the patient's response to your treatment by periodically asking questions such as:
   1. How are you feeling?
   2. Is it tender here?
   3. Is this pressure OK?
C. Length of application. Varies from 5 min for one body part to 45 min for the entire body
D. Frequency of application
   1. Depends on the purpose of the massage.
   2. Clinicians must use massage when massage is indicated as part of a treatment regimen—not whenever an athlete wants a rubdown.

E. Duration of therapy. As long as massage continues to have a positive impact on the resolution of the injury; however, don't abuse it.

STEP 4: POSTAPPLICATION TASKS

A. Equipment removal. Remove any remaining massage lubricant.
B. Instructions to the patient
   1. Schedule the next treatment.
   2. Instruct the patient about the level of activity and/or self-treatment before the next formal treatment.

C. Record of treatment, including unique patient responses
D. Replace soiled towels and sheets with clean ones.

STEP 5: MAINTENANCE

A. Keep your hands free of calluses.
B. Make sure massage tables are in good working order.
C. Make sure you have plenty of massage lubricants on hand for future use.

CLOSING SCENE

It is midway through the track and field season. Your clinical instructor approaches you and tells you she has received many compliments regarding your athletic training skills, particularly with giving massages. "I'm especially impressed," she adds, "that you don't let the athletes abuse massage as a modality. You always remind the runners to do a proper cool-down, including jogging and stretching, and you limit their massages to when their muscles are tight, not just when they want a rubdown." You think to yourself, "Massage can be a great modality when it is used appropriately." You thank your supervisor for the compliment and feel good inside because you just had your ego massaged.

CHAPTER REFLECTIONS

1. Read and ponder each of the following points. Do you feel you have a clear understanding of each concept? If not, reread the appropriate section of the chapter.
   - Define effleurage and explain why it is used.
   - Define pétrissage and explain why it is used.
   - Define friction massage and explain why it is used.
   - Define myofascial release and explain why it is used.
   - Define percussion and explain why it is used.
   - Define vibration and explain why it is used.
   - What is a typical format for a sports massage?
   - Describe the physiological effects of massage.
   - Compare and contrast the reflexive and mechanical effects of massage.
   - List the indications for massage.
   - Name the contraindications for massage.
   - What are the advantages and disadvantages of common lubricants used during massage?
   - Explain the difference between a therapeutic massage and a rubdown.

2. Write three to five questions for discussion with your class instructor, clinical instructor, classmates, and clinical colleagues.

3. Get together with classmates and quiz each other on the concepts of this chapter. Use the points in exercise 1 and questions you wrote for exercise 2 as a beginning. Explaining concepts out loud to others requires a deeper grasp of the material than feeling you understand it as you read.

4. Once you feel you understand the principles of application of therapeutic massage, practice applying them using the five-step approach with a classmate or clinical colleague. Alternate applying the modalities to each other. When it is being applied to you, listen and observe carefully to determine whether your classmate is using proper application. Consult your notes when the modality is applied to you and for the first few times you apply the modality to another person. Continue practicing the application until you can do so without using your notes.

CRITICAL THINKING RESPONSES

Critical Thinking 17.1

Pétrissage, using the kneading, lifting, and wringing techniques, is the most effective stroke for relaxing the knot.

Critical Thinking 17.2

Friction massage does not require a lubricant. Because the goal is to break up adhesive scar tissue, your thumbs or fingers need to remain in contact with the skin, not glide or slide over it.

REFERENCES

1. Andrade C-K, Clifford P. Outcome-Based Massage. Baltimore: Lippincott Williams & Wilkins, 2001.
2. Hinds T, McEwan I, Perkes J, et al. Effects of massage on limb and skin blood flow after quadriceps exercise. Med Sci Sports Exerc 2004;36:1308–1313.
3. Tiidus PM. Manual massage and recovery of muscle function following exercise: A literature review. J Orthop Sports Phys Ther 1997;25:107–112.
4. Sevier TL, Wilson JE. Treating lateral epicondylitis. Sports Med 1999;28:375–380.
5. Woodman R, Pare L. Evaluation and treatment of soft tissue lesions of the ankle and forefoot using the Cyraix approach. Phys Ther 1982;62:1144–1147.
6. Boone T, Cooper R, Thompson WR. A physiologic evaluation of the sports massage. Athl Train 1991;26:51–54.
7. Hemmings B, Smith M, Graydon J, Dyson R. Effects of massage on physiological restoration, perceived recovery, and repeated sports performance. Br J Sports Med 2000;34:109–114; discussion 115.
8. Shoemaker JK, Tiidus PM, Mader R. Failure of manual massage to alter limb blood flow: Measures by Doppler ultrasound. Med Sci Sports Exerc 1997;29:610–614.
9. Tiidus PM, Shoemaker JK. Effleurage massage, blood flow, and long term post-exercise strength recovery. Int J Sports Med 1995;15:478–483.
10. Harmer PA. The effect of pre-performance massage on stride frequency in sprinters. Athl Train 1991;26:55–59.
11. Dirckx JH. Stedman's Concise Medical Dictionary for the Health Professions. 4th ed. Baltimore: Lippincott Williams & Wilkins, 2001.
12. Draper DO, Karns PB, Sokolowski MS. Chronic ankle and foot injuries in professional ice hockey players: Jumpstarting inflammation to re-direct healing. J Athl Train 2001;38:S90.
13. Holey E, Cook E. Therapeutic Massage. London: Saunders, 1997.
14. Fritz S. Fundamentals of Therapeutic Massage. St. Louis, MO: Mosby-Lifeline, 1995.
15. Tappan FM. Benjamin P. Tappan's Handbook of Healing Massage Techniques. 3rd ed. Stamford, CT: Appleton & Lange. 1998.
16. Salvo SG. Massage Therapy. Philadelphia: Saunders. 1999.
17. Loving J. Massage Therapy. Stamford, CT: Appleton & Lange, 1999.

Spinal Traction

A 47-year-old college professor has had episodes of back pain about every 6 months for the past few years. The pain used to last 2 weeks and then disappear, until the last episode. After 5 weeks of pain, an MRI study was done on his back. The MRI revealed a herniated disk between vertebrae L3 and L4 and a bulging disk between L5 and S1 (Fig. 18.1). These irregularities explained the buttocks pain and radiating pain down his right leg. He was offered several solutions, including extension exercises, painkilling drugs, and traction. The medication and exercises helped, but the radiating pain still bothered him. He wondered if lumbar traction would help his situation.

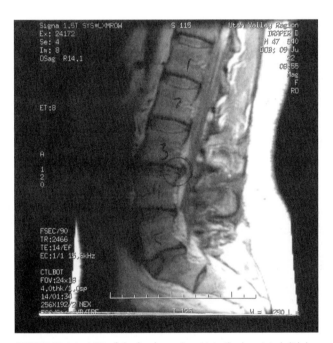

FIGURE 18.1 An MRI of the lumbar spine. Note the herniated disk between L3 and L4 and the bulging disk between L5 and S1. Manual, mechanical, and inversion traction were applied to this patient.

Cervical Pain and Lumbar Pain

The scenario in the opening scene is not uncommon; in fact, it happened to one of us (DD). As we get older, degenerative changes occur in the spine. Our intervertebral disks become thinner and lose elasticity, whereas small boney outgrowths (calcium deposits), called **osteophytes**, form on the vertebrae. These changes often put pressure on nerve endings, resulting in neck or back pain.

Cervical pain, or neck pain and stiffness, is a common problem that affects up to 30% of people 25–29 years of age. Among working people >45 years of age, the percentage increases to 50%.[1] Pain that is referred to the arm may indicate irritation or entrapment of a cervical nerve root. Common causes are a bulging or herniated disk or

degenerative changes, including apophyseal joint or ligamentous hypertrophy and osteophytes.[1]

Approximately 80% of the population will experience lumbar pain, or low-back pain, at some time in their lives; of these, 90% will resolve in 2–4 weeks, but 60–80% will recur within 1 year.[2] In the workplace, low-back pain is the leading cause of employee morbidity, disability, and lost productivity. Medical care is sought by 15–20% of those with back pain, making it the second most common reason for all physician visits.[3]

CRITICAL THINKING 18.1 *Why do you think more people suffer from low-back pain than do suffer from neck pain?*

The Intervertebral Disk

Between each of our cervical, thoracic, and lumbar vertebrae is an **intervertebral disk** that functions to resist compressive forces and shock, provide flexibility, and provide adequate space between vertebrae. The outer layer of the disk is the **annulus fibrosus**, a series of interlacing cross-fibers that are attached to adjacent vertebral bodies. The inner layer is the **nucleus pulposus**, a protein gel between the cartilaginous end plates of the vertebrae and the annulus fibrosus.

The nucleus pulposus is watery; as we age, it loses fluid (from 85–90% at birth to 70% by age 70) and fullness. Another cause for a disk to lose its full size and normal shape is via injury. The stretched or weakened annular fibers (annulus fibrosus) can protrude from the pressure of a bulging nucleus pulposus. For example, a bulging or **herniated disk** might look like what happens when you overinflate a bicycle tire inner tube that has a weak spot in it (Fig. 18.2).

If the disk is damaged, and you move into a weight-bearing position, the nucleus pulposus will shift according to fluid-dynamic principles. For example, if you bend to the right side, the vertebrae squeeze the nucleus to the left. If tears develop in the annular fibers, the nucleus will tend to take the path of least resistance and move in that direction (Fig. 18.3).

Traction increases the separation of the vertebrae, decreases the central pressure in the disk space, and encourages the nucleus pulposus to return to a central position. The mechanical tension of the annulus fibrosus and ligaments surrounding the disk (especially the posterior longitudinal ligament) help push the nucleus pulposus back into its proper place.[4]

Traction as a Therapeutic Modality

Several modalities are used to treat cervical and lumbar pain, including heat, cold, electrical stimulation, and exercise. In the United States, it is estimated that lumbar traction is used 21% of the time as part of a regimen to treat patients with low-back pain.[5]

Traction, from the Latin *tracio,* for "drawing or pulling apart,"[6] is a technique in which a pulling force is applied to body segments to stretch soft tissues and separate joint surfaces or bone fragments. Generally limited to the cervical or lumbar regions, traction has been used to treat fractures, dislocations, and spinal disorders for over 3000 years.

The Physiological Effects of Traction

Results of scientific studies show that when 25 lb of traction are applied to the cervical spine, it elongates 2–20 mm, resulting in widening of the neural *foramen,* an opening for the passage of nerves or blood vesssels.[7] It is believed that fatigue or relaxation of the cervical paraspinal muscles occurs with cervical traction. The lumbar spine also elongates with traction when a force of about 50% of the body weight is used.[7]

Although scientists have demonstrated that traction can cause vertebral separation, it is short lived. Once the traction force is removed and the patient sits or stands, the separation is reduced. However, traction can break the pain–spasm–pain cycle and muscle guarding and thus plays a valuable role in the overall treatment plan.

In one study, scientists used CT to study the effects of traction on disk herniation in 30 patients.[8] The herniated nucleus pulposus material retracted during traction in 78.5% of median herniations, 66.6% of posterolateral herniations, and 57.1% of lateral herniations. Other mechanical changes were noted, including widening of disk spaces, separation of apophyseal joint facets, increase in neural foramina, and thinning of the ligamentum flavum. The authors attributed the retraction of the herniated nucleus pulposus during traction to a suction effect of negative intradisk pressures and a pushing effect of the posterior longitudinal ligament. After 1 month of conservative treatment (heat, exercises), including traction, 28 of 30 subjects had significant pain relief.[8]

Pain relief is the main reason spinal traction is used. Traction appears to relieve pain by:[6,9–12]

- Increasing the space between vertebrae
- Separating the apophyseal joints
- Widening of the intervertebral foramina

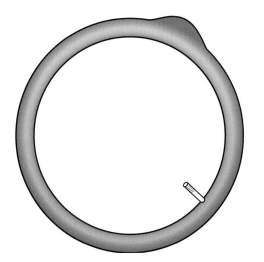

FIGURE 18.2. The weak spot of an overinflated bicycle tire inner tube resembles a bulging or herniated disk.

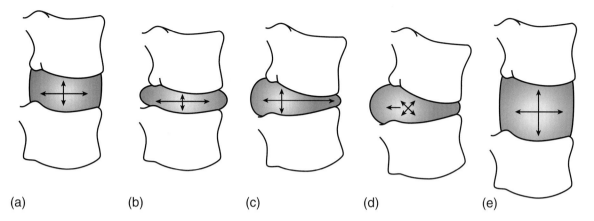

FIGURE 18.3. Intervertebral disk movement. **(a)** A disk that is not bearing weight. **(b)** A normal weight-bearing disk. **(c)** A damaged disk; movement in a weight-bearing position shifts the nucleus pulposus. **(d)** Bending to the right side causes the vertebrae to squeeze the nucleus to the left. Tears in the fibers of the annulus fibrosus cause the nucleus to move in this direction. **(e)** Traction separates the vertebrae, decreases the central pressure in the disk space, and returns the nucleus pulposus to a central position. The mechanical tension of the annulus fibrosus and ligaments surrounding the disk help push the disk back into place.

- Removing pressure or contact forces on injured tissue
- Increasing peripheral circulation
- Stretching muscles and ligaments
- Reducing muscle spasm
- Relaxing muscles
- Changing intervertebral disk pressures
- Tensing the posterior longitudinal ligament to exert force at the back of the vertebrae
- Creating suction to draw protruded disks toward their center
- Flattening of an abnormal lumbar curvature

Other than pain relief, spinal traction results in physiologic adaptations to various structures around the spine:

- *Bone:* Increases spinal movement, overall and between each vertebra. Reverses immobilization-related bone weakness by increasing or maintaining bone density.
- *Ligament:* Creates ligament deformation, thereby increasing movement and decreasing impingement problems (long-term effects).
- *Articular facet joints:* Increases the separation between joint surfaces. Decompresses articular cartilage, allowing synovial fluid exchange to nourish the cartilage. May decrease degenerative changes. May decrease pain perception
- *Muscles:* Lengthens tight muscles and allows better muscular blood flow. Activates muscle *proprioceptors*, further decreasing pain.
- *Nerves:* Decreases compression forces on nerves.

Guidelines Before Applying Traction

Before deciding on traction as a modality, a qualified clinician should study the results of the patient examination.

The history, diagnostic test results, and current symptoms will determine whether traction is indicated or contraindicated. It is important that you, as a student, observe several traction techniques performed by a qualified clinician before performing any techniques by yourself. You should be supervised until you become proficient at the traction techniques you employ.

Indications for Traction

Traction might be indicated for a patient, when he presents with any or all of the following signs and symptoms: local or radiating pain, tightness, muscle spasm, weakness of limbs, or decreased deep tendon reflexes. Many of these signs and symptoms are associated with pressure on spinal nerves or connective tissue contractions. Traction is rarely used alone; it is part of a treatment regimen involving exercise, massage, electrical stimulation, and thermal modalities. The main effects of traction are mechanical. Therefore, the use of traction should be limited to conditions of the spine where the *mechanical effects* of traction would be expected to produce results. These include

- Compression of nerve roots
- Disk protrusion
- Joint hypomobility
- Adhesions
- Muscle spasm
- Disk generation
- Foraminal stenosis
- Contracted connective tissue
- Apophyseal joint impingement
- Radiating pain that does not improve with trunk or neck movement

Contraindications for Traction

Traction is contraindicated in some conditions. In general, traction is contraindicated after acute trauma to the neck or back. By *acute,* we mean that excessive force caused the symptoms. Also, when traction increases **radicular pain,** or pain along the pathway of a spinal nerve, this technique should be avoided. Specific contraindications for cervical and lumbar traction include:

- Malignancy, either primary or metastatic
- Infectious diseases of the spine, such as tuberculosis
- Uncontrolled hypertension
- Rheumatoid arthritis
- Spinal cord compression
- Osteoporosis
- Cardiovascular disease
- Aortic aneurysm
- Acute neck or low-back pain
- Frail older adults
- Severe respiratory disease
- Hypermobile vertebrae (e.g., spondylolisthesis)
- When traction increases radicular pain

    Specific contraindications for lumbar traction include:

- Pregnancy
- Hiatal hernia
- Abdominal hernia
- Active peptic ulcers
- Glaucoma (inversion gravity method)

Do not substitute traction for a more beneficial treatment (e.g., McKenzie extension exercises for a posterior disk protrusion).

Commonly Used Traction Devices

In general, there are two types of traction: manual and mechanical. With **manual traction,** a distraction force is applied by another person. **Mechanical traction** involves the use of a machine or other apparatus to apply the distractive force.

Cervical Traction

There is more support for cervical traction than for lumbar traction.[4,6,9,13–16] Cervical traction is generally applied with the patient in a supine or sitting position. The supine position is preferred over sitting, because it eliminates the effects of gravity. This allows for increased relaxation of the patient, decreased muscle guarding, more separation between vertebral bodies, and less force having to be applied by the clinician.[13] There are three main types of cervical traction: manual cervical traction, mechanical traction, and motorized intermittent or sustained traction.

MANUAL CERVICAL TRACTION

Manual cervical traction is the technique that is most readily available to the clinician because, usually, no equipment is needed except the hands. It enables the clinician to feel the patient's reaction to the treatment.

Manual traction should always be applied before mechanical traction when treating the neck. This approach lets you carefully control the applied force and head position to maximize the relief of symptoms. To perform this technique, have the patient lie down in a supine position on a padded treatment table. Sit or stand at the head of the table facing the patient. Cradle the head in your hands, or with a towel, in a position that allows distraction of the cervical vertebrae without causing any discomfort to the patient (Fig. 18.4). Begin with gentle traction of 10–15 lb, then slowly increase the force up to 25 lb, which is necessary to overcome the resistance of the head and soft-tissue structures.[7,13] As you apply traction, slowly move the head into a position of greatest relaxation and comfort as follows:

- Neutral position for pain affecting the upper cervical vertebrae
- Flexed 30° for pain affecting the lower cervical vertebrae
- Lateral flexion for pressure on spinal nerves with radiating pain into the arms or hands

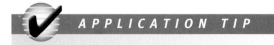

APPLICATION TIP

START WITH MANUAL TRACTION. *When treating the neck, always start with manual traction before you perform mechanical traction. In this way you can rapidly stop a motion that might be troublesome to the patient.*

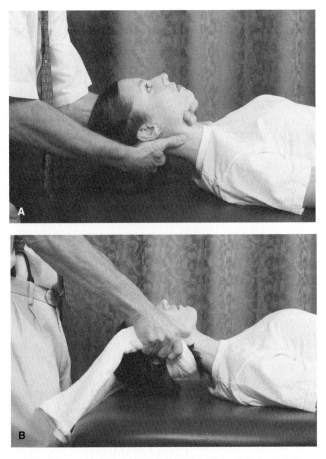

FIGURE 18.4. When performing manual traction, the clinician sits or stands at the head of the table facing the patient. The head is cradled in **(a)** the hands or **(b)** in a towel to allow distraction of the cervical vertebrae without hurting the patient. As traction is applied, the head is slowly moved to maximize relaxation and comfort.

MECHANICAL TRACTION

For mechanical traction, a harness cradles the patient's head. The patient uses a pulley to adjust the tension, the force of which applies sustained traction and separates the vertebrae (Fig. 18.5).

MECHANICAL INTERMITTENT OR SUSTAINED TRACTION

Mechanical intermittent or sustained cervical traction uses a head harness attached to a mechanical device at the end of a table. The device can pull sustained traction, or intermittent traction (usually 30 sec on; 10 sec off) (Fig. 18.6). Moeti and Marchetti[17] applied mechanical intermittent cervical traction to 15 patients who had radiating pain from pressure on spinal nerves. Those who had been experiencing pain for 12 weeks or less demonstrated a reduction in pain and disability.[17]

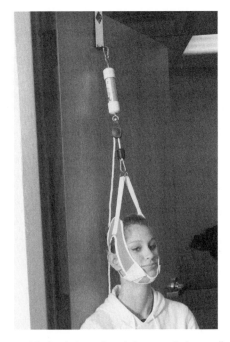

FIGURE 18.5. Mechanical traction. A harness device cradles the patient's head. The patient adjusts the force and applies sustained traction and separates vertebrae.

Lumbar Traction

There are more types of lumbar traction than of cervical traction available to the clinician. The following are some of the most commonly used techniques.[18]

MANUAL LUMBAR TRACTION

Similar to manual cervical traction, this technique is the most readily available to the clinician, allows the clinician to feel the patient's reaction to the treatment, and can be used as an examination technique. The clinician uses her hands or a belt to pull on the patient's legs and separate the vertebrae (Fig. 18.7).

Single-Leg Traction

One type of manual traction for the lumbar area is single-leg traction (Fig. 18.8). To apply this technique, two clinicians are required. The patient can lie prone or supine on the table. One clinician supports the patient's torso while the other clinician puts traction on the leg. After a series of five, 30 sec bouts of traction, the patient lies supine at the edge of the table and stretches the affected hip flexors, which are usually tight with radicular pain.

Unilateral Leg-Pull Manual Traction

Another type of manual lumbar traction is referred to as unilateral leg-pull traction. In this technique, the patient

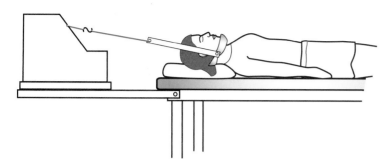

FIGURE 18.6. Cervical traction using a head harness attached to a mechanical device at the end of a table. This technique can provide sustained or intermittent traction.

lies supine. The clinician puts traction on one leg with the patient's hip in 30° of flexion, 30° of abduction, and maximal outward rotation.

> *CRITICAL THINKING 18.2 A patient comes into the clinic complaining of radiating pain all down his right leg from the buttocks to the foot. What type of traction might give him some immediate relief?*

MECHANICAL LUMBAR TRACTION

Mechanical lumbar traction uses a specialized table that can be separated when adequate forces are applied. The patient's head and torso are on one half of the table, and the legs are on the other half. One end of a strap, belt, or harness is firmly attached to the patient, and the other end is attached to a mechanical device that applies a traction force that slowly elongates the lower spine (Fig. 18.9). There are two types of mechanical lumbar traction: sustained and intermittent.

Sustained Traction

Sustained traction involves a sustained force that is about 50% of the patient's body weight. The force is slightly less than intermittent traction because there is no rest period. Treatment time is typically 10–30 min.

Intermittent Traction

The intensity of intermittent traction is slightly greater than sustained traction, but the treatment can last longer because there is a rest period (when the unit is off). This technique uses a mechanical device to alternately apply and release the traction force at preset intervals. The typical intervals are 30 sec on and 30 sec off. Longer on periods of up to 60 sec are recommended for disk injury, whereas shorter on periods of 15 sec are recommended for joint facet dysfunction.

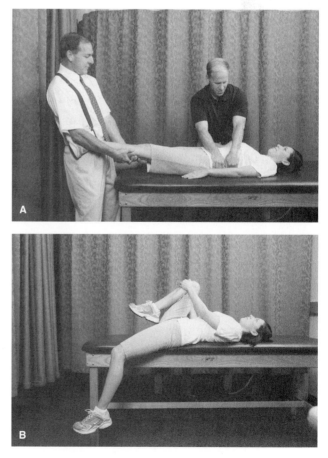

FIGURE 18.8. Manual single-leg traction. The patient lies on a table in the prone or supine position. **(a)** One clinician supports the patient's torso while the other clinician puts traction on the leg. **(b)** After the traction, the patient lies at the edge of the table and stretches the hip flexors, which are usually tight with radicular pain.

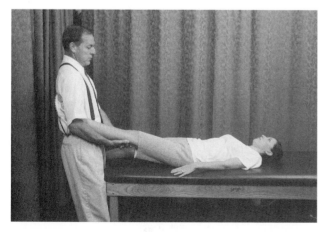

FIGURE 18.7. For manual lumbar traction, the clinician pulls, with his hands or a belt, on the patient's legs to separate the vertebrae.

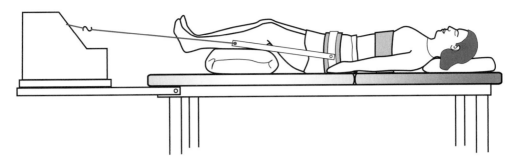

FIGURE 18.9. Mechanical lumbar traction uses a special table, which has two sections that can separate. This facilitates elongation of the lower spine when torso movement is restricted and adequate force is applied to the torso.

AUTOTRACTION

Autotraction uses a specially designed table divided into two sections that can be individually tilted and rotated. Patients can apply the traction force by holding on to, or pulling on, overhead bars (Fig. 18.10). Because of the cost of the table and the difficulty patients with low-back pain have experienced with this technique, the use of autotraction has recently declined.

POSITIONAL LUMBAR TRACTION

The idea behind positional lumbar traction is to place the patient in a position in which the body can pull traction on itself. This is accomplished by using bolsters or rolled-up towels to maintain flexion and rotation of the spine to achieve distraction of a specific vertebral segment. The goal is to alleviate pressure on an entrapped spinal nerve, thus decreasing pain and promoting muscle relaxation. The most common technique is to have the patient lie on the nonpainful side (Fig. 18.11). The bolster is then placed under the side of the trunk, producing lateral trunk flexion. This should lead to increased spacing between the vertebrae on the painful side, thereby releasing pressure on the spinal nerve

THE 90/90 TRACTION TECHNIQUE

The 90/90 traction technique is self-administered and convenient for home treatment. The patient is positioned with the hips and knees flexed to 90°. The patient then tilts the pelvis and flattens the lumbar lordosis by pulling on a rope that traverses the unit's frame and attaches to a pelvic harness.

POOL TRACTION

Pool traction is applied in an aquatic setting and uses the buoyancy of the water to reduce weight on the spine.

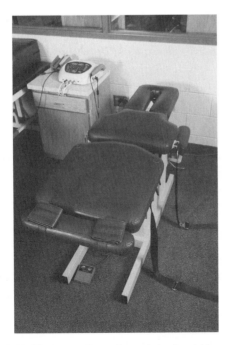

FIGURE 18.10. The two sections of an autotraction table can be individually tilted and rotated.

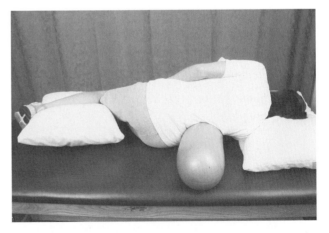

FIGURE 18.11. Positional lumbar traction. The patient is lying on the nonpainful side with a bolster under the side of the trunk, causing lateral trunk flexion. This increases the spaces between the vertebrae on the painful side, releasing pressure on the affected spinal nerve.

CRITICAL THINKING 18.3 *How could a water flotation belt or water ankle cuffs be used to assist someone who has low-back pain? Answer the question, and then look at Fig. 18.12.*

INVERSION TABLE TRACTION

Inversion table traction is an inexpensive, effective way to gain the benefits of traction. The patient is suspended upside-down or at a variety of angles by the ankles or thighs (Fig. 18.13). This position allows the weight of the upper body to act as a traction force. Because it causes a significant increase in blood pressure, the technique is contraindicated for patients with hypertension. It also increases pressure to the eyes, so patients with glaucoma should not use inversion traction. Guvenol et al.[19] compared inversion traction with mechanical traction on patients with herniated lumbar disks. The was no difference in the alleviation of patient symptoms between the two devices.

One of us (DD) has used both mechanical and inversion table traction. The preference is the inversion table. It is inexpensive and can be purchased at warehouse stores for <$200, making it ideal for home use. The table is easy to use, and it works; the straps don't slip and give you a wedgie like they often do on hori-

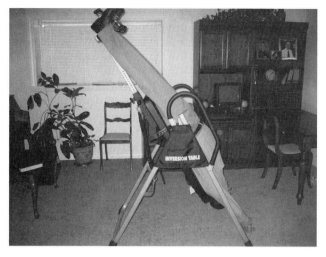

FIGURE 18.13. Inversion table traction. When the patient is suspended upside-down, the weight of the upper body acts as a traction force.

zontal mechanical traction tables. For a step-by-step procedure on how to use an inversion traction table, see Box 18.1.

Remember, when traction is applied to the low back, it increases the separation of the vertebrae and decreases the central pressure in the intervertebral disk spaces. By immediately performing prone extension after traction, the posterior longitudinal ligament helps push the nuclear material of the disks back into proper position (Fig. 18.14).[4]

THE EFFECTIVENESS OF LUMBAR TRACTION

Of the techniques of lumbar traction described in this chapter, most of the research has been performed on sustained and intermittent mechanical traction. The results of these studies are mixed. For example, research by Beurskens et al.[20] showed that lumbar traction was no more effective than placebo. However, Meszaros et al.[21] report that when an adequate traction force is applied, lumbar traction significantly reduces pain. Harte et al.[22] performed a systematic review of randomized clinical studies on lumbar traction, concluding that the variability in the results of lumbar traction studies might be owing to poorly designed studies and limited applications of traction in clinical practice.[22]

Based on the observations that many patients with intractable pain obtain rapid relief with the application of an adequate load, traction is given intermittently. In both intermittent and intermittent pulsed traction (which allows a gradual increase and decrease of the traction force), the brief periodic nature of the application permits the use of larger loads without significant stress to the patient. No form of traction is entirely without discomfort.

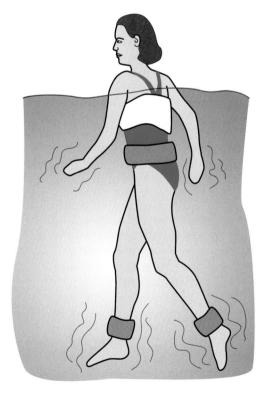

FIGURE 18.12. A flotation belt and water cuffs cause drag, resulting in traction on the lumbar vertebrae.

BOX 18.1 *USING INVERSION TABLE TRACTION*

1. Set the length adjustment by pulling the spring-loaded pin at the bottom of the table and setting it at the patient's height.
2. Adjust the strap on the bottom of the table to determine the angle at which you want to unload the spine. For example, many people find that it is difficult to start hanging directly upside-down and prefer to start at a 45° or 60° angle until they get used to the table.
3. Adjust the padded leg clamps so that the ankles will slide comfortably into place.
4. Have the patient step into the padded leg clamps. Some people go barefoot; others prefer to wear shoes as extra padding.
5. The patient then lies supine on the table. You may place a lumbar roll into the small of the patient's back for added support.
6. Tell the patient to reach both arms over her head, and the table should slowly invert. If the table inverts too quickly for comfort, she should simply grasp onto the side rails and slow the table down.
7. Remember, separation of the joint surfaces is resisted by the muscles and other soft tissues surrounding the joints. While in the inverted position, the patient should try to relax her muscles and breathing rate as much as possible. If she does this, she will be able to take the pressure off her nerves and intervertebral disks. At first the patient might be comfortable in this position for only 1–2 min, but eventually she can train herself to relax and enjoy the inversion for 10–15 min.
8. Tell the patient to slowly bring her arms back to her waist, grasp hold of the side rails, and bring the table to a horizontal position to let the blood return to the lower limbs.
9. Repeat the process. The patient should try for three sets of 5 min each.
10. When the patient is finished with the last set, she should slowly return to the starting position.
11. The patient should then get off the table, and lie prone on the floor. It may help to use a 12-in. firm wedge. The patient remains in this position for 30 min while reading a book or relaxing.

Treatment Parameters

The treatment parameters for traction are as follows:

- Patient position
- Treatment mode
- Traction force
- Duration
- Frequency

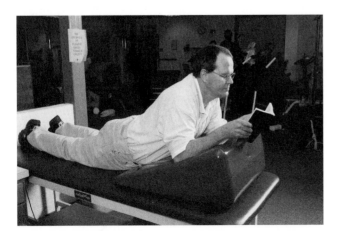

FIGURE 18.14. Lying prone and using a wedge after undergoing inversion traction helps readjust the position of the intervertebral disks.

PATIENT POSITION

For cervical traction, the patient can be sitting or supine. When lumbar traction is applied, the patient can be standing, sitting, supine, prone, and horizontal or inclined.[18] One way of determining the appropriate patient position for lumbar traction is to first find out what position decreases the pain when standing. For example, if the patient hurts while sitting but the pain goes away while he is lying or during trunk extension (such as would happen with a posterior bulging disk), he will probably respond best to traction in the prone position. If the patient hurts while lying down or in trunk flexion but the pain decreases while sitting, he will probably respond best to traction in the supine position. The most important thing to remember is that muscle relaxation is considered essential to achieving the optimal effects of traction.[18] Therefore, the patient should be positioned so that muscle relaxation is maximized.

TREATMENT MODE

Treatment mode refers to applying traction in either the sustained or the intermittent mode. There are various opinions regarding which mode is better to use. Some believe that sustained traction is essential to fatiguing the muscles and allowing the traction force to act on the joints, whereas intermittent traction creates a stretch reflex and is ineffective in reducing disk problems.[9]

Others are of the opinion that the same result can occur with both modes of traction, although patients are more able to tolerate higher forces when traction is intermittent. Still others state that the diagnosis should determine which mode to follow.[6] For example, if the diagnosis is a disk protrusion, the sustained method (or longer hold–rest periods) should be employed. If the diagnosis is degenerative disk disease or joint hypomobility, the intermittent mode (with shorter hold–rest periods) should be used.[6]

TRACTION FORCE

A force of sufficient magnitude and duration must be exerted to separate the vertebrae. This can be done by weights and pulleys, and mechanical devices or manually. The direction of the traction force may be either vertical, horizontal, or at an angle. The magnitude of the needed force depends on the frictional resistance to traction and the resistance to stretch by the muscles and soft tissues. A small additional force will bring about separation of the vertebrae. During traction, movement of the body by the external force must be resisted by an equal and opposite force—either body weight or friction with the surface that is in contact with the body. The friction force is approximately equal to one half the body weight. Gravity may either assist or resist traction.[23]

When frictional resistance is not sufficient to prevent movement, an additional counterforce must be added. This force also dissipates some of the desired traction force and hence some of the effectiveness. The part of the force that is lost as a stretch force must be reclaimed by applying a heavier traction force unless the frictional resistance can be overcome or eliminated. This can be done with a split traction table or by applying the force in a vertical position.

Separation of the joint surfaces is also resisted by the muscles and other soft tissues surrounding the joints. The traction force must then be increased by a force sufficient to overcome this additional resistance to stretch before distraction of the joint surfaces can take place. In clinical practice, the patient's tolerance and response to stretch must be the ultimate guide in the therapeutic use of traction.

The minimum traction force to get separation in the cervical spine is about 25 lb, although there is general disagreement about the minimum force needed for effective treatment. The angle of pull also plays a significant role in the cervical spine. For example, when the neck is flexed to 20°–30°, the anterior curve of the cervical spine is decreased. Traction force applied at between 20° and 30° of flexion has been shown to give moderate to complete pain relief.

For lumbar traction, there are similar disagreements about the necessary and sufficient force to obtain clinical relief. Meszaros et al.[21] studied patients with low-back pain and found significant decreases in pain when 30% and 50% of the patient's body weight was used as the traction force. When only 10% of the patient's body weight was used as a traction force, there was no reduction in pain.[21]

The resistance to stretch the lumbar muscles provide is considerable. We recommend starting with 25% of the body weight, and if this is easily tolerated, increase the force to 50% of the patient's weight. Elimination of the lumbar lordosis has been suggested as a method of reducing the traction force needed to obtain separation of the vertebrae. It is apparent, then, that the proper angle of pull is just as important in lumbar traction as it is in cervical traction.

APPLICATION TIP

USE THE ONE THIRD GUIDELINE WHEN SETTING UP INTERMITTENT TRACTION FORCE CYCLES. With intermittent traction, the force applied at rest is typically one third of the force applied during the on setting. For example, if the force during the on cycle is set at 90 lb, the force during the off cycle should be set at 30 lb.

DURATION

Recommended treatment times for sustained or intermittent traction range from a few minutes to 40 min. The important thing to remember is during the first session, apply traction for just a short time, and then assess the patient's response to the treatment.[23]

FREQUENCY

Although some clinicians advocate daily treatment sessions, there have been no scientific studies to suggest that traction performed daily is any better than traction performed every other day. Because many health insurance companies limit the number of reimbursable visits, many clinicians schedule their patients to be treated every other day.

As previously stated, traction should not be administered until a full evaluation has been completed, a definitive diagnosis has been made, and specific indications for traction have been established.[23] Taking a careful history, a physical examination, and diagnostic x-rays of the spine are all necessary. Traction is usually administered in conjunction with heat, massage, and immobilization. Exercises may also be used if indicated.[23]

Space will not allow us to describe how to apply all of the types of traction. Thus we have limited our scope to one manual and one mechanical traction technique of the cervical and lumbar spine:

- Manual cervical traction
- Mechanical cervical traction (intermittent or sustained)
- Manual lumbar traction (unilateral leg pull)
- Mechanical lumbar traction (intermittent or sustained)

STEP 1: FOUNDATION

A. Definition. Traction is a technique in which a pulling force is applied to body segments to stretch soft tissues and separate joint surfaces or bone fragments.
B. Effects
   1. Spinal movement. Increases spinal movement, overall and between each vertebra
   2. Bone. Reverses immobilization-related bone weakness by increasing or maintaining bone density
   3. Ligament. Creates ligament deformation, thereby increasing movement and decreasing impingement problems (long-term effects)
   4. Articular facet joints
      a. Increases separation of joint surfaces
      b. Decompresses articular cartilage, allowing synovial fluid exchange to nourish the cartilage
      c. May decrease degenerative changes
      d. May decrease pain perception
   5. Muscular system
      a. Lengthens tight muscles
      b. Allows better muscular blood flow
      c. Activates muscle proprioceptors, further decreasing pain
   6. Nerves. Decreases compression forces on nerves
C. Advantages. See Effects.
D. Disadvantages
   1. Manual traction can become physically tiring for the clinician to perform.

2. For some techniques, special equipment is required.
3. Once the traction force is removed and the patient sits or stands, the vertebral separation is reduced.
E. Indications
   1. Compression of nerve roots
   2. Disk protrusion
   3. Joint hypomobility
   4. Adhesions
   5. Muscle spasm
   6. Disk generation
   7. Foraminal stenosis
   8. Contracted connective tissue
   9. Apophyseal joint impingement
   10. Radiating pain that does not improve with truck or neck movement
F. Contraindications
   1. Cervical and lumbar traction
      a. Malignancy, either primary or metastatic
      b. Infectious diseases of the spine, such as tuberculosis
      c. Uncontrolled hypertension
      d. Rheumatoid arthritis
      e. Spinal cord compression
      f. Osteoporosis
      g. Cardiovascular disease
      h. Aortic aneurysm
      i. Acute neck or low-back pain
      j. Frail older adults
      k. Severe respiratory disease
      l. Hypermobile vertebrae (e.g., spondylolisthesis)
      m. When traction increases radicular pain
   2. Lumbar traction
   3. Pregnancy
   4. Hiatal hernia
   5. Abdominal hernia
   6. Active peptic ulcers
   7. Glaucoma (inversion gravity method)
G. Precautions. Do not substitute traction for a more beneficial treatment (e.g., extension exercises for a posterior disk protrusion).

STEP 2: PREAPPLICATION TASKS

A. Make sure traction is the proper modality for this situation.
   1. Re-evaluate the injury or problem. Make sure you understand the patient's condition.

2. Check for contraindications.

3. Confirm that the objectives of therapy are compatible with the use of traction.

B. Preparing the patient psychologically

1. Explain that a pulling sensation should be felt, but it should not cause discomfort.

2. The force should relieve pressure and decrease any radiating pain owing to pressure on nerves.

C. Preparing the patient physically

1. Remove clothing, earrings, bandages, tape, braces, and so on as necessary.

2. Secure the head harness (cervical traction) or chest and pelvic harness (lumbar traction) to the patient.

3. Position the patient

   a. Manual cervical traction

     i. Supine on padded treatment table

     ii. Head is cradled in the clinician's hands by placing one hand under the patient's chin and the other hand supporting the back of the head starting at the occiput.

     iii. Head is flexed 20°–30°

   b. Mechanical cervical traction

     i. Supine on padded treatment table

     ii. Attach the harness to the mechanical unit so the maximum pull is placed on the occiput, not the chin.

     iii. Neck is flexed 20°–30°

   c. Unilateral leg-pull manual traction (lumbar)

     i. Supine

     ii. Hip flexion of 30°

     iii. Hip abduction of 30°

     iv. Maximal outward rotation

   d. Mechanical lumbar traction. Depends on technique used.

D. Preparing the equipment

1. For mechanical traction, see the user manual for specific setup

2. Make sure the machine is operating properly

3. Make sure the displayed traction is correct

4. Make sure the duty cycle is operating properly, if using intermittent traction

3 ▪ STEP 3: APPLICATION PARAMETERS

A. Procedures

1. Manual cervical traction

   a. With the head supported, the clinician gently applies a force (20–25 lb) toward him.

   b. An intermittent force is applied lasting 5–10 sec on with a very short rest period.

   c. Total treatment time is 3–10 min.

2. Mechanical cervical traction

   a. With the head supported in the harness, the machine gently applies a force (20–25 lb).

   b. An intermittent force is applied with an on–off ratio of 3:1 or 4:1. For example, if the on time is 12 sec, the off time would be 3 or 4 sec.

   c. Total treatment time is 20–25 min.

3. Manual lumbar traction (unilateral leg pull). A steady pull is applied until a noticeable distraction is felt.

4. Mechanical lumbar traction

   a. Intermittent or sustained

   b. Select force of traction

   c. Select duty cycle (if intermittent)

   d. Select number of progressive steps (if intermittent)

   e. Select treatment time

B. Dosage

1. Cervical

   a. Sustained: up to 25 lb

   b. Intermittent: up to 25 lb

2. Lumbar

   a. Sustained: Start with 25% of body weight, then work up to 50% of body weight

   b. Intermittent: Start with 25% of body weight, then work up to 50% of body weight

C. Length of application

1. Cervical

   a. Sustained: 10 min

   b. Intermittent: 20 sec on, 5 sec off for 20–25 min

2. Lumbar

   a. Sustained: 4 min or more

   b. Intermittent: 15 sec on, 10 sec off for 20–25 min

D. Frequency of application. Every day, if possible

E. Duration of therapy. Traction can be used daily, as long as it helps decrease pain.

4 ▪ STEP 4: POSTAPPLICATION TASKS

A. Equipment removal

1. Remove harness or belts from the patient.

2. Make sure the machine is turned off.

B. Instructions to the patient

1. Schedule the next treatment.

2. Instruct the patient about the level of activity and/or self-treatment before the next formal treatment.

3. Instruct the patient about what she should feel after treatment.

C. Record of treatment, including unique patient responses

D. Clean up. Clean off the table (if used).

STEP 5: MAINTENANCE

Periodic check of belts, harnesses, and so on to ensure they are in good working order.

CLOSING SCENE

The professor in the chapter opening scene had a herniated disk and a bulging lumbar disk that were causing pain. He tried extension exercises, walking, cardio glide at the gym, intermittent traction tables, and massage. Each of these provided only temporary relief from the radiating pain. After 3 months, he purchased an inversion table traction unit for his home. He used this two or three times a day for 5–10 min each time and ended each session with extension exercises. This routine provided the most relief, and slowly (over 4 weeks) the radiating pain began to centralize (returned to the origin) and diminish.[24,25] The patient did end up undergoing partial surgical removal of the disk between L3 and L4. However, the disk between L5 and S1 was saved, probably owing to traction, extension, exercise, and luck.

CHAPTER REFLECTIONS

1. Read and ponder each of the following points. Do you feel you have a clear understanding of each concept? If not, reread the appropriate section of the chapter.
   - Define traction.
   - List the physiological effects of traction.
   - Describe the difference between manual and mechanical traction.
   - Identify the parameters for delivering cervical traction.
   - Name the parameters for delivering lumbar traction.
   - List the indications for traction.
   - List the contraindications for traction.

2. Write three to five questions for discussion with your class instructor, clinical instructor, classmates, and clinical colleagues.

3. Get together with classmates and quiz each other on the concepts of this chapter. Use the points in exercise 1 and questions you wrote for exercise 2 as a beginning. Explaining concepts out loud to others requires a deeper grasp of the material than feeling you understand it as you read.

CRITICAL THINKING RESPONSES

Critical Thinking 18.1

People have more low-back pain than neck pain for a couple of reasons. One reason is poor mechanics from lifting; we should bend more at the knees and use our legs, not our back. Another reason is that our lumbar region supports much more weight than the cervical spine.

Critical Thinking 18.2

An irritation of the sciatic nerve is probably causing the pain to radiate from the buttocks down the patient's entire right leg. Manual single-leg traction applied to the right leg can increase intervertebral disk space of the lumbar vertebrae and decrease pressure on this nerve.

Critical Thinking 18.3

A flotation belt or ankle cuffs could be worn as the patient swims in a horizontal position, causing drag and thereby creating traction on the vertebrae.

REFERENCES

1. Shakoor MA, Ahmed MS, Kibria G, et al. Effects of cervical traction and exercise therapy in cervical spondylosis. Bangladesh Med Res Counc Bull 2002;28:61–69.
2. Hides JA, Richardson CA, Jull GA. Multifidus muscle recovery is not automatic after resolution of acute, first-episode low back pain. Spine 1996;21:2763–2769.
3. Cypress BK. Characteristics of physician visits for back symptoms: A national perspective. Am J Public Health 1983;73:389–395.
4. Ellenberg MR, Honet JC, Treanor WJ. Cervical radiculopathy. Arch Phys Med Rehabil 1994;75:342–352.
5. Jette AM, Delitto A. Physical therapy treatment choices for musculoskeletal impairments. Phys Ther 1997;77:145–154.
6. Saunders H, Saunders R. Evaluation, Treatment and Prevention of Musculoskeletal Disorders: Spine. Vol 1. 3 ed. Bloomington, IN: Educational Opportunities, 1995.
7. Geiringer SR, deLateur BJ. Physiatric therapeutics. 3. Traction, manipulation, and massage. Arch Phys Med Rehabil 1990;71:S264–266.
8. Onel D, Tuzlaci M, Sari H, Demir K. Computed tomographic investigation of the effect of traction on lumbar disc herniations. Spine 1989;14:82–90.
9. Cyriax J, Russell G. Textbook of Orthopaedic Medicine. Vol. 2: Treatment by Manipulation, Massage and Injection. 10 ed. London: Bailliere Tindall, 1980.
10. Cailliet R. Low Back Pain Syndrome. Philadelphia: Davis, 1988.
11. Goldish G. Lumbar Traction. Interdisciplinary Rehabilitation of Low Back Pain. Baltimore: Williams & Wilkins; 1989.
12. Krause M, Refshauge KM, Dessen M, Boland R. Lumbar spine traction: Evaluation of effects and recommended application for treatment. Man Ther 2000;5:72–81.
13. Cameron M. Physical Agents in Rehabilitation: From Research to Practice. St. Louis: Saunders, 2003.
14. Swezey RL, Swezey AM, Warner K. Efficacy of home cervical traction therapy. Am J Phys Med Rehabil 1999;78:30–32.
15. Tekeoglu I, Adak B, Bozkurt M, Gurbuzoglu N. Distraction of lumbar vertebrae in gravitational traction. Spine 1998;23:1061–1063; discussion 1064.
16. Lee MY, Wong MK, Tang FT, et al. Design and assessment of an adaptive intermittent cervical traction modality with EMG biofeedback. J Biomech Eng 1996;118:597–600.
17. Moeti P, Marchetti G. Clinical outcome from mechanical intermittent cervical traction for the treatment of cervical radiculopathy: A case series. J Orthop Sports Phys Ther 2001;31:207–213.
18. Pellecchia GL. Lumbar traction: A review of the literature. J Orthop Sports Phys Ther 1994;20:262–267.
19. Guvenol K, Tuzun C, Peker O, Goktay Y. A comparison of inverted spinal traction and conventional traction in the treatment of lumbar disc herniations. Physiother Theory Pract 2000;16:151–160.
20. Beurskens AJ, de Vet HC, Koke AJ, et al. Efficacy of traction for nonspecific low back pain. 12-week and 6-month results of a randomized clinical trial. Spine 1997;22:2756–2762.
21. Meszaros TF, Olson R, Kulig K, et al. Effect of 10%, 30%, and 60% body weight traction on the straight leg raise test of symptomatic patients with low back pain. J Orthop Sports Phys Ther 2000;30: 595–601.
22. Harte AA, Baxter GD, Gracey JH. The efficacy of traction for back pain: A systematic review of randomized controlled trials. Arch Phys Med Rehabil 2003;84:1542–1553.
23. Hinterbuchner C. Traction. In: Basmajian J, ed. Manipulation, Traction and Massage. Baltimore: Williams & Wilkins; 1985.
24. Draper D. Inversion table traction as a therapeutic modality, Part 1. Athl Ther Today 2005;10(3):42–43.
25. Draper D. Inversion table traction as a therapeutic modality, Part 2. Athl Ther Today 2005;10(4):40–42.

Laser and Light Therapy

KENNETH L. KNIGHT AND TY HOPKINS

CHAPTER OUTLINE

Alex was stumped when his professor asked, "What do an athletic trainer, a cancer surgeon, a plastic surgeon, an air force general, a computer printer, a robot in a Detroit auto factory, a college professor, a telephone, and a TV have in common?" He was more stumped by the answer: "Each uses lasers to do his job." Surely, Alex thought, the simple-looking device he saw in the athletic training clinic was not the same as the devices that are used to shoot down missiles in outer space, point to important (and sometimes dull) elements on a lecture room screen, print computer-generated text and pictures, carry telephone and television signals in an optic fiber, weld car parts, and so on. And how could the same device be used in medicine to perform microsurgery, cauterize ruptured blood vessels, assist in a variety of diagnostic tasks, and reduce pain and stimulate healing?

Light Therapy

Light therapy, also known as *phototherapy*, is a broad term that refers to the application of light by a variety of devices for a variety of therapeutic purposes. Devices include lasers, light-emitting diodes (LEDs), super-luminous diodes (SLDs), fluorescent lamps, infrared lamps, ultraviolet (UV) lamps, diachronic lamps, and very bright incandescent light bulbs. They are used to treat orthopedic injuries, skin conditions, and psychological problems such as depression and seasonal affective disorder and to tan the skin. In this chapter we are concerned only with the therapeutic use of lasers and LEDs, but we will briefly mention ultraviolet radiation.

Light therapy began with lasers in the 1970s. **Laser,** an acronym for light amplification by stimulated emission of radiation, is a device that transforms electromagnetic energy of various frequencies, in or near the range of visible light, into an extremely intense, small, and nearly nondivergent beam of monochromatic radiation with all its waves in phase. The therapeutic theory is that specific wavelengths of laser light, when absorbed, cause specific physiological responses in the body. Although the therapeutic value of these responses has been debated, the industry continues to grow. Numerous factors, including technological advances, have led to the use of nonlaser devices, such as LEDs, SLDs, and polarized polychromic light, to deliver light of specific wavelength to the body.[1]

As with any emerging technology, there is much confusion in terminology.[1,2] Light therapy is today where electrotherapy was in the early 1980s (see Chapter 9). Terms and acronyms used to describe light therapy include phototherapy, cold laser, soft laser, low-energy laser, low-level laser therapy (LLLT), low-energy laser therapy (LELT), low-intensity laser-activated biostimulation (LILAB), low-power laser irradiation (LPLI), low-power laser therapy (LPLT), low-intensity laser (LIL), and monochromatic infrared energy. It is easy for clinicians to become confused when reading the professional literature. Leaders in the field are now calling for clinicians, scientists, and corporate professionals to begin using the terms *light therapy* or *phototherapy*.[1,2]

LASER AND NONLASER DEVICES

Both laser and nonlaser devices (LEDs, SLDs) deliver light of specific wavelengths, although the way the light is generated and some of its characteristics are different. There is no consensus about the relative merits of these two technologies, and it is difficult to discuss their therapeutic value. The major problem is with terminology. Some lasers use LEDs, so the discussion cannot be lasers vs. LEDs. Some scientists use the terms *laser and nonlaser light*,[1] whereas others use *coherent and noncoherent light*[3] to distinguish the two technologies. To understand the difference, you must understand how each is produced.

Characteristics of Lasers

To produce laser radiation, a laser device must have an energy source, a mechanical structure, and a **lasing medium,** either gas, liquid, crystal, chemical, or semiconductor (such as LEDs). The difference in lasing medium will result in differing wavelengths, levels of light coherence, and levels of light divergence.

Laser light is different from normal light. Laser light is monophasic, monochromatic, coherent, and nondivergent (directional)—meaning it is composed of particles of

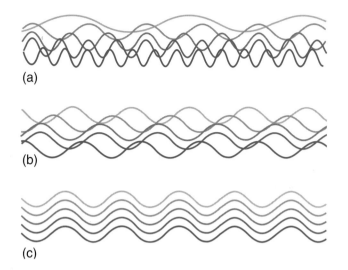

(a)

(b)

(c)

FIGURE 19.1. Wave patterns of three types of light. **(a)** Light from a common light bulb is composed of waves with different frequencies. **(b)** An LED emits light with waves of the same frequency (monochromatic) but out of phase (incoherent). **(c)** A laser emits light with waves of the same frequency (monochromatic) and in phase (coherent).

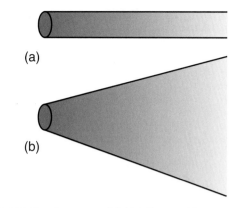

(a)

(b)

FIGURE 19.2. The divergence of light is illustrated by contrasting **(a)** a nondivergent beam with **(b)** a divergent beam.

light with equal energy and of a single phase and color that move in step with each other (Fig. 19.1). The following list of terms and definitions further describes the characteristics of lasers.

- **Light:** Electromagnetic radiation that can produce a visual sensation
- **Amplify:** To increase in size, volume, or significance
- **Stimulate:** To excite or invigorate; to encourage or provoke something to grow, develop, or become more active
- **Emission:** A flowing forth, such as the release of electrons from parent atoms
- **Radiation:** The transfer of energy in the form of rays, waves, or particles, often from a central source; also called radiant energy
- **Electromagnetic energy:** One of the fundamental forms of energy in the universe. Its characteristics change radically, depending on frequency and wavelength, which tend to correlate closely with each other (see Chapter 11).
- **Frequency:** The rate of vibration of a force or wave, usually measured relative to local time
- **Visible light:** An electromagnetic wave that is divergent, multichromatic, incoherent, and multiphasic
- **Nondivergent:** Incapable of separating or widening. Contrast the light from a laser pointer (nondivergent) with that coming from a flashlight (divergent). Nondivergent light is also known as directional light (Fig. 19.2).
- **Monochromatic:** Having a single frequency and a single color (if it is in the light spectrum (Fig. 19.1b,c)

- **Coherent:** Logically ordered or integrated; a quality of electromagnetic waves that have the same wavelength and a fixed phase relationship (Fig. 19.1c)
- **Fixed phase:** The unified launching of the wave fronts of all light particles of a laser beam

A laser is not a single device but rather a variety of devices, each with a specific frequency, amplification, and focus of its emitted beam. The therapeutic modality used to treat wounds could not be used to control your TV or weld car parts, and vice versa. Some therapeutic lasers have applicator heads with a variety of diodes (laser-emitting devices) so they can deliver a variety of frequencies or laser beams.

The word *laser* is used as part of several related concepts:

- *Laser device:* A machine or device that produces, or generates, and emits a laser beam. This is generally what is meant when the word *laser* is used by itself.
- *Laser beam:* The output of a laser device; highly amplified, single-frequency, single-colored, nondivergent, coherent light
- *Laser light:* The light of a laser beam
- *Laser energy:* The energy of a laser beam

THE NATURE OF LIGHT

Lasers are possible because of the dual nature of light: Light is both a wave and a particle.[4] In most situations, including when it travels from one point to another, light acts as a wave of oscillating electrical and magnetic fields (see Fig. 11.3). When it is absorbed or emitted by atoms, however, it acts as a particle. The particles, or packets of energy, are called **photons.** The amount of energy of a given photon is a function of its wavelength, or frequency, because each photon has a unique wavelength and a unique frequency (see Chapter 11).

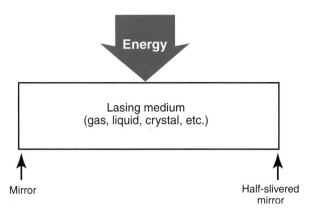

FIGURE 19.3. The basic components of a laser.

LASER ENERGY PRODUCTION

The production of laser energy requires four components (Fig. 19.3):

- An amplifying chamber, or resonating cavity in which the stimulation and amplification take place
- A lasing medium (gas, liquid, crystal, chemical, or semiconductor), which is placed in the amplifying chamber
- An external source of energy (electrical, chemical, or optical)
- A pair of mirrors at either end of the amplifying chamber, one of which is a **half-slivered mirror**, meaning it reflects only half the light and allows the other half to pass through

When external energy is applied to a lasing medium, some of the lasing medium atoms absorb the energy. The absorbed energy excites the atoms, causing them to move to higher-energy orbits. This is an abnormal or unstable state, however, so the electrons return to their normal state. As they do, the absorbed energy is released as a photon, a particle of light.

Photons are part of our daily life. Atoms release energy as photons of light all the time. The light from light bulbs; TV picture tubes; fire; and the heating coils on electric stoves, ovens, and toasters are all caused by the release of photons as atoms change orbits. Unlike laser energy, however, these photons are released at a variety of wavelengths and, therefore, appear and behave very differently from laser energy.

Lasers are designed to control the excitation (stimulation) of atoms and the subsequent release (emission) of this stimulated energy. Identical atoms with identical states of excitation will emit photons of identical wavelengths. Thus, by using a specific lasing medium and controlling the process, the released photons are monochromatic and coherent.

A pair of mirrors, one at each end of the lasing medium, is essential to laser energy production. The majority of the photons are lost. As shown in Figure 19.4 photons P1, P2, and P3 exit the amplifying chamber without striking the mirrors. Photons P4 and P5 strike the mirrors and are reflected out of the amplifying chamber. Photon P6, however, strikes the mirror at a right angle and is reflected back toward the second mirror. As photons bounce back and forth between the two mirrors, through the lasing medium, they stimulate electrons of excited atoms to return to their normal state, giving up energy in the form of additional photons. Thus a cascade effect occurs in which more and more photons are emitted. The photons that pass through the half-slivered mirror become the laser beam (light). This process may be affected by the type of lasing medium. For example, lasers

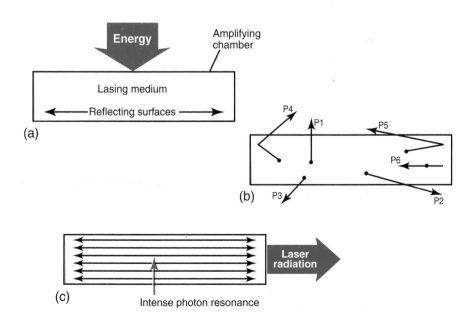

FIGURE 19.4. The production of laser energy. **(a)** The application of external energy to the medium causes **(b)** the spontaneous release of photons, some of which (P6) reflect back and forth between the two mirrors. **(c)** This leads to intense photon resonance, part of which is released as laser light through the half-slivered mirror. (Adapted with permission from Baxter.[5])

with a semiconductor medium do not emit purely mono-chromatic light, and the coherence length is shorter than that of lasers with a chemical medium. So, although LED-based lasers produce light at a wavelength in a therapeutic range, the differences in the energy and other light characteristics (e.g., coherence) cause some researchers to question the effectiveness of semiconductor-based devices.

ENERGY LEVEL DETERMINES EFFECTS

The effects of a laser are largely determined by the amount of energy it emits. High-energy lasers produce great amounts of heat, which is useful in welding and shooting down satellites. In the human body, tissue is destroyed if high levels of energy are applied. Although this may be desirable to a surgeon, it is not the goal of an athletic trainer.

Therapeutic modality lasers emit low levels of energy (<500 mW) that do not heat body tissue. These are called low-level lasers, also referred to as *cold lasers* or *soft lasers* (Fig. 19.5).

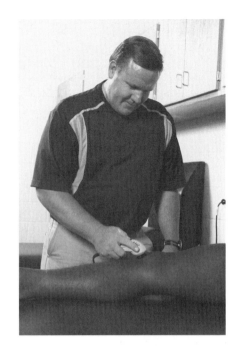

FIGURE 19.5. A low-level laser, or cold laser.

MODALITY MYTH

COLD LASERS DO NOT PRODUCE HEAT

It is only partially true that cold lasers do not produce heat. They are said to be athermic, meaning they do not directly heat tissues. However, because low-level lasers increase blood flow to the treated area, there is a slight measurable increase in tissue temperature as a result of their use.

LASER CLASSIFICATION

The wide variety of lasers are commonly classified in two ways: according to the type of lasing medium they employ (Table 19.1) and according to their safety (Table 19.2). The following list summarizes the five types of lasers and their lasing medium:

- *Gas lasers:* Use gas as a lasing medium. Helium and helium neon (HeNe) are the most common gas lasers.
- *Diode or semiconductor lasers:* Use semiconductors as the lasing medium; they can be either small and low powered or large and high powered. Low-powered semiconductor lasers are those used in laser pointers, laser printers, and CD players. In fact, the 780 nm aluminum gallium arsenide (AlGaAs) laser diode, used in CD players, is the most common type of laser in the world. Large industrial diode lasers are capable of generating great amounts of heat and are used for cutting and welding.
- *Dye lasers:* Use large-molecule organic dyes in a liquid solution as the lasing medium. They can be "tuned" to produce laser beams over a broad range of wavelengths.
- *Solid-state lasers:* Use minerals as their lasing medium. Examples are the ruby and neodymium:yttrium-aluminum-garnet (YAG) lasers.

TABLE 19.1	Types of Lasers		
LASER TYPE	**LASING MEDIUM**	**WAVELENGTH (NM)**	**SAFETY CLASSIFICATION**
Gas	HeNe	633	I–IV
Gas	CO2	10,600	IIIb–IV
Gas	Argon	488–514	IV
Diode or semiconductor	AlGaAs	600–1000	IIIb
Dye	Tunable dye	577	IV
Solid state	Ruby	694	IV
Solid state	HdYag	1060	IV
Excimer	Dimer	351	IV

TABLE 19.2	*Safety Classifications of Lasers*		
CLASS	**POWER (MW)**	**VISIBILITY***	**SAFETY CONCERNS**
I	<0.5	Either	None
II	<1	Visible	Safe for momentary viewing
IIIa	<5	Either	Photochemical effect
IIIb	<500	Either	Photobiomodulation, no photothermal effect, no harm to skin or clothing, potential damage to eye
IV	>500	Either	Photothermal effect; harmful to skin, eyes, and clothing; use with extreme caution

*Either means there are both visible and nonvisible laser beams in this class.

- *Excimer lasers:* Use a dimer as the lasing medium. (A dimer is a pseudo-molecule created by electrically stimulating a mixture of reactive gases, such as chlorine and fluorine, with inert gases, such as argon, krypton, and xenon.)

Safety is determined by the amount of energy applied to the lasing medium and the subsequent amount of energy released in the form of light—in other words, the power of the laser. The greater the power of the laser, the greater the potential danger (see Table 19.2).

Two other factors to consider when discussing types of lasers are wavelength and color. Although neither wavelength nor color is used to classify lasers, these terms are important when discussing and applying lasers. The body's response to laser application is specific to the laser's wavelength. A laser of one specific wavelength will cause a certain tissue reaction, whereas a laser of another wavelength will cause a different reaction or no reaction at all. This specificity of response makes understanding and using lasers complex and at times confusing. Clinicians must always identify the specific wavelength of a laser when discussing its effects with patients.

Lasers are often referred to by their color, such as a red laser or a violet laser. This practice is imprecise, though, and we recommend against it. For example, all lasers with wavelengths of 150–380 nm are ultraviolet (Table 19.3). But the tissue response to a 150 nm laser is different from that to a 380 nm laser, so each laser should be referred to by its specific wavelength, rather than calling them both ultraviolet lasers.

Characteristics of LEDs and SLDs

A light-emitting diode (LED) is a special type of semiconductor diode that emits visible light when an electric current passes through it.[4,6] As its name implies, a super-luminous diode (SLD) is a brighter LED. Like normal diodes, SLDs consist of a semiconducting material (such as silicone or germanium) that is impregnated, or *doped*,

with impurities to create a structure called a p–n junction. In crystalline form, silicone and germanium are electrical insulators, but the impurities turn them into electrical conductors. Although they are not strong conductors like metal, they will conduct electricity adequately.

The p–n junction of the diode consists of two pieces of a semiconductor material, each doped with a different substance (Fig. 19.6). After the doping material on the n-side of the junction chemically bonds with the semiconductor material, there are extra free electrons. This results in the semiconductor being negatively charged, hence the *n*. The doping material on the p-side does not have enough electrons to fully bond with the semiconductor material, so the result is a positively charged material, hence the *p*. The interaction of the two sides of the p–n junction gives the diode some unique characteristics, such as allowing electrical current to flow in one direction but blocking it in the opposite direction and generating light.

As electricity passes through it, the diode gives off energy in the form of photons. The wavelength of the energy given off, and thus the color of the emitted light, is determined by the chemical composition of the doping materials. LEDs and SLDs typically are covered by plastic cases of varying colors. The plastic case has no bearing on the color of the light; it simply is used to indicate the specific

TABLE 19.3	*Tissue Penetration of Various Wavelengths*	
WAVELENGTH (NM)	**COLOR RANGE**	**DEPTH OF PENETRATION (MM)**
150–380	Ultraviolet	<0.1
390–470	Violet to deep blue	~0.3
475–545	Blue to green	~0.3–0.5
545–600	Yellow to orange	~0.5–1.0
600–650	Red	~1.0–2.0
650–1000	Deep red to infrared	2.0–3.0
1000–1350	Near to mid infrared	3.0–5.0
1350–12000	Infrared	<0.1

*Adapted with permission from Baxter.[5]

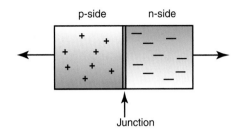

FIGURE 19.6. The p–n junction of a diode.

wavelength of energy emitted by the diode and, therefore, the color of the light.

Light emitted from an LED or SLD is monochromatic but not coherent. This means its light will be more scattered than that of a laser and, therefore, less of the light will strike the target. Thus less energy is imparted to the tissue.

DIFFERENCES BETWEEN LIGHT THERAPY LASERS AND DIODE DEVICES

Since both semiconductor-based lasers and diode devices use LEDs and SLDs, one might think that the light delivered from the two devices is the same. Not true. The p–n junction of the diode device emits energy directly to the patient.[4] With a semiconductor laser, however, the emission from the diode is further processed by the laser to stimulate additional photons. When the photons escape via the laser's half-slivered mirror they are coherent but also have a greater photon density—that is, more photons per area. The clinical implications are that diode devices will take much longer to deliver the same amount of energy to the target tissue, and the energy they deliver probably will not penetrate the tissue as effectively as laser light.

Although many insist that coherence is essential for clinical effectiveness, others argue that light is light, and it is the wavelength and the dose that matter.[7] It also should be noted that SLDs and/or clusters of SLDs have been effective in the treatment of some cells and tissues.[1]

Lasers in Medicine

Various forms of lasers are used in medicine.[8,9] Applications include surgery (cutting tissue or cauterizing bleeding vessels), diagnosis, imaging, and physical medicine and rehabilitation. The lasers, LEDs, and SLDs used in rehabilitation are very different from the laser therapies used in other areas of medicine—primarily, the power is much lower. The maximal output of these devices is <500 mW.

The relatively low power output of light therapy makes it athermic. This does not mean that no thermal reactions take place in treated tissues, rather that the temperature rise is so small that it is virtually undetectable.

The U.S. Food and Drug Administration (FDA) has not approved light therapy for rehabilitation, but it has cleared specific machines for specific therapeutic uses. The FDA believes that more evidence (from controlled clinical trials) is necessary for approving light therapy. To date, light therapy has been cleared for use in the temporary relief of neck and shoulder pain of musculoskeletal origin, wrist and hand pain associated with carpal tunnel syndrome, and iliotibial band syndrome pain.[10] Light therapy devices may also be used in controlled clinical trials with approval from the Institutional Review Board, a committee at universities and research institutions that reviews research proposals involving human subjects to ensure that the research does not expose those subjects to undue risk or harm and that their rights are protected.

Many clinicians feel that once a low-level laser has been purchased it can be used to treat about any medical condition.[10] There are no "laser police" to prevent such actions, but this does not relieve the clinician of liability for any damages that might result from the improper use of the device.[10] Use lasers with caution.

When used properly, light therapy is relatively safe. Although many electrical modalities have extended lists of contraindications and precautions, light therapy appears to be safe for patients who have pins, metal plates, plastic implants, growth plates, and pacemakers and for treating the gonads.[5]

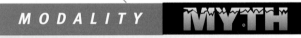

MODALITY **MYTH**

LASER THERAPY HAS GOVERNMENT APPROVAL

It is true that in the United States, the federal government has given limited approval for laser therapy. The FDA has cleared specific models of low-level lasers from certain manufactures for treating particular musculoskeletal conditions. Thus the use of lasers other than the specifically approved models is illegal. In addition, the use of an approved model for treating of any condition other than the approved condition is illegal.

THE EFFECTS OF LIGHT THERAPY ON TISSUE

Laser and nonlaser devices vary in the depth of penetration, the type of tissue that is affected, and the types of molecules within the tissue that are affected. Water and organic molecules, such as amino acids, nucleic acid bases, hemoglobin, and melanin, account for absorption rates of radiation in body tissues. Skin color may thus play a role in how much light is absorbed by the tissue and to what depth it penetrates during treatment.

Photobiomodulation

Photobiomodulation is the act of modifying biological processes with light. That's exactly what laser therapy does—it stimulates tissue in a way that modifies pain and/or the healing processes. Some clinicians continue to use an older term, *biostimulation,* but this term is only half right.[10] Lasers sometimes inhibit biological processes, as in reducing pain.

Mechanisms of Action

When light is absorbed by tissues, it acts at the molecular level by one or a combination of the following three mechanisms (Fig. 19.7):

- Excitation of electron bonds within molecules, which can result in molecules breaking or undergoing structural changes
- Excitation of atoms to higher levels of oscillation (movement) in relation to each other within the molecule, which could lead to low levels of heat production
- Rotational changes of atoms within the molecule, which could also lead to changes in temperature

The exact mechanisms by which laser light affects tissues have not been decisively determined. The energy of any electromagnetic wave is a photon. The accepted theory is that photons are absorbed by photoreceptors in tissue cells,[11] causing a change in the photoreceptors' molecular configuration (called the primary reaction). This change in configuration alters the cells' molecular processes (called secondary reactions).

In vitro studies, in which cellular or tissue cultures are used to model living human tissue, support this theory, including these secondary reactions:

- Photobiomodulation of cellular events
- Stimulated/optimized tissue repair
- Pain relief

More research is needed to confirm that these effects occur **in vivo**—within the tissues when lasers are applied to the body directly.

Many components of the body's metabolic pathway may be primary photoreceptors, absorbing laser light and inducing changes in cellular homeostasis, ultimately enhancing healing by promoting the synthesis of adenosine triphosphate (ATP) molecules for energy and numerous cellular activities related to the proliferation (spread or increase) of new cells.[11,12] Fibroblasts do increase after HeNe irradiation of tissue cultures.[13–16] Furthermore, light therapy seems to increase collagen production by fibroblasts.[17] The conversion of fibroblasts to myofibroblasts also appears to be a positive effect of light therapy.[18] (Myofibroblasts are modified fibroblasts that help contract or pull the margins of wounds closer together during wound healing.) Although these findings support the use of light therapy, the results have not always been duplicated owing to variations in treatment parameters and tissue culture types.[19,20] Therefore, more research is needed to support the positive effects of light therapy and identify the specific mechanisms that mediate those effects.

Light therapy may be effective in increasing lymphocyte proliferation[21] and their ability to bind pathogens.[22,23] However, results of other studies suggest that light therapy has the opposite effect: a decrease or inhibition of lymphocyte proliferation.[24,25] It appears that these effects may depend on the wavelength and power output used in treatment. The data may help support the idea that lasers assist in healing chronic wounds by suppressing the immune system. Again, more research is needed to support these potential effects of light therapy on the immune system.

Tissue Healing

The cellular and molecular effects just described help explain why light therapy may strengthen tissue healing. Enhanced ATP synthesis would lead to increased fibroblast proliferation, so fibroblasts would produce increased levels of collagen, and as a result, fibroplasia (production of fibrous tissue) would theoretically be facilitated and wounds would contract more quickly.

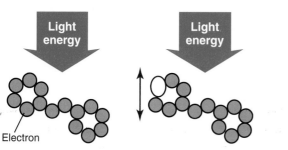

(a)   (b)   (c)

FIGURE 19.7. Three possible mechanisms by which molecules absorb light. **(a)** Excitation of molecular electron bonds. **(b)** Excitation of atoms to higher levels of oscillation (movement). **(c)** Rotational changes of atoms within the molecule. (Adapted with permission from Baxter.[5])

This idea is supported in the research. Light therapy enhances wound contraction of experimental wounds on human skin,[26] the healing of skin ulcerations in humans,[27–29] peripheral nerve regeneration,[30] and various skin injuries in animals.[22,31] It should also be noted again that other studies using animal and human wounds have shown light therapy to have no effect on healing.[32–34] In fact, there is a much greater discrepancy in these studies than in the previously reported in vitro studies.

It is possible that light therapy enhances tissue healing during three phases of tissue healing as follows:[5]

1. *Cellular phase:* Increased mast cell release, interleukin 6 (an inflammatory regulatory substance) formation, and decreased dermal necrosis
2. *Collagenization phase:* Enhanced collagen formation, degranulation, and myofibroblast conversion
3. *Remodeling phase:* Wound contraction and tensile strength/stress

With an increase in fibroblast proliferation and collagen activity during the repair phase of healing, some clinicians suggest that light therapy may result in oversize scarring. Although this is certainly something the clinician should pay attention to, there is currently no evidence to suggest that light therapy results in hypertrophic scars or keloids. In fact, light therapy has been shown to flatten and soften existing keloids.[13]

Pain Relief

Opinions are varied concerning the affect of light therapy on acute and chronic pain. Much of the support for reducing pain with light therapy is from anecdotal claims rather than from controlled, blinded investigations or randomized clinical trials, although there have been at least five randomized clinical trials of neck pain.[35] Controlled research has been split: some indicating light therapy is effective in reducing pain,[35,36] and others indicating it is not.[37–39] Much of the debate centers on the optimal parameters for the application of light therapy to reduce pain and the elusive mechanism by which light therapy occurs.

Several studies support the use of light therapy in treating the following painful conditions:

- Acute musculoskeletal trauma[36]
- Myofascial pain[40,41]
- Rheumatoid arthritis[42]
- Carpal tunnel syndrome[43]
- Low-back pain[44]
- Trigger points[40,41]
- Neck pain[35]

Conversely, other controlled studies indicate that light therapy had no effect on the following conditions:

- Musculoskeletal pain[39]
- Lateral ankle sprains[38]
- Plantar fasciitis[45]
- Delayed-onset muscle soreness[46]

Several theories have been suggested to explain how light therapy works to relieve pain. Although there is no concrete evidence supporting one specific mechanism of action, these theories collectively point to some possibilities:

- Increased serotonin,[38] which, if released in the central nervous system (CNS), may inhibit pain transmission
- Decreased cholinergic release[5] and, therefore, reduced pain transmission in the CNS
- Inhibition of prostacyclin,[47] a key player in pain during the inflammatory process of healing
- Increased sensory nerve transmission time of superficial nerves,[48,49] potentially decreasing overall pain transmission over time; however, other studies failed to replicate these findings.[50]
- Increased CNS pain perception threshold[51]
- Placebo effect

Treatment Parameters

The treatment parameters for light therapy are

- Delivery technique
- Dosage and duration
- Tissue penetration

DELIVERY TECHNIQUE

Light therapy can treat a variety of different sites, including a lesion, wound, or area of pain; nerve roots and trunks; trigger points or acupressure points; and lymphatic and blood vessels. Most lasers use a **single laser probe** to deliver light of a specific wavelength to tissues. However, in recent years **cluster probes** have been used to apply multiple wavelengths to a larger area during treatment (Fig. 19.8).

For optimum delivery of laser light, the laser probe should be in contact with the skin, to minimize divergence and reflection. In the case of open wounds, the probe may be held close (<1 cm) to the wound without touching it. Some clinicians use a sterile transparent film placed over the open wound so that the probe can be placed in contact with the damaged tissue.

Obviously the cluster head is the best option for treating a large area. However, when a cluster head is not avail-

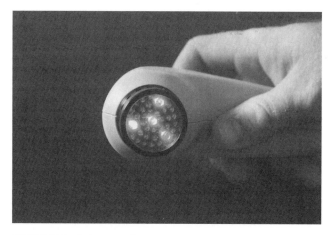

FIGURE 19.8. A cluster probe.

able, a single probe can be used in one of two ways: sequential application to multiple areas of tissue, called **grid application**, or moving the head across the area like an ultrasound head, a technique called **scanning**.

To use the grid application, imagine the treatment area as a series of 1 cm² segments. Systematically treat each segment with the appropriate dosage for the condition. Scanning consists of moving the laser probe back and forth over the treatment area at a slow and steady rate. Each pass progresses across the wound until the treatment area has been covered. Then the entire area is treated a second time, with the probe moving at 90° to the first pass. The entire treatment area and the machine's output should be considered to formulate the duration of treatment. Dosage is much less accurate using the scanning method.

For treatment over trigger points or acupressure points, slowly move the laser probe and apply more pressure for a massage effect. Ask the patient to let you know if the pressure is too great.

DOSAGE AND DURATION

The dosage depends on three factors: average output power, time of light exposure, and treatment area. These factors are represented in the following formula:

$$\text{Dosage} = \frac{(\text{average power} \times \text{Tx time})}{\text{Tx area}}$$

where:

- Dosage is given in joules per centimeter squared (J/cm²)
- Average power is the average output power of the machine (in mW)
- Tx time is the length of treatment (Tx) (in min)
- Tx area is area of the laser beam or area to be treated (in cm²)

The power output of a laser is fixed, and the only way to alter the dosage is to alter the time of application. Treatment time must be computed for each specific device, because the output differs for each device. Treatment time is computed from the total output of the specific device.

Manufactures report the total output power of their individual devices, and many of those who offer multiple pulse rates report the average power for each of their pulse rates. If, however, average power is not given, you must compute it using the following formula:

$$\text{Average power} = \text{pulse rate (Hz)} \times \text{peak power (mW)} \times \text{pulse width (sec)}$$

Dosage ranges for specific conditions have been derived from available research and mathematical theory. Some of these are presented in Tables 19.4 and 19.5. The differences in these two tables reflect the lack of precise knowledge about this modality. Consult the application

TABLE 19.4	Musculoskeletal Conditions and Their Approximate Laser Dosages	
CONDITION	**DOSAGE***	**NOTES***
Superficial wounds	0.5–4.0 J/cm²	Increase dosage as the wound bed develops over time
Trigger points	8 J/cm²	Use a laser probe; treat each trigger point with 1 J
Nerve root application	8–24 J/cm²	Use a laser probe (1–3 J/point)
Tendinitis	1–3 J/point	
Capsulitis	1 J/point	
Epicondylitis	2–3 J/point	
Muscle strain	1–2 J/point	
Patellofemoral problems	1–2 J/point	
Ligament strain	2–4 J/point	
Plantar fasciitis	1–3 J/point	

*Point denotes an area the size of the laser probe.
Adapted with permission from Baxter.[5]

TABLE 19.5	Basic Recommendations for Laser Treatment Dosages				
	ACUTE (J)			**CHRONIC (J)**	
CONDITION	**Per Point**	**Dosage Total**		**Per Point**	**Dosage Total**
Muscle strain	3–4	25–35		5–6	35–45
Tendinitis	3–6	24–30		5–8	35–45
Ligament sprain	3–4	25–30		5–6	35–45
Stress fracture	7–8	25–30		8–10	35–40
Open wounds	0.5–1.5	*		1–4	*
Myofascial trigger point	1.0 J	†		1.0	†

>*Depends on the size of the wound.
†Because of their focalized nature, myofascial trigger points are treated once at the most tender location.
Reprinted with permission from McLeod.[9]

manual for the unit used in your clinic for additional dosages.

Compute treatment time using the following formula:

$$\text{Tx time} = \frac{(\text{dosage} \times \text{Tx area})}{\text{power}}$$

where

- Dosage is the value (in J/cm^2) obtained from a table
- Tx area is the area (in cm^2) you want to treat
- Power is the peak power (if you are treating with a continuous wave) or average power (if you are treating with a pulsed wave), per the manufacturer's data or the average power calculated via the formula

For example, if the desired dosage for a specific condition is $1.5\ J/cm^2$, the average power of the laser is 0.5 mW, and the surface area of the laser beam is $0.1\ cm^2$, then:

$$\text{Tx time} = \frac{(1.5\ J/cm^2 \times 0.5\ cm^2)}{0.5\ mW}$$

Because 1 joule = 1 W·sec and 0.5 mW = 0.0005 W, the formula can be rewritten as:

$$\text{Tx time} = \frac{(1.5\ W\text{·}sec/cm^2 \times 0.5\ cm^2)}{0.0005\ W}$$

Tx time = 300 sec or 5 min

To deliver $1.5\ J/cm^2$ it would take 5 min. However, if the treatment area were larger than the laser probe, then the time to treat the entire area could be computed using a scanning method. If the grid application were to be used, then treatment would be delivered using the treatment time calculated for the laser probe, and each grid would be treated for that time period.

TISSUE PENETRATION

Depth of penetration is a major issue with light therapy. No matter how effective the light is on specific tissue,

its effect is of no value if it does not reach the target tissue with appropriate dosage. As light is absorbed by various tissue cells, the depth of penetration is reduced.

Laser penetration is a function of its wavelength and power. Although wavelength is probably the most important factor in determining depth of penetration, there must also be a driving force. The driving force is the power or amount of energy that is being applied. A good analogy is that of a short nail and a long nail. The shorter nail represents a shorter wavelength and hence a lower depth of penetration; the longer nail represents a longer wavelength. If we were to drive the shorter nail into a piece of wood with a heavy blow and were to gently tap the longer nail, common sense dictates that the shorter nail would be driven deeper into the piece of wood. Despite the fact that the longer nail is capable of penetrating more deeply, the lack of force results in a shallower depth of penetration. Keep in mind that no matter how hard either nail is hit, the total depth of penetration is limited. The same is true for lasers—for any given wavelength, there is a maximum depth of penetration, and to elicit responses up to and including the maximum depth of penetration, an appropriate amount of energy must be used.

Tissue penetration of lasers is only superficial, at best 5 mm (see Table 19.3). It is even less with LED and SLD devices. Most wavelengths penetrate <1 mm, however. This partly accounts for the difference between results of in vitro studies and in vivo studies: Cells in a culture dish are irradiated directly, whereas those in tissue are irradiated only after the beam is partially absorbed in skin and other tissues.

Depth of penetration is wavelength dependent. The near to middle infrared spectrum (1000–1350 nm) appears to penetrate deepest: 3–5 mm.[5] These depths may be affected by the power or intensity of the incident light, however, so it is debatable whether light therapy has enough dosage to treat deeper tissues.

It appears from the literature that light therapy may be beneficial to superficial wounds and pain originating from superficial tissues. Because light energy is absorbed by only superficial tissues, its use is limited.

 CRITICAL THINKING 19.1 Compare and contrast diathermy and laser therapy. In what ways are they alike? In what ways are they different?

Skin Color

Melanin, a pigment that contributes to skin color, absorbs light in the visible spectrum very well.[5] Therefore, patients with darker skin may absorb more light in the cutaneous layers, preventing light from penetrating to deeper tissues. In addition, the production of melanin is triggered by light in the near-ultraviolet range. This could result in darkening of skin or scar tissue as more melanocytes are produced.

Obesity

Considering the issues related to depth of penetration of therapeutic light, the thickness of subcutaneous fat should be considered when treating conditions that exist deep to the subcutaneous layers. It seems debatable whether light therapy can reach deeper tissues at a dosage appropriate for treatment. When the subcutaneous fat layer is excessively thick, the likelihood of therapeutic dosages reaching deeper tissues is even more questionable.

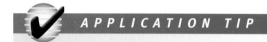

APPLICATION TIP

WEAR SAFETY GOGGLES. *Even with the low-power output of therapeutic lasers, the light is sufficient to cause damage to the eyes. You and your patients must wear protective goggles during laser applications to prevent accidental exposure of the eyes to the light. Goggles are equipped with light filters aimed at reducing the incident light.*

Application of Light Therapy

STEP 1: FOUNDATION

A. Definition. Light therapy is the application of light for therapeutic purposes.
B. Effects
  1. Photobiomodulation of tissue healing
  2. Pain relief
C. Advantages
  1. Relatively safe
    a. No side effects
    b. Athermic
  2. Easy to use
  3. Cost-effective
    a. Therapist time
    b. Patient recovery
D. Disadvantages
  1. Effects of light density on eyesight
  2. Limited depth of penetration
E. Indications. The indications for light therapy are numerous. Although conclusive data do not exist to support all reported indications for light therapy, the following are supported:
  1. Activating cells into a healing mode
  2. Wound healing
  3. Pain relief
  4. Increasing tensile strength of scar tissue
F. Contraindications
  1. Irradiation directly into the eye
  2. Irradiation of the uterus during pregnancy
  3. Cancer
  4. Organ transplant patients
G. Precautions
  1. Be cautions when applying light therapy to a patient who:
    a. Is photosensitive
    b. Suffers from epilepsy
  3. Has had a recent steroid injection
  4. Is taking anti-inflammatory medication
  5. Has an acute infection
  6. Suffers from a thyroid condition

STEP 2: PREAPPLICATION TASKS

A. Make sure light therapy is the proper modality for this situation.
  1. Reevaluate the injury or problem. Make sure you understand the patient's condition. Question the patient about any abnormalities resulting from the previous treatment.

2. Check for contraindications.
3. Confirm that the objectives of therapy are compatible with the use of light therapy.
B. Preparing the patient psychologically. Explain that no sensation should be felt.
C. Preparing the patient physically
  1. Remove clothing, earrings, bandages, tape, braces, etc. as necessary.
  2. Clean and dry the skin of the treatment area.
D. Preparing the equipment
  1. Check the manual for the average power output of the unit.
  2. Calculate the treatment time based on desired dosage, average power output, and the area to be treated.
  3. Make sure the machine is operating properly.
  4. Make sure the displayed time is correct.
  5. If applicable, make sure the pulse rate is set appropriately for the treatment.

STEP 3: APPLICATION PARAMETERS

A. Procedures
  1. Turn on the machine (if necessary).
  2. Adjust the output parameters as needed (pulse rate and treatment time).
  3. Wear safety goggles.
  4. Application technique
    a. Direct contact with the skin, with the exception of an open wound
    b. Treat large areas with one of the following:
      i. Cluster probe
      ii. Grid application, treating 1 cm^2 areas consecutively
      iii. Scanning technique, criss-crossing the wound area
B. Dosage
  1. Tables 19.4 and 19.5 provide approximate dosages for various musculoskeletal conditions.
  2. Consult the manual for more recommendations on dosages.
C. Length of application. Treatment time is calculated from:
  1. Desired dosage
  2. Average power output
  3. Area to be treated
D. Frequency of application: Daily
E. Duration of therapy: As long a discernible progress is being made.

4 STEP 4: **POSTAPPLICATION TASKS**

A. Equipment removal; patient cleanup
B. Instructions to the patient. These should be written if they are extensive or complicated.
 1. Schedule the next treatment.
 2. Instruct the patient about the level of activity and/or self-treatment before the next formal treatment.
 3. Instruct the patient about what she should feel after treatment.

C. Record of treatment, including unique patient responses
D. Equipment replacement; area cleanup

5 STEP 5: **MAINTENANCE**

A. Regular equipment cleaning. Clean the laser head with a disinfectant if it was applied directly to the skin.
B. Routine maintenance
C. Simple repairs

Ultraviolet Radiation

Ultraviolet modalities were once part of athletic training clinics, but this no longer the case. It now is generally applied by dermatologists. This brief section is intended to inform you of the effects so you understand the treatment given when one of your patients sees a dermatologist.

Ultraviolet (UV) radiation is a portion of the electromagnetic spectrum that produces chemical reactions in microorganisms and in the epidermis and dermis. Its effects are superficial and mainly chemical, and it is used therapeutically to destroy superficial infectious organisms and other microorganisms.

UV radiation is easy to misuse. Incorrect application can lead to numerous dermatitis conditions, such as local ulceration, impetigo, folliculitis, and herpes simplex. Overexposure can lead to increased sensitivity to ordinary sunlight. It can also lead to cancer.

Caution must be exercised when treating patients with generalized dermatitis (eczema, psoriasis, herpes simplex, etc.), freckles atrophy, keratoses, or prematurely senile skin; diabetes, or hyperthyroidism and those who are highly nervous.

CLOSING SCENE

Alex now understands how lasers are used by a variety of people for a variety of reasons and that, although they are similar in principle, lasers differ in the type of lasing medium they use to produce their beam and in the wavelength and power of their output. He understands that the laser a surgeon uses to burn tissue generates more power than the one an athletic trainer uses to stimulate tissue healing. Alex also knows that although light therapy appears to be powerful therapy for some conditions, it is no more than a placebo for others. He is eager to follow the future writings of scientists and master clinicians as they more fully determine when it is most appropriate to use lasers.

CHAPTER REFLECTIONS

1. Read and ponder each of the following points. Do you feel you have a clear understanding of each concept? If not, reread the appropriate section of the chapter.
 • Define *laser*.
 • Describe how a laser beam is generated.
 • Define each of the following terms as they relate to lasers: light, amplify, stimulate, emission, radiation, electromagnetic energy, frequency, visible light, nondivergent, monochromatic, coherent, fixed phase, lasing medium, half-slivered mirror, and photon.
 • Explain what is meant by this statement: Lasers are not a single device but rather a variety of devices.

- Describe how lasers are classified, and name some of the levels within the classification.
- Explain how laser safety is determined.
- Explain the roles of wavelength, color, and energy level in the body's response to laser therapy.
- Explain the difference between laser therapy and light therapy using an LED or SLD. What are the implication of this difference?
- Explain the differences between the lasers used by surgeons and athletic trainers.
- Describe what happens at the molecular level when lasers are applied to the tissue.
- What is photobiomodulation, and what role does it play in laser therapy?
- Differentiate between in vitro and in vivo research, and relate these concepts to laser therapy.
- What does light therapy mean, and how is it related to laser therapy?
- What are the primary indications for laser therapy?
- Define the three primary delivery techniques used to apply laser therapy.
- Explain how dosage is determined for treating orthopedic injuries with laser therapy.

- Discuss the depth of penetration of lasers in human tissue, and explain the implications this has on laser therapy.
2. Write three to five questions for discussion with your class instructor, clinical instructor, classmates, and clinical colleagues.
3. Get together with classmates and quiz each other on the concepts of this chapter. Use the points in exercise 1 and questions you wrote for exercise 2 as a beginning. Explaining concepts out loud to others requires a deeper grasp of the material than feeling you understand it as you read.
4. Once you feel you understand the principles of application of light therapy, practice applying them using the five-step approach with a classmate or clinical colleague. Alternate applying the modalities to each other. When it is being applied to you, listen and observe carefully to determine whether your classmate is using proper application. Consult your notes when the modality is applied to you and for the first few times you apply the modality to another person. Continue practicing the application until you can do so without using your notes.

CRITICAL THINKING RESPONSE

Critical Thinking 19.1

Diathermy and laser therapy are alike because both are electromagnetic and the photon is the basic unit of both modalities. Differences include diathermy generates heat, laser does not; diathermy penetrates deep, laser is only superficial; laser waves are visual, diathermy waves are not.

REFERENCES

1. Enwemeka CS. Low level laser therapy is not low. Photomed Laser Surg 2005;23:529–530.
2. Smith KC. Laser (and LED) therapy is phototherapy. Photomed Laser Surg 2005;23:78–80.
3. Vladimirov YA, Osipov AN, Klebanov GI. Photobiological principles of therapeutic application of laser radiation. Biochemistry (Moscow) 2004;69:81–90.
4. Quimby RS. Photonics and Lasers. Hoboken, NJ: Wiley, 2006.
5. Baxter GD. Therapeutic Lasers: Theory and Practice. Edinburgh, UK: Churchill Livingstone, 1994.
6. Harris T. How Light Emitting Diodes Work. Available at: www.electronics.howstuffworks.com/led1.htm. Accessed July 2006.
7. Enwemeka CS. Light is light. Photomed Laser Surg 2005;23: 159–160.
8. Berlien H-P, Müller GJ, eds. Applied Laser Medicine. New York: Springer, 2005.
9. Müeller G (ed). Laser applications in medicine, biology, and environmental science. Proceedings of the International Conference on Lasers, Applications, and Technologies, Moscow, Russia, 2002.
10. McLeod IA. Low-level laser therapy in athletic training. Athl Ther Today 2004;9:17–21.
11. Karu TI. Molecular mechanism of the therapeutic effect of low intensity laser irradiation. Lasers Life Sci 1988;2:53–74.
12. Karu T, Pyatibrat L, Kalendo G. Irradiation with He-Ne laser increases ATP level in cells cultivated in vitro. J Photochem Photobiol B 1995;27:219–223.
13. Abergel RP, Meeker CA, Lam TS, et al. Control of connective tissue metabolism by lasers: Recent developments and future prospects. J Am Acad Dermatol 1984;11:1142–1150.
14. Boulton M, Marshall J. He-Ne laser stimulation of human fibroblast proliferation and attachment in vitro. Lasers Life Sci 1986;1:125–134.
15. Poon VK, Huang L, Burd A. Biostimulation of dermal fibroblast by sublethal Q-switched Nd:YAG 532nm laser: Collagen remodeling and pigmentation. J Photochem Photobiol B 2005;81:1–8.
16. Pourzarandian A, Watanabe H, Ruwanpura SM, et al. Effect of low level Er:YAG laser irradiation on cultured human gingival fibroblasts. J Periodontol 2005;76:187–193.
17. Lyons RF, Abergel RP, White RA. Biostimulation of wound healing in vivo by helium neon laser. Ann Plastic Surg 1987;18:47–50.

18. Pourreau-Schnieder N, Ahmed A, Soudry M, et al. Helium-neon laser treatment transforms fibroblasts into myofibroblasts. Am J Pathol 1990;137:171–178.

19. Colver GB, Priestly GC. Failure of HeNe to affect components of wound healing in vitro. Br J Dermatol 1989;121:179–186.

20. Hallman HO, Basford JR, O'Brien JF. Does low energy HeNe laser irradiation alter in vitro replication of human fibroblasts? Lasers Surg Med 1988;8:125–129.

21. Stadler I, Evans R, Kolb B, et al. In vitro effects of low-level laser irradiation at 660 nm on peripheral blood lymphocytes. Lasers Surg Med 2000;27:255–261.

22. Mester E, Mester A, Mester A. The biomedical effects of laser application. Lasers Surg Med 1985;5:31–39.

23. Young S, Bolton P, Dyson M, et al. Macrophage responsiveness to light therapy. Lasers Surg Med 1989;9:497–505.

24. Inoue K, Nishioka J, Hukuda S. Altered lymphocyte proliferation by low dosage laser irradiation. Clin Exp Rheumatol 1989;7:521–523.

25. Ohta A, Abergel RP, Vitto J. Laser modulation of human immune system: Inhibition of lymphocyte proliferation by gallium-arsenide laser at low energy. Lasers Surg Med 1987;7:199–201.

26. Hopkins JT, McLoda TA, Seegmiller. Low-level laser therapy facilitates superficial wound healing. J Athl Train 2004;39:223–229.

27. Chromey PA. The efficacy of carbon dioxide laser surgery for adjunct ulcer therapy. Clin Podiat Med Surg 1992;9:709–719.

28. Gogia PP, Hurt BS, Zirn TT. Wound management with whirlpool and infrared cold laser treatment. A clinical report. Phys Ther 1988;68: 1239–1242.

29. Schindl A, Schindl M, Schindl L. Successful treatment of a persistent radiation ulcer by low power laser therapy. J Am Acad Dermatol 1997;37:646–648.

30. Gigo-Benato D, Geuna S, Rochkind S. Phototherapy for enhancing peripheral nerve repair: A review of the literature. Muscle Nerve 2005;31:694–701.

31. Dyson M, Young S. Effect of laser therapy on wound contraction and cellularity in mice. Lasers Med Sci 1986;1:126–130.

32. Allendorf JD, Bessler M, Huang J, et al. Helium-neon laser irradiation at fluences of 1, 2, and 4 J/cm^2 failed to accelerate wound healing as assessed by wound contracture rate and tensile strength. Lasers Surg Med 1997;20:340–345.

33. Hunter J, Leonard L, Wilson R, et al. Effects of low energy laser on wound healing in a porcine model. Lasers Surg Med 1984;3:285-290.

34. Lundberg T, Malm M. Low-power HeNe laser treatment of venous leg ulcers. Ann Plastic Surg 1991;27:537–539.

35. Chow RT, Barnsley L. Systematic review of the literature of low-level laser therapy (LLLT) in the management of neck pain. Lasers Surg Med 2005;37:46–52.

36. Enwemeka CS, Parker JC, Dowdy DS, et al. The efficacy of low-power lasers in tissue repair and pain control: A metanalysis. Photomed Laser Surg 2004;22:323–329.

37. Beckerman H, de Bie RA, Bouter LM, et al. The efficacy of laser therapy for musculoskeletal and skin disorders: A criteria-based meta-analysis of randomized clinical trials. Phys Ther 1992;72:483–491.

38. de Bie RA, de Vet HCW, Lenssen TF, et al. Low-level laser therapy in ankle sprains: A randomized clinical trial. Arch Phys Med Rehabil 1998;79:1415–1420.

39. Gam AN, Thorson H, Lonnberg F. The effect of low-level laser therapy on musculoskeletal pain: A meta analysis. Pain 1993;52: 63–66.

40. Simunovic Z. Low level laser therapy with trigger points technique: A clinical study on 243 patients. J Clin Laser Med Surg 1996;14: 163–167.

41. Simunovic Z, Trobonjaca T, Trobonjaca Z. Treatment of medial and lateral epicondylitis—tennis and golfer's elbow—with low level laser therapy: A multicenter double blind, placebo-controlled clinical study on 324 patients. J Clin Laser Med Surg 1998;16:145–151.

42. Brosseau L, Welch V, Wells G, et al. Low level laser therapy for osteoarthritis and rheumatoid arthritis: A metaanalysis. J Rheumatol 2000;27:1961–1969.

43. Naeser MA, Hahn KK, Lieberman BE, Branco KF. Carpal tunnel syndrome pain treated with low-level laser and microamperes transcutaneous electric nerve stimulation: A controlled study. Arch Phys Med Rehabil 2002;83:978–988.

44. Basford JR, Sheffield CG, Harmsen WS. Laser therapy: A randomized, controlled trial of the effects of low-intensity Nd:YAG laser irradiation on musculoskeletal back pain. Arch Phys Med Rehabil 1999;80: 647–652.

45. Basford JR, Malanga GA, Krause DA, Harmsen WS. A randomized controlled evaluation of low intensity laser therapy: Plantar fascitis. Arch Phys Med Rehabil 1998;79:249–254.

46. Craig JA, Barlas P, Baxter GD, et al. Delayed-onset muscle soreness: Lack of effect of combined phototherapy/low-intensity laser therapy at low pulse repetition rates. J Clin Laser Med Surg 1996;14: 375–380.

47. Gür A, Karakoc M, Nas K, et al. Efficacy of low power laser therapy in fibromyalgia: A single-blind, placebo-controlled trial. Lasers Med Sci 2002;17:57–61.

48. Snyder-Mackler L, Bork CE. Effect of helium-neon laser irradiation on peripheral sensory nerve latency. Phys Ther 1988;68: 223–225.

49. Vinck E, Coorevits P, Cagnie B, et al. Evidence of changes in sural nerve conduction mediated by light emitting diode irradiation. Lasers Med Sci 2005;20:35–40.

50. Basford JR, Daude JR, Hallman HO. Does low intensity helium-neon laser irradiation alter sensory nerve action potentials or distal latencies? Laser Surg Med 1990;10:35–39.

51. Ferreira DM, Zangaro RA, Villaverde AB, et al. Analgesic effect of He-Ne (632.8 nm) low-level laser therapy on acute inflammatory pain. Photomed Laser Surg 2005;23:177–181.

Review Questions

Chapter 17

1. Which massage technique is also known as kneading?
   a. tapotement
   b. vibration
   c. pétrissage
   d. Rolfing
   e. effleurage

2. Which of the following is *not* a physiological effect of massage?
   a. wringing out lactic acid
   b. decreasing pain
   c. increasing flexibility
   d. stimulating circulation
   e. facilitating healing

3. Which of the following is a contraindication for massage?
   a. postacute edema
   b. pain
   c. muscle spasm
   d. embolism
   e. sore muscles

4. Which of the following is *not* a reflexive effect of massage?
   a. decreased pain
   b. elongated fascia
   c. increased circulation
   d. increased metabolism
   e. relaxation

5. Which massage stroke is used to stimulate the muscles for competition?
   a. pétrissage
   b. friction
   c. effleurage
   d. percussion
   e. tapotement

6. Which type of massage technique is used to break up adhesions?
   a. pétrissage
   b. friction
   c. effleurage
   d. tapotement
   e. raindrops

7. Which of the following is *not* a contraindication for massage?
   a. fractures
   b. arteriosclerosis
   c. pain of no known origin
   d. acute edema
   e. none of the above

8. Which massage technique is used to relieve soft tissue from the abnormal grip of surrounding tissue?
   a. pétrissage
   b. friction massage
   c. Hoffa technique
   d. myofascial release
   e. deep effleurage

Chapter 18

1. Which of the following is *not* a treatment parameter for traction?
   a. patient position
   b. treatment mode
   c. traction force
   d. device needed
   e. frequency

2. Which of the following refers to whether or not the traction is sustained or intermittent?
   a. patient position
   b. treatment mode
   c. traction force
   d. device needed
   e. frequency

3. In general, what percentage of the patient's weight should be applied when performing lumbar traction?
   a. 30
   b. 40
   c. 50
   d. 60
   e. 70

4. In general, no more than how many pounds of force should be applied when performing cervical traction?
   a. 25
   b. 35
   c. 45
   d. 55
   e. one quarter of the body weight

5. Which of the following requires a special split table to apply traction?
   a. manual traction
   b. autotraction
   c. single-leg manual traction
   d. pneumatic mechanical traction
   e. inversion table traction

6. Which of the following is contraindicated by someone with glaucoma?
   a. manual traction
   b. autotraction
   c. single-leg manual traction
   d. pneumatic mechanical traction
   e. inversion table traction

7. Which of the following is a contraindication for traction?
   a. adhesions
   b. apophyseal joint impingement
   c. muscle spasm
   d. radiating pain that does not improve with trunk movement
   e. acute neck pain

8. Which of the following is not a way in which traction appears to relieve pain?
   a. widening the intervertebral foramen
   b. creating suction to draw protruded disks toward their center
   c. relaxing muscles
   d. decreasing space between vertebrae
   e. two of the above

9. Benefits of the inversion table traction device include _____.
   a. it can be purchased at a wholesale outlet store for about $200.00
   b. it is easy to use
   c. there are no belts to slip, thus constant traction is applied the whole time
   d. the patient can control the level (in degrees) of traction desired
   e. all of the above

Chapter 19

1. Light therapy is a form of _____.
   a. electromagnetic energy
   b. mechanical energy
   c. superficial heat
   d. deep heat
   e. none of the above

2. Which of the following is not a characteristic of laser?
   a. monophasic
   b. monochromatic
   c. radiant
   d. coherent
   e. divergent

3. Lasers are commonly classified according to _____.
   a. the type of lasing medium they use
   b. their safety
   c. the intensity of their color
   d. both a and b
   e. both b and c

4. The safety of a laser is primarily a function of its _____.
   a. color
   b. divergence
   c. energy
   d. lasing medium
   e. coherence

5. The difference between a surgical laser and a therapeutic laser is primarily owing to its _____.
   a. color
   b. divergence
   c. energy
   d. lasing medium
   e. coherence

revolve around carefully limiting the choices to accomplish a goal, assessing the outcome of a modality, and then possibly adding an additional modality to address the other symptoms the modality did not relieve.

The approach taken may be more effective if the patient is involved in the process. For example, if a patient recently read an article in a magazine about the benefits of icing for pain reduction, he might respond better to ice treatments than electrical stimulation. Or if a patient saw an advertisement on television about the benefits of portable, long-lasting heat, she might use the product at home as an adjunct to heat used in the clinic.

EVIDENCE SUPPORTING THE MODALITY

Before you employ any modality, ask yourself: Is there evidence to support the use of this modality in this situation? Perhaps the most important consideration is whether a modality actually does what the product brochure says. If there is little or no evidence to support the use of the modality, don't waste your time and the patient's money in a purely placebo treatment. Familiarize yourself with the research regarding the modalities you use the most. Also, if there is ample support for the use of a particular modality, consider sharing these positive research results with the patient. This may lead not only to improved treatment outcomes but also to better patient compliance.

PATIENT COMPLIANCE

Patient compliance means following the treatment orders or instructions given by the clinician. **Patient noncompliance** is the failure to fully follow the treatment orders or instructions given by the clinician, including home treatment and returning for clinic treatments. Many factors are involved in whether a patient will comply with your treatment orders. Compliance on the part of the patient's family or spouse is important, too. Your patients will never reach 90–100% of their preinjury status if they are not supportive of what you are trying to accomplish.

An example of noncompliance to a home treatment is a junior high school basketball player who suffered an acute ankle sprain in Friday's game. The athletic trainer prescribed rest, ice, compression, elevation, stabilization (RICES) over the weekend. Unfortunately, the athlete found the cold treatment to be uncomfortable. His parents gave in to his complaints and allowed him to omit the ice treatments. In this way, noncompliant parents supported a noncompliant patient. The result was that the athlete returned to school on Monday with an ankle that was still swollen and painful.

Poor treatment in the clinic often results in noncompliance—the patient fails to return for follow-up treatments. If the clinician doesn't seem to take much of an interest in the

patient or if the treatments are painful, the patient might not return as often as possible to obtain optimal results. For example, when one of us (DD) was running cross-country at a junior college, he had knee surgery that required his left leg to be in a straight-leg cast for 4 weeks. The week the cast was removed, he reported to physical therapy. The therapist noted very little range of motion (ROM) in knee flexion and attempted to restore it in one treatment. The therapist had the patient lie down on the table and said, "Now this is going to hurt." She then grabbed the leg and tried to flex it as far as possible in one quick motion. He cried out in pain as he slid forward on the table. He never returned to that physical therapist or clinic. Patient compliance could have been achieved if the therapist provided some form of heat therapy to the patient's knee and then performed graded joint mobilizations.

CLINICIAN COMPLIANCE

Another component of therapeutic intervention leading to patient compliance or noncompliance is **clinician compliance**—the reliability, knowledge, confidence, and professionalism of the clinician. If the clinician approaches the patient with an unsure attitude such as, "Well, I'm not sure if this piece of equipment will help, but let's give it a try," the patient loses faith in the clinician. Also, if several modalities are used in a shotgun manner, the patient might question whether the clinician knows what he is doing. A patient who is made to feel like a guinea pig will often refuse to return for follow-up treatment.

Another reason for noncompliance in returning for treatment is improper use of modalities. If the treatment protocol doesn't make sense to the patient (and isn't helping the condition improve), the patient may not return for follow-up treatments. For example, a 14-year-old girl was diagnosed with temporomandibular joint (TMJ) syndrome. The physician prescribed a heat-and-stretch routine for the jaw and referred her to a nearby clinic. Ultrasound was correctly applied with the proper protocol to heat the tissues (3 MHz; continuous; 1 W/cm^2; 5–6 min). Unfortunately, the therapist did not begin to stretch the mandible until 30 min after the ultrasound treatment. By that time, the tissue was cooled, and the modality had little effect on the stretching. After two additional similar sessions, the parents took the girl out of therapy. The therapist either did not understand the role of the ultrasound treatment in preparing the tissues for the stretching or was too complacent to care.

It is imperative that clinicians have a firm knowledge of therapeutic modalities. Those who understand the modalities tend to use them to the patient's benefit. On the other hand, clinicians whose only modality is their hands probably do not understand how these valuable tools can prepare tissues for the therapist's hands.

CLOSING SCENE

Recall from the chapter opening scene that you were seeing Andrew, who sprained his ankle; because he thought it was a minor injury, he did nothing to care for it. A week later it is swollen and painful when he walks. Your clinical instructor asks you what your first goals are. Then she asks you how you plan to accomplish these goals and what therapeutic modality should you use. Differential application of modalities refers to the process of determining the optimal modality to use under specific circumstances. You decide that your first goal should be to remove swelling and restore pain-free range of motion. You employ a lymphedema pump and elevation twice a day to help remove the edema. When the athlete is not in the pump, he wears a compression sock on the ankle.

CHAPTER REFLECTIONS

1. Read and ponder each of the following points. Do you feel you have a clear understanding of each concept? If not, reread the appropriate section of the chapter.
   - What is meant by differential application of therapeutic modalities? How does this concept differ from the way modalities have been taught in this book? How is it more like real life than the approach taken in the previous chapters of this book?
   - Describe several situations in which you would use certain modalities in different phases of injury.
   - List several treatment goals and what modalities would be appropriate to use to reach those goals.
   - Provide several examples of patient compliance.
   - Provide several examples of patient noncompliance.
   - Provide several examples of clinician compliance.
   - Provide several examples of clinician noncompliance.

2. Write three to five questions for discussion with your class instructor, clinical instructor, classmates, and clinical colleagues.

3. Get together with classmates and quiz each other on the concepts of this chapter. Use the points in exercise 1 and questions you wrote for exercise 2 as a beginning. Explaining concepts out loud to others requires a deeper grasp of the material than feeling you understand it as you read.

CRITICAL THINKING RESPONSE

Critical Thinking 20.1

The following are factors that could hinder you from properly using the differential application process in choosing therapeutic modalities:

- Inadequate understanding of the anatomy, pathophysiology, and mechanism of specific injuries. Each of these elements is necessary to make a correct diagnosis. And without a correct diagnosis, you cannot develop a proper treatment plan.

- Inadequate understanding of the indications, contraindications, and limitations of each modality. Constant reading of the latest research, including randomized clinical trials, is a prerequisite to properly selecting and using therapeutic modalities.

- Limited availability of a specific therapeutic modality. Knowing that a specific modality is the best modality for the job is of no value if you don't have access to the modality.

REFERENCES

1. Behrens BJ, Michlovitz SL. Physical Agents: Theory and Practice for the Physical Therapist Assistant. Philadelphia: Davis, 1996.

2. Draper DO, Harris ST, Schulthies SS, et al. Hotpack and 1 MHz ultrasound treatments have an additive effect on muscle temperature increase. J Athl Train 1998;33:21–24.

Case Studies Using Therapeutic Modalities

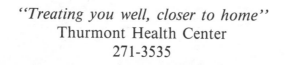

"Treating you well, closer to home"
Thurmont Health Center
271-3535

Clinical Case Studies

The case studies in this chapter will help you apply the differential application principles introduced in Chapter 20. In these case studies, we present a brief history (Hx) and diagnosis (Dx) as they would come to you on a referral slip. (Table 21.1 provides definitions for common abbreviations physicians use on therapy referral slips.) Based on this information, decide what therapeutic modality would be best suited in each situation and why you feel it is best. As you read each case, keep in mind the pathology, the effects of each physical agent, and the precautions that must be addressed. Our opinions about the preferred modality are presented later in the chapter.

If there are differences between your opinions and ours, try to determine why by doing the following:

- Refer to the chapter(s) in which the modalities are presented.
- Discuss the differences with fellow students, your professor, and a clinical instructor.

CASE STUDY 1: LUMBOSACRAL PAIN

Referral	
Hx:	22 y/o overweight offensive lineman, c/o diffuse LBP x 2 week. Pain is nonradiating and increases c̄ strenuous lifting
Dx:	Lumbosacral muscle spasm c̄ 1° strain of quadratus lumborum

CASE STUDY 2: PIRIFORMIS SYNDROME

Referral	
Hx:	20 y/o ♀ volleyball player c/o (L) buttocks and LBP, x 6 week
Dx:	Piriformis syndrome c̄ sciatica

CASE STUDY 3: CHRONIC SUPRASPINATUS TENDINITIS

Referral	
Hx:	44 y/o ♂ painter, c/o pain in R shoulder, and limited shoulder ROM owing to pain
Dx:	Chronic supraspinatus tendinitis

CASE STUDY 4: HYPOMOBILE RADIAL CARPAL JOINT

Referral	
Hx:	22 y/o ♂ soccer goalie, x 3 month p/o bone graft for avascular necrosis of the (L) scaphoid
Dx:	Hypomobile radial carpal joint in all motions owing to prolonged cast immmobilization

TABLE 21.1 *Abbreviations Commonly Used on Referrals*

ABBREVIATION	DEFINITION	ABBREVIATION	DEFINITION
AA	active assistive	MMT	manual muscle test
Bil	bilateral	NN	nerve
c̄	with	OA	osteoarthritis
c̄/o	complains of	p	post
Dx	diagnosis	p/o	postoperation
ER	emergency room	pt	patient
EXER	exercise	RA	rheumatoid arthritis
F or ♀	female	ROM	range of motion
fx	fracture	RUE	right upper extremity
Hx	history	Rx	prescription
LBP	low-back pain	s	without
LLE	left lower extremity	s/p fx	status postfracture
L-S	lumbosacral	Tx	treatment
M or ♂	male	x 6 mo	for 6 months (or 6 months' duration)
MM	muscle	y/o	year old

CASE STUDY 5: FIRST-DEGREE INVERSION ANKLE SPRAIN

Referral	
Hx:	16 y/o ♀ basketball player c/o pain on R lateral ankle, c̄ swelling 24 hr postinjury
Dx:	1° inversion sprain of R ankle

CASE STUDY 6: CARPAL TUNNEL SYNDROME

Referral	
Hx:	37 y/o R-handed ♀, employed as a computer operator, c/o tingling and numbness in R hand c̄ loss of ROM and grip strength
Dx:	Early stages of carpal tunnel syndrome in R hand

CASE STUDY 7: ACHILLES TENDINITIS

Referral	
Hx:	30 y/o ♂ marathon runner, c/o chronic pain in area of (L) Achilles tendon
Dx:	Achilles tendinitis

CASE STUDY 8: MILD SPASM OF R/L UPPER TRAPEZIUS

Referral	
Hx:	40 y/o ♂ c/o pain in the cervical region, c̄ muscle spasms. X-rays ruled out fx
Dx:	1° spasm of R/L upper trapezius

CASE STUDY 9: SECOND-DEGREE QUADRICEPS STRAIN

Referral	
Hx:	20 y/o ♂ soccer player c/o pain on L mid-portion of quadriceps, c̄ swelling 30 min postinjury
Dx:	2° strain to the L quadriceps

CASE STUDY 10: PATELLAR TENDINITIS

Referral	
Hx:	20 y/o ♂ collegiate miler, c/o chronic pain in area of (R) patellar tendon
Dx:	Patellar tendinitis

CASE STUDY 11: LATERAL EPICONDYLITIS

Referral	
Hx:	18 y/o ♀ tennis player, c/o chronic pain in area of (R) elbow
Dx:	Lateral epicondylitis

CASE STUDY 12: ACROMIOCLAVICULAR (AC) SEPARATION

Referral	
Hx:	21 y/o ♀ rugby player c/o pain on R AC joint, c̄ swelling 2 hr postinjury. No visible or palpable step-off deformity
Dx:	1° AC sprain of R shoulder

CASE STUDY 13: HAMSTRING CONTUSION

Referral	
Hx:	20 y/o ♂ soccer player c/o pain on L midportion of hamstring, c̄ swelling 30 min postinjury
Dx:	Moderate contusion to the L hamstring

Possible Treatment Regimens

Following are possible treatment regimens for the case studies presented in this chapter. Compare your suggestions with the ones we provide. Are there differences? If so, does that mean that you (or we) are wrong? Not necessarily. Discuss these cases with classmates, clinical instructors, or your professor. If differences exist, try to determine why.

CASE STUDY 1: LUMBOSACRAL PAIN

This injury is chronic. The goal is to decrease muscle spasm and increase circulation to assist healing. Possible modalities to decrease muscle spasm:

- Interferential current: Use a rapidly moving sweep or dynamic vector; intensity adjusted to contraction level to fatigue the muscle spasm. This large treatment area can easily be bracketed with four electrodes.
- Pulsed shortwave diathermy: Deep heat may help relax the muscle spasm, plus this modality will cover a large area.
- Massage: Especially pétrissage; the kneading will help reduce the spasm.
- Traction: Lumbar traction may help decrease the spasm.

A possible modality to increase temperature and blood flow and assist with healing is pulsed shortwave diathermy, which provides deep heat to a large area. If you don't have access to PSWD, try one of the following:

- Warm whirlpool: Superficial heat, yet the warm water will surround the entire area.
- Hot packs: Superficial heat, yet a large pack will cover the entire area.

CASE STUDY 2: PIRIFORMIS SYNDROME

This injury is chronic. The goal is to decrease muscle spasm and pain and to increase hip internal rotation by stretching the piriformis. Possible modalities to decrease muscle spasm and pain:

- NMES: Setting of 5–10 sec on, 5–10 sec off; intensity adjusted to contraction level to fatigue the muscle spasm.
- TENS: Setting of 5–10 sec on, 5–10 sec off; intensity adjusted to contraction level to fatigue the muscle spasm
- Massage: Especially pétrissage; the kneading will help reduce the spasm.

Possible modalities to heat the area before stretch include pulsed shortwave diathermy, which provides deep heat to a large area. If you don't have access to PSWD, try one of the following:

- Warm whirlpool: Superficial heat, yet the warm water will surround the entire area.
- Hot packs: Superficial heat, yet a large pack will cover the entire area.

CASE STUDY 3: CHRONIC SUPRASPINATUS TENDINITIS

This injury is chronic. The goal is to decrease muscle spasm and pain. Possible modalities to decrease muscle spasm and pain:

- NMES: For muscle spasm, use a setting of 5–10 sec on, 5–10 sec off; intensity adjusted to contraction level to fatigue the muscle spasm. For pain, use a continuous setting with intensity adjusted to sensory level for stimulation of large myelinated nerve fibers. This large treatment area can easily be bracketed with four electrodes.
- TENS: For muscle spasm, use a setting of 5–10 sec on, 5–10 sec off; intensity adjusted to contraction level to fatigue the muscle spasm. For pain, use a continuous setting with intensity adjusted to sensory level for stimulation of large myelinated nerve fibers.
- Pulsed shortwave diathermy: Provides deep heat to a large area, which may help relax the muscle and reduce the spasm.

- Massage: Especially pétrissage; the kneading will help reduce the spasm.
- Hot packs: Superficial heat, yet a large pack will cover the entire area.

CASE STUDY 4: HYPOMOBILE RADIAL CARPAL JOINT

The goal is to increase ROM of the radial carpal joint. A heat and stretching regimen and heating the area before joint mobilizations are the best options. To heat the tissues before stretching or joint mobilization:

- Ultrasound, 3 MHz: Continuous setting to patient tolerance; the wrist structures are superficial, which is in the heating range for 3 MHz ultrasound.
- Paraffin: Superficial heat that will form a glove surrounding the treatment area.
- Hot pack: Superficial heat, applied to the dorsal aspect of the hand to focus on the scaphoid.
- Whirlpool: Superficial heat, yet the warm water will surround the entire area.

CASE STUDY 5: FIRST-DEGREE INVERSION ANKLE SPRAIN

The goal is for immediate care, reduce pain, and prevent secondary metabolic injury. Then decrease the swelling and increase function during transition care. To prevent secondary metabolic injury and reduce pain, use RICES for 30 min. Reevaluate the injury. If the diagnosis is still a first-degree sprain, begin transition care. If the injury seems more severe, continue RICES until the next day.

To decrease swelling and increase function, use cryokinetics to gain an increase in function as per patient progress.

To decrease swelling during transition care:

- Cryokinetics: Preferred treatment
- NMES: For muscle pumping to get rid of edema, use a setting of 5–10 sec on, 5–10 sec off; intensity adjusted to contraction level.
- Sequential lymphedema pump: This will assist with lymphatic drainage, but is not as effective as cryokinetics.

CASE STUDY 6: CARPAL TUNNEL SYNDROME

The goal is to reduce pain and inflammation on the median nerve. Possible modalities:

- Ice pack: When applied to the ventral and dorsal aspects of the wrist, it will cover the entire treatment target.
- Ice water immersion: This will cover the entire treatment target and allow for active ROM exercises.
- Cold whirlpool: This will cover the entire treatment target and allow for active ROM exercises).

CASE STUDY 7: ACHILLES TENDINITIS

The goal is to break up scar tissue and stretch the triceps surae. A heat-and-stretch regimen, to break up adhesions, is best here. To heat the tissues before joint movement:

- Ultrasound 3 MHz: Use a continuous setting to patient tolerance. The Achilles tendon is superficial, which is in the heating range for 3 MHz ultrasound.
- Paraffin: Superficial heat that will form a glove surrounding the treatment area.
- Warm whirlpool: Superficial heat, yet the warm water will surround the entire area.
- Hot packs: Superficial heat, yet a large pack will cover the entire area.

To break up adhesions, use cross-friction massage. Going perpendicular to the fibers will aid in breaking up scar tissue.

CASE STUDY 8: MILD SPASM OF R/L UPPER TRAPEZIUS

The goal is to reduce muscle spasm. Appropriate modalities:

- Cryostretch: After several minutes of cold application, the area will become numb, thus reducing the pain and muscle spasm.
- Cervical traction: Gentle distraction will take pressure off of nerves and help reduce muscle spasm.
- TENS: This small treatment area is easily targeted with TENS. For muscle spasm, use a setting of 5–10 sec on, 5–10 sec off; intensity adjusted to contraction level to fatigue the muscle spasm. For pain, use a continuous setting with intensity adjusted to a sensory level for stimulation of large myelinated nerve fibers.
- Interferential current: This small treatment area can easily be bracketed with four electrodes. For muscle spasm, use a rapidly moving sweep or dynamic vector; intensity adjusted to contraction level to fatigue the muscle spasm. For pain, use a continuous setting with intensity adjusted to sensory level for stimulation of large myelinated nerve fibers.

CASE STUDY 9: SECOND-DEGREE QUADRICEPS STRAIN

The goal is to reduce pain and swelling and prevent further secondary metabolic injury. Then transition into functional activity. Use RICES for 30 min. The treatment is repeated every 2 hr. Keep a compression wrap on and the limb elevated during and between ice pack applications.

To increase function during transition care:

- Cryostretch: Cold applications and stretching will break the muscle spasm.
- Cryokinetics: Transition into after muscle spasm is reduced.

In addition:

- NMES: For muscle pumping to get rid of edema, use a Setting of 5–10 sec on, 5–10 sec off; intensity adjusted to contraction level.
- Sequential lymphedema pump: This will assist with lymphatic drainage, but is not as effective as cryostretch and cryokinetics.

CASE STUDY 10: PATELLAR TENDINITIS

The goal is to break up adhesions associated with the tendinitis and increase pain-free ROM. A heat-and-stretch regimen and heating the tissues before breaking up adhesions are good options. To heat the tissues before joint movement:

- Ultrasound, 3 MHz: Use a continuous setting to patient tolerance. The patellar tendon is superficial, which is in the heating range for 3 MHz ultrasound.
- Warm whirlpool: Superficial heat, yet the warm water will surround the entire area.
- Hot pack: Superficial heat, and a small pack will cover the entire area.

To break up adhesions, use cross-friction massage. Going perpendicular to the fibers will aid in breaking up scar tissue.

CASE STUDY 11: LATERAL EPICONDYLITIS

The goal is to break up adhesions associated with the epicondylitis and increase pain-free ROM. A heat-and-stretch regimen and heating the area before breaking up adhesions are good options. To heat the tissues before joint movement:

- Ultrasound, 3 MHz: Use a continuous setting to patient tolerance. The attachment of the wrist extensors on the lateral epicondyle are superficial, which is in the heating range for 3 MHz ultrasound.
- Warm whirlpool: Superficial heat, yet the warm water will surround the entire area.
- Hot pack: Superficial heat and a small pack will cover the entire area.

To break up adhesions, use cross-friction massage. Going perpendicular to the fibers will aid in breaking up scar tissue.

CASE STUDY 12: ACROMIOCLAVICULAR (AC) SEPARATION

The goal is immediate care, reduce pain, and prevent secondary hypoxic injury. Then decrease swelling in the area during transition care. To prevent secondary hypoxic injury and reduce pain:

- RICES (30 min): Treatment repeated every 2 hr. Keep a compression wrap on and the limb elevated during and between ice pack applications.
- TENS: This small treatment area is easily targeted with TENS. Use a continuous setting with intensity adjusted to sensory level for stimulation of large myelinated nerve fibers.

To decrease swelling in the area during transition care, use cryokinetics or NMES. For muscle pumping to get rid of edema, use a setting of 5–10 sec on, 5–10 sec off; intensity adjusted to contraction level.

CASE STUDY 13: HAMSTRING CONTUSION

The goal is immediate care, reduce pain, and minimize secondary metabolic injury. Then decrease swelling in the area during transition care. To minimize secondary hypoxic injury and reduce pain, use RICES for 30 min. The treatment is repeated every 2 hr. Keep a compression wrap on and the limb elevated during and between ice pack applications.

To decrease swelling in the area during transition care:

- Cryokinetics
- NMES: For muscle pumping to get rid of edema, use a setting of 5–10 sec on, 5–10 sec off; intensity adjusted to contraction level.
- Sequential lymphedema pump: This will assist with lymphatic drainage, but is not as effective as cryokinetics.

Review Questions

Chapter 20

1. The process of determining the optimal modality to use under certain circumstances is referred to as _____.
   a. indication
   b. contraindication
   c. differential application
   d. compliance
   e. noncompliance

2. A patient follows the treatment orders given by the therapist is an example of _____.
   a. indication
   b. contraindication
   c. noncompliance
   d. compliance
   e. differential application

3. Which of the following would be the *best* modality to use to heat a large joint (such as the knee) before stretching?
   a. shortwave diathermy
   b. ultrasound
   c. whirlpool
   d. hot packs
   e. cryokinetics

4. Which of the following is *not* a limiting factor to modality use?
   a. availability of the modality
   b. time available for treatment
   c. evidence supporting the modality
   d. patient compliance
   e. none of the above, all are limiting factors

5. *Clinician compliance* refers to the _____.
   a. reputation of the clinician
   b. reporting to work on time
   c. reliability and professionalism of the clinician
   d. clinician using the same modality day after day

Answers to Review Questions

Part I

CHAPTER 1

1. d
2. b
3. b
4. a
5. c

CHAPTER 2

1. b
2. d
3. e
4. b

CHAPTER 3

1. e
2. e
3. b
4. d
5. d
6. b

Part II

CHAPTER 4

1. a
2. b
3. e
4. e
5. d
6. e
7. a

CHAPTER 5

1. c
2. c
3. c
4. d
5. a
6. e

CHAPTER 6

1. c
2. e
3. e
4. b
5. e
6. e

Part III

CHAPTER 7

1. b
2. b
3. a
4. d
5. a
6. d
7. a
8. a
9. d

CHAPTER 8

1. c
2. e
3. b
4. e
5. a
6. c
7. c

Part IV

CHAPTER 9

1. a
2. d
3. a
4. c
5. d
6. c
7. a
8. c
9. a
10. d
11. b
12. b

CHAPTER 10

1. d
2. e
3. a
4. e
5. a
6. a
7. b
8. e
9. e
10. b

Part V

CHAPTER 11

1. a
2. c
3. b
4. a
5. a
6. e
7. c
8. d
9. a
10. d

CHAPTER 12

1. b
2. e
3. e
4. b
5. b
6. e
7. b
8. a

CHAPTER 13

1. b
2. e
3. b
4. a
5. c
6. a
7. b
8. a

CHAPTER 14

1. a
2. d
3. d
4. d
5. c
6. b

CHAPTER 15

1. b
2. a
3. c
4. b
5. e
6. e
7. a
8. e
9. a
10. c
11. d
12. b

CHAPTER 16

1. b
2. c
3. e
4. e
5. b
6. e
7. c
8. e
9. a
10. b

Part VI

CHAPTER 17

1. c
2. a
3. d
4. a
5. d
6. b
7. e
8. d

CHAPTER 18

1. d
2. b
3. c
4. a
5. b
6. e
7. e
8. d
9. e

CHAPTER 19

1. a
2. e
3. a
4. c
5. d
6. d
7. b
8. e
9. c

Part VII

CHAPTER 20

1. c
2. d
3. a
4. e
5. c

Glossary

absorption The action of electromagnetic waves being immersed or taken in by a substance.

AC train A continuous repetitive series of pulses at a fixed frequency (or a segment of AC).

acoustic microstreaming The unidirectional movement of fluids along the boundaries of cell membranes resulting from ultrasonically induced pressure waves.

acoustic waves Waves produced by sound and ultrasound. Also known as sound waves.

action potential A change in electrical potential between the inside and outside of a nerve cell membrane.

active electrode The electrode under which the current density is great enough to elicit the desired response. See also DISPERSIVE ELECTRODE.

acute care Treatment of an acute injury during the first 4 days after the injury.

acute injury An injury of sudden onset, caused by high-intensity, short-duration forces; examples are sprains, strains, and contusions.

acute pain Rapid-onset pain of brief duration, caused by the activation of nociceptors from external sources, such as a contusion, or internal sources, such as a muscle strain.

advantages In the context of the five-step application procedure, the benefits of a specific modality that make it more effective in treating a specific injury than other modalities.

A-delta fiber A peripheral nerve that carries sensations, including nociceptive stimuli that result in acute pain; larger and faster-acting than C fibers.

afferent nerve A sensory nerve; it enters the spinal cord via the dorsal horn.

A fiber The largest (1–22 μm in diameter) nerve fiber; conducts action potentials the most rapidly (5–120 m/sec). Some A fibers are sensory; others have a motor function.

agility A combination of speed of movement and coordination; developed as skill patterns are performed quickly, usually with sport-specific team drills.

alternating current (AC) A continuous flow of electrons that rhythmically changes direction because the two generator terminals alternatively change from positive to negative.

ampere (amp) A unit of current flow, equal to the passage of 1 coulomb (i.e., 6.28×10^{18} electrons) per second.

amplify To increase in size, volume, or significance.

amplitude The amount of current flowing through the circuit; also known as intensity.

ampmeter A device that measures the rate of current flow.

analgesic balm An externally applied drug that has a topical analgesic, anesthetic, or anti-itching effect by depressing cutaneous sensory receptors or a topical counterirritant effect by stimulating cutaneous sensory receptors.

annulus fibrosus The outer layer of an intervertebral disk, consisting of a series of interlacing cross-fibers attached to adjacent vertebral bodies.

Arndt-Schultz principle There is an optimal amount of energy absorption per unit of time that is beneficial. Less than this amount will not cause a reaction, and more than this amount will be detrimental.

arthrogenic muscle inhibition (AMI) An ongoing reflex inhibition of muscles surrounding a joint, caused by distension or damage to that joint.

artificial ice pack A vinyl pouch filled with water and enclosed in a nylon covering, frozen in a freezer at 1°F (~17°C).

asymmetrical pulse A pulse with differing phases.

atom A single unit of an element; composed of protons, electrons, neutrons, and other smaller substances.

adenosine triphosphate (ATP) The major source of energy in muscles.

attenuation A decrease in energy as an ultrasound wave is transmitted through various tissues owing to scattering and dispersion.

autonomic motor nerve A nerve that transmits impulses from the CNS to the periphery of the body and terminates in smooth muscle, cardiac muscle, glands, and organs; controlled involuntarily.

autonomic nervous system (ANS) The part of the peripheral nervous system that regulates smooth muscle, cardiac muscle, organs, and glands; consists of sympathetic and parasympathetic branches.

average current The average magnitude of a pulse.

balanced pulse A pulse containing equal phase charges.

beam nonuniformity ratio (BNR) An indicator of the amount of intensity variability within an ultrasound beam; the ratio between the average intensity of the ultrasound beam across the soundhead divided by the highest intensity of the ultrasound beam.

beat frequency An adjustable frequency; the difference between two intersecting currents of different frequencies.

B fiber Between A and C fibers in size (1–3 μm) and in rate of conduction (3–14 m/sec); autonomic motor nerve.

biofeedback A process of measuring a biological mechanism using an objective means and then telling the patient his scores. The feedback helps the patient progress more quickly.

biphasic A pulse with two phases; current flows in both directions.

bipolar technique The application of electrodes of equal size, resulting in essentially equal current density under them; both electrodes are, therefore, active.

BNR See BEAM NONUNIFORMITY RATIO (BNR).

brief-intense TENS A modality used to treat chronic pain before rehabilitation by stimulating C fibers; beat frequency varies between low and high and changes periodically; intensity higher than sensory mode TENS (to the patient's tolerance). The patient reports a burning, needling sensation and twitch and tetanic muscle contractions. Also known as noxious TENS.

burst A finite series of pulses (or a finite interval of AC at a specific frequency) flowing for a limited time period, followed by no current flow (e.g., turning a pulse train or AC on and off).

burst interval The time during which a burst occurs, usually measured in milliseconds.

capillary arcade A series of capillary arches that eventually develop throughout the entire wound area, providing abundant circulation, which is necessary to support collagenization.

capillary arch The process in which adjacent capillary bud sprouts migrate toward one another, meet, and form together creating an arch.

capillary budding A process where endothelial cells of existing vessels at the edge of the wound begin to divide. The new cells crawl away from, but keep contact with, the existing vessel. New cells force themselves between existing cells, thus forcing the end cells to advance into the wound area.

capillary filtration pressure The mathematical sum of a number of forces, known as Starling forces.

capillary hydrostatic pressure (CHP) Pressure that forces fluid out of the capillary.

capillary oncotic pressure (COP) Pressure that pulls fluid into the capillary.

capsaicin A derivative of the hot pepper plant; an irritant included in analgesic balms to provide a sensation of heat.

cardiorespiratory endurance The ability of the heart and lungs to supply exercising muscles with adequate oxygen to produce the energy needed to maintain the activity.

carrier frequency The preset frequency built into a machine.

cavitation The formation of gas-filled bubbles that expand and contract owing to ultrasonically induced pressure changes in tissue fluids.

cellular phase In the repair process, the same as leukocyte migration and phagocytosis in the inflammatory response. Macrophages scavenge the cellular debris. The circulatory and lymphatic systems (mostly lymphatic) drain away the liquefied cellular remains, which are mostly small particles of free protein.

central control A theory that previous experiences, emotional influences, sensory perception, and other factors could influence the transmission of pain signals and thus the perception of pain.

central control trigger theory A modification of the gate control theory of pain.

central nervous system (CNS) The brain and spinal cord

cerebral cortex The outer part of the brain; coordinates pain signals and determines pain location and intensity. The cerebral cortex initiates descending pain control mechanisms.

C fiber A peripheral nerve that carries sensations, including nociceptive stimuli that result in chronic pain; smaller and slower-acting than A fibers. The smallest (<1 μm) and slowest (<2 m/sec) nerve fiber; sensory nerves.

chemical mediators Chemicals, such as histamine, bradykinin, and cytokines, that mobilize the body's resources after injury to neutralize the cause of the injury and to begin removing the cellular debris so that repair can take place. Chemical mediation is one of eight events in the inflammatory response.

chronic inflammation A cellular response to long-term, low-intensity forces; not to be confused with recurring acute inflammation.

chronic injury (1) An injury caused by low-intensity, long-duration forces, in tendinitis or bursitis. (2) A recurring acute injury, such as a chronic sprained ankle.

chronic pain Pain that lasts a month beyond the usual course of an acute disease or a reasonable time for an injury to heal; also associated with a chronic pathological process that causes continuous pain or in which the pain recurs at intervals for months to years.

circuit breaker A safety device that protects equipment and body structures against excess current by opening the circuit when too much current is flowing.

clinician compliance The reliability, knowledge, confidence, and professionalism of a clinician.

closed circuit A complete circuit, allowing flow; there are no breaks in the circuit.

clotting A multistage process that results in fibrin and platelets closing a damaged blood vessel.

cluster probe A laser applicator with multiple probes that can apply multiple wavelengths to a larger area during treatment.

coherent Logically ordered or integrated; a quality of electromagnetic waves that have the same wavelength and a fixed phase relationship.

cold The absence of heat or something that has less heat than one would desire; the sensation produced by low temperatures.

cold hypersensitivity Intense pain during ice or cold pack application.

cold-induced vasodilation (CIVD) An increase in the circumference of blood vessels as a result of cold applications.

cold pack A generic term that refers to crushed ice packs, gel packs, artificial ice packs, and crushable chemical packs.

collagen A fibrous protein found in all types of connective tissue; the primary solid substance of ligaments, tendons, and scar tissue.

collagenization The process of manufacturing and laying down collagen in the wound space.

collimated beam A focused, less-divergent beam of energy. Both ultrasound and laser energy are transmitted as collimated beams.

compliance The extent to which a patient follows a prescribed treatment regimen. Also called adherence or maintenance.

compression A region of high molecular density and high pressure as the molecules in a longitudinal wave are squeezed together. See also RAREFACTION.

conduction A process of heat transfer that occurs when two objects of uneven temperatures come into contact with each other. Heat is transferred from the object with the higher temperature to the object with the lower temperature, causing the warmer object to cool and the cooler object to warm.

conductor A substance that can transport electrical charge (or current) from one point to another; it must have free electrons that can be pushed along (e.g., metal, water).

connective tissue stretch A combination of heat application, long-term passive stretch, and cold applications, used to increase joint flexibility after prolonged immobilization during which connective tissue contractures have developed.

constant stimulation pattern Stimulation in which amplitude of successive pulses (or cycles) is the same.

continuous ultrasound An ultrasound mode in which the sound intensity remains constant throughout the treatment and the ultrasound energy is being produced 100% of the time.

contraction Collapsing of the capillary arcade toward the end of repair. Makes the scar smaller and paler.

contraction and restructuring phase In the repair process, two processes that cause scar tissue to become smaller and paler (in light-skinned people); a new scar will appear red (in a light-skinned person) and mounded or raised above the surrounding tissue.

contraindications Situations in which a specific modality should not be used—that is, situations in which it may do more harm than good.

contrast bath therapy The alternating immersion of an injured body part in hot and cold water baths.

convection The transfer of heat to or from an object by the passage of a fluid or air past its surface.

conversion A process that occurs when a form of energy other than heat (electricity, chemical, mechanical, etc.) is converted to heat within the body.

cookbook approach to rehabilitation A treatment approach in which the clinician follows a specific "recipe" or protocol for each injury, consisting of phases with specific time periods and therapeutic interventions. All patients with the same or similar injury are treated the same, without regard for individual patient differences.

cosine or right-angle law The optimum radiation occurs when the source of the radiation is perpendicular to the center of the surface of the area to be radiated.

coulomb The basic unit of charge, produced by 6.28×10^{18} displaced electrons (6280 quadrillion).

counterirritant A substance that irritates the skin, causing mild skin inflammation, which causes a gating effect and thereby relieves mild pain in muscles, joints, and internal organs.

coupling medium In ultrasound, a substance that facilitates the transmission of ultrasound energy by decreasing impedance at the air–skin interface. In electrotherapy, a substance that facilitates the transmission of electrical current from the electrodes to the skin; also called couplant.

critical thinker approach to rehabilitation An organized procedural outline that includes fairly broad guidelines to help the clinician choose the most appropriate modality and mode of applying that modality.

crushable chemical pack A thin-walled vinyl pouch of a liquid packaged within a stronger, larger vinyl pouch of dry crystals. Squeezing breaks the smaller pouch, and fluid leaks into the larger, outer pouch. Fluid and crystals combine in a chemical reaction that cools the fluid.

crushed ice pack Crushed ice, typically from an ice machine, in a plastic or cloth bag.

crutch palsy A temporary or permanent loss of either sensation or the ability to move or control movement.

cryokinetics Alternating cold application and active graded exercise for rehabilitating acute joint sprains.

cryostretch Alternating cold application, passive stretch, and resistive muscle contraction for rehabilitating acute muscle strains.

cryosurgery A surgical technique that uses ultra-low-temperature probes (−4 to −94°F [−20 to −70°C]) to freeze tissue and thereby destroy it.

cryotherapy The therapeutic use of cold; the application of a device or substance with a temperature less than body temperature, thus causing heat to pass from the body to the cryotherapy device.

crystal An ultrasound transducer.

current density A measure of the quantity of charged ions moving through a particular cross-sectional area of an electrode.

current electricity A stream of loose electrons passing along a conductor.

current flow The flow of electrical charge from one point to another, from an area of higher electron concentration (the negative pole or cathode) to an area lacking electrons (the positive pole or anode).

current modulation Manipulating, regulating, and adjusting of the input current to create a variety of specific output wave forms.

cycle In an alternating current, two impulses: current flowing from the baseline to the maximum in one direction and back to the baseline.

daily adjustable progressive resistive exercise (DAPRE) technique An aggressive, four-set system of isotonic weight lifting that takes advantage of the fact that strength can be redeveloped more quickly than it was developed initially. Patients perform maximal repetitions during their third and fourth sets, and the number of repetitions performed is used as a basis for adjusting the resistance during the fourth set and on the next day, respectively.

decay time The time from maximal amplitude to the end of a phase.

deep thermotherapy The application of modalities that cause a tissue temperature rise (TTR) in deeper tissues.

dermatome The area of skin innervated by a particular spinal nerve.

descending endogenous opiate system (DEOS) A system operating at supraspinal levels that contains opiate secreting neurons to assist in pain control.

diathermy The therapeutic use of high-frequency electromagnetic waves to heat deep tissues.

differential application of modalities The process of determining the optimal modality to use under specific circumstances.

direct current (DC) A steady or continuous, unidirectional flow of electrons between the anode and the cathode of a battery; also known as galvanic current.

direct (galvanic) wave form Pure DC, used for iontophoresis.

direction of current flow The flow of current from the positive pole to the negative pole.

disadvantages In the context of the five-step application procedure, the possible negative effects a specific modality might cause or the benefits that might be lost by not using another modality.

discharge note A type of SOAP note written when treatment is discontinued.

dispersive electrode The electrode under which the current density is not great enough to elicit the desired response. See also ACTIVE ELECTRODE.

dopamine A neurotransmitter in the brain used by the body to synthesize norepinephrine and epinephrine; affects brain processes that control movement, emotional response, and the ability to experience pleasure and pain.

dorsal horn The posterior portion of the gray matter of the spinal cord; also called posterior horn.

dry cell A battery that uses electrolyte paste rather than a solution. One example is a zinc-carbon battery in which a zinc tube is filled with electrolyte paste and a carbon rod is inserted into the middle.

duty cycle The percentage of time that ultrasound is being generated (pulse duration) over one pulse period.

dynamic vector In IFC therapy, two intersecting, moving currents used to treat large areas.

edema An accumulation of the fluid portion of blood in the tissues.

effective radiating area (ERA) The part of the surface area of a soundhead in an ultrasound device that transmits a sound wave from the crystal to the tissues.

effects In the context of the five-step application procedure, the physiological and/or pathological changes the modality evokes, both locally and systemically (throughout the body).

efferent nerve A motor nerve; it exits the spinal cord via the ventral horn.

effleurage A gliding manipulation performed with light or heavy pressure (directed toward the heart) that deforms subcutaneous tissue down to the deep fascial layers; also called stroking.

electrical charge The net sum of the charges of electrons and protons in an atom or molecule; the difference between the number of protons and electrons.

electrical circuit A system of conductors that allows electrons to move between the two poles of a battery or generator.

electrolyte A substance that contains ions and can, therefore, conduct electricity.

electromagnetic energy One of the fundamental forms of energy in the universe; consists of electrical and magnetic waves.

electromagnetic induction The process of converting mechanical power into electrical power (electrical generator) and for converting electrical power into mechanical power (electrical motor).

electromagnetic wave A combination of oscillating electric and magnetic fields at right angles to one another that travel in wavelike fashion through space at a speed of about 186,000 mi./sec (300 000 km/sec); also known as radiation. Forms include heat, light, electricity, x-rays, cosmic rays.

electron A subunit of an atom, orbiting the nucleus, with a negligible mass and an electrical charge of -1.

element The primary substance of matter (e.g., oxygen, copper, carbon).

emergency care Care given after a serious or life-threatening injury, such as CPR or transportation to a hospital.

emission A flowing forth, such as the release of electrons from parent atoms.

endogenous Developed or produced within the body.

endorphin A drug that inhibits pain signal transmission and decreases the amount of chemical irritants present in the CNS.

endothelium The wall of a blood vessel.

enkephalin A drug that blocks pain by interfering with A-delta and C fiber signal transmission to T cells.

epinephrine A hormone secreted by the adrenal glands in response to stress; a neurotransmitter that stimulates the fight-or-flight response. Also known as adrenaline.

evidence-based practice Health care that is based on scientific evidence rather than tradition and experience alone. Its goal is to improve the quality and effectiveness of health care.

extracellular space The space between cells.

extrapyramidal system A neural network in the brain that controls and coordinates movement.

facilitation Enabling a neural response.

faradic wave form Induced asymmetrical AC.

five-step application procedure A standardized framework for applying any therapeutic modality. It is rigid enough for quality control yet flexible enough to allow the clinician to use modalities in the context of a critical thinking approach to rehabilitation.

fixed phase The unified launching of the wave fronts of all photons of a laser beam.

fluid dynamics The movement of fluid between capillaries and tissue.

frequency *(1)* The rate of passage of crests on a wave form, expressed in cycles per second or hertz (Hz). *(2)* The rate of vibration of a force or wave, usually measured relative to local time.

friction massage A repetitive, specific, nongliding, shearing technique that produces movement between the fibers of dense connective tissue, increasing tissue extensibility and promoting the alignment of collagen fibers.

functional progression The performance of functional activities in an ordered sequence, beginning with unloaded, single-plane, slow-speed, slow-transition activity and progressing to overloaded, multiple-plane, high-speed, quick-transition activities. Accomplished by graded exercise, it facilitates the acquisition or reacquisition of skills needed for the safe, effective performance of complex skills. Also known as progressive reorientation.

fused response A sustained sensory response that feels like pins and needles, in response to moderate-amplitude, high-frequency pulsed or AC stimulation.

galvanometer A device that measures the electromagnetic effects of currents.

gate control theory of pain A theory that proposes a gating mechanism in the dorsal horn of the spinal cord that allows only one sensation at a time to pass through to the brain.

gel pack A reusable type of cold pack, made with water, antifreeze, and a gel in a vinyl pouch. Cooled in a freezer at 1°F (~17°C), but does not freeze.

generator A device that converts an input electrical current (AC or DC) into various output currents (AC, DC, or pulsed).

glycolysis The conversion of glucose to lactic acid when sufficient oxygen is not available. The primary mechanism of anaerobic metabolism.

graded exercise A series of exercises of increasing complexity and difficulty used to progressively reorient a patient to full functional activity following injury. See also FUNCTIONAL PROGRESSION.

graphic rating scale A pain-rating scale that uses a horizontal line with anchor points at each end and descriptors spread along the line; administered and scored the same as the VAS.

grid application A technique of applying a single laser probe to a large area by dividing the treatment area into a grid and treating each area separately.

ground-fault interrupter (GFI) A device that senses very small ground-fault currents, such as current flowing through the body of a person standing on damp ground while touching a hot AC line wire. The GFI quickly trips the circuit breaker, thereby limiting the total energy flow through the body to a safe value.

half-slivered mirror A mirror that reflects only half the light and allows the other half to pass through.

heat The kinetic energy of atoms and molecules; a form of energy that is transferred by a difference in temperature. All substances with a temperature above absolute zero ($-273°C$) possess heat.

heat sink An area of the body that can accept and dissipate great amounts of heat.

hemarthrosis The presence of blood in a joint.

hematoma An accumulation of hemorrhaged blood and cellular debris.

hemodynamic changes Vascular changes that mobilize and transport defense components of the blood to the injury site and secure their passage through the vessel wall into the tissue.

hemorrhaging Bleeding.

herniated disk Disruption of the annulus fibrosus of an intervertebral disk.

high-volt pulsed current (HVPC) A twin-peak, monophasic, pulsed current driven by a high electromotive force or voltage for the purpose of pain modulation, edema reduction, muscle reeducation, spasm reduction, and wound healing.

hot pack A form of moist superficial heat that can be heated and reused.

hot spot An area at tissue interfaces that is overheated from too much energy being concentrated in one area.

hunting response An oscillating in surface temperature during prolonged (>15 min) ice water immersion. It is caused by the build up and interruption of a thermal gradient—not to cold-induced vasodilation.

hydrocolator pack A canvas pack that encases silica gel and that can be heated and reused.

hydrostatic pressure Pressure exerted by a column of water.

hypothalamus The brain's central monitoring and control station; regulates autonomic nervous system functions, and plays a role in mood and motivational states.

hypoxia Inadequate oxygen in body tissue, often resulting from prolonged ischemia. Not as severe as anoxia, a total lack of oxygen.

ice massage Stroking a body part (usually a muscle) with a large ice cube or ice cup (ice pop).

ice water immersion The use of a container filled with cold water and ice 32–34°F (0–1°C) for numbing extremities before exercise; also called ice bath immersion and sometimes inappropriately called ice water submersion.

immediate care Treatments within the first 12 hr after an orthopedic injury; a subset of acute care.

impedance Resistance or opposition to the flow of AC.

impulse AC current flow in a single direction.

indications In the context of the five-step application procedure, situations in which a specific modality should be used; conditions that would benefit from application of a certain modality.

inflammation The local, or tissue, response of the body to an injury or irritant. Also known as the inflammatory response.

infrared (IR) lamp A form of superficial heat that radiates from a heat lamp.

inhibition Restraining or repressing a neural response.

initial note A type of SOAP note written after the initial assessment.

insulator A nonconductor; something that resists the flow of electrons because they have no free electrons to move (e.g., rubber, glass, wood).

intensity A measure of the rate at which energy is being delivered per unit area.

interburst interval The time between bursts, usually measured in milliseconds.

interferential current (IFC) therapy The interference or superimposition of at least two separate medium-frequency sinusoidal currents on one another, mainly used to relieve pain.

interferential wave form Symmetrical, sinusoidal, high-frequency (2000–5000 Hz) AC. Two channels, with different frequencies, used simultaneously, causes a current amplitude modulation in the tissue.

interim note A type of SOAP note that includes periodic documentation of the results of the treatment plan. Also known as progress note.

interpulse interval The time between successive pulses.

interrupted DC wave form Unidirectional current flow caused by rapid and repeated turning of the current on and off.

intervention A medical treatment; an action taken to improve a medical disorder.

intervertebral disk A structure between two vertebrae that functions to resist compressive forces and shock, provide flexibility, and provide adequate space between vertebrae.

inverse square law ($I - 1/d^2$) The intensity (I) of radiation is inversely proportional to the distance squared (d^2).

in vitro In cellular or tissue cultures.

in vivo Within the tissues.

ion An atom or molecule that has lost or gained one or more electrons and is, therefore, positively or negatively charged.

ion migration Ions move through the tissue in response to continuous DC stimulation.

iontophoresis The application of a mild direct electrical current (DC) to transport negatively or positively charged ions from a drug solution into a patient's skin and underlying tissues.

ischemia A deficit in blood supply to an organ or body part, usually owing to functional constriction or actual obstruction of a blood vessel. If prolonged, ischemia leads to tissue hypoxia.

joint flexibility The ability of a joint to move through its full range of motion.

knobology A tongue-in-cheek term referring to the study of application without theory. Knobologists are students and clinicians who want to know only which knobs on a therapeutic modality to turn but are uninterested in why they are doing so.

laser Acronym for light amplification by stimulated emission of radiation, a device that produces and emits a highly amplified single-frequency and single-colored beam of nondivergent coherent light.

lasing medium A substance (gas, liquid, crystal, chemical, or semiconductor) that is activated and subsequently gives off photons during laser light production.

latent heat of fusion The amount of heat energy needed to convert a substance from a solid state to a liquid state without changing its temperature.

law of Grotthus-Draper Electromagnetic waves must be absorbed to be beneficial.

leukocyte A white blood cell; contains and kills foreign substances and cellular debris.

leukocyte migration The movement of leukocytes from blood vessels to the injury site.

light Electromagnetic radiation that produces a visual sensation.

light therapy The application of light by a variety of devices for a variety of therapeutic purposes; also known as phototherapy.

light-emitting diode (LED) A special type of semiconductor diode that emits visible light when an electric current passes through it; used in both laser and nonlaser devices.

lock and key A metaphor for the way neurotransmitter shapes fit specific receptors on dendrites.

longitudinal wave The primary wave form in which ultrasound energy travels in soft tissue, with molecular displacement along the direction in which the wave travels. See also TRANSVERSE WAVE.

low-level laser A low-power laser, also referred to as a cold laser or soft laser.

lymphedema pump A device consisting of a pump attached to a boot or sleeve that intermittently forces air or chilled water into the sleeve for the purpose of decreasing lymphedema; formerly known as intermittent compression device, cold compression device, and pneumatic compression pump.

lysosome A cellular organelle containing enzymes that digest foreign matter.

macrophage A long-lived leukocyte that is the primary scavenger after tissue damage occurs.

macrotrauma An injury that results in immediate tissue disruption. Also called impact injury or contact injury. Injuries that result from macrotrauma are classified as acute injuries.

magnetic field The force field that develops between the two poles

manual traction A distraction force applied by another person.

massage lubricant A lotion, oil, cream, or powder used to decrease friction and control the amount of glide and drag that occurs between the clinician's moving hands and the client's skin.

matter Anything that has weight and occupies space.

McGill Pain Questionnaire A pain-rating scale that uses pictures, scales, and words to help patients describe the sensory and affective aspects, as well as magnitude and changes, in their pain.

mechanical nociceptor A lightly myelinated A-delta fiber, activated primarily by strong mechanical displacement of the skin; also called high-threshold mechanoreceptor.

mechanical traction A distraction force applied by a machine or other apparatus.

menthol An alcohol obtained from oil of peppermint and derived from mint plants; an irritant included in analgesic balms to provide a sensation of cold, or cool burning.

methyl salicylate Wintergreen oil, produced synthetically or from distilled sweet birch leaves; an irritant that causes redness on the skin, included in analgesic balms to provide a sensation of heat.

microcurrent electrical nerve stimulation (MENS) The therapeutic use of constant (direct) and pulsed (interrupted) currents by which the stimulus amplitude is in the microamperage (millionth of an ampere) range.

microtrauma An injury caused by overuse, cyclic loading, or friction. Injuries that result from microtrauma are classified as chronic injuries.

microwave diathermy (MWD) The therapeutic use of high-frequency (usually 2450 MHz) electromagnetic waves, similar to radar, to heat tissues.

modified square wave form Monophasic, rectangular, pulsed current.

molecule Two or more atoms held together in a chemical bond.

monochromatic Having a single frequency and a single color (if it is in the light spectrum).

monophasic A pulse with one phase; current flows in one direction only.

morphine A drug that blocks pain by filling receptors so that neurotransmitters cannot occupy them.

motor point The point at which a motor nerve enters a muscle, usually located at the beginning of the muscle belly; the place where a given amount of current will elicit the greatest muscular contraction.

motor skill The integration and coordination of many muscles acting in concert to produce a desired movement; developed only by practicing sport-specific skill patterns.

motor TENS A TENS application used to treat chronic pain by stimulating small-diameter afferent nerves; beat frequency is low (1–5 pps) and intensity higher than sensory TENS (to the patient's tolerance). The patient reports some burning, needling sensation, and a slight muscle twitch.

motor unit A motor nerve and all the muscle fibers with which it synapses.

muscle cramp A sudden, intense, painful, tetanic muscle contraction that is short-lived, usually lasting <20 sec; commonly called charley horse.

muscle guarding An involuntary process of splinting an injured limb by inducing a low-grade (mild) muscle spasm of antagonistic muscle groups.

muscle spasm *(1)* A muscle tightness of gradual onset, usually not very painful. *(2)* A sudden, involuntary contraction of one or more muscles. A low-grade spasm manifests as tightness, as opposed to a muscle cramp or charley horse.

muscular endurance The ability of a muscle to contract repeatedly without becoming fatigued.

muscular power The combination of strength and speed of movement; must be developed after those performance attributes.

muscular speed The speed at which a muscle contracts. Explosive-type activities (short duration, maximal power) develop muscular speed.

muscular strength A measure of the ability of a muscle to exert force. Regularly performed progressive resistive exercises will increase muscular strength.

myofascial release A technique that combines traction with varying amounts of stretch to produce a moderate sustained force on the muscle and its associated fascia.

myoglobin An oxygen-transporting and storage protein in muscle cells. Similar in function to hemoglobin in the blood.

naloxone A drug that reverses the effect of morphine.

negative feedback Activity on a nerve fiber that eventually is returned through a neural network, thereby inhibiting further activity on that neuron.

negative terminal The terminal into which the current enters the battery or generator from the body.

nerve A bundle of nerve fibers that transmits information via electrical signals among the brain, spinal cord, and other parts of the body.

nerve excitability The amount of electrical current applied to the surface necessary to elicit an action potential in a specific nerve

nerve fiber An axon of a single neuron, or nerve cell, and its multiple dendrites.

nerve palsy The partial loss of motor function in a local area; may be permanent or temporary.

neural inhibition The decreasing or stopping of neural activity, thus retarding or preventing normal musculoskeletal functioning. (Derived from the Latin *hibitus*, "to keep back.")

neuromatrix theory of pain A theory of pain that involves a gating mechanism in the spinal cord, as in the gate control theory, but that emphasizes a much larger role of the brain in interpreting and responding to painful stimuli. It is regarded as the most complete explanation of pain and pain management.

neuromuscular electrical stimulator (NMES) A therapeutic device that delivers current to the body to cause sensory and motor nerve depolarization. Its purpose is to cause muscle contraction.

neuron The basic functional unit of the nervous system; main components are the cell body, dendrites, the axon, and branches that end in axon terminals. Also called nerve cell.

neurotransmitter A chemical released by axon terminals that transmits an impulse across a synapse. Neurotransmitters fit into receptors on the cell body or dendrites of the postsynaptic neuron, where they either stimulate or inhibit a response.

neutron A subunit of an atom, located in the nucleus, with a mass of 1 and an electrical charge of 0.

neutrophil A short-lived leukocyte that forms the first line of defense against pathogens. Also called a polymorph.

nociception The ability to feel pain; also known as pain sense, algesia, algesthesia, and nociperception.

nociceptor A peripheral nerve that receives and transmits painful or other noxious stimuli.

nondivergent Incapable of separating or widening. Contrast the light from a laser pointer (nondivergent) with that coming from a flashlight (divergent). Nondivergent light is also known as directional light.

non-weight-bearing gait A crutch walking gait used when the objective is to completely remove weight from one leg or foot. The injured limb is lifted and the patient walks alternatively on the good leg and the two crutches. Also known as the swing-through gait.

norepinephrine A hormone secreted by the adrenal glands; the principal neurotransmitter of sympathetic nerves supplying the major organs and skin. It increases heart rate, blood pressure, the rate and depth of breathing, and blood sugar level, and decreases digestive functions. Also known as noradrenaline.

noxious stimulus A harmful, unhealthy stimulation. Pain is caused by noxious stimuli.

noxious TENS TENS applied with a high enough intensity to be painful.

nucleus pulposus The inner layer of an intervertebral disk, composed of a protein gel between the cartilaginous end plates of the vertebrae and the annulus fibrosus.

number scale A tool for measuring pain intensity that consists of a range of numbers and descriptors. Patients select the number that best describes their pain.

ohm A unit of resistance or opposition to the flow of DC: 1 ohm (Ω) is equal to the resistance caused by a column of mercury 1 mm^2 in cross-section, 106 cm high at a temperature of 0°C. It is equal to 1 V/amp.

Ohm's law The relationship between current, force, and resistance (current = force/resistance; amp = volt/ohm).

ohmmeter A device that measures resistance to current flow.

oncotic pressure Pressure resulting from the attraction of fluid by free protein. Also called colloid osmotic pressure.

open circuit An interrupted or broken circuit; flow ceases.

opiate A substance that numbs or decreases pain; its synthetic form is known as an opioid.

organelle A specialized structure within tissue cells.

orthopedic injury A sprain, strain, fracture, or contusion caused by excessive stress.

osteophyte A small, bony calcium deposit that forms on the vertebrae.

overload The concept of challenging the body to greater function by pushing it beyond its comfort zone to near its limits. The body adapts by increasing its capacity.

pain An unpleasant sensory and emotional experience associated with actual or potential tissue damage or described in terms of such damage.

paraffin bath A form of moist superficial heat applied by forming a wax glove around the affected body part.

parasympathetic nervous system The branch of the ANS that regulates the "rest and digest" responses, such as decreased heart rate and secretion of digestive enzymes.

partial conductor A substance that allows some flow of electricity under certain conditions (e.g., dry wood, paper, tap water, moist air, kerosene).

partial-weight-bearing gait A crutch walking gait in which the patient walks as with a normal gait, except for using the crutches to remove just enough weight from the injured limb to eliminate pain and limping. Also called the three-point gait.

patient compliance The act of following the treatment orders or instructions given by a clinician.

patient noncompliance The failure to fully follow the treatment orders or instructions given by a clinician.

peak area of the maximum BNR (PAMBNR) An ultrasound beam profile.

peak current The highest magnitude of a pulse.

percussion Repeated, rhythmical, light striking of the skin. Techniques include gentle tapping, pounding, cupping, hacking, and slapping the skin; also called tapotement.

performance attributes Specific neuromuscular functions necessary for sport or work performance, such as pain-free movement, muscular strength, and motor control. Injury disrupts one or more of the performance attributes, and rehabilitation should systematically reestablishes them.

periaqueductal gray (PAG) matter Gray matter in the brain whose neurons are excited by endorphins and opiate analgesics. It plays a role in the descending modulation of pain and in defensive behavior.

peripheral nervous system (PNS) The cranial nerves and spinal nerves.

pétrissage A group of related techniques that repetitively compress (squeeze), shear (wring), and release muscle tissue with varying amounts of drag, lift, and glide.

phagocytosis The process of digesting cellular debris and other foreign material into pieces small enough to be removed from the injury site via lymph vessels.

phagolysosome A sac in a leukocyte, formed by lysosomes spilling their digestive enzymes into a phagosome; digests pathogens and debris from an injury site.

phagosome A sac within a leukocyte, formed as the leukocyte engulfs pathogens or debris from an injury site.

phantom limb pain Pain that a person interprets as coming from an amputated limb.

phase A period of unidirectional charged particle movement (current flow).

phase change A change from one state (solid or liquid or gas) to another without a change in chemical composition.

phase charge The total electrical charge of a single phase, expressed as coulombs (microcoulombs for MNES). It is the time interval (area under the curve); the result of both amplitude and width (duration).

phase duration The time during which current flows in a single direction.

phase shape The shape of an output current after being modulated (e.g., rectangular, spike, triangular, sawtooth).

phonophoresis A technique in which ultrasound is used to help move a topical medication into the tissues. See also SONOPORATION.

photobiomodulation The act of modifying biological processes with light.

photon A particle of light; the basic unit of radiant energy. The amount of its energy is a function of the frequency of the electromagnetic wave.

physiatrist A physician who specializes in physical medicine, the medical subspecialty relating to the treatment of injury and disease by physical agents, such as heat, cold, light, electricity, and exercise.

physical agent An external form of energy, such as heat, cold, light, electricity, or exercise.

physical medicine Treating injury or disease by physical agents, such as heat, cold, light, sound, electricity, and exercise.

physical medicine and rehabilitation The medical subspeciality relating to the treatment and rehabilitation of physical conditions.

piezoelectric effect The contracting and expanding of a crystal, when an alternating electrical current is passed through it.

placebo A medicinally inactive substance or mock intervention administered to bring about a desired response and satisfy the patient's demand for medicine.

placebo effect The measurable, observable, or felt improvement in health not attributable to treatment; occurs in response to many types of interventions.

plateau The time during which electrical pulses remain at maximum preset intensity.

polarity The positive or negative voltage on an active electrode compared to the voltage on a dispersive electrode. Polarity applies only when a unipolar placement technique is used.

polymodal nociceptor An unmyelinated C fiber, activated by several different types of stimuli, such as heat, mechanical pressure, or inflammatory chemical mediators produced by tissue injury.

polyphasic A pulse with many phases. Current flow with many phases.

positive feedback Activity on a neuron that eventually is returned through a neural network, thereby facilitating further activity on that neuron.

positive terminal The terminal from which the current leaves the battery or generator to enter the body.

postacute care Treatment of an acute injury after 14 days after the injury.

power A function of both pulse width and pulse frequency, measured in watts. Also called intensity.

precautions Situations that could cause harm if the clinician is not careful. For example, failure to move the soundhead during ultrasound treatment could damage tissue or cause extreme pain.

primary injury Cellular damage caused by an acute traumatic force.

progress note A type of SOAP note that includes periodic documentation of the results of the treatment plan. Also known as interim note.

progression The practice of inducing incremental increases in a performance attribute by sequentially overloading the body as it adapts to a training load.

progressive reorientation See FUNCTIONAL PROGRESSION.

proprioceptive neuromuscular facilitation (PNF) Techniques that help maintain joint flexibility, such as hold–relax (static stretch interspersed with isometric contraction of the involved muscle) and contract–relax (static stretch interspersed with isometric contraction of the antagonistic muscle).

proton A subunit of an atom, located in the nucleus, with a mass of 1 and an electrical charge of +1.

pulse A finite period of charged particle movement separated from other pulses by a limited time during which no current flows. Consists of one or more phases.

pulse charge balance The relationship between the charges of two phases of a biphasic pulse, independent of whether or not the phases are symmetrical.

pulse charge The amount of electrical charge of a single pulse; the sum of phase charges.

pulsed current Interrupted or noncontinuous electron flow.

pulsed shortwave diathermy (PSWD) The therapeutic use of high-frequency (10–100 MHz) electromagnetic waves, in pulsed form, to produce nonthermal and thermal effects in deep tissues.

pulsed ultrasound An ultrasound mode in which the intensity is periodically interrupted, with no ultrasound energy being produced during the off period. With pulsed ultrasound, the average intensity of the output over time is reduced.

pulse period The beginning of a pulse to the beginning of the subsequent pulse; pulse duration plus interpulse interval.

pulse rate The number of pulses per second (pps).

pulse symmetry The relationship between the shapes of the two phases of a biphasic pulse.

pulse width The time required for each pulse to complete its cycle; also known as pulse duration.

quadripolar technique The application of four electrodes of equal size; generally they crisscross the target tissue.

radiating pain Pain that originates from an irritated nerve root and travels along that nerve's dermatome.

radiation Energy that is transmitted in the form of rays, waves, or particles, often from a central source; also called radiant energy. See also ELECTROMAGNETIC WAVE.

radicular pain Pain along the pathway of a spinal nerve.

ramp down The time during which the intensity of an electrical surge decreases.

ramp up The time during which the intensity of an electrical surge increases.

randomized clinical trial (RCT) A controlled research study of a specific medical intervention on patients with a specific disease or injury.

raphe nucleus A group of neurons in the center of the brainstem that release serotonin, making them part of brain's pain relief system.

rarefaction A region of lower molecular density in a longitudinal wave, as the molecules are pulled apart. See also COMPRESSION.

Raynaud disease A circulatory disorder caused by cold or emotion, in which the hands, and less commonly the feet, become discolored and painful.

reconditioning Conditioning again. Often improperly used as a synonym for *injury rehabilitation*. Although rehabilitation and conditioning share many principles, there are fundamental differences. Rehabilitation is much more than conditioning again, and the terms should not be used synonymously.

reconstitution The process of replacing damaged cells with healthy cells of the same type as those that were injured.

record keeping The process of writing and storing accurate and detailed information about individual injuries, treatments given, and how the patient responded to the treatments.

recurring inflammation Acute inflammation that is reinitiated before the previous episode of acute inflammation has finished.

referred pain Pain at a site other than the location of a trauma; usually projects outward from the torso and distally along the extremities.

reflection The bending back of electromagnetic waves when they hit a substance. The angle of reflection is determined by the angle of the strike.

refraction The bending of electromagnetic waves when they pass through a substance. The amount of bending depends on the frequency of the waves.

refractory period The time during which the nerve membrane repolarizes; divided into relative and absolute refractory periods.

rehabilitation The process of restoring an individual to a normal or optimal state of health. (Derived from the Latin *rehabilitare,* "to make fit again.")

repair The process of replacing dead or damaged cells with healthy ones.

replacement The process of replacing damaged cells with simpler cells, as in connective tissue, muscle tissue, and CNS tissue and in any area where the damage is extensive enough to disrupt the basic cellular framework. Replacement results in scar tissue formation. Also called repair by connective tissue.

residual pain Pain that develops after an unaccustomed activity, generally occurring the next day. It indicates that the previous day's activity was too rigorous.

resistance Opposition to the flow of electricity, caused by a conductor.

response A reaction, such as contraction of a muscle or secretion of a gland, that results from stimulation.

restructuring Collagen fibers are reorganized from the haphazard way they were laid down to a parallel arrangement, causing the scar to become more compact. Occurs near the end of repair.

RICES Acronym for rest, elevation, ice, compression, elevation, and stabilization: the prescription for immediate care.

rifle approach Treating a patient with one or two specific modalities, targeted to achieve a particular goal. It is more focused than the shotgun approach.

rise time The time from the beginning of a phase until it reaches maximal amplitude.

Russian wave form A medium-frequency polyphasic, symmetrical, sinusoidal, burst wave form generated in 50 bursts/sec envelopes.

SAID principle Acronym for specific adaptation to imposed demands. The body responds to a given demand with a specific and predictable adaptation. Specific adaptation *requires* that *specific* demands be imposed.

scanning A technique of applying a single laser probe to a large area by moving the head across the area like an ultrasound head.

secondary enzymatic injury Tissue damage resulting from enzymes, such as those in lysosomes, released from damaged cells.

secondary injury Cellular injury caused by enzymatic action and metabolic deficiency.

secondary metabolic injury Tissue damage resulting from a metabolic imbalance secondary to an acute traumatic orthopedic injury.

semiconductor A substance with poor conductivity at low temperatures; conductivity increases when other substances are added, or by the application of heat, light, or voltage. Used to regulate the flow of electricity (e.g., carbon, silicone, germanium).

sensory nerve A nerve that transmits impulses from the periphery of the body to the CNS.

sensory TENS A TENS application with a high beat frequency (80–200 pps) and intensity adjusted to the point at which the patient reports a buzzing or tingling sensation; used to treat acute pain by stimulating large-diameter sensory nerves.

sensory twitch Repetitions of brief isolated sensory ticks in response to moderate-amplitude, low-frequency pulsed stimulation. This response is not used therapeutically.

sequela An effect that follows, or results from, an injury, disease, or treatment.

serotonin A biochemical messenger and regulator, found primarily in the CNS, GI tract, and blood platelets; mediates several physiological functions, including neurotransmission.

shortwave diathermy (SWD) The therapeutic use of high-frequency (10–100 MHz) electromagnetic waves, similar to radio waves, to heat deep tissues.

shotgun approach Treating a patient with every possible modality, with the hope that one will be effective. It gives the impression that the clinician's only goal is to reduce the patient's symptoms. See also RIFLE APPROACH.

single laser probe An applicator of laser light.

sinusoidal wave form Pure AC. A biphasic, symmetrical, balanced wave form with a gradual rise in the amplitude followed by a gradual decline in the amplitude.

SOAP note A type of problem-oriented medical record. S = subjective, information gathered primarily from questioning the patient on his present condition; O = objective, reproducible information from tests or evaluative measures; A = assessment, the clinician's professional judgment or impression of the injury; P = plan, the course of action to rehabilitate the patient.

somatic motor nerve A nerve that transmits impulses from the CNS to the periphery of the body and terminates in skeletal muscle; controlled voluntarily.

somatic nervous system (SNS) The somatic motor nerves and sensory nerves.

sonoporation A process in which ultrasound increases cell membrane permeability, thereby facilitating the delivery of molecules of a medication to precise locations in the body. See also PHONOPHORESIS.

soundhead A ceramic, aluminum, or stainless-steel plate attached to the crystal that transfers the acoustic energy (sound waves) from the crystal to the tissues.

spatial average intensity (SAI) The intensity of an ultrasound beam averaged over the area of the soundhead.

spatial peak intensity The highest intensity in an ultrasound beam across the soundhead's surface.

spatial summation Summed over space; occurs when a number of subthreshold stimuli from different axons converge on one cell body simultaneously.

specific heat The amount of heat energy required to raise 1 kg of a substance 1°C.

spinal adaptation syndrome A theory that nociceptive impulses from traumatized tissue inhibit motor functions and tissue repair but that voluntary activity can reestablish central control and prevent this inhibition. Prolonged inactivity after an injury will lead to neural inhibition that could become permanent.

stabilization The act of supporting or holding steady, with or as if with a brace. After injury, it allows surrounding muscles to relax.

standard operating procedures (SOPs) Specific guidelines and protocols for performing a specific task. Having SOPs is a form of quality control because they promote consistency. They help you remember the specific steps and ensure that all essential elements are performed.

Starling forces Forces that cause capillary filtration: capillary oncotic, capillary hydrostatic, tissue oncotic, and tissue hydrostatic.

static electricity Frictional electricity created by rubbing two objects together; one object gains electrons and the other one loses electrons.

static vector A vector that stays centered where two interferential currents cross.

stimulate To excite or invigorate; to encourage or provoke something to grow, develop, or become more active.

stimulation pattern The structure of the pulses used in the current.

stimulus The action of one agent on another (e.g., nerve, muscle) that evokes activity in the receiving structure or agent.

stretching window The time period of vigorous heating when tissues will undergo their greatest extensibility and elongation.

structural integrity The health of a patient's anatomical structures, such as bones, muscles, ligaments, and tendons.

subacute care Treatment of an acute injury during days 4–14 after the injury. An injury in this stage is moving beyond acute but is still somewhat or bordering on acute.

substantia gelatinosa (SG) The location of the pain gate in the dorsal horn of the spinal cord, according to the gate control theory of pain.

subthreshold stimulus Stimulation below the threshold level; does not evoke a response but causes a change in the electrical activity of the tissue.

summation A process by which subthreshold stimuli add together to evoke a response.

superficial thermotherapy The application of modalities that heat primarily the surface tissues.

super-luminous diode (SLD) A very bright LED.

surged stimulation pattern Stimulation in which amplitude of successive pulses (or cycles) gradually increase from zero to a maximum preset intensity.

swelling An increase in tissue volume owing to extra fluid and cellular material in the tissue.

symmetrical pulse A pulse with identical phases.

sympathetic nervous system The branch of the ANS that regulates the body's fight-or-flight responses, such as increased heart rate.

synapse The junction between two neurons; the space between the axon terminal of a presynaptic neuron and the cell body or dendrite of a postsynaptic neuron.

systems approach to rehabilitation An approach to rehabilitation based on the philosophy that each patient and each injury is unique, so treatment must be individualized, dynamic, and interactive. Intervention is based on the patient's initial signs and symptoms and is altered according to patient progress. The systems approach is based on 11 principles of rehabilitation and consists of 10 core goals related to performance attributes.

T cell Transmission cell; a group of cells in the dorsal horn of the spinal cord that determines which impulse will continue up or down the spinal cord and to other parts of the body.

temperature The measure of an object's ability to spontaneously give up energy; indicates the level of molecular motion associated with heat.

temporal average intensity (TAI) The power of ultrasonic energy over a given period of time.

temporal summation Summed over time; occurs when a number of subthreshold stimuli from the same axon are repeated one after another before the effect of the previous stimulus has dissipated.

TENS See TRANSCUTANEOUS ELECTRICAL NERVE SIMULATOR (TENS).

tensile strength The amount of longitudinal stress a wound can withstand before tearing apart.

terminal (pole) The output device of a battery or generator.

tetanic contraction A sustained muscular contraction in response to repetitive high-frequency, high-amplitude pulsed or AC stimulation of at least 20–30 pulses per second; occurs in individual muscle fibers or in entire muscle groups.

tetany The point at which muscle fibers, as a result of increased frequency of stimulation, do not have time to relax between stimuli so that the contraction becomes steady, as opposed to a series of individual twitches; occurs when stimulation exceeds 20–30 pps, depending on the type of muscle fiber.

thalamus The brain's relay center. Signals from the sense organs (except the nose) are sent to the thalamus, which relays the information to the cerebral cortex.

therapeutic goal An aim or desired result of a therapeutic regimen.

therapeutic massage The systematic manual manipulation of the body's tissues to restore normal function.

therapeutic modality A device or application that delivers a physical agent (heat, cold, light, electricity, exercise) to the body for therapeutic purposes.

therapeutic purpose A goal of using physical agents in treating orthopedic injuries; examples are promoting wound healing, relieving pain, and increasing flexibility or range of motion.

thermal gradient A gradual change in temperature from the interior of one object to the interior of the other object as heat is exchanged by conduction; also known as temperature gradient.

thermoreceptor A sensory receptor that responds to heat and cold.

thermotherapy The therapeutic use of heat; the application of a device or substance with a temperature greater than body temperature, thus causing heat to pass from the thermotherapy device to the body.

threshold The minimal point at which a stimulus begins to produce a gross response (psychological or physiological).

time off The time during which the current does not flow; the time between surges.

time on The time during which the current flows from the beginning to the end of a surge.

tissue hydrostatic pressure (THP) Pressure that forces fluid into the capillary.

tissue oncotic pressure (TOP) Pressure that pulls fluid out of the capillary.

tract A bundle of nerve fibers with a common origin, termination, and function; also called pathway.

traction A technique in which a pulling force is applied to body segments to stretch soft tissues and separate joint surfaces or bone fragments.

transcutaneous electrical nerve stimulator (TENS) A therapeutic device that delivers current to the body to cause sensory nerve depolarization. Its purpose is to stimulate sensory nerves to modulate pain.

transducer A device that converts variations in a physical quantity (such as pressure or brightness) into an electrical signal, or vice versa

transition care Treatment of an acute injury between 12 hr and 4 days after the injury; a subset of acute care.

transmission The action of an electromagnetic wave passing through a substance.

transverse wave A wave form occurring only in bone, in which the molecules are displaced in a direction perpendicular to the direction in which the ultrasound wave is moving. See also LONGITUDINAL WAVE.

trauma A physical injury caused by physical force.

trigger point The site of referred pain.

trigger point pain A hypersensitive area or site in muscle or connective tissue; usually associated with myofascial pain syndromes.

triphasic A pulse with three phases of current flow.

twin pulse wave form Monophasic, pulsed, twin spiked form; common wave form of high-volt muscle simulators.

twitch contraction Repetitions of isolated brief muscular contraction followed by relaxation in response to low-frequency, high-amplitude pulsed stimulation; occurs in individual muscle fibers or in entire muscle groups.

ultrasound Inaudible, acoustic vibrations of high frequency that produce thermal and/or nonthermal physiologic effects.

ultrasound applicator The housing for the crystal and soundhead plus a handle that facilitates application of the ultrasound to patients.

ultrastructural changes The breakdown and disruption of cell membranes and cellular organelles.

ultraviolet (UV) radiation A portion of the electromagnetic spectrum that produces chemical reactions in microorganisms, epidermis, and dermis; usually used therapeutically to kill microorganisms.

unbalanced pulse A pulse containing unequal phase charges.

unipolar technique The application of electrodes of unequal size, thus creating active and dispersive electrodes; the active electrode(s) is (are) applied to the treatment area and the dispersive electrode is applied to a remote location.

urticaria A noncontagious, short-lived allergic reaction characterized by wheals on the skin. It is caused by cold or exercise or from eating certain foods or taking certain medicines. Also known as hives.

vascular phase In the repair process, a transient phase of 4–6 days during which new blood vessels are formed to deliver oxygen and nutrients to the wound area.

ventral horn The anterior portion of the gray matter of the spinal cord; also called anterior horn.

verbal rating scale A pain-rating scale that consists of a group of descriptors but no numbers. Patients rate their pain as absent, mild, moderate, or severe, and their pain relief as none, slight, moderate, or good.

vibration Repetitively moving soft tissue (usually muscle) back and forth over the underlying bone with minimal joint motion; also called shaking.

visible light An electromagnetic wave that is divergent, multichromatic, incoherent, and multiphasic.

visual analog scale (VAS) A pain-rating scale that consists of a line of specific length, usually 100 mm (4 in.), with contrasting descriptors ("no pain" and "severe pain") on the two ends. Patients make a vertical slash on the line indicating pain level. The clinician measures from the left side of the scale to the slash to assess pain level.

volt A unit of force required to push a current of 1 amp through a resistance of 1 ohm.

voltage The force created by an accumulation of, or an absence of, electrons on an atom or body.

voltmeter A device that measures voltage.

wave form The shape of an electrical current, created when the current is graphed with amplitude on the vertical axis and time on the horizontal axis.

wavelength The distance of one repetition of a sinusoidal wave, expressed in meters or centimeters; often defined as the distance from the crest of one repetition to the crest of the next repetition of the wave.

wet cell A battery that consists of two metals and an electrolyte solution; also called a galvanic cell.

wheal A smooth, slightly raised, rounded, or flat-topped area of skin, usually accompanied by burning or intense itching. Also known as a welt or a hive.

whirlpool A large body of either hot or cold water that is forcibly circulated or "whirled" about in its container.

Index

Page numbers in *italics* denote figures; those followed by t denote tables; those followed by b denote boxes.

Index **389**